STUDIES IN SANTAL MEDICINE AND CONNECTED FOLKLORE

STUDIES IN SANTAL MEDICINE AND CONNECTED FOLKLORE

PART I, II and III

P.O. Bodding

GYAN

Published by

Gyan Publishing House
5, Ansari Road
Daryaganj, New Delhi-110002
Phone: 011-47034999, 9811692060
E-mail: books@gyanbooks.com

Distribution Network
gyanbooks.com
India, USA, Canada, UK, Australia, France

ISBN: 978-81-212-1365-3 (HB)

Reprint in India, 2024
First Published, 2017

Printed at: Gyan Press, Delhi.

Studies in Santal Medicine and Connected Folklore
Author: P.O. Bodding

CONTENTS

PART I

THE SANTALS AND DISEASE

APPENDIX I.

The Santal *ojha* (from within)

APPENDIX II.

APPENDIX III.

PART II

SANTAL MEDICINE

Page

PART III

HOW THE SANTALS LIVE

CLASSIFIED LIST OF SANTAL "PRESCRIPTIONS."

FOREWORD

Rev. P. O. Bodding's *'Studies in Santal Medicine and Connected Folklore'* was first published by the Asiatic Society in three parts between 1925 and 1940. It was republished in 1986. It is now out of print. The merit of this book lies in the fact that it has revealed the connection of Santal Folklore with the unique attitude of the Santals towards various diseases and their treatment. Santals embrace a belief that diseases are caused by malevolent powers who are to be satisfied and appeased through various attempts made by professional medicine-men, generally called *Ojhās*. Bodding has collected the folksongs current in the Santal community, with the chanting of which the Santal-people try to pacify the spirits who are believed to be the originators of diseases. Bodding has thoroughly travelled the places inhabited by the Santals, learnt Santali language, gathered experience about the social and religious customs of the Santals and all these are reflected methodically in this book. It is amazing that a man from far off Norway had come to India and mixed himself closely with the people having a distant culture and home-bred language. Bodding's deep dedication to the study of the socio-religious fabric of the Santal people has resulted in the composition of this valuable book which the Asiatic Society took up for publication. Repeated demands of academicians from different corners have enthused us to publish the book for the third time. Some pages have been recomposed to maintain the quality of production.

The Asiatic Society
Dated the 27th August 2001

Manabendu Banerjee
General Secretary

PART I

THE SANTALS AND DISEASE

INTRODUCTORY

'Studies in Santal Medicine and connected Folklore' consists mainly of two parts, one treating of the medicines used by the Santals, their administration and application, and one called The Santals and Disease, dealing with the general attitude of the Santals when they have to face disease, their ideas as to the origin and causation of disease, their superstitions and fears, their various attempts to appease and satisfy the malevolent powers supposed to be responsible for disease, the professional medicine-men, especially the *ojha* and his doings, his magic and religious endeavours; it is further told, how they act when disease is thought to have become a matter of public concern. In an appendix is described, how a Santal becomes an *ojha*; a description is given of the annual village-course in *ojha*- science and of various matters connected with this; a number of songs used when this course is finished off are recorded; specimens of the *ojha's mantars* and *jhaṛnis* are also given. The table of contents will show what is found in this paper and its appendices.

There is one matter to which I should like to draw attention here. It has been touched on in the paper itself in several places and is of interest, as it may possibly contribute towards showing, how certain religious ideas may change, especially how people belonging to the stage of development found amongst the Santals may adopt and transform the beliefs and practices of others. My remarks, which shall not be many, concern the attitude of the Santals towards the spirits, *boṅga*, as they are called (the Supreme Being, differently styled and sometimes called the *boṅga* of the *boṅgas*, being here always left out of consideration).

The ordinary Santal attitude is shortly as follows. They believe in the existence of a large number of *boṅgas*, all more or less malevolent, often immoral and downright bad. They worship these *boṅgas*, that is to say, they offer sacrifices to them; they do so, not because they love them or respect them or expect anything good from them, but because they fear them. The sacrifices are a kind of tribute, or payment, to ensure the non- interference of these spirits with the Santals, with their health and their substance.

Any grown-up male Santal may perform a sacrifice, provided he knows the 'ritual,' i.e., the manner of proceeding, the invocation *(bakhẽṛ*, as it is called), the kind of sacrificial animal required and the name of the *boṅga*, and provided he dares to act. No *sid* is necessary. To perform sacrifices for the community they have in every village two priests; for the annual hunt, they also have a special priest. No *sid* or initiation is necessary to become such a priest; they are really chosen by the community and appointed. In the case of the hunt-priest *(dihri)*, they make sure that he has the requisite knowledge, and in the case of one of the village priests (the *ato naeke*, the village priest, but not in the case of the *kuḍam naeke* whose special work is to worship the spirits, supposed to reside on the village borders, and some others) the priest is formally 'chosen' by the *baṅgas* themselves. The village people, in the case of a vacancy, go to the holy grove and call on the *baṅgas*, whereupon a man is 'possessed' (*rum*, see p. 34) by one of the spirits, and in this state goes and embraces one of those present, and in this way selects a priest. It is not called *sid*; the *baṅgas* are in this way supposed to show by whom they will be pleased to be served.

There is no special course of training to be enabled to worship, it is free to everyone who wants, and knows, so far as all private worship is concerned, apart from the public functions referred to.

They do not use any *mantars*, only invocations (*bakheṛ*).

With the *ojha* the attitude seems to be considerably different. His work is confined to a particular sphere, and due allowance must be made for this.

He has to go through a course of training, and after having passed a couple of preliminary ceremonies, he has to receive a formal initiation or *sid*.

Whilst the ordinary Santal stands in fear of his *baṅgas*, the *ojha* does not show fear, whatever he may feel. So far as one can see, it would be contrary to his profession and work to fear those whose assistance he engages. His constant 'association' with his *boṅgas* may breed familiarity. The specimens of *ojha*-invocations quoted speak for themselves. There is no reverence in the *ojha*'s way of addressing his *boṅgas*; he tries to use one *boṅga* against another, appealing to the knowledge and grace of his tutelary *boṅgas*, more especially the first and original *ojha-guru*, now a *baṅga*.

On the whole the *ojha* acts as one familiar with the *boṅgas*, and as one able to enlist the use of the power of certain *boṅgas*. This is obviously foreign to the Santal mind.

The *ojha* is in supposed communication with a large number of *boṅgas* and spirits not generally known to the Santal, anyhow not invoked by the ordinary Santal. The nature of his *boṅgas* does not seem to be much different from that of the ordinary Santal ones. Hindu ideas have, however, influenced the *ojha* mind to some extent, especially when the greater Hindu deities are referred to. But it is not the holiness or righteousness of the *boṅgas* that are thought of (even if such qualities should be found); it is the power of the *boṅgas* to which they appeal, and which they try to secure for their purpose. They will appeal to the *boṅga*'s trustworthiness, and threaten or cajole them to be honest in their transaction with the *ojha*.

There are two special matters that should be mentioned, the *mantar* and the *saket*, peculiar to the *ojha*.

It has in the paper all along been taken as a matter of course, that the *ojha* has originally received his 'science' from Hindu sources, and there does not seem to be any reasonable doubt as to this. Now a faultlessly recited *mantra* is supposed to have power over the gods; the one who knows and is able to recite faultlessly a *mantra* is supposed to be able to obtain his object.

Santali *mantar* is the same word as *mantra*, and with the word the thing itself has been borrowed; but I am under the impression that the Santal *ojha*'s use of his *mantars* is different from what was stated above. It is naturally necessary, that the *ojha* knows the appropriate *mantar*; but it does not seem necessary that the wording and the recitation of the *mantar* should be faultless or according to some acknowledged formula. What is considered essential seems to be a knowledge of, and the proper use of the names of the appropriate *boṅgas* and some matters connected with the disease in question. Any one knowing the Santals will here recognize a peculiar trait of theirs, their need of having to do with concrete realities.

Further, there does not seem to be any thought of a *boṅga* being compelled to do the bidding of an *ojha* by his uttering a *mantar* alone. It rather seems to be that the *ojha* stands in a particular relation to the *boṅgas* concerned and, by the *mantar* and special means, is able to enlist the assistance of these, provided the inducement is sufficient. It is a remodelling of foreign tenets to suit Santal conceptions.

The *ojha* is generally exhorted to make sure the *saket*. To the Santal, *saket* means a sacrifice vowed to a *boṅga* by an *ojha*, to be performed when the patient recovers. It is also used as an adjective, meaning the particular *boṅga* to whom the *ojha* makes such a vow, and whose assistance the *ojha* is supposed to secure. These *saket boṅgas* are many and different, invoked according to the predilection and faith of the *ojha* (see p. 64). The *saket* consequently is the power behind the scene, known to and engaged by the *ojha*, supposed to be available on certain conditions, the *ojha*'s spiritual power. That the appeal is ineffective does not cause any difficulty; it is easy to find a plausible explanation.

Saket is not an original Santali word; I do not think one is mistaken in connecting it with Hindi *śakt*, able, powerful, *śakit* (a part. form meaning capable), comparing it with Hindi (Sanskrit) *śakti*, ability, power, etc., also the energy or active power of a deity personified as his wife. Etymologically *saket* can scarcely be the same as *śakti*; there is no reason why this word, except for the sibilant, should not in this case be reproduced in Santali; besides, a *saket boṅga* may be either male or female, so the idea of female energy does not apply. But it is not impossible that the idea mentioned of *śakti* may in some vague and unreflected way have taken hold of *ojha* imagination and transformed itself into what is actually observed. This would be in keeping with the nature of other loans.

If the supposed origin is correct, we consequently have here an example of how Santals adopt a foreign idea, and adapt this to their own system of thought and belief or superstition, so that it ultimately becomes something different from what it was or is in its own sphere.

What is said about the *saket* also applies to the *mantar*. The idea is borrowed but what has been felt to be impossible to the Santal has been permitted to become non-essential, whilst other points have been made essential, or even added to the original idea, as mentioned above. It would be of considerable interest to know, whether a similar line of development might be found with other peoples than the

Santals, whether aboriginals or people now belonging to the lower strata of the large Hindu system, when they borrow in this way.

To sum up, so far as the 'spiritual' side of the *ojha*'s work is concerned, he seems to be dealing in imitations. His attitude towards the *boṅga*-world is influenced by the ideas of those from whom he has originally borrowed.

The *ojha* is a Santal, living in his village in constant intercourse with his compatriots and, apart from his professional work, following the same pursuits as the other villagers; whilst he himself is influenced by his origin and his surroundings, he may also to some extent influence the mental vision of his fellows, on the one hand by lessening the fear of the *boṅgas* and altering the common view of these, on the other hand by assisting in turning the Santal mind away from his old *boṅgas* towards the Hindu pantheon. The influence of the *ojha* in this respect should not be overestimated, his own position or the estimation in which he is held, does not count for much; but his influence works in the direction mentioned, and it falls into line with the process of development that may be observed among the present-day Santals.

MOHULPAHARI, SANTAL PARGANAS.
22nd June, 1925.

THE PRONUNCIATION OF SANTALI.

Vowels:

a like in father.

e like in German *See*, or in English men.

i like in police or bit.

o like in Norw. stor or sort.

u like in moon or put.

ẹ is the open vowel, like in Engl. air.

ọ is the open vowel like in Engl. law or not.

ạ, a vowel sound peculiar to Santali, sounds to an English ear somewhat like *u* in hut; it is, however, a different sound.

All vowels may be nasalized, this is shown by the circumflex (ˆ) above the vowel.

The consonants are pronounced as follows:

h like in house (never mute).

k, *kh*, *g*, *gh* like the corresponding gutturals in Hindi.

ṅ is the velar nasal, like ng in song.

c, *ch*, *j*, *jh* like the corresponding palatals in Hindi (practically).

ń is the palatal nasal, like the Spanish *ñ*.

y is always the open medio-palatal fricative, like in Engl. yes.

ṭ, *ṭh*, *ḍ*, *ḍh*, *ṛ*, *ṇ* are the so-called cerebral sounds, pronounced very much like the corresponding Hindi ones.

t, *th*, *d*, *dh*, *n*, *r*, *l* like the corresponding consonants in Hindi.

p, *ph*, *b*, *bh*, *m* like the corresponding labials in Hindi.

v, *w* practically like in English.

s like in Engl. sink; Santali *s* is always voiceless.

k̕, *c̕*, *t̕*, *p̕* are sounds peculiar to Santali, checked consonants, without the off-glide. The consonant is formed in the mouth, but checked, just as the off-glide should ordinarily come.

THE SANTALS AND DISEASE.

By THE REV. P. O. BODDING, *Mohulpahari, Santal Parganas.*

I.

The general attitude. Beliefs as to life and death, God and the spirits.

The Santals look upon illness and disease as something unnatural, and make their own deductions from this proposition.

They have an idea, perhaps never well defined, found out more by deduction than from any direct statement of theirs, that a human being has a natural right to health and life, and that consequently he ought to live to old age. Disease is something foreign and inimical to man. How is it then that all are liable to be attacked by disease and carried off by death at any time? That is the problem, also to the Santals.

On the other hand, they theoretically profess to believe, that just as man is brought into the world and given what is necessary for support by the Creator or Supreme Being, so man is also carried away by His order. God, *Ṭhakur*, as He is called by the old *gurus*, "measures out to every one his seer," as they express themselves, at the time of birth (more will be found on this subject later on), and as long as this lasts, no one can take us away. The life of man is, according to this belief, predestinated by God. And man is not immortal, although his soul is believed to be so.

Now, if they acted up to this belief, the logical consequence would be, that death comes according to the will of God, and not according to the will of any other being, specially not the will of evil spirits and witches. If this is so, the next deduction might be that whatever ends in death must also be caused by God. But to this they do not agree.

They reason as follows: God is good; it is ordinarily unnecessary to worship Him, *i.e.*, to make sacrifices to Him. God is thought to be fairly well satisfied with the Santals and will not distress them, except when it may be absolutely necessary. Famine, the result of unseasonable weather (according to Santal belief, God is the giver of rain), is thus deemed to be a sign of the displeasure of the Supreme Being. This implies that man is not always good and may be punished by God. As a matter of fact, also certain diseases are considered to be the direct punishment for certain acts estimated especially sinful.

Besides in a Supreme Being the Santals also believe in a numbers of spirits, without exception evil and enemies of man. These *boṅgas*, as they are called, are supposed to harrass humanity, to 'eat' people (as the Santals express it), because they are hungry, displeased, hurt or envious, and this 'eating' is the devouring of the health and substance of the person exposed to the displeasure of the spirits. These spirits may further be used by, or themselves use, the witches who are always women.

It is strange that, except in connection with the evil eye which either sex may have, men are not suspected of exercising an evil, not natural or, in a way, supernatural influence; only women. It is one of the many silent testimonies to their distrust of, but also to their acknowledgement of, the qualities and powers of woman. As is known, the Santals are not alone in this attitude.

In short, it will be understood that the Santals believe in a good power who gives life, provides the necessaries for life and allots the span of life; and in destructive, inimical powers; and that man is exposed to the action of the latter.

II.

General beliefs as to the origin of disease.

To understand the Santal attitude towards disease it is necessary to bear in mind what has just been stated. They acknowledge natural causes of illness; they cannot avoid seeing effect and immediate cause; as a rule they can also see the material nature of a disease. But there is always a suspicion that the natural cause is not the original one, but that evil influences are at work in the first instance.

If any illness or disease is of a commonly known nature and runs its course, and a person is well again within a reasonable time (*i.e.*, within a few days), they will naturally let the matter rest there and not trouble themselves further. Even if they have had suspicions, it would serve no purpose to give heed to such, and it would entail unnecessary expense, to mention only one thing, if they would move in the matter.

But if there is a recrudescence, if the disease won't cease, if it commenced suddenly and is of an unusual character, not known, or anyhow, not understood, and above all, if death ensues, the always latent suspicion will assert itself. Nature should run its course; any disturbance must be due to extraneous malevolent influence. The origin cannot be found with man, nor, except as mentioned above, with the Supreme Being (in this case not malevolent, but acknowledged as just retribution).

Even when there is an evident immediate cause, as with accidents, who knows?—there may be something behind. To take an example: it is not by one's own will that one falls down from a tree; it is legitimate to climb a tree; if one climbs a tree and tumbles down, breaking his neck, have they not seen over and over again, that such a tree has dried up and died within a year of the accident?—A sure sign that the tree has been cursed. And why? I have heard this kind of reasoning over and over again; it apparently does not enter their minds, that part of the happenings might be explained by the fact that the tree was in a decaying condition, even if there were no external signs of this.

If, to take another example, a boy accidentally kills another boy by shooting him with an arrow, there is no doubt that the arrow is the immediate cause of death; but as the one boy had no intention of hitting the other one, and as a matter of fact was aiming at something else, is there not a possibility that some inimical power had something to do with the fatal direction of the arrow? The natural cause is there, undoubtedly; but there is, according to their mind, room for something more.

In cases like those described action against anybody is excluded, except that they will take up for investigation whether the shooting boy intended to do harm or not.

Left to themselves the Santals will let a matter of this kind rest with a secret suspicion.

If their suspicion in case of disease becomes directed towards a concrete object, or if their natural affections are specially touched (as when children or grandchildren die), they will as often as not take action, and the *ojhas* will egg them on, as we shall hear further down.

III.

The supernatural influence. The qualities of the boṅgas. *Medicines against all ills provided by the Creator.*

How the supernatural influence is brought into action, on this they do not much reflect. They are satisfied with the supposed fact.

As this supernatural influence is always inimical and evil, and according to their ideas, there is no possibility of the malevolent influence being turned to a benevolent or good one, the only practical question for them is, how to stop it, and, in the case of witches, how to stop and punish it.

It is believed and freely acknowledged by the Santals that the *boṅgas* can work only evil, and that they have no power to make good again what they have committed of evil. The only thing they can do, and the only thing that can be expected of them is, that they may be induced to cease doing mischief. It will be seen from the specimens of invocation given further on, that there is no thought of asking for positive help from these spirits.

Santals may be heard to express themselves like this: "It is not sufficient to 'make *boṅga*' (*i.e.* to worship the spirits called *boṅga* with animal sacrifices) in order to bring about recovery. *Boṅgas* and witches know how to 'eat'; they do not know how to make well. They only know how to cause distress. It is with them, as it is with us: we are able to fell a tree, but we do not know how to join the tree on to the stump and make it a living tree again. In the same way the spirits know how to fell, but not how to restore."

Cando (a name often used by the Santals for the Supreme Being who is confounded with *cando*, the sun), the Creator, is the only one who can give and restore life, and He has created the trees and plants that contain remedies against all ills. He has 'sown' the seeds of these all over the earth. To bring about recovery from any disease it is necessary to find the medicine which suits or is intended for any particular disease or illness. If, to use a common expression of theirs, "medicine and disease meet one another," a patient will recover.

From their point of view this is not bad reasoning. If we were to follow up their thoughts on the different subjects here mentioned to their logical ends, we would likely be able to point out some contradictions. It will not, however, serve our present purpose to say more on this subject. What has already been said will furnish some explanation of the Santal attitude towards the matters here referred to.

As mentioned above, disease is something foreign and inimical to man. Their language shows their attitude. They will not say, as we do, that somebody catches a cold, or gets measles, etc. It is always the other way: it is the disease which catches, makes a commencement with, attacks or overpowers man.

Now we also frequently make use of similar expressions; people suffer from an attack of fever, gout, lumbago, etc. Whatever our expressions may have originally implied, we do not now combine with them thoughts of malevolent action. We should not, perhaps, put too much meaning into the Santal expressions either. One gets, however, an impression that the Santals attribute to certain diseases a kind of separate existence. One may hear them talk of somebody having gone to some place or other, and there having met with and been caught by some disease or other. How much their ideas amount to, I have not been able to fully ascertain. They do not look upon disease as a kind of spirit with a will of its own, but perhaps as a kind of concrete, localized, specific influence. Their language is to be taken more literally than we can do our own.

Like other people the Santals divide disease into several categories, besides having different names for a great number of ailments (on this subject more is written in another place).

They naturally also have the many different kinds of complaints commonly supposed to be of no consequence. The Santals treat these very much as we do. A very few hypersensitive persons are met with also among them; but the rule is to look upon such things as negligible. They do not reflect on such matters, or think that such complaints have any other than a natural explanation, provided they do not come as the commencement of some serious disease.

IV.

Santal philosophy on bodily health.

As among us we may hear a chill or a cold mentioned as something to be treated with respect, so the Santals think something analogous with regard to what they call *haḍi*. This is with them the name for a swelling of certain muscles of the neck and back. It is very common and is painful, but soon cured when they use their excellent massage. They have a saying, that *hạḍi* is the *raebarič* (lit. marriage broker) of disease; from *hạḍi* many kinds of disease will arise according to their belief.

I have heard a Santal give the following explanation: "Our body," he said," is like a *kọl gạḍi* (lit. a machine carriage, any vehicle propelled by an engine). This moves by the power of the engine. As long as the engine works, we can go and come as we like; because of our machinery we can stretch or bend our arms and legs. Our machinery is made up by *sirs* (by *sir* the Santals understand the muscles and sinews, the nerves, arteries and veins; if not specified, the *sir* may be any of these; generally there is an idea that blood is found in the *sir*). When any part of a machine is out of order, the machinery will not move, but stands still, until it is repaired. In the same way, if any of the *sirs* of our body gets out of order, we first feel out of sorts; we stretch ourselves and say, 'To-day I feel unwell in my body.' Some *sir* or other has been sprained or dislocated or twisted. If you get massage quickly, well and good; if not, some disease or other will commence. People say, that the blood flows along in the *sirs*, and if these are twisted or dislocated or sprained, the blood cannot flow along. And then there you are. It is mostly from the *sirs* of the back that disease arises. In the back such a lot of *sirs* meet together. One goes from the neck above the ear to the forehead; if this gets out of order, you get a headache. From the neck again another *sir* goes forward and down through the opening behind the collar-bone and into the lungs; that gives you a cough. One *sir* goes from the back below the shoulder-blade and inside; that gives *betha* (pain in the breast, pleuresy or pneumonia). Another one goes in between the ribs on the side; that gives rise to certain kinds of convulsions.

"Further, if you lift or carry anything heavy, you may suddenly feel a sharp pain in the middle of the back; you get lumbago. There is also a *sir* below the ribs, just above the hip-bone; if this gets out of order, you get spleen.

"When a *sir* gets bad, if you do not get medicine quickly, it will gradually become worse; then some day the *sir* will suddenly stand like a cord, and convulsions will 'get hold of you'; the *sir* will be drawn tight, and then your soul will depart (*i.e.* you will die, death being due to the departure of the soul from the body)."

So far the Santal "authority." It will be seen, that part of his explanations and speculations cannot be of any great antiquity; otherwise his statements fairly well represent the Santal ideas concerning these matters. I suppose, their ideas about *sir* are more or less founded on the observations of those who practise massage.

The Santals are aware that the stomach plays a great rôle with regard to health. The man cited above is responsible also for the following speculations: "People say, we have a body like a railway engine. We eat food; that is the coal. Just as they feed an engine with coal and water, so we also feed our body. We break wind; that is the smoke that gets out. What we eat, they say, first passes into the belly; there the food is diluted. If there is too little water, we feel thirsty and have to drink. Finally it all turns into the substance of rice-water, and this is turned into blood. When we sneeze, they say, this fluid is drawn up through some narrow *sir*, and as it passes through the liver and lungs, it becomes blood. The water is squeezed out and becomes urine, and what dries uselessly becomes excrement and is expelled. In this way disease may come through the medium of food and drink."

They are aware that errors of diet will produce trouble. The Santals generally live on a vegetable diet, because they cannot afford to eat meat often. When they get meat, they may take too much, or the meat may be bad or not properly prepared, with the unavoidable result. They speak figuratively of this, saying that 'the pig has rooted him up,' 'the ram has battered him,' 'the buffalo has struck him (with his horn),' the meaning being that a person has got a disordered stomach through eating curry prepared from the kind of meat mentioned. It is, however, astonishing to observe what kind of meat and food a Santal can eat with impunity.

They are not, however, very apt at distinguishing between serious and indifferent symptoms. They may become rather exercised in their minds, when their stomachs rumble or 'sound,' as they express themselves, or when their urine becomes 'like that of a goat,' as it generally will during the hot season; but they may go with really serious complaints for a long time without paying much attention to them.

V.

The tejo *theory.*

The Santals have some curious ideas about several diseases being due to what they call *tejo*, by which name they ordinarily understand larvæ, worms, etc.; a *tejo* may be fairly large, but may apparently also be so small as to be invisible to the naked eye.

To give some examples: rabies they believe to be caused by some infinitely small *tejo*; they have their medicine against this disease; when giving it they admonish the patient to look at his urine. If something like oil is seen floating on the surface, they are sure the *tejos* have come out; the patient is out of danger.

People are supposed to have two *tejos* at the root of their nose. If these work their way up into the brain in the forehead and commence to butt one another, the person gets an attack of epilepsy.

Caries of the teeth is caused by *tejos* which are 'demonstrated,' when they endeavour to smoke them out. The proceeding is described elsewhere.

Leprosy and cancer of the jaw are caused by some specific *tejos*. Indeed, our whole body is supposed to be full of *tejos* of sorts. If you feel the need of scratching yourself, it is because *tejos* are eating you. There are the *tejos* of scabies, ringworm, eczema, and so on.

With such ideas one might think that they should be more understanding than they really are as to infection. They are, of course, aware of the contagious nature of some skin diseases, of the venereal diseases, and to a certain extent also of the infectiousness of epidemic diseases; but their views with regard to most other infectious diseases are hazy.

The following description given by a Santal will give some idea of their beliefs in certain cases: "If any one eats oneself full, or eats without measure, cholera is apt to ensue. When a person has overeaten himself, he gets pain in the stomach; the food is not digested; there are eructations, and the stomach rumbles, and he passes stools incessantly; sometimes this will empty him out and finish him. Now his stools will dry up; when this takes place, a kind of vapour arises from the place; if any one goes there and inhales this vapour, the disease will get into his body, and so you have it in the country."

They have also an idea that stools of such and like patients may dry up and lie innocuous anywhere; but when the rains come, the dry stuff becomes fresh again and is carried along by the water; if any one drinks such water or bathes in it, he is sure to get the disease. Cholera may also come, they say, from eating new (fresh) grain.

As already mentioned, the Santals believe that leprosy is caused by a *tejo*; some, however, say that this disease and paralysis (hemiplegia) are the direct punishment by the Creator for some unrighteousness committed before Him, and that they consequently are incurable. Leprosy is, moreover, passed from parents to children for generations. But infection, they say, may be avoided, if one does not eat food touched or left by the leper.

Tuberculosis, they say, runs in the families; they do not, however, understand the nature of this disease, so they do not take any measures that might help to check its spreading.

In connection with many different diseases and infirmities they have theories of a gross superstitious nature. As it would necessitate going into a number of details, we shall not here make any lengthy mention of these.

They have a superstition that witches every year go to a place called *Kuṇḍli pukhri*[1]; from this tank they bring back with them the germs of certain diseases, specially epidemic ones, and in accordance with what they bring any year the people will have to suffer.

They further believe that a certain kind of pain in the back (lumbago) is caused by direct witch-action (the same belief must have been common in certain parts of Europe, to judge from the name given to the same complaint, cf. Norwegian 'hexeskud,' lit. witch-shot). They also believe, that witches cut out and eat the liver of people, whereby these get some disease or other, not by any means always, or even generally, in the liver; from such disease no one will recover, if the witch is not forced to make restitution.

Other ideas are, that people mostly get disease through carelessness with their body. If we eat anything in an unclean way, we get into trouble. Mist and fog cause

---

1 *Kuṇḍli pukhri*, lit. the Ring tank, is in these parts reported to be somewhere to the north-east. The Santa witches do not, like their European 'sisters,' travel riding on broomsticks, which are unknown, but go along sitting on the branches of the pipol tree (Ficus religiosa, L.), or, as some tell, in a *matkom* tree (the *mahua*, Bassia latifolia, Roxb.); at their behest the tree rises up into the air and flies along with the witches. One tree is supposed to be sufficient for a large number of them.

cough, and bathing in dirty water when the first rain falls, gives rise to ophthalmia, and so on.

On the whole, sense and superstition are curiously mixed up together, with a premium on superstition.

VI.

The Stamina of the Santals. Influence of fear and supposed calls from the other world. Optimism and despair.

Before commencing to describe the attitude of the Santals during illness and disease, there are a few matters that might be conveniently mentioned here.

First as to their physical strength. They are accustomed to a life of exposure and many privations; they are from childhood inured to hardship. So long as they can go about their daily work without serious hindrance, they do not think it necessary to make any fuss. I should say, they act very much as a good many of us would do.

Whilst they are apparently able to bear up for a long time against disease, one is often surprised to see, how little is required to take them off.

A Santal may be seen sitting, right up to the time of death; they make use of the expression 'to sit down to die,' equivalent to what we would call to be lying on one's death bed. I have actually seen a man sitting on his bed *in extremis* a few minutes before death. It might be remarked, that I have never heard such behaviour having anything to do with the superstition found among certain other peoples, that if one lies down, it means that one throws up the sponge.

Some may pull through the most serious diseases; others get a little fever and 'a little headache,' and die in a very short time, according to Santal ideas, without sufficient or reasonable cause.

This apparent lack of stamina may be caused by lack of proper nutrition, something very common with them; but it may perhaps also have something to do with their mind. It is sometimes quite patent that they give up fighting for existence; they make up their mind that they are going to die—and die. The cause may be self-suggestion; they have been frightened; they are sure that they have been exposed to the deadly enmity of witches, or they believe that they have run foul of *boṅgas*. It is not so astonishing, as it may seem at first sight; their lack of knowledge and a proper estimation of the natural causes of disease will easily lead them to exaggerate or to admit the thought and conviction of evil spirits being at work.

They may sometimes believe, that they have got a call from the other world, and start on the long journey, often at a previously specified time. Any one who has had to do with the Santals will have met with, or heard of, examples of this kind. These phenomena are of considerable psychological interest. One may be tempted to think, that their simple minds are in nearer contact with nature, than ours are.

The Santals may be optimistic with regard to illness, or more or less careless, until they think it is serious. If they do not get the idea that supernatural powers are at work, it will, as a rule, as already mentioned, take a lot to make them believe that something really serious is the matter with them.

This should not, however, be taken as meaning that they do not care what happens. If their children are ill, they will watch over them constantly, and will often leave everything, even most necessary work, to attend to those who suffer. It is a pitiful sight to see them, when they come and sit round the bed of a relative, in despair and hopelessness, especially when they harbour suspicions that evil spirits or witches are at work. The behaviour of the frightened and hopeless surroundings must affect the patient very seriously.

The carelessness mentioned is probably mostly due to a lack of knowledge of the real nature of the complaint, combined with an idea that there is no hurry. One may find among them any number of neglected cases, often serious and even hopeless, where it might have been easy to help, if they had come in time for proper medical aid.

VII.

First attitude on being faced by disease. The medicine-man and the ojha.

We shall then proceed to see how a Santal generally acts when faced by illness and disease.

When somebody in a family falls ill,—if it is not something unquestionably of a serious nature which demands immediate assistance by a 'doctor,'—they will not as a rule call in a medicine-man at once. They prefer to wait and see how it will go. There is the question of expense and bother, although this is not permitted to play any large rôle with them, if any rôle at all, in case of disease. They have also an idea, that they should let the disease 'become tired,' as they express themselves, exhaust itself, so to say.

In the meantime the people of the house will apply the household remedies, *sekao*, and *iskir*, and if the nature of the complaint seems to call for such, then *tobak* and *sǫsǫ*. The nature and the manner of application of these remedies have been described in the Introductory remarks to the paper on Santal Medicine (sect. IX) to which the reader is referred.

As a rule the average Santal 'knows' one or more of what they call *rẹhẹt ran*, lit. 'root-medicine,' and the responsible head of the household will, if he thinks it will answer, try to make use of his knowledge, or, may be, some friend or relative may, in a friendly and unprofessional way, be able to assist.

If, however, the disease is of a pronounced nature, or does not give way to the household remedies, or if it does not stop of itself in a few days, they will call in a 'doctor,' a medicine-man or an *ojha*, from the village or the neighbourhood.

Both these are 'physicians,' the difference between them being, that the first named gives only medicine, whilst the *ojha* in addition to giving medicine, or rather previous to the administration of it, will try to drive away the disease by magic, incantations, etc., *i.e.* by the assistance of his special *boṅgas* whom he knows how to make to work; the *ojha* professes to know how to find out and deal with the possible supernatural powers at work. The last mentioned abilities are the qualifications on which the *ojha* rests his claims as a 'physician,' just as much as, or perhaps more than, on anything else.

Among the medicine-men there may sometimes be found persons with a natural gift for 'medical' work, and with quite a remarkable amount of knowledge of medicinal plants, etc.

The Santal name for this kind of 'doctor' is *raranič*, one who administers *ran*, their name for medicine, a Santali word. Sometimes, specially in more recent time, one hears them called *kubṛaj*, the Santal way of pronouncing *kaviraj* or the Bengali কবিরাজ. This is perhaps thought to be much grander.

There are, of course, no 'schools' for them; any one having an inclination for such work must try to acquire wherever possible whatever knowledge he may be able to pick up. Any one wishing to learn will arrange to follow and learn from some known *raranič*. It might be mentioned, that many Santals seem to take an interest in 'medicine.'

The *ojha* requires to be mentioned somewhat more fully.

First as to the name used: *ojha* is a Hindi word (ओझा); in Hindi it is used for 'a diviner, soothsayer, sorcerer, wizard, enchanter, conjurer, exorcist, magician;—one who pretends to cast out evil spirits, to cure snake-bite, etc., by means of charms and incantations' (Platts, Dictionary of Urdu, Classical Hindi and English). The word is derived from the Sanskrit उपाध्याय, a sub-teacher who instructs in a part only of the Veda,—a spiritual teacher, a teacher in general (Monier Williams, Sanskrit Dictionary.) The old idea of deriving the word from Hindi *ojh*, entrails, comparing *ojha* with the Latin *haruspex*, is likely abandoned. There does not seem to be any foundation for such a construction in Indian practice.

As the name is Hindi and undoubtedly adopted by the Santals from Hindi-speaking peoples, and as the work of a Santal *ojha* in nature partly resembles that of the Hindu *ojha*, it is most probable that they have received the 'institution' also from the Hindus. Incidentally it might be mentioned, that the special *boṅgas* invoked by the Santal *ojhas* all have names of Hindi origin (in addition to their special *boṅgas* they also invoke the common Santal godlings). Although, taking all circumstances into consideration, this cannot be said to be conclusive proof, it goes far towards making the here mentioned supposition probable.

A comparison between the Santal *ojha* and his Hindu confrère, as he lives in his village at the present day, might be interesting, but cannot be given here. Much of the practices of the Santal *ojha* seems to be essentially outside the Hindu fold. On the other hand the *ojha*'s special *boṅgas* seem to be of a nature somewhat different from that of the ordinary Santal *boṅgas*.

VIII.

More about the ojha.

As mentioned in Appendix II, the Santals themselves have a tradition that they have learnt to be *ojhas* from a personage called *Kạmbru* or *Kạmru guru*, probably a Hindu, whether he was a person so named, or, as is possible, a man from Kamrup. There is no cause whatever to doubt the correctness of their statement that they have learnt this 'craft' from an outsider, only as already pointed out, this should not be taken to mean, that Santal *ojhas* and Hindu ditto are, at the present time, or for that matter have ever been, the same.

A Santal *ojha* is supposed to be able to perform certain things that are outside the knowledge and power of ordinary people. These things are mainly six, according to the Santal traditions as told by *Kolean guru*, viz.:

(1) To consult the oracle, or, divination by leaves and oil (described later on, see Sec. X).

(2) To 'sow' rice (described Sec. XII, *adwa caole* and *bul mãyãm*).

(3) To make disease gather at one point of the body and to get the evil out by biting and sucking (see Appendix I).

(4) To remove *boṅgas*, or rather their symbols, by digging (see below Sec. XVI).

(5) To exorcise *boṅgas* (described below, Sec. XVI).

(6) To administer medicine.

To this should be added that the *ojha* is also able to perform sacrifices, when required, and that he knows the necessary *mantars* and *jhạṛnis* and how to use these (see below, and Appendix I).

To become an *ojha* it is necessary to become a disciple with such a one, to learn from him the different *mantars*, *jhạṛnis* and invocations, formulæ, songs, etc., that have to be used at the different occasions, and also to learn the medicines and their application. When his course is thought completed, the disciple asks the old *ojha* for, and receives, what is called *sid*, the final touch or initiation.

There are at the courses mentioned two classes of disciples, some (and these are by far the majority) who only learn some *mantars* and songs, so as to be able to go the rounds and beg Indian corn in the villages at the time of the *Dasãe pọrọb*, the Santal name for the Durga festival; and a few others who take up *ojha*-work as a serious business. These last ones ask for and receive the *sid*, the others not.

In Appendix I there will be found a description of the Santal *ojha*, how he is taught and initiated, and how he works his magic, a number of things that cannot conveniently find a place in this part of the paper.

With regard to the *ojha* and the medicine-men it may in a general way be said that, so far as medical knowledge and skill are concerned, they are about equal. Among the medicine-men are found perhaps the best; they are generally honest according to their lights and have a strong belief in their craft. Among the *ojhas* many are rank humbugs; perhaps an even stronger expression might fit them better.

Whenever these *ojhas* are unable to effect a cure, the bad result is not, of course, due to their own lack of ability, or the insufficiency of their remedies. The responsibility is elsewhere, with the powers behind the scenes. The 'eaters' (that is to say the destructive powers, whether they are *boṅgas* or witches) have gained the upper hand, the *ojha* will say, and he considers himself free from all responsibility.

Sometimes they may very likely believe that they have not been able to appease the malevolent powers; but very often they play on this string to make money and also to get some good food. The spirits are appeased through sacrifices; the *ojha* will perform these or, at least, participate in them, and consequently get his portion of the flesh of the sacrificed animals and of the perquisites. It is thus in a double way to the *ojha*'s interest to bring the supernatural in: they are relieved of responsibility, and benefit by the sacrifices.

All honour is due to those who try to do their best according to their lights. An up-to-date physician and surgeon can do very much that a Santal *ojha* would never dream of being able to do; but there is also very much that no modern doctor is able to do, any more than an *ojha*. The criticism of the *ojha* comes rightly in where he acts as a humbug.

IX.

The ojha *commences.*

After this description of the professional we shall come to his work. When an *ojha* or medicine-man is called in, he will act more or less as he, according to his lights and the rules of his profession, ought to do. He will start with asking the messenger calling him, and then the head of the household, or the person responsible, about the patient, to get a general idea of the state of matters, and also to get an inkling of the opinion of all concerned as to the nature and cause of the complaint. He will enquire how long the patient has suffered, and also whether other *ojhas* have been called in.

They will tell him what they have done, and say that they have tried to apply what they know themselves; but that they as this had no effect have called him, the professional, in. The *ojha* is careful all along to act, not as one who seeks employment, although he indirectly does all he can to persuade the people concerned to engage one of his craft. He endeavours to make it look, as if he undertakes the task only after much imploring and persuasion.

After these preliminaries the *ojha* will approach the patient, question him, look at his face and tell him to put out his tongue. Thereupon he will sit down on his haunches beside the sufferer snapping the ground several times with his fingers, preparatory to feeling his pulse, first of the right hand, then of the left. Whilst he with one hand (the index finger) feels the pulse at the wrist, he takes loosely hold of the fingers with his other hand, all along exhibiting an attitude of the most profound attention and thought. While feeling the pulse he must not let himself be distracted, and therefore looks down and away from the patient. It is meant to be impressive and solemn.

The *ojha* can make much more out of the pulse than his European confrere will ever be able to do. He has no watch to count by and has no certain knowledge of the nature of the blood circulation; but this, of course, is no impediment; on the contrary it leaves him a good deal more latitude. I have heard it told that some *ojhas* can distinguish as many as 23 different kinds of pulse in each of the arms, and if the *ojha* is at the top of his profession, he is expected to know from the pulse, what ails the patient, where the seat of his complaint is, and so on.

If, according to their idea, the pulse comes towards the thumb or the index finger, it is a sign, that *boṅgas*, the *oṛak boṅga* (that is, the house *boṅga*) or some of the other *boṅgas* are at work (are 'hungry,' as it is called). If the pulse comes towards the middle finger, the *abge boṅga* (a kind of tutelary, but rather uncertain and feared *boṅga*) is 'hungry'; if towards the ring or little finger, a spirit of the field or of the village outskirts is at work. The pulse is further supposed to reveal, whether the complaint is due to 'sudden fright', to inflammation, to poison, and so on.

Having felt the pulse, the *ojha* will come away from the patient to be questioned by the people of the house. He will tell them that the complaint will likely take some time to run its course, will urge them to get hold of some *ojha*, and not on any account to delay taking the necessary steps, until the patient becomes so weak that no *ojha* will be able to do anything. Besides, an *ojha* may, by exercising his specific knowledge and powers, be able to drive away the trouble immediately. In any case, to start with a complaint, he tells them, may be nothing more than a local thing or some muscular pain; but, he explains, a small and insignificant thing may become anything and grow into the most formidable disease.

The head of the house, or the person responsible, will, of course, tell the *ojha* that they have called him in to avail themselves of his services; the lady of the house chimes in and implores the *ojha* to do his best. He need have no fear; they will provide him with the necessary fowls and animals for sacrifices, without fail. The *ojha* gets what he wants, an unqualified assertion that he is engaged, and commences to act.

The preliminaries will not always be so many and circumstantial as those just described; often the *ojha* starts work without any further prelude. But according to what the writer has been told, the dignity of the 'profession' should really demand something of the kind described.

The first thing an *ojha*, after the preliminaries mentioned and after having 'diagnosed' the case, will do, is to try to drive away the complaint or disease by uttering a *mantar*, as they call it (a kind of magic formula), or singing a *jhaṛni* over the patient. These, which differ according to disease, will be found described in Appendix I. Having finished the *mantar* (it is always very short) the *ojha* blows over the patient, commencing at the head and finishing downwards and towards the back. This blowing comes immediately at the end and as the finishing touch of the *mantar*. A *mantar* followed by blowing is never repeated. If once is of no help, it is useless to try again.

In certain cases (principally when the case is due to poison, as in cases of snake-bite, or when a person has been bitten or touched by some snake, lizard, frog, etc., supposed to be poisonous, further when the patient suffers from convulsions, giddiness, has swooned off, in cases of pneumonia and some other complaints) in addition to, or instead of, uttering a *mantar*, they practise what is called *jhaṛ*. The patient is kept lying down, ornaments, as *e.g.* earrings, necklaces, armlets, anklets, etc., are taken off, the *ḍora*, a string always worn round the waist by men, is cut off, the hair-top of a woman (or of a man, if he wears one) is loosened, everything is removed that is artificial or foreign to nature and might act as a hindrance; in cases of snake-bite the person is put on his back on the ground naked, so that there is nothing between him and the earth, and with only just enough cloth to cover the middle part of the body in front.

The *ojha* now takes in his left hand a feather of the adjutant bird, a peacock feather or a straw or two of a broom (in these cases the broom must have been made of *sirom*, Andropogon muricatus, Retz., or *saparọm*, Nyctanthus arbor-tristis, L.), and moving this just above or just touching the body of the patient from the head downwards towards the fingers or extremities, he sings a kind of *mantar*. It may be the same words as the spoken *mantar;* generally the words are different. This 'song' is called *jhạṛni*. The *jhạṛni* itself is not sung more than once, but the *jhaṛ* with the melody whistled is sometimes repeated.

The general contents of both the *mantar* and the *jhạṛni* are apparently an attempt at pacifying, or commanding the disease (or whatever may be supposed to be behind) to cease or to come out of the patient. The whole is a rigmarole, enumerating supposed possible causes, etc., with few exceptions ending in a reference to *Kạmru guru* or some other *guru* or godling, by whose authority and with whose power the *ojha* is supposed to act. Whatever may be their personal convictions the *ojhas* act, as if they have an implicit belief in the magical power of the *mantar* and the *jhạṛni*, the words of which they often do not understand, perhaps one reason for belief in their efficacy. It does not trouble them, that they are never effective; the cause of this is, as mentioned, found with the powers behind.

Mantar, *jhaṛ* and *jhạṛni* are Hindi words; the *mantar* is generally in some corrupt Bihari or Bengali, sometimes with some Santali interspersed; the *jhạṛni* is sometimes in a kind of Santali. As already mentioned, the Santal *ojha* generally has only a very limited understanding of the contents, and on account of his lack of knowledge of the language in question, the language of the *mantar* or *jhạṛni* used is often very far from correct. One might, taking all into consideration, think oneself justified in supposing that the whole method has been originally borrowed from the Hindus.[1]

[1] The writer has sometimes been wondering, whether the practice of *jhaṛ* might possibly originally have had some thing t° do with hypnotism, that is to say, whether the present practitioners might, through any number of intermediary

It was forgotten to mention above that the *jhaṛ* is also concluded by blowing over the patient treated. The idea seems to be that the personality, or the life principle, of the *ojha*, as represented by blowing, or of those he represents through his invocations, etc., is thought strong enough to drive the foreign influence away, or something similar. In this connection cf. the supposed vitiating influence of one's breath, kept back during the application of certain medicines. In this case the natural breath of a person will interfere with the effect of the 'medicine'; it is obviously different with the *ojha* whose personality is not supposed to be antagonistic. Cf. also the common practice of blowing into the ears, etc., of persons fainting or believed dying.

After this digression we return to the doings of the *ojha*.

When the *mantar*, or *jhaṛ*, or both, have no effect, as they naturally never have in cases of disease, the next thing the *ojha* will do is to call for some *sal* leaves and a little oil, to perform what is called *sunum boṅga* or *khaṛi* (or *khaṛi maṭi*). He is by this means to verify the correctness of his diagnosis, arrived at by feeling the pulse, or otherwise, and more especially to ascertain the ultimate cause and origin of the disease, if at all necessary. This process will be found described in detail below.

When this is done he will give what he considers the necessary instructions with regard to food and treatment, and himself bring or order to be brought the ingredients wanted for the medicines he is going to give, and will then administer these according to his custom and knowledge. This part of an *ojha*'s or medicine-man's work is treated of in detail in the part of the present work called 'Santal Medicine,' to which the reader is referred for information on this point.

It is perhaps unnecessary to mention that the *ojha* is careful not to let other people know all the secrets of his profession, for instance, not all the ingredients of his medicines.

The *ojha* is optimistic; to be so is one of his tenets. He knows how important it is that a doctor should be cheerful. Except in obviously hopeless cases he will announce that there is no need of anxiety or fear; he will cure the patient in the course of a few days.

If this does not come about, it must not be acknowledged that the remedies of the *ojha* are at fault. He guards himself against being judged incompetent by always presupposing the possibilities of inimical and malevolent powers behind the scene. The blame rests anywhere else than with the *ojha*.

As elsewhere remarked, the Santals expect a speedy cure. If the case develops favourably, it is all right; if not, it will not be long before they will find it necessary

---

links, have received something, the nature and proper practice of which they have never known or understood, but which originally was some kind of hypnotic passes or the like. I do not know, but I should not wonder to learn that some form of hypnotism has been known in old India. If this should be so, one might possibly think that persons having knowledge of hypnotism may have attempted to use their knowledge to counteract the collapse so frequently supervening, *e.g.*, in cases of real or supposed snake-bite, and often due to sheer fear. There are examples of persons having died in the course of a couple of hours after having been bitten or touched by absolutely harmless lizards from collapse due to fright. It is possibly a wild idea; but it is difficult to get any satisfactory explanation of how anything like *jhaṛ* should have come to the Santals, or be practised by them.

to call in some other *ojha*. On the whole, the people will take a generous view of the *ojha*. They may doubt his ability, and whether through his means 'medicine and disease have met.' But it is probably more his ability to appease the *boṅgas* that they will doubt.

Whilst the *ojha* acts as stated, the medicine-man will take a similar course, that is to say, he will feel the pulse and do all he knows to diagnose the case, he will give instructions as to treatment and prescribe or himself prepare medicines, very much like the *ojha;* but being only a medicine-man and not an exorcist of spirits he confines himself to the remedies of nature, omitting all dealings with the supernatural.

The ideas in vogue among the people being what they are, it is not strange that the people themselves generally want an *ojha;* they want to make sure against all possibilities. They will think it wise, perhaps a necessary precaution, to have sacrifices performed to appease the supernatural powers, and to have the powerful assistance of the *ojha*'s special *boṅgas*.

I have heard of otherwise really sensible medicine-men who had a fair knowledge of Santal medicine and used their knowledge according to their best ability, and did not care to mix themselves up in performing sacrifices and so on, but who were forced by the superstitions of their clientèle to add *boṅga*-worship to their medical practice, partly not to lose this, partly to keep their patients at ease. It is quite an interesting phenomenon to observe, how the parties in question influence one another.

One gets the impression that the *raranko*, *i.e.*, the medicine-men, are honest according to their lights and abilities, and really know more than the *ojha* whose work may be more or less spoilt by his double activities.

X.

Divination by leaves described.

Before proceeding further we shall hear how the divination by leaves is performed. It plays a rather important rôle with the Santals when they wish to find out the final cause or origin of disease and death. As already mentioned, the Santals call this process *sunum boṅga* (lit. oil offering), or *khaṛi* or *khaṛi maṭi* (lit. chalk earth).

To perform this the *ojha* needs some leaves, the leaves nearly always used being those of the *sal* tree (Shorea robusta, Gärtn.); but also the leaves of Bauhinia Vahlii, W. and A., are thus used. Besides he needs a little (mustard) oil and a little water. The ingredients are always brought by the person who engages the services of the *ojha*.

Having received the leaves and the oil (in a leaf-cup) and the water the *ojha* sits down on his haunches, facing any direction, a little away from those who have asked him to 'divine,' not further, however, than so that his every act may be observed.

He first jerks his head a couple of times upwards to the right side. Thereupon he dips his right-hand index-finger in the oil, and filliping sprinkles a few drops about, more specially in the direction of the sun. Then he puts a mark of oil on the ground with the same finger, this last being for *Dhạrti mae* (lit. earth mother, a goddess not otherwise much recognized by the Santals and not worshipped by others than *ojhas*, a sign that the here described proceedings are not of unmixed Santal origin. *Dhạrti mae* or only *mae* seems to be mixed up with *Kạli* sometimes).

The *ojha* now takes the *sal* leaves and looks first at the one, then at the other with an intense look, keeping them high up. The rib of the leaves may be torn off, and the two leaves are often folded and creased, so as to make marks across the surface. This assists in localizing, as will be seen.

On one of the leaves he now commences to put oil-marks. A *sal* leaf has a number of strong ribs or veins, dividing the surface into a number of 'compartments.' In separate places the *ojha* with his right-hand index- or middle-finger puts a drop of oil, saying at the same time, what each oil-mark is to stand for, *viz.*, the supposed possible cause or origin of the patient's disease or trouble.

The possibilities are supposed to be found among four classes: natural causes, human beings, *boṅgas*, and the Ancestors.

The natural causes are mostly counted into two headings, natural disease and *disom duk*, *i.e.*, an epidemic with high mortality; *disom duk* is mentioned elsewhere in the Introductory Remarks to the Santal Medicine to which the reader is referred; *disọm duk* is somewhat doubtful as to its natural or other origin, hence it is kept separate for possible later investigation.

The human beings who cause disease are the witches, and as every woman is considered a potential witch, separate marks are put down for the women of the household of the patient, of the wife's father's household, and of the wife's mother's original household. Individual beings are not sought for at this stage, only the household in which a possible witch may be found. A mark, or several, may also be put down for the village households.

The *boṅgas* are several; the most commonly suspected are the family *boṅga* of the patient, or of his wife's father (if the patient is a grown-up and married person), the *simạ boṅga* (the spirit of the village boundary), the *boṅgas* supposed to reside outside the village, those invoked in the rice-fields and on the threshing-floor; on the whole *boṅgas* who have a reputation for being particular, exacting, easily hurt, and for being specially malevolent.

The fourth class consists of the forefathers, *hapṛamko*. They might be classified as *boṅgas*; there is, however, a decided difference, to mention one thing, sacrifices to *boṅgas* are performed by beheading the sacrificial animal, whilst to the *hapṛamko* it is always done by a stroke of an axe-head on the neck. The Ancestors are seldom brought in, perhaps mostly when the *ojha* has a suspicion that some recently dead person in the family may have a grudge of some kind.

The *ojha* in this way puts marks here and there on the leaf, at the same time muttering to himself, that this is for such and that for such, and a third for something else, and so on, whereupon he commences to rub each mark in with his finger. This should be particularly noted, because here the *ojha* has an opportunity of using his 'art' and discretion. It is not wholly accidental when this or that cause is finally shown up.

Whilst rubbing in the oil as described, the *ojha* mutters the following *mantar* or incantation: *Tel tel, rae tel, man tel, kusum tel, kocṛak tel, aṛnḍik tel, bherṇḍak tel, rae rui tel, i tel poṛhaete ki uṭho? ḍan uṭho, bhut uṭho, jugin uṭho, bis uṭho; kẹ poṛhẹz guru poṛhẹ; guru giã, mae poṛhẹ, poṛhasrẹ kaḥri giã, Kạmru guru dohaere dohae poṛhẹ.*

The meaning of this rigmarole is about as follows: 'Oil oil, mustard oil, *man* oil (oil from some kind of mustard seed), *kusum* oil (from the seeds of Schleichera trijuga, L.; the Santali name of the tree is *bạru*), *kocṛak* oil (from the seeds of the *mohua* tree, Bassia latifolia, Roxb.; the name of the tree is in Santali *matkọm*, of the fruit *kũiṇḍi*, hence also of the oil in Santali *kũiṇḍi* oil), castor oil (the name of the tree, Ricinus communis, L. used by the Santals is *eraḍọm*), *bherṇḍak* oil (oil of Jatropha curcas, L., in Santali generally called *bherṇḍa*), *rae rui* oil (meaning uncertain, *rae* is mustard, *rui* is the cotton of the Bombax malabaricum, D.C.; the expression is possibly meant to give a general name for oils expressed by the Hindu *tili* caste, an explanation offered by Santals), this oil reading over (or, to read), what will appear? a witch may appear, a *jugin* (female demon, sorceress or witch) may appear, an imp may appear (*bhut* in Santali is supposed to be the spirit of a child, dead before getting a name, or before birth; it may be something a little different here), poison may appear; who reads? the *guru* reads, the *guru*'s knowledge (*giã* is possibly a corruption of *gyan*, a form, in Santali pronounced *gean*, that is also sometimes heard; another explanation heard is that *giã* is the same as *aggya*, command, order), *mae* (see above, perhaps a name for *Kali*) reads, do read (or, reads, as the word is also heard pronounced *poṛhẹ siri*), by *Kạhri's* knowledge; by *Kạmru guru*'s grace, grace he reads.'[1]

The *mantar* is finished off by the *ojha* blowing on the leaf. Having muttered the *mantar* the *ojha* takes the other leaf and places this on the top of the one marked with oil nips off the tips and presses the two leaves together and rubs them against one another. He salutes the leaves and mutters a fresh *mantar*, of which the follow-

[1] The translation of this and other *mantars* reproduced is as literal as possible, but always in accordance with the ideas the Santals themselves combine with the words; the text is, however, often obscure. I might mention that I have not succeeded in finding any Santal, *ojha* or others, able to explain certain words and phrases in these formulæ. They simply state that they are repeating what they have learnt from their *gurus*. That the text is corrupted from what it may have originally been, is only what may be expected. On the one hand these *mantars* are in a language foreign to, and not always understood by a Santal; on the other hand the method of teaching is far from perfect. The writer has heard several *ojhas* reeling off these *mantars*, and it has been very difficult to make out exactly what was said. The words come tumbling on the top of one another, reeled off in a great hurry, spoken, not freely, but with bent head, muttered into the clothes, indistinctly. If the *mantars* are pronounced in a similar way, when the *ojha* disciples learn, it will not be strange, if they do not catch all that is spoken; it must be difficult for them to get the words correctly. It must also be difficult for the *ojha guru* to hear whether the disciples repeat his wording correctly. The experience of the writer has been, that the *ojhas* have difficulty in remembering the words of a *mantar* or *jhạrni*, if they are to be pronounced fairly slowly; in such cases they are liable to leave out several words and are often unable to say how it should be; they have to start the rigmarole again from the beginning and reel it off at top speed to get all properly out. This is, of course, a phenomenon not unknown with people who cram without understanding or reflecting on the meaning. It is naturally not the sense of it that interests, but its supposed inherent magic. The meaning of *Kạhri* is obscure. See below, Appendix I, p. 48, footnote 2.

ing is a sample: *Pat pat, sal pat, cihũṛ pat, bhelar pat, ki ki uṭhe? ḍạn uṭhe, jugin uṭhe, dhargaṛ uṭhe, debṭa uṭhe; kẹ dẹkhẹ? guru dẹkhẹ, dekhasẹ uṭhạs.*

Translated it runs something like this: 'Leaf leaf, *sal* leaf, *cihũṛ* leaf (here is meant the leaf of Bauhinia Vahlii, I am informed, and not of what the Santals call *cihũṛ*, Spatholobus Roxburghii, Benth.), *bhela* leaf (leaf of what the Santals call *sọsọ*, Semecarpus anacardium, L.): what, what appears? A witch may appear, a female demon may appear, some demon may appear, some godling may appear; who sees? thẹ *guru* sees; let yourself be seen, come out.'

Making a fresh obeisance to the leaves he puts them for a short while on the ground; he just presses them down and leaves them there; if there is any wind, he puts a small clod of earth or a small stone on top to prevent the leaves being blown away. Then again saluting the leaves he picks them up and keeps them like a shield for a moment up against the sun or sky, whereupon he removes the covering leaf and proceeds to investigate the result, which is judged according to the way in which the oil spots are found in the different parts of the leaf marked off as mentioned above. In one place the oil may look like a ring, in another there is a streak, and so on.

Above is a description of the practice followed by most *ojhas*. There are, as might be expected, variations in detail. The *mantars* may differ a little, and the whole may be a little more or a little less circumstantial.

Some *ojhas* are in the habit of offering a short invocation (*bakhẽṛ*), before the leaves are taken up for inspection, this to secure the benevolence of those invoked. This *bakhẽṛ* (nearly all of it in Santali) runs somewhat like this: *Johar tọbẹ, am Siń boṅga ar Dhạrti mae, ẹnḍẹkhan nui hoṛ cet lekate nãṛã piṛiń ńam akal, niạge acarke, bicạrkeapẹ, dud kẹ dud, pạni kẹ pạni, Gosãe bạpu Ṭhạkur tiń dọ.*'

Translated this means: 'Hail then, thou *Siń boṅga* (lit. day-spirit, i.e., the sun, often confounded with the Supreme Being) and *Dhạrti mae* (see above): now then, how this person has acquired this troubling matter may you (it might be noted that the plural is used, and not the dual, as might be expected) judge and settle, milk for milk, water for water, *Gosãe bạpu Ṭhạkur tiń dọ.*'[1]

Another form of the invocation may be translated as follows: 'Hail then, thou *Siń boṅga*, I am offering oil in the name of so and so. If it is to be true, let the true show up. Do not let anything false show up.'

This last to some extent reminds one of certain oaths taken by the Santals, when the Supreme Being is invoked to be a witness to the truth.

As already remarked, these invocations are not always, or even frequently used.

Before leaving this matter it might be mentioned that the *mantar* '*Tel, tel, etc.*'

---

1 The last words, sometimes omitting *gosãe*, are a stereotype ending of nearly every Santal *bakhẽṛ* or invocation, addressed to the *boṅgas*. It is an address. *Gosãe* is the Hindi word and is borrowed from the Hindus; the Santals have a female deity, worshipped in their 'holy' groves, called *Gosãe era*, Gosãe's wife. *Bạpu* is rustic Bengali for 'father'; *Ṭhạkur* is a word met with in late Sanskrit, likely of Sanskrit origin, used by the Santals, specially by their *gurus*, as their name for God. *Tiń* means 'mine', *dọ* is a particle not generally translatable. The whole might thus be rendered; 'Lord, Father, my God.'

or something like it, sometimes is 'read' over oil in a leaf-cup, when the oil is to be used as an embrocation. This is called *sunum paṛhao*, to 'read' oil.

When in the *mantars* so many different names of oils and leaves, etc., are used, it may be explained by a wish to have any possibly used kind of oil mentioned. Only one kind is used at the time, but there is no objection to any kind of oil. If the particular kind used should not be mentioned in the *mantar*, the magic would be spoilt.

In addition to the above described *sunum boṅga* the *ojha* will sometimes make use of the following means to ascertain the nature of the disease and the name of the *boṅga* who is making mischief.

Sitting down he makes, with a twig or the handle end of a *sirom* broom, three long lines on the ground, drawing a number of short lines across the three long ones, consequently getting a figure with a number of squares. When the figure is ready he fixes the twig in the ground inside one of the squares (or if he uses a broom, he keeps this in a vertical position, handle down, for a little while); he then takes the twig (or broom) and raises it to his forehead, as if he were saluting it, whereupon he destroys the figure. He repeats this operation a couple of times, every time destroying the figure drawn. When saluting the twig, a disease is mentioned; if the hand trembles, it is the disease then just named.

This is called *tạrik*, this word being in Santali used in the meaning, not only of a date, but also of ascertaining, finding out; here one might call it diagnosing by divination. The *tạrik* operation is, as will be understood, to find out what kind of disease it is.

Next he takes a broom (of *sirom*, Andropogon muricatus, Retz., straw). With the handle end of this he draws a circle on the ground. The *ojha* sits on his haunches facing the east. Having drawn the circle he puts the handle end of the broom down in the centre. Taking the broom up to his forehead he salutes it; naming the name of a *boṅga* he puts the handle end down again in the middle of the circle and keeps the broom there in a vertical position for a few moments. He keeps on saluting, mentioning a *boṅga*'s name and putting down the broom again, until his hand holding the broom commences to tremble, of course, involuntarily. Then he knows, it is the *boṅga* just named that is making the mischief.

It is strange to meet with practices of this kind among people like the Santal *ojhas*.

The marks made on the ground are in all cases obliterated by spitting on them and then rubbing them out with the heel of the left foot. They are never left for others to see.[1]

---

1 Divination is not something peculiar to the *ojha's* mental attitude; it is resorted to even by Santal boys at an early age, as the following examples will show, also called *khạri*.

Santal boys are from infancy, one might say, accustomed to use the bow and arrow. A small bow is one of the earliest playthings a Santal father will give his son; the small boys often spend their time shooting at whatever may suit. If—as sometimes happens—an arrow cannot be found, in spite of all search, the boys sit down, and one of them, takes a bow, strung tight and bent, and puts one end down on the ground; keeping the bow upright with one hand on its upper end he makes the bow spin round and round, whilst he pronounces the following *bakheṛ*: *Tope uṛič*

XI.

The result of the divination. Alleged causes of disease.

Whether the *ojha* believes in the possibility of any revelation by the above described supposed supernatural means, it is difficult to say. It is scarcely likely, and many have confessed to the whole being done to keep people satisfied, for show. There may possibly be found some *ojhas* who have a belief. It is in any case to the *ojha*'s interest to keep this thing going; it is also part of his profession.

As to the result of this 'divination': the *ojha* will, without great difficulty, be able to get an inkling of the mind of those whom he is called in to serve. There are also some points which it is always safe and profitable to bring out. The desired result is, as suggested above, obtained by more or less rubbing when applying the oil. And even if all should not be exactly as expected, this might be taken as a special 'revelation.' Except when invited by the *ojha*, no one will look at the leaves; he is at liberty to declare what he sees, and very few would think of challenging his 'vision'; this might involve disrespect of the supernatural and taking responsibility on oneself.

According to circumstances the *ojha* finds out that the origin of the trouble is a natural one, or is to be sought with witches, or some *bońga* or other, and so on. Frequently a mixed cause is 'found.'

It is a general belief among the Santals that the several *bońgas* supposed to reside on the outskirts of the village are more than ordinarily malevolent and very difficult to propitiate. It is not within the competence of everybody to perform the necessary here; but the *ojha* knows.

As previously mentioned, the *bońgas* are all looked upon as evil and malevolent. If they are in any way 'hurt' (e.g., if a sacrifice has not been offered; or, offered, but not with a faultless liturgy, and so on), or they are 'hungry' (for a sacrifice), they may cause disease: how, is not reflected on.

---

bạṇḍiạ kakṛa, ńamok̆ khan dǫ ńamok̆ ma, bań khan hǫpǫnme lań dal gǫjea, that is, Tailless uṛic̓ (a small bird, supposed to give omen), lizard without a tail, if it is to be found, may it be found; otherwise we two (inclusive dual, as commonly used in threatening language) shall strike thy young one dead.

The boy then suddenly takes his hand off, the bow turns round a few times and falls down. The direction in which the bow falls indicates where they are to look for the arrow.

Another proceeding of a similar kind is the following. When boys are playing together it will happen that some one breaks wind. The matter is taken up, and the offender is asked to confess. All deny any knowledge, but the offender must be found. The boys sit down in a circle; one boy takes a small twig and breaks it to the requisite length; standing in the middle of the circle he spits in his left hand, and putting one end of the small bit of the twig in the spittle he presses it down, so it will stand upright for a moment, when he takes his right hand off. When the twig falls, the one towards whom it points is the culprit. He is at once charged with the offence, and if he does not confess, they all of them commence to slap him, so he has to confess! If he does not confess, the others will not let him play with them. The oracle cannot fail!

Some time ago I read about a famous assyriologist who had been digging in vain to find something he thought must surely be somewhere there. Then he closed his eyes, turned himself round several times, and having lost all sense of direction he threw a potsherd or something, whereupon he gave orders to dig where this was found, and right enough, that was the place!! Nihil sub sole novi.

Having performed the divination, the *ojha* will tell those who have employed him what is needed. He will say something like this: 'Such and such a *boṅga* (mentioning a tribal or family *boṅga*) comes out on the oil leaf. Somehow he has been offended or hurt. Please satisfy him and make him friendly again. Libate water to him (this is done, coupled with a promise of a sacrifice on recovery). Do something yourselves; do not trust in the *ojha* alone. However, there are also signs, that some spirit of the outskirts is at work. I myself shall take care of him. You look after your own. And if you have any doubt, please seek corroboration elsewhere. It will sometimes happen, that the divination points in a wrong direction. It is satisfactory to get corroboration from elsewhere; then all doubt vanishes.'

It is felt necessary to take this last reservation. The *ojhas* have plenty of evidence that their divinations have pointed the wrong way. The cause is, of course, not that the whole is humbug, but (what is always suspected) that witches have been at work. These are supposed to have power to prevent the divination of an *ojha* from exposing them (the witches), and to throw the blame on others. But to tell the Santal beliefs on this point belongs to elsewhere.

XII.

The ojha *propitiates the spirits of the outskirts of the village.* Bul māyām *performance.* Kombro sim. Bulau.

The *ojha* will next call for some *adwa caole* (*i.e.*, rice husked without having been previously boiled in the husk; only *adwa* rice is used for sacrificial purposes, and the husking is, for this purpose, done by grinding the *adwa* grain in a winnowing fan with a *guṛgu*, a cylindrical stone used ordinarily for grinding spices, etc.), and for a little *sindur*, the red lead or vermilion stuff, which he packs in a leaf and first takes to the patient, instructing him to touch this with his left hand. This *sindur* is taken along if they intend to perform a sacrifice.

Having got these things the *ojha* and the head of the house go out a little way off. Here the *ojha* with a thorn pricks himself on his thigh and on his stomach, so that blood comes out (by pressure). If the patient is very ill, he will do the same on his breast (the nipple), the tongue and the scrotum. He has up to thirty-three (some say a hundred) places on his body where he may prick himself. The blood extracted is smeared on the rice and all well mixed; whereupon he scatters this rice on the ground (without first making any *kǫṇḍ* or magic circle) as an offering to the *boṅgas*, one portion for each *boṅga*, as they are mentioned. The first to be mentioned at this occasion is the *bahre boṅga* (the spirit of the outskirts); then *Maraṅ buru* (lit. the great mountain, the principal national Santal godling), and so on.

This offering of blood is called to administer *bul māyām ; māyām* is the Santali word for blood, *bul* is a word otherwise used for a drunken, unconscious state; the word seems also to mean 'impregnated with, infused with' in a few expressions. As this does not seem to give any good meaning, it might be suggested to compare the word with the Hindi *bali* which may mean an oblation, offering. In support of this *bal kaṭi* might be mentioned ; the *ojha*'s fee for this special work is called so.[1]

In explanation of this act of the *ojha* it might be suggested that it is meant to be vicarious, or possibly to induce the *boṅga* to believe that the patient is dead. Anyhow, the object is to make the *boṅga* satisfied.

Blood is given to satisfy a malevolent spirit. As they express themselves: Seeing or tasting blood the *boṅgas* are very pleased and are quickly ready to listen. It will be told further on, how they try to deceive certain deities by having a funeral *in effigie*. It might possibly be that something of the same kind is intended here also, and that the expression is meant to convey the idea, that it is blood of a person *in extremis*. This is, however, only a conjecture.

When strewing the blood-soaked rice, the *ojha* will at the same time invoke the *boṅga*. The following is a specimen of such an invocation: "Now then, thou so and so (name of *boṅga*) ; for some reason or other thou hast been filled with covetousness and desire and hast run foul of and set thyself against this house : or, who knows, perhaps somebody has engaged thee and egged thee on, and thou hast therefore caused illness and transgression to commence and be started in this house.

"To-day we two (*i.e.*, thou and I) have caught thee, have clutched thee like a fish, like a crab ; wherever thy place, thy abode may be, thither thou wilt go, thou wilt start. From to-day may the pain, the suffering cease and give way. From to-day mayest thou leave alone, keep clear of the house of this so and so (name of householder) ; also may a thief commit adultery with thy mother.

"Now then, if I see thy trustworthiness, in some days I shall give thee, hand to thee thy dues, thy sacrifices and thy offerings. May a thief commit adultery with thy mother.

"Now then, look here, you of the holy grove, you Five-Six, thou Lady of the grove, *Gosãe* lady, Great mountain, Pargana, *Mạñjhi haṛam* (the different national godlings or *boṅgas* who are ordinarily worshipped in the villages), do not assist, do not support this (name) *boṅga*. Wherever his place, wherever his abode, thither you will lead him and follow him. From to-day may he leave alone, keep clear of this one's house. You also, may you warn him, may you rebuke him.

"Now then, look here, within the surrounding boundaries of this (name) village as many as ye are found, big big ones on hills and hillocks, in roots and stumps, in pits and holes, to all of you I give and hand this offered blood, this soaked blood (*bul māyām siṭkạ māyām*). May ye warn, may ye rebuke this (name) *boṅga*.

---

[1] I have not succeeded in getting a satisfactory explanation from any Santal as to what they really understand by the expression, except, of course, that it is their name for this specific sacrificial performance. In the *bakhẹ̃ṛ* (invocation), cited below, they use as a kind of synonym the word *siṭhạ* (*bul māyām*, *siṭkạ māyām*) ; now these *bakhẹ̃ṛ* have nearly always doublets to express their meaning ; the doublets are really about the same, but may each lay stress on a different side of the same idea or action. *Siṭhạ* is their name for fever (in females) combined with strong thirst, specially also for puerperal fever. I may mention that I have heard a Santal *ojha* give the following explanation of this last mentioned : *siṭhạ māyām* is the blood of menstruation ; witches soak rice in this and give it to *boṅgas* and in this way seduce them. How this should fit the *ojha*, the man could not explain.

"Now then, look here, ye Bhuyas, Nayas, Doms, Hadis, Jolhas, Dhunyas (these castes and races, all of a low order and living in the country, here stand for their respective godlings), ye naked males, ye naked females, have a care, to all of you I give and hand this *bul māyām siṭkạ māyām.* This one (name) is ill; may he get well, may he recover.

"Now then, ye who draw near, come near; ye who do not come near, from a distance give witness to it, give splendour to it with your presence.

"Now then, *Patcirạ* (lit. torn leaf, name of a *boṅga*), be greeted. Look here, to thee also I am giving, I am handing this here. If any widow, or woman of ill omen, has selected this one for destruction, has put a stop like a dried leaf, a rolled up leaf, drive her away like the dust of the road; like a whirlwind may she be carried off."

Truly a very comprehensive invocation. Here is another specimen, addressed to only one *boṅga*, the name of which is supposed to have been found out by repeated divination by leaves. Some of the expressions have been considerably toned down in the translation, because they would be impossible of literal rendering.

"Now then, look out, *Kal Cạṇḍi* (name of a female *boṅga*, as the name shows, borrowed from other races), thou hast set thyself against, hast run foul of (some one) in the house of such and such a Santal. Some widow, some ill-omened woman whoever it may be, has hired thee, invited thee. Therefore thou hast become fixed, become nailed down in so and so's house. Now look here, like a fish, like a crab I have caught thee, have clutched thee. From countryside to countryside, everywhere it was made evident, it was proved that it is thou (*i.e. sunum boṅga* has been performed in many places, and this *boṅga* has been shown up).

"Now look here, on that account, with buffaloes, with rams I give thee, I hand to thee *bul māyām, siṭkạ māyām*, broken grain, rice grain. From to-day mayest thou hiss at, mayest thou drive away (ill) in the house of so and so. Wherever thy place, wherever thy abode, thither thou wilt start, wilt go. From to-day if any widow, any one who has lost her husband, destines for perdition, shuts up any one on a torn leaf, a folded leaf (hints at the procedure followed in performing *sunum boṅga*, see above), then thou wilt rub, wilt scour the principal stool, the principal sitting board. If from to-day thou wilt not listen to this, thou and I shall dishonour thy mother, thou and I shall buy twelve *gurus* and pierce thee with twelve thorns; root and branch thou shalt be eradicated, be left without descendants. Like salt thou shalt melt away; like ashes thou shalt be blown away. If thou art living with, committing incest with thy father, with thy brother, thou wilt not in any way listen to this, certainly not; but if thou livest innocent in righteousness, thou wilt listen to this."

An invocation like the above reveals a good deal, both as regards the *ojha* and as regards the conception he, and the others, have of the nature of the *boṅgas*.

As the *ojha* mutters his invocation, he strews the rice soaked with blood on the ground; having finished this he goes to where there is water, to wash the parts where he has pricked himself. He also sprinkles a little water on his head. Those who are with him (there will naturally always be some besides the person who has engaged him) also sprinkle water on their heads, whereupon the *ojha* expresses himself to the effect, that now he has done this thing and his part, and exhorts the person responsible to do his part; then they will see that all will be well.

Before, or after, the *bul māyām* performance the *ojha* may take some other precautions. He calls for a *kombṛo sim*, a thieving fowl. They bring him a speckled fowl or a *risą* fowl (*risą sim* is their name for a fowl with the feathers standing the wrong way; these are considered to be of special merit for certain purposes; it must not, however, be white, if intended for a sacrifice to a *boṅga* other than *Marań buru*).

The proceedings are as follows: The *ojha* gets some charcoal and some earth or burnt clay (called *eṭko hasa*), scraped from the inside of a fireplace; these two stuffs he grinds to powder and puts temporarily aside wrapped up in two leaves (they are not mixed).

He has brought with him a leaf of the *sal* tree on which he has performed *sunum boṅga* (see above Sec. X; it might be remarked that whilst *boṅga*, when used as a verb, generally means to sacrifice, and also figuratively is used for beheading, it is here used for rubbing oil on a leaf, whilst invoking spirits); the covering leaf is there, it has not been thrown away.

As a rule, the *ojha* performs what is here mentioned inside the house, where the patient is, not far from the door; some say it must be done here; apparently it may also, if thought more satisfactory, be performed at some place away from the houses.

Sitting on his haunches the *ojha* first with a small bit of wood, a twig or the like makes a circle on the floor, some ten to twelve inches in diameter. Thereupon he takes the two *sal* leaves mentioned in his left hand, removes the covering leaf, and keeps the other up in the air, looking intently at the 'figures' or marks seen on it. Inside the circle drawn on the floor he now with the twig makes a number of marks, so far as possible resembling those on the leaf; thereupon he spits on the marks made on the floor and puts his left heel heavily down on the circle, and finally with the same left heel rubs out the marks he has drawn.

This performance is repeated several times from beginning to end; it is called *ãk rapuṭ* (to break the figure, *i.e.* the marks supposed to be caused by a witch). The *ojha* does not say anything during the operation. The object is to undo the deception of a possible witch.

When ready with this he gets a leaf-plate (of the same kind as those used to eat from). Putting this down on the ground he makes a circle on it by dropping down on it the above mentioned *eṭko hasa* (burnt clay from a fireplace). He takes a little between his fingers and lets it gradually fall down, as he moves his hand in a circle; thereupon he makes cross marks inside the circle in the same way, only that he for these makes use of the powdered charcoal. The cross lines (diameters) may be two or four, dividing the circle into four or eight sections or sectors. These cross-lines are called *ḍhera dag*, *ḍhera* mark; *ḍhera* is their name for the wooden cross-pieces of a hand-spindle.

He next turns over the leaf-plate, and so most of the figures made are destroyed

4

by the powdered stuff falling down (it is all dry). He repeats the process two or three times; then he puts his left heel down in the centre of the figure on the leaf-plate, and ultimately bites the plate with his teeth and in this way turns it over.

Thereupon he makes a last figure on the leaf-plate, just like what has been described. They give the *ojha* some *adwa* rice; he takes a little with his fingers and lets it fall in a couple of the sectors of the figure, also making some *sindur* marks in the middle of the plate.

Now the above-mentioned fowl is given into his hand, and the *ojha* applies *sindur* to its head. He then calls for the patient who is brought and sits down in front of the *ojha*. The *ojha* is facing towards the east, the patient consequently more or less towards the west. The *ojha* has the fowl in his left hand; at his command the patient touches the fowl, also with his left hand, whereupon the *ojha* makes the fowl feed on the rice put on the leaf-plate.

After this the *ojha* performs what is called *bulạu* with the patient. He takes the fowl and moves it thrice round the patient (to do this the *ojha* must stand up), making a circle alternately from right to left, and alternately thrice the opposite way passing the fowl on its way between his legs from behind and forwards; the fowl is first taken in the right hand round the patient, passed between the *ojha's* legs from behind underneath the right thigh; here the *ojha* takes hold of the fowl with his left hand and passes the fowl round the sitting patient and beneath his left thigh, when he again changes hands.[1]

The fowl is made to feed on the rice three or five times, and the *bulạu* is performed as many times.

Hereupon the *ojha* takes some cowdung and with this obliterates the traces of the circle he at first made on the floor with the twig. With his left-hand little-finger he makes a small circle or square at the spot; from this he pinches off a little earth; this he mixes with the remnants of the cowdung used and rolls it all into a ball. This ball he puts into a cup with water, at the same time dipping his fingers well so as to clean them a little. A leaf-cup with water is also brought; in this he throws some ashes (some say, also some salt, sometimes one cup is made to suffice for all).

The *ojha* then takes the leaf-wrappers (in which the charcoal and *eṭko* were), and wrapping these and whatever else he has used, up in the leaf-plate used for making figures on, he walks out (or if outside, away from the place) with the fowl in his hand. He must not look back. When he passes out, all people belonging to the house enter and go well inside (people not belonging to the household may be staying in the court-yard, it does not matter). The people inside the house now take the cup with the cowdung-mixed water and throw the water after the *ojha*; the same is done with the leaf-cup with ashes and water, only in this case the cup it-

---

[1] It is of no consequence; but as the proceedings have been described a little differently by the late Dr. Campbell in his Santali dictionary, specially remarking that the fowl is taken by the right hand underneath the left thigh, which is only possible if the fowl is passed between the legs from the front side, I may remark that the *ojhas* in these parts expressly deny that so is done. There are also other differences.

self is also thrown out. Hereupon they take a broom and sweep any water that may have been spilt on the floor or on the threshold, out and away, and quickly close the door. They remain inside shut up in this way for a few minutes, long enough to let the *ojha* get away from the house. The *ojha* apparently takes the 'difficulty' along with him.

Followed by some of the village men the *ojha* goes straight off to the forest or to some other place away from people. Here he sacrifices the fowl in the name of some *bonga* of the outskirts (the name has been ascertained by *khaṛi* previously), offering a *bakhẽṛ* (invocation) similar to those cited above.

Some decapitate the fowl and eat it forthwith (*i.e.*, the *ojha* and those who have followed him). Others perform the sacrifice by wringing the fowl's neck; in this case they do not eat the fowl; it is left at the spot with some stones thrown over it. This last procedure is likely the most common.

The *ojha* after having done all this returns to the house of the patient, where he 'brings down oil and *sindur*' (*ãṛgo*), as it is called. He makes in the court-yard some marks with *sindur*, at the same time making vows of offering sacrifices to some special *bonga* of his, when the patient recovers (this is the *saket*).

Now the *ojha* is ready to commence administering medicines.

It might be remarked, that the performances just described are generally only gone through when the state of the patient is considered grave or difficult.

XIII.

Behaviour awaiting results. Saket. *Proceedings on recovery of patient.*

The *ojha* has now done what is required of his profession, and the man responsible will invite him to come home along with him. Here he is well fed, treated with great consideration and flattered; he is told, that they now look to him for help. He is particularly asked to bring medicinal roots and prepare the necessary medicine. "It is not enough," they repeat, "to make *bonga* (*i.e.*, to worship the spirits with sacrifices) in order to bring about recovery," and so on (*vide supras*).

To this the *ojha* answers that "this is the truth, and according to this I shall bring the proper medicine. But as the saying is : it is God who makes well, so even if I do my utmost, it may happen, that the, patient does not recover." "However, I shall exert myself to the extent of my knowledge of medicine. But I am no God, that I should be able to make the patient well and sound at once. We must try by Medicine as far as we can ; whatever *Bidhi Bidhaṇta* have written on our foreheads that happens. There is also something written about life and death; and when we reach that we die." [1]

[1] The belief here referred to is as the two names at once show, not of Santal origin, but has some time or other, perhaps in a not very remote antiquity, been adopted from the Hindus, and thereupon adapted to suit Santal ideas. The Santals have a hazy kind of belief that life and life's happenings are predestined. This belief does not play any great

After this or some similar harangue the *ojha* goes home; but for the next three days or so he will exert himself, all he can, in administering medicine.

The people who have called in the *ojha* will, if they have not already done so, now say to him: "Please make sure the *saket* and then administer medicine." The *saket* is the sacrifice to be offered to the special tutelary *bonga* of the *ojha* (referred to in the previous chapter); the meaning of the above is that the *ojha* shall give a formal vow to sacrifice to his *bonga* when the patient recovers. The object is double, to make the *ojha* exert himself and to secure the co-operation of the *bonga*.

The *saket bonga* varies; the different *ojhas* often have different *bongas*.

The *ojha* will then make a vow of sacrificing a goat or a ram, or pigeons, or a pig; and so administer medicine.

With the beliefs a Santal has, it is possible to understand the "remedies" resorted to.

Provided the patient recovers, there is nothing more to do than what has been described, except that they have to fulfil their vows and pay the *ojha*. They will wait a couple of months after recovery, and when they feel sure that there will be no relapse, they approach the *ojha* and say that they will give him the *saket* sacrifice, whatever he may have promised to give to his special *bonga*. When the *ojha* has told what animals will be required, they procure these, if they have no suitable ones in the house; they also brew some beer. When they have all ready, they tell the *ojha* that at such and such a time he must not go anywhere; they want to settle and get finally rid of the 'difficulty of some time ago.' A day is then appointed on which the *ojha* is fetched. The headman and the deputy headman of the village are also invited.

---

rôle in the ordinary life of a Santal, but may be brought out as a kind of solace or explanation at times of death or calamities. There is with many a belief in fate, accepted as a matter of course, but not reflected on.

The following is told by Santal *gurus*:—

Ṭhạkur, the Supreme Being, previous to the creation of man, created two beings, *Bidhi* and *Bidhạnta*, and appointed them to be his *muhril* (the Santali form of the Hindi word *moharrir*), *i.e.*, writers. When a human being is born these two beings have to attend at once, immediately after birth, to write on the forehead of the newborn babe what is to be his or her fate. At the same time they measure out the seer to the newborn (see above, p.1).

It is further told that at the birth of every human being all diseases appear, elbowing each other to reach the babe first. It is just like what is to be seen when a crowd of people attempt to get a sight of anything strange; all try to push their way to the front. Whichever disease is able to come first gets a kind of proprietary right in the child from the *Bidhi* and *Bidhạnta*. When your seer is finished or eaten, *i.e.*, when your time for dying is come, this disease will catch hold of you and carry you off. Do whatever you like, there is no rescue.

To modify this, so far as possible, the following is done:—When labour has commenced with a woman, some one of the household, such as the husband (it must be a man, not a woman) lights a fire in the court-yard just outside the door. As soon as the child is born, some one comes hurriedly out of the house (this time a woman, as men do not attend at labour) and strikes the roof of the house heavily with a stick. The cause of these actions is said to be the following: A human being will in any case have to 'go away' by fire, *i.e.*, his dead body will be cremated. So let the fire here called *Borma Ṭhạkur*, be the first to attend. The beating of the roof is meant to frighten the different diseases away.

It might, however, be noted, that the commonly given explanation of the roof-beating is that it is done to prevent the newborn child from becoming timid. If it is omitted, the child will, they say, be frightened and startled even at the least sound.

A variant of the preceding is as follows:—Immediately after birth all kinds of animals, specially tigers and snakes, urther trees, water, fire, in short all beings and natural objects that may kill or be the cause of death, appear before *Ṭhạkur* and put in their claim to getting possession of the child. The one succeeding in coming first will take the life some day. The fire is lighted to ensure that the person when dead shall be burned, *i.e.*, that death shall not take place when the body cannot be recovered. The last variant sounds like an attempted improvement.

They commence their 'business' with rice-beer. Then the *ojha* goes to bathe (bathing is always necessary before performing a sacrifice); after returning he prepares a *kõṇḍ*, a small place levelled and 'cleaned' with cowdung, puts a few handfuls of *adwa* rice in the *kõṇḍ* and makes some marks (always an uneven number) with mustard oil and *sindur*.

The sacrificial animals are then brought to the *ojha* who sprinkles some water on their front-heads and paints their front-heads and shoulders with *sindur*, whereupon he lets them feed on the rice in the *kõṇḍ*. He then invokes the *boṅga* to whom he made his vow somewhat like this:

"Now observe, thou so and so (name of *boṅga*), when so and so (person is named) was ill, I called on thee and made a vow to thee. Now here to-day I am giving thee, handing to thee twice thrice of what I promised. Don't ask questions; don't make difficulties; mayest thou stand it, like it. Some day in the future I may again call on thee, invoke thee in a like way. Then also be quick to stand up."

Having invoked the *boṅga* in this way he performs the sacrifice by cutting off the heads (as is invariably the custom, see remarks above). The sacrificed animals are then prepared for eating. They do not flay the animal, but put the decapitated body on a smouldering fire and singe off all the hair whereupon it is cut open; the stomach is taken out, all the intestines are 'milked' empty and the flesh is cut into small pieces (it should be remembered that as the fingers only are used when eating, everything has to be of such a size that no cutting is necessary). The head is put aside (the head of a sacrificed animal can never be eaten by others than males, often only by the sacrificer alone). The liver and lungs are cut into bits and cooked in rice together with the head (a process called *suṛe*, the result being something like a meat and rice hash). This last mentioned stuff is on this occasion eaten by four men, *viz.*, the *ojha*, the village headman and his deputy (the *mạṅjhi* and the *paranik*) and the head of the household. All the rest is divided into three equal parts, of which the *ojha* gets one and the head of the house one. The third part is given to the village people who happen to be present. The meat falling to the head of the house is made into *utu* (*i.e.* curry); rice is also prepared, and the whole is eaten by the people assembled.

After having eaten they start afresh drinking rice-beer. Whilst this is going on the head of the house gives the *ojha* Re. 1-4-0, called *dạdni* (fee). Of this the *ojha* gives the village headman four annas; the rest he keeps for himself. In this way all concerned get their dues and more, and there is great jollification, no one thinking of anything else than the happy cure.

When one year has passed without relapse, the *ojha* often gets a final fee of five rupees and a loin cloth.

XIV

Proceedings in case of continued disease. More ojhas. *Mock funeral.* Jib dan.

Now this was all under the supposition that the patient gets better and is cured. If this does not happen within a few days, if the patient continues the same or gets worse, the *ojha* will profess to be astonished and give pretty broad hints that all is not as it should be. A common Santal belief, referred to above, is that the witches, when having set into action their evil influence, are able to prevent their activities being shown up in the oil-leaf divination. This, of course, leaves the gate open to suspicion; something has been seen; but there is the possibility that something wrong, something else than the truth, has been shown on the leaf through the influence of a witch who is the real culprit.

If no betterment comes, the *ojha* will offer to withdraw and will advise the calling in of others, not so much people who might know a little more medicine than he himself (has not *he* cured any number with the same symptoms ?), as some one who might perhaps know a little more about reducing *boṅgas* to sense. "It will not come to anything through me," he will say.

In some cases the relatives of the patient may have some doubts as regards the *ojha*, both as regards his medicinal knowledge and as regards his ability to accurately recognize the nature of the disease. Consequently it may be advisable to call in another man; but they will generally ask the first man also to remain.

The new *ojha* will start work on the same lines as the first one. According to circumstances he may either praise the work of the first man or act so as to show that they, in his opinion, were foolish to engage the services of a person like the first one. Whereupon they have the whole over again. And so they may go on, until the patient dies, or until they have called in all the *ojhas* they know or have heard of, have spent in medicines and sacrifices all their worldly possessions, and have on the top of this got inextricably involved with the money-lenders. So long as the fight against the disease and the malevolent spirits go on, there is, with the Santals, generally very little thought of the after-effects of borrowing. Such extreme cases may be comparatively rare, although they are to be met with; but it is not rare to come across people who have suffered seriously in a pecuniary way, in the manner described.

Before proceeding further, mention shall be made of a curious, in parts revolting, attempt to bring about recovery. It is of rare occurrence.

After having performed *sunum boṅga* (as described above) they make a tiny model bedstead. The legs of this bed are made of the leaf stalk of the *Ricinus*-tree, cut to a length corresponding to the length of the two outer joints of one's little finger; the two end pieces of the bed-frame are 'the length of the index finger,' and the two long pieces are the 'length of the index finger and down to the root of the thumb.' The bed-bottom is woven with thread.

A figure is then made from the stalk of a banana, cotton or Ricinus leaf, the length of the figure being as that of the middle finger.

A leaf is found with three or five ribs (*i.e.* a palmate leaf); on this the spaces between the ribs are painted alternatively red (with *sindur*) and black (with soot).

Now they draw magic marks on the floor (as previously described), and catch a fowl which is made to feed on the *adwa* rice put down in the magic spot (*kǫ̃ṇḍ*) after having let the patient touch it.

Thereupon they draw a bedsted on the floor with a *tirsuṛ* (trident) at the head. They now again let the fowl feed on the rice in the *kǫ̃ṇḍ*, first making it face towards the East; whilst doing this they break its left leg. Then they make it face towards the West and break its right leg, and whilst making it face towards the North and South they break its wings. The fowl is made to feed in the name of the *Jǫmraj* (*i.e.* the king of death).

They also catch two grasshoppers (of a large kind, resembling locusts) which are made to 'feed' on rice put on the leaf painted red and black, these two in the name of *Dhạrti mae.* The rice and *sindur* for the grasshoppers are kept separate. Before they let the grasshoppers 'feed,' they 'exorcise' the patient by blowing upon him, whereupon they cover him up.

The magic marks are destroyed in the way previously described; ashes and salt are also put in water and poured out.

Thereupon they go out some distance away from the houses and build a tiny funeral pyre. The fowl mentioned is sacrificed, but the two grasshoppers are buried in a small hole dug for the purpose.

The above-mentioned 'bedstead' with the figure on it is put on the pyre; the *ojha* takes off his *bhagwa* (*i.e.* the piece of cloth worn between the legs and fastened in the *ḍora* or loin-string at front and back) and, naked, sets fire to the pyre. As soon as the smoke rises, he says: "Now *Jǫmraj*, having seen this smoke, depart."

Hereupon they return to the house and the *ojha* gives the patient what is called *jib dan* (*jib dan* is a Hindi or Bengali word meaning gift of health or life). This is done as follows: They catch a black chicken (other colours are believed to be of no use), cut it open and take out the liver from the living fowl. The cut is sown up again and they let the chicken go, only, of course, to die immediately. The liver thus procured is mixed with a little blood, a bit of the nest of white ants and a new shoot of *dhubi ghās* (Cynodon dactylon, Pers.), all ground together. With part of this the *ojha* rubs the patient on the breast; some of it he gives him to eat.

Some say there is no invocation combined with this revolting procedure, and they will call it medicine. Others say that this fowl is sacrificed to *Kạli mae.* The whole horrible performance, combined with the name given to it, makes it reasonable to suppose that the *jib dan* is meant partly as a vicarious act. The liver is a vital part; it is also the part of the body which the witches are reputed to 'eat.'

Both performances, the mock funeral and the *jib dan,* are resorted to when nothing seems to avail.

XV.

Inimical influence of malevolent spiritual powers suspected (witches). Public called upon to assist. Village takes action.

If the patient does not recover, and the medicines and exertions of the *ojha* do not avail, the suspicions always latent gain strength. The relatives of the patient feel that the case has become so serious, that they ought not any longer to try to tackle the disease alone; they need the help of the community; moreover the case has possibly become one of public interest; it may, of course, be that the cause of it all is witchcraft in their midst, a public danger that must be put down.

The responsible relative of the patient will therefore go to the village officials, the headman and his deputy, and request them to take action, as nothing they themselves have been able to do has had any effect. It might be noted, that the whole village is always more or less interested in cases of illness in their midst; every family will make constant enquiries how the patient is progressing.

The headman orders the *goḍet* (village headman's messenger) to call together the village people (naturally only the men) at the house of the patient, whereupon he (the headman) makes some remarks to the assembled men that 'they' (*i.e.* somebody or other) have made so and so very ill.

The village people reply that they must all of them help and get the proper *ojha* for whom they promise to be surety that he gets his dues, etc. At the same time they exhort the relative of the patient to 'follow the case up.' The responsible relative implores the headman to do so for him. This is really the point for which he has applied to the village people.

Hereupon the headman arranges to send people out to seek 'enlightenment.' The people thus sent take *sal* leaves and a little oil with them, and go in pairs (never only one alone) to a number of known *ojhas* in the vicinity, to make these consult the oracle (divine by leaves) and find out the cause of the disease.

When they find the *ojha*, they give him the leaves and the oil, asking him to perform *sunum boṅga*. The *ojha* asks, in whose name he is to do this, and thereupon does what is required, in the way previously described, tells the messengers what he has seen in the leaves, and gives advice and warning.

In the evening when all the messengers have returned, the village people (that is, the men) again come together in the house of the patient to hear the results. The messengers are called on to report, and do so one after the other. As a rule they all have very much the same to tell; there may be a few differences in the minor details, but the essentials are the same. That this should be so is not strange The *ojhas* follow the system of the fraternity; there are only a few classes of causes to choose between (see above, Sec. X); there are certain causes of disease, according to the beliefs of the people, which are safe to be mentioned. And naturally in the course of their talk with the *ojha* the messengers will let out the general idea of the village people as to what is at the bottom of the matter, specially whether they suspect anybody of having practised witchcraft. The *ojha* will listen for any utterance, however small, which may give him a clue to follow.

The result, as a rule, is that when the messengers come back they tell that the *ojhas* have found the cause of the disease to be that some *bongas* are at work, being hurt or hungry, the family-*bongas* a little, those of the outskirts very much. Or, they have ceased to worship a peculiar *bonga* which their father or grandfather specially worshipped; or they may have neglected one of the Ancestors, and so on. The message generally ends with a more or less strong admonition to take the necessary and proper precautions at once. They must engage a first class *ojha*.

The assembled men then speak to the person responsible, saying that he now can see the result of their help; he must himself look after the family-*bongas*, and not trust in the *ojha* alone. To the already engaged *ojha* they will address some words, instructing him to make sure of his *saket* (the godling who gives him, or is, his power), and assuring him that they shall be responsible for his getting the necessaries for his work. "They will not let his legs be broken," as they express themselves.

The *ojha* acts at once. They bring him water in a *loṭa* and a little cowdung. Having washed his hands and feet he 'cleans' a small bit of the ground with cowdung. He first stands up in front of this facing the East with the *loṭa* in his hand. Then he takes a piece of cloth, twisted like a rope, round his neck, the two ends being twisted together in front (an ancient custom, signifying submission), puts three marks of *sindur* on the spot plastered with cowdung, and standing with his hands 'folded' together over the *loṭa* he offers an invocation to *Siń bonga*, promising a sacrifice as soon as the patient is well. He then obliterates the plastered and *sindur*-marked place, feels the pulse of the patient (as previously described) and proceeds to bring and prepare medicine. And the whole goes on as previously described, with sacrifices by the head of the household and the *ojha*, only that now the case has become a public affair with the village officials, as representing the community, in cooperation.

XVI.

Propitiating the naihaṛ bonga. *Sending away the* kisāṛ bonga. *Buried* bongas.

If all continues to be in vain the various *ojhas* engaged will take counsel together and find out that since nothing avails, specific treatment of the *bonga* in question must be resorted to.

There are two or three kinds of *bongas* that can be treated in this way. One is the so-called *naihaṛ bonga*, the spirit of the father-in-law's household, which is believed sometimes to follow the bride to her new home. The *naihaṛ bonga* is a difficult and much feared personage, really belonging to another subsept and accustomed to some treatment different from what is customary where he has come. He has followed the girl, because there was something or other to which he was attached and would not be parted from, or for any other reason. As soon as a Santal is convinced, that the *naihar bonga* has come along, he will either make yearly sacrifices to him, or, as there is some risk connected with that, as one does not know the requirements of this 'foreign' *bonga*, he will make arrangements to send him back at once. Of himself he will not return.. If either is not done the consequences are disease and death in the house.

If in cases of disease divination by leaves shows this *bonga* up, imminent danger is proved, and the only remedy is to make him return to his old place. To bring this about it is necessary first to send back everything that the bride has brought with her from her father's house, and then to take two animals to the *naihar*, there to be sacrificed to this *bonga*.

Another *bonga* that must be exorcised, if leaf-divination shows him to be responsible, is the so-called *kisãr bonga*, a spirit somewhat akin to the hobgoblin, or the *nisse* of Scandinavian folklore. The *kisãr bonga* is of a rather uncertain character. A man who has got such a one into his house, will be made wealthy through the *bonga* who steals from others and carries all to the house of his 'master,' but if he is offended, there is no end to the mischief he will make. If on his account disease is brought into a family, the whole of it will be eradicated, if the *kisãr bonga* is not effectually sent away from the house.

How this has to be done, is told by the old *Kolean guru*, as follows: They first collect all the necessaries: a silk cloth, a small box of red lead, a tassel, a long plait of horse or cow's hair, an iron hairpin, a small box of eye-paint, a winnowing fan, a wide flat basket, an iron stick, five chains, five iron nails, a pair of wooden clogs, a wooden stool, a miniature cart, a straw bundle containing a little of each of all the crops cultivated by the Santals, five rupees, two cows, a pig, a goat, a ram and five fowls. They tie a bell to the ram. When they have completed collecting all the above, they fetch the *ojha* who knows the proceedings.

Thereupon the *ojha* summons the *kisãr bonga* spirit, that is, he causes a man there present to be possessed by the spirit. The *ojha* puts an old and worn winnowing fan in front of the man to be possessed (generally one who has been through an *ojha*'s course)[1]; putting a handful of sun-dried (*adwa*) rice in the winnowing fan he says: "Come, my lord (*Gosãe*), come thou, such and such a spirit, to the house of so and so. I am calling upon thee; I am crying unto thee, come running, hurry up, the disciple, the pupil is sitting, is waiting" (*i.e.*, the one to be possessed).

---

1 The Santals believe that *bongas* may possess people. The external sign of this possession is a many times repeated, violent turning of the head from one side to another. The hair must be loosened (it is not so very long ago, that the Santal men also were in the habit of keeping their hair long, tied up in a knot). It seems strange that a person can sit quietly down performing this operation; they must have found a method of twisting their head and neck that does not give too much giddiness. To be possessed in this way is called *rum*. When a man is 'possessed,' he loses his own identity and is for the time of 'possession' supposed to be the possessing spirit, is addressed as such and speaks and acts as such. The Santals believe that *rum* in olden times was genuine. Now-a days they apparently believe in its possibility, but have doubts as to any special occasion. The custom is, however, kept up. Many 'rascals' act being *rum* to make people give them beer and the like; such persons have, *e.g.*, observed that all was not absolutely according to ritual at a festival (with sacrifices); shortly afterwards they go to the place, sit down and become *rum*, telling the people that they are such and such a *bonga* who has come being offended at their doings; the people thereupon give them drink etc., to make them satisfied. See further on the subject of *rum* in Appendix I, p. 57 and p. 59.

The man soon becomes possessed, when they ask him: "Well, my lord, now thy master has come to an end with serving and worshipping; well then, he will not keep thee any longer, what hast thou to say?" The *boṅga* thereupon gives a grunt and says: "If he won't keep me, I shall take myself off; let him give me all that is mine."

They thereupon bring all the necessary things out to him and say: "Here are thy belongings, art thou pleased or not?" He says: "Pleased," whereupon he enters the cowshed to choose cows for himself. He slaps two on the back and comes out again, whereupon the others ask him: "Well, hast thou got everything?" "Yes, I have," he replies. The sliding bars at the entrance to the cowshed are then let-down, and the two cows selected by the *boṅga* come out of their own accord, it is told; the two cows are tied together with a rope. Hereupon the people take all the requisite things and say to the *boṅga*: "Come along, lead us to where thy dwelling place, thy abode is." At this stage the *boṅga* leaves the man possessed.

The two cows lead the way of their own accord, the people following behind. The *ojha* takes the winnowing fan along, carrying it under his arm. Wherever the two cows come to a stand and lie down, there the sacrificial animals are beheaded. The ram's head is strung on the chains and nailed to a tree. The flesh of the sacrificed animals is cooked with rice and eaten there on the spot by the people assembled. All the things brought are left behind at this place. No one will touch them; should any one do so, the *kisāṛ boṅga* will follow his goods home to such people. The man from whom the *boṅga* has been driven away will be impoverished before the expiry of a year; his cattle and buffaloes will all die, his paddy and rice will somehow or other disappear; in fact, the family will become paupers.

So far old Kolean who adds: "This has been actually seen. Wealth unrighteously acquired will not remain."

Even now-a-days such proceedings take place; but according to what is told, the *ojha* is not afraid of taking possession of the things left.

Sometimes the *ojha* tells that he has seen in the divination leaf that a '*boṅga*' is buried in their house, and that this is the cause of the disease they have.

The patient's relatives then send people round to other *ojhas* to get this vision verified. It is serious, because witches are supposed to be at the bottom of this. It isalso, by its nature, a public affair (see below, Sec. XVII, where the witches are mentioned); the person affected therefore seeks the assistance of the village community.

A day is fixed for doing the necessary, that is, for removing the buried (*thapna*) *boṅga*, as it is called. An *ojha* who is reputed to understand this, is brought; he comes accompanied by one or two assistants, generally his *paṭ cela* (a disciple of the *ojha*'s, who is fairly advanced in *ojha* science and has passed the preliminary degrees; see below in Appendix I, p. 51 and p. 59), anyhow somebody who may be used. The village people also come together to assist.

First the *ojha* ascertains through divination (*sunum boṅga*) that a *boṅga* is buried in the house. They are supposed to be buried just in front of or inside the *bhitạr* (the ancestors' stall), in front of the fire-place, just inside the threshold, or also just outside, and in the cattle-shed or outside this. The site apparently depends on what or where the suspected enemy works to hit.

The *ojha* now sits down in the court-yard or in the cattle-shed; in front of himself he has a large brass cup with a little oil in it. At his side some of the village people sit down to watch. Looking at the oil he sees that *bongas* have been buried in several places; he orders his assistant to go in and show the places (the *ojha* himself remains seated). The assistant points out the places making a circle with a stick or with a sickle, whereupon the people commence to dig with, preferably, a *khonta* (a wooden bar with a flat iron at one end); the earth dug up is taken outside, crushed and sifted, but nothing is found. The *ojha* continues to look at the oil and exclaims, that he sees the *bonga*; it is moving. The *ojha*'s assistant then goes in with his stick; this should be what is called *ṭaini ṭhenga* (see below, Appendix I, p. 69), a bamboo stick with an iron 'crown' as a head; but as these are seldom found, an ordinary bamboo stick will do. Going inside the assistant stamps the ground with the stick (this is called *ṭak ṭaki*), until it suddenly stops by itself, a sure sign that it is above the buried *bonga*; as it stops, he hawks loudly, and shortly afterwards the *ojha* declares, that now he sees in the oil that the *bonga* will be found. They consequently again dig, and the *bonga* is found. This is generally a small bit of stone (quartz or the like), painted with *sindur* and with human hair tied round it. It may also be some other object; see below.

The secret is, that the *ojha* has brought the '*bongas*' with him; when the assistant performs the *ṭak ṭaki* he has one of these in his hand with which he holds the stick, and lets it drop where convenient. Inside the house there is no difficulty, because a Santal house is dark; outside it is more difficult; the crowd is, however, ordered to keep away, as they might have an adverse influence on the *ṭak ṭaki* operation. I have been told, that *ojhas* or rather their assistants have been caught in the act when digging for such *bongas*. When they are unable to 'plant' the thing, no *thapna bonga* is found, and the *ojha* has to explain this as best he can.

The holes dug are not small, often half a yard deep and as broad.

When the *bongas* have been found, the *ojha* takes possession of these, and the whole company goes to the nearest forest or somewhere away in the open field, and the *ojha* here performs the necessary sacrifices of he-goats, rams or pigs; these are eaten in the usual way; nothing is brought back to the house.

The *thapna bonga* digging described concerns one household only, that has been exposed to the enmity of witches who are believed to be at the bottom.

For the sake of completeness it might be mentioned, that it also happens that a whole village is believed to have been exposed to the same kind of evil action. Such is believed to be the case when a previously prosperous village becomes poor, when the cattle die, when the cows cease to give milk, when the crops, for some reason not understood, deteriorate or fail, and so on.

The proceedings are similar to what has been described; the village people, headed by the village chief, seek enlightenment with an *ojha* who performs the leaf divination; when *thapna bonga* is shown, the matter is verified from other *ojhas*, whereupon the village people collect the money necessary for the expenses *(ojha's* fee and sacrificial animals). An experienced *ojha* is brought; performing *sunum boṅga* he sees in the oiled leaf, that '*boṅgas*' have been buried in several places, as, *e.g.* at the end of the village street *(i.e.* at the entrance to the village), in the middle of the village street, at the *mañjhi than* (where the original village headman has his place of worship), at cross-roads, in the *jaher* (the holy grove of the village), and so on.

In this case the buried *boṅgas* are considerably more elaborate; they may be the shell of a large snail, a silk cocoon, the horn of a ram, of a goat, or even of a bullock, a hollow bone, or something similar to serve the purpose. This is the receptacle for sundry goods; such as a sample of all cultivated cereals, milk, ghee, or anything that may be the cause of the envy of enemies. It is believed that the burying of such goods as those mentioned (with the self-understood accompanying imprecations and in the names of *boṅgas)* will cause injury to the vicinity and its inhabitants.

It should be mentioned that the shells, etc., also have some *sindur* inside, generally painted on a small bit of stone, and that these shells, etc., may also be buried when used against individual households.

As mentioned the *boṅgas* are located through divination by oil-leaf, here not in a cup of oil; but I have heard it said, that if the diggers do not find the buried *boṅga* quickly, the *ojha* moves excitedly about looking into a small mirror (they are up-to-date, the mirror takes the place of the oil), calling out that he sees it is there and there.

He does not always himself dig, and the man who digs has to do so naked; women are kept away during this operation. When the *baṅgas* have been found the *ojha* takes them along, and they all go to the forest, or somewhere away, with the animals that are to be sacrificed. The proceedings here are as described above ; but the *boṅgas* dug out are here burnt to ashes. Being for the whole village the sacrifice is larger and more costly.

This last described *boṅga* digging is called to 'clean the village' *(ato saphae).*

How the *boṅgas* are 'planted' in this case I am unable to say; it cannot be done as in the first case. There is, of course, the possibility that some *ojha* or some one hired by the *ojha*, has done it some time previously to the here described operation. There is also the possibility that witches have buried the things. In such case the object would be to cause mischief by working on the fears of the superstitious people. They will naturally let it be known. I have heard of such cases, and have had such *boṅgas* brought to me, where it seems to have been proved that women (supposed to be witches, see Sec. XVII) have with evil intent buried *boṅgas*. It is not the place to take this matter up for discussion here; I have heard several circumstantial stories of buried *boṅgas*, and whatever may be thought of the *ojha*, the village people have been very excited and in great fear.

When the name *boṅga* is used for the buried things, it is likely because they believe that the powers of a *boṅga* may be joined to the buried stuff; the buried things art a concrete manifestation of the power of a *boṅga*. When such a thing is found, it is a sure sign to the ordinary Santal mind, that a witch has prevailed upon a *boṅga* to do mischief.

The old *guru* Kolean says, that the sacrifices on such occasions were : one ram, one pig, one goat, five fowls and one pair of pigeons.

The result of these exertions to overcome disease is — to follow the Santal course of thought — always doubtful; sometimes the patient recovers, sometimes he gets worse. If *boṅgas* are at the bottom, it is not so easy to make them give up their enmity. They are malevolent and it may be outside the powers or knowledge of man to satisfy them to the full. Then what can man do?

The character of the *ojha* does not come out well here. It is strange that the people with all they have to show them the humbug of the proceedings just described still will practise them.

XVII.

The witches. Proceedings against them. Locating the witch. The withering branch oracle. Testing the verdict.

As has been mentioned several times, there is according to Santal ideas, another possible cause that may be at the bottom of all the trouble. This is witchcraft.

We shall not here enter on the very large subject of witchcraft among the Santals, but tell how the Santals try to combat and overcome this source of disease. Witchcraft is a very real thing to the Santals. Many have tried to pooh-pooh the whole; but more is required to get rid of this nuisance. If we define a witch as a woman who belongs to a secret "society," the members of which meet at certain places and at certain times, have their own secret songs and *mantars* and very likely also their own worship, there is among the Santal villages scarcely one where some such are not to be found. Most of these are likely quite innocuous; but some are bad and downright evil; they know it, believe themselves to be in collusion with evil spirits and try to exert an evil influence. They may possibly also themselves believe that they have magic powers and are able to influence supernatural beings. I have heard them assert this. They are, of course, powerless to do anything, except through suggestion and putting people under the influence of fear, and through giving poison.

There is no genuine Santal who does not believe in witches. This being so, it is not strange that a suspicion is always present that witches may be at work when people fall ill and do not recover. If they have got, to them satisfactory, proof that a woman may be a witch (*e.g.*, by observing any woman out at night where she has no business to be, or a woman who has shown traits of character which ought not to be found in any good woman, and so on), the suspicion materializes and gets an object. Although they are very careful and reticent, this will leak out. I take it that such felt suspicion is the most common cause of *ojhas* 'seeing' witches in the divination leaf.

We have previously heard about the leaf divination. If witchcraft comes out, it is, of course, very serious, not only for the patient, but for the whole community, and no one would think of tackling a matter of this magnitude on his own responsibility. The village authorities are called in, and the headman takes action. Followed by the village men he walks at evening time (when all are supposed to be at home) through the village street, calling out outside every house in a loud voice, "Beware, *phalna* (lit. so and so, no name is mentioned, or could be mentioned here): so and so is ill; may he recover. We have caught thee; if he does not recover, we shall certainly not call thee good."

As will be observed, it is a threat at random. They have no doubt that a witch is at the bottom of it; but they do not know, or have so far no 'proofs,' whatever their suspicions may be, who may be the actual witch; she may be in any house in the village; it is consequently advisable and politic to warn all; then possibly the guilty one may think better of it and leave off.

If the patient after this should recover, well and good. It is to nobody's interest to go further into the matter. Wife, daughter, sister or mother of any of the men of the village might be 'proved' to be a witch. The headman's wife is more often than not suspected.

If, on the other hand, there is no improvement, the headman sends men out in pairs, as previously described, to get other *ojhas* to divine by leaves, what is the cause of the disease. If the verdicts do not agree, they next day send to other *ojhas*. If the messengers bring the same verdict of witchcraft from three different *ojhas*, all doubts are thrown away.

The next thing is to find out, or rather, to 'prove' by divination, where the witch is. There is likely not one of those concerned who does not suspect a certain person; but suspicion is not enough, and as there is no possibility of direct evidence, they have to rely on divination again. But now it is not the *sunum boṅga* that is brought into operation.

Under the leadership of the village headman (it will be remembered, that the community has taken the matter up) they proceed as follows: Going to a place where there is water they plant along the edge of the water a number of fresh-cut small branches. First of all they plant a branch in the middle as a 'witness,' then in succession one for the house-god (*oṛak boṅga*) of the patient's household, then one for the house-god of his father-in-law's household, then one for each of the several fraternal relatives, one for daughter and for sister, one for the unrelated part of the village and one for *disom duk* (epidemic disease). The number of branches will vary according to the number of relatives, and they may sometimes plant one for each house-hold, also unrelated, in the village. As each branch is planted, *sindur* is applied to it.

After having scattered *adwa* rice over the place the following invocation is made: "Greeting then, Day-god of the heavens! Thou art spread out like a mat, thou hast overspread the four corners, the four worlds; here then, as thou seest, we have planted branches to ascertain the delinquent; what is guilty thou wilt pronounce guilty, let that dry up and wither—thou wilt bring out witness,—and if it be otherwise, thou wilt bud fresh, thou wilt remain unaltered and sound" (this to the witness branch).

It will be observed that they have planted twigs also for *boṅgas*; even if the leaf-oracle has pronounced the culprit to be a witch, here the appeal is made to the Supreme Deity, and no possibility must, in justice to all, be left unnoticed. Hence these twigs. They also address these *boṅgas*, somewhat in the following strain:

"Take care then, if thou art a *boṅga*, let this one dry up and wither, and if it be not thou, remain unaltered and sound. Thou wilt bring out witness." This formula is repeated over each branch. Having done all this they return home. Some five hours afterwards (when they think that withering may have commenced), or if the 'planting' takes place in the evening, then early next morning, they return to have a look at the branches. Whichever branch is dead, the one in whose name it was planted is understood to be proved responsible. If it is 'proved' to be a witch, the female occupants of as many households as the representative branches of which have died are considered possible witches.

To be adjudged a witch is a serious matter; they do not therefore rest satisfied with doing this twig-planting only once. They repeat it twice or thrice, and each time inside the boundary of another village. It may, of course, happen that the oracle gives a different verdict in the different places; in such cases there is to the Santal mind no doubt that the witches have been at work to hinder them in finding out the truth. However, they continue, until they are satisfied.

It will have been observed that they do not always put more than one branch down for all the houses in the village occupied by other people than blood relations of the patient. In such cases they work on the supposition, that one's enemies are those of one's own house or family. If the one branch planted for the non-related houses should wither, they proceed to repeat this divination by planting branches for every house in the village.

Sometimes they try to test the result by putting a leaf with some *adwa* rice wrapped up in it in a white-ant hill. If the white ants attack the leaf and the rice, the case is clear; if not, there is something wrong. The house is innocent.

Some people will let the matter end here; it is no small responsibility to carry it further. The parties moving in the matter may be sure to expose themselves to the bitter enmity of the 'witches' themselves, and of their husbands and near relatives.

As has been seen, the divination proceeds by eliminating the various possibilities. The whole has by this time been narrowed down to a certain household. The individual has not been singled out as yet, although there is pretty little doubt in their minds.

It should be specially noted, that the operations undertaken by the *ojhas* and the village people, *viz.*, the *sunum boṅga* and the other kinds of divination, do not profess to single out any individual (except, of course, *boṅgas* who are specifically mentioned when they consult the oracle). So far as human beings are concerned, they do not go further than pointing out certain limits within which the culprit is to be sought. They do not attempt the responsibility of naming individuals.

XVIII.

Identifying the witch. The jan, *or witchfinder.*

To name the individual is the business of the *jan* (the soothsayer, also a word borrowed from Hindi). He is the man who 'knows,' *viz.*, by revelation. 'The *jans*,' says old Kolean from whose description much of the following is gleaned, 'are our High Court in witchcraft matters. Those which the *jans* pronounce to be witches, we deem witches. Whether they really find them out, or the whole is humbug,—we believe that they find them out.'

If the patient or his relatives decide to carry the matter to a *jan*, they always go along in quite a crowd. If the whole village is down with some disease, the headman will go along; if not, he only gives advice as to who ought to go. There are, as a matter of course, a couple of men representing the patient, the husband and male relatives of some woman clearly suspected, and half a dozen or so for the village people as witnesses. They go together and never lose sight of one another to prevent any one from secretly informing the *jan* about their business. The mutual trust is never very great.

They will, as a rule, go to a *jan* living at a distance who cannot be supposed to have personal knowledge of the matter or of the persons concerned. When they reach the *jan's* village, they camp outside and are careful not to tell anybody any particulars as to why they have come or who they are. They go to the village headman and ask him to introduce them to the *guru*, which he does, whereupon the headman tells them to bring out the things necessary for divination, viz., one betel nut, one leaf-cup, some *adwa* rice, mustard oil, *sindur*, resin of the *sal* tree, and some leaves of the bael tree.

The *jan* tells them to come to him at a specified time, and they return to their camping place. If any one asks them any question, they either do not answer, or if they do, they purposely give wrong answers.

At the fixed time they return to the *jan*, who will transact his business with them either in his own house, in the *jaher* (the holy grove of the village), or somewhere outside the village. The clientèle sit quiet and look on. The *jan* puts down small handfuls of the *adwa* rice in a number of places in the name of different *boṅgas*, puts alongside all these heaps of bael-leaves, and finally, having mixed the oil and *sindur*, puts *sindur* marks in front of the rice. He then throws the resin on burning coals, blows the shell, sounds the *boṅga* bell and worships his *boṅgas*. (It will be noted, that the proceedings are entirely different from the ordinary Santal worship; much is obviously directly adopted from Hindu practice.)

Next he becomes 'possessed' by the spirit of divination and in this state commences to utter incessantly incoherent words. He ultimately first names the part of the country where they come from, then their village, then tells how the village street runs, the name of the headman, of the person at whose behest they have come, the names of his uncles, brothers, sisters, sons, daughters, and how many they are. All to prove that he has knowledge, outside the ordinary.

It is very impressive, and when the *jan* asks: "Well, gentlemen, have I told you this right or not?" they answer: "Absolutely correct; we are convinced; now let us hear the oracle."

The *jan*, however, first demands his fee, one rupee, and if they have made any vow before starting, then the full amount of this in addition. When he has received all, he tells them who is at the bottom of their troubles, a *boṅga* or a witch, and also reveals the names of these.

To confirm them in their faith the *jan* next asks them, whether they have not planted branches in so and so many places, and whether they did it properly. The answer is, of course, in the affirmative. And the *jan* dismisses them saying: "If you are not satisfied, seek confirmation with seven soothsayers. If any such should tell anything else than what I have told, I shall return you the fees you have paid."

Hereupon the deputation returns home. If the *jan* has mentioned a *boṅga*, the patient will promise sacrifices. If he has declared any woman to be a witch, this woman is harrassed in every possible way, is ill-treated and fined (that is to say, the nearest male relative, father, brother, husband, son, will have to pay), or the 'witch' is driven ignominiously out of the village, and her home, being often treated in a most revolting way.

Sometimes the relatives of the woman pronounced a witch will try their luck with another *jan*; but it is futile, says Kolean; every *jan* will tell the same. However, there are a few witches (according to their belief) who are able to muddle up things even for a *jan* through their magic.

The present-day *jans* are, according to Santal belief, not like the old righteous ones. The *jans* of old were, according to tradition, not possessed by a divination spirit; they got their knowledge through dreams at night or through visions in the day time. The *boṅgas* appeared to the old *jans* and told them what to reveal.

Now-a-days the *jans* are, according to *Kolean guru*, rank humbugs; they have no visions, but keep informers who find out and tell them all particulars, and if they cannot manage to find out all at once, the *jans* will tell that there is a 'hindrance' that must be got rid of, and they instruct them to get the informer to make a sacrifice for this purpose of a fowl, a grasshopper, a pig, a white cat, or the like. This person will, of course, naturally ask for whom he is to perform this sacrifice, and so all comes out. The informer is careful not to go to the *jan*; but when he has found all out, his wife takes the tale to the *jan*'s wife.

Sometimes, when a *jan* thinks it possible, he will sit in front of the deputation and look well at their faces whilst he, pretending that he talks 'possessed,' mentions the first syllable of names. A look will betray them, if he has mentioned the first part of the name of their village, etc.

It is strange that the Santals with their lack of belief in the present-day *jans* will keep on going to them. But it requires some strong-mindedness to leave such an old custom, so long as they keep to the beliefs and superstitions which they have.

In many cases what makes them seek the *jan* may possibly be, that they want to get a kind of 'moral' support for doing what they want to do, but for which they otherwise cannot find a proper pretext; it may also possibly be an attempt to free themselves from a responsibility which they would otherwise have.

It may be that the *jans* have during latter years commenced to find it safer to fix the blame on some *boṅga* or other in preference to on a witch. They have been, and undoubtedly still are, the cause of much unjust suffering and hardship. They are unmitigated scoundrels who have not even got their own superstition as an excuse.

Jans are now-a-days seldom met with; they are also careful, as they may make themselves liable to imprisonment. Many have been sentenced to jail for their doings.

It is not here the place to tell about the fate of women pronounced witches. The wives of influential persons, specially of village headmen, may manage to keep their position or even to turn the tables on their accusers. Others have, as mentioned, suffered horribly. Even now women, both young and old, are found in the country who have been driven away from husband, home and children, because a *jan* has called them a witch.

It should be added, that the prosecution of a supposed witch will be continued after the death of the patient, partly in revenge and as a punishment, partly as a public duty, to save the community from such dangerous individuals. Strangely enough, they do not seem to reflect, that if these women really had such powers, or anyhow, could make use of the powers of the spiritual world, it would seem likely, that they might use these against their oppressors, and 'eat' them.

The story of witchcraft among the Santals has to be told elsewhere. So much has here been recorded, because it is tied up with their superstitious beliefs in connection with the causation of, and remedies against disease.

XIX.

Concluding remarks.

From what has been told in the preceding chapters it will be seen that the Santals, whilst accepting disease as possibly natural, that is to say, as due to natural causes, are always liable to suspect or believe that the ultimate cause of disease and death may be found with evil spirits and witches, or, very rarely, with dead persons.

These beliefs of theirs naturally influence their attitude. On the one hand, they have to take steps to counteract the inimical influence of the powers behind the scenes, partly to pacify, propitiate, or satisfy these, partly to fight, and punish them (in the case of witches). How this is done has been told in the preceding chapters.

To do what is deemed needed they resort to the *ojhas* and the *jans*, the first ones professionals in combating disease, the last ones in finding out the witches.

They do not, however, let a matter rest with taking only so-to-say 'religious' precautions. They believe, that the Creator has furnished remedies against all ills, if they can only find them. This belief does not always seem to be compatible with their belief in the doings of the evil spirits; but they exert themselves to cure also by natural means. They make use of symptomatical remedies, such as fomentation, massage and blistering. They administer medicines, made up from a large number of plants and trees and also other natural objects. Many of these are undoubtedly worthless, not to use a stronger expression; many of them are very much of the same class as that found in vogue with other peoples of the same stage of development as that of the present-day Santals. Many of their remedies may likely have little or no value, but it may be that proper pharmacological investigation might show a few to have some real worth.

This side of the subject will be found described in detail in the part of this work, called Santal Medicine.

APPENDIX I.

The Santal ojha (*from within*).

I.

In the following pages very many details are found, possibly of no great interest to the ordinary reader. Among the reasons for recording so much, the following may be mentioned:—It has been the writer's wish to give a full description of the functions and customs here reported, with everything that appertains to them. The ideas and beliefs underlying these are of considerable interest from an ethnological and psychological point of view.

A full description will assist in elucidating the origin of these practices. It is not likely that they are originally, all of them, the property of the Santals. The details will to some extent show, how the property of others may, without permission and not properly, have been taken over, and thereupon adapted, transformed and often added to, in accordance with the ideas and understanding of the adopters.

The present-day Santals are religiously, ethnologically and linguistically under the influence of the peoples surrounding them, specially of the Hindus. What is here told, will, as far as it goes, show in part, how this development or change is taking place.

The origin of the name of *ojha* and the probable origin of the institution have been mentioned above, see Sec. VII, and Appendix II, to which the reader is referred. Whatever the origin may be, the institution has been adapted and is kept up by the Santals according to their own ideas, and is propagated among themselves, an *ojha guru* or authority transmitting his 'knowledge' and 'power' to a *cela* or disciple.

Much has already been told about the *ojha* and his doings. Leaving out what has been already stated, I shall here try to give an account of how a Santal becomes an *ojha*, how he is initiated, and also give samples of his *mantars* and *jhaṛnis*, and how an *ojha* makes use of these; a description of the yearly *ojha*-course and its conclusion is also given.

One might say that two classes of *ojhas* are met with among the Santals, amateurs and professionals, those who take the work up in earnest, and those who only play at it, and are never finally initiated; a special object with these last ones being to be able to participate in certain begging ceremonies that will be mentioned below. Apparently it is thought proper for a Santal man to have some knowledge of the *ojha*'s 'science'; and there are in fact a large number of Santals who have been in contact with *ojha*'ism and have got a smattering of this particular 'knowledge'; they soon forget what they may have learnt and are not styled *ojha*, but, as long as the course lasts, *cela*, disciple, or *cela caṭiạ*, disciple pupil, and when the course is finished, then by the village people *Dasãe koṛa*, that is, *Dasãe* boys. Those who take the matter up as a kind of profession are comparatively few.

The first beginning is generally the same both for the amateur and for the professional, and as this beginning also plays some small rôle in Santal village life, we shall describe it here.

As mentioned, to become an *ojha* one has to become a *cela* with a *guru*, one who already is an *ojha*. It is customary, although in no way compulsory or obligatory, with the Santals that young men (naturally never women) have once yearly a course in *ojha* 'science.' The course lasts ordinarily from one of the last days of May up to the end of September, or the beginning of October, that is, to the day of *belbọrọn*, with the Hindus the fifth day in the *Dasãe pọrọb*, as the Santals call the Durga puja (*Dasãe* is their name for the month of *Aswin*, September to October; *pọrọb* means festival), with the Santal *ojha*, practically always, a couple of days earlier. That day the *guru* may also give his disciples (only those who may want it) the *sid*, that is, the initiation as *ojha*. The same day *ojha* and disciples commence their begging in the villages.

To return to the beginning: Towards the end of the hot season custom reminds the young men, that they should learn this *bidią*, science, as they express themselves. They consult together, and having made up their mind they go to the *ojha* and ask him to teach them, at the same time intimating that they are prepared to meet all expenses and otherwise pay what is customary.

There is an *ojha* in practically every village, so there is no need to go outside, and it is not done, according to what is told. This lack of interaction will naturally to some extent influence the teaching both as to form and as to contents.

The *ojha* agreeing, they commence the course at the time of *ruhni*, the first day of which falls on the 13th day of the month of *Jheṭ*, as the Santals call Jaishtha, that is, ordinarily one of the last days of May their first sitting being on a Sunday, or, in some cases, on a Friday.

They go to the *guru* after having had their evening meal in their respective homes; so the first day and all along. They sit in the *guru*'s court-yard. Having commenced the course they come daily, till it is finished, as stated above.

The *ojha* has in his court-yard a small *than*, a place for the worship of his *bońgas*. Sacrifices are also performed here. The *than* itself is a small mound of earth, a foot or so high and half a yard or a little more long and broad, square or rectangular in shape. At the head of this is planted a *tursi* plant (Ocymum sanctum, L., the same as the *tulsi*, the holy basil, worshipped by Hindus).

When the rains come the *guru* and *celas* will require some shelter. For this purpose the disciples erect a small shed in the court-yard not far from the *than*; the shed is called *caṛi*. It is generally built in the *bańgla* fashion, that is, with a gable-roof, some three yards long and about two broad, just sufficient to seat and shelter 10–12 persons. According to size the shed has six or nine posts, one at each corner, one at each end in the middle, and, if large, one post in the middle of each side and at the centre. The posts are fixed by unmarried *celas*; married ones must not have anything to do with the erection of the shed. The posts are of *sal*; a wood like that of *terel* (Diospyros tomentosa, Roxb.) is not permissible, because the *boṅgas* are believed to be afraid of this. The shed is thatched with straw of some sort; the whole is open on the sides; it is only meant to be temporary, just to last out the course, somehow. In the middle of the shed a hen's egg and a *chiṛ sakǫm*, a thin kind of iron wristlet or arm ornament, are kept. This is meant to prevent witches from molesting them.

Some may leave, before the course is finished, others may join the party 'after the work,' that is, when they have finished their work of planting rice, or any time up to the ripening of the Indian corn; these are not, however, considered proper or real *celas*; their object is to learn a number of songs and some kind of dancing and acting, so as to be able to join the others in the fun when they go begging in the villages (the so-called *Dasãe daṛan*, the *Dasãe* wandering).

The first act of the *ojha* when they have come together is to do what is called *akhṛa raṛa*, that is, to perform the opening ceremony to ensure that all may go well and without hindrance. *Akhṛa* is a place of performance, also the (single) performance itself, and *raṛa* means to untie, release, set free, open.

It is done in the following way. The *ojha* has certain special *boṅgas* whom he is in the habit of invoking. The first evening the disciples bring along with them some *sindur* which is given to the *guru*. In five different places in the court-yard the *ojha* makes *sindur* marks in the name of five different *boṅgas*, viz., *Kạmru guru* (the reputed first teacher of *ojha*-science to the Santals, now considered a *boṅga* and worshipped as such by all *ojhas*), *Serma siṅ Ṭhạkur* (lit. heaven, or sky, day *Ṭhạkur*; also called *Siṅ boṅga*, the day god, the sun, representing the Supreme Being), *Kạli mą̃i* (the Hindu goddess Kali), *Dibi mą̃i* (the Hindu goddess Durga), and *Gaṅga mą̃i* (the Ganges goddess). In the three last names sometimes the form *mą̃i*, in Santali meaning 'girl' is used, sometimes *mae*, the Hindi pronunciation, meaning 'mother.'

To each of these he offers the following invocation (a kind of *bakhẹ̃ṛ*), only changing the name for each *boṅga*:

Nǫ̃k̓ǫ̃e, Kạmru guru (or, as the case may be, *Serma siṅ Ṭhạkur*, etc.), *amiṅ ṭikạwam kana; nǫ̃k̓ǫ̃e cela koṛako duṛup̓ akana; adǫ ṅindạ ṅutạ ko hi̊juka calak̓ako; ṭobẹ bạdi bạiri noko cela alo baṛẹ lagaoako ma, alo jẹmǫn hǫe husil, ṭaṭka biṛki hoyok̓ ma; nae napae baṛẹko hijuk̓ calak̓ mako!*

That is, translated: "Here you see, Kamru guru, I am making a mark for thee; here you see, disciples are sitting; they will come and go at night in darkness; then may malevolence and enmity not come in contact with these disciples; may there be no spell of an evil eye, no sudden fright; in perfect safety may they come and go!"

There may with different *ojhas* be small variations in the wording of the invocation, but the meaning is the same. It should be noted that the language of the invocation is Santali, whilst most of the *mantars* and *jhạṛnis*, etc., are in some corrupt form of Bengali or Bihari, frequently not understood, and scarcely ever fully understood, by the *ojhas* themselves.

It might be noted that the *sindur* is used only this first evening, with consequent invocation of the *boṅgas* mentioned; some say, however, that *sindur* may be applied also at the time of the Monsa and Jithia festivals. The *boṅgas* are, as will be remarked, mostly of Hindu origin, intermixed with genuine Santal, or aboriginal ones, an interesting fact from which some deductions as to the origin of the craft are possible. Something will be found on this point later on.

After having invoked the *boṅgas* mentioned, the *guru* utters the opening *mantar* which, with variations, runs as follows:[1]

Akhṛa khollom, makṛa khollo, piṛ khollo, kẹ khollom? Guru khollo, guru giã; mae khollo, khollom siri Kạhri giã, Kạmru dohae khollo.

This may be rendered as follows: "I have opened the place of performance, I have opened the site of performance (*makṛa* is only a jingle to *akhṛa*, a word not otherwise heard); I have set free the stools to sit on. Who has set free (or opened)? The *guru* has set free, by the *guru's* knowledge (or possibly 'command,' see p. 18; a Santal understands it, as if a 'by' were spoken); the Mother (likely Kali) has set free; I have opened by the knowledge of Sri Kahri (or, knowing the fortunate wording), by the grace of Kamru I have opened"[2]

---

[1] It might, once for all, be remarked that the *mantar*, *jhạṛni*, etc., here and elsewhere cited, are invariably written down as muttered by the *ojhas* from whom I have received them, or as written down for me by Santals. It has never been attempted to polish them or in any way to correct the often very faulty, partly unintelligible language. I have attempted to transcribe them exactly as heard. The Santal *ojha* does not himself know the foreign language properly, if he knows it at all. In pronouncing the *mantar*, etc., he invariably follows the phonetic law of his own language, makes free use of what has been called the resultant vowels (not met with in the surrounding Aryan languages), and the open vowel sounds. In writing these I have followed the system of transliteration used by us in writing Santali.

The Santali language does not, in the verb distinguish the persons formally, otherwise than by making use of the personal pronouns. Very likely this peculiarity influences the *ojha*, so he does not always distinguish the person of the verb he utters. It has been elsewhere mentioned that the form of the third person may be meant to be that of the first. I have as a rule translated the verbal form ending in *-e* or *-ẹ* as being third person. I am, however, inclined to think that the first person is often meant. It is the *ojha* himself who is operating and speaking. The same may be said about the form *-lo* that is used alternatively with *-lom* (the *o* is pronounced as if it were resultant); here the first person is generally meant. See also p. 52.

In the *mantars* verbal forms ending in *-ae* have generally been taken to be a Beng. causative form, although a similar form in Bihaṛi is simple Present.

The language used seems originally to have been a form of Bihari or rustic Bengali, but forms belonging to Hindi are occasionally met with. This mixing may perhaps be partly due to the *ojha's* personal knowledge of any particular foreign language; unconsciously this may influence him.

In support of the above suggested interpretation of *e*, the following story may be told. Many years ago now, a large number of Santals emigrated from these parts and settled to the south, in Birbhum. Some of our preachers once on a tour down there came across a Santal whom they had known here; the man, however, refused to be recognized. They spoke to him in Santali; he affected not to understand and said: *ami deko bọtẹ!* (that is, literally, I is a deko), according to what the Santals told me.

To examine these matters properly must be left to others.

I shall only add that the translations given are in accordance with what the Santals believe they understand by the words cited; in one or two places the misunderstandings have been pointed out; it has been thought to be of more interest to hear what the persons concerned think they are saying, than to get a possibly correct rendering.

[2] The meaning of *siri kạhri* is very uncertain, and not understood by the Santals. *Siri* cannot well be anything else than the same word found in Hindi and also used in Santali; the question is whether it is to be taken as a noun or as an attribute to *Kạhri*. *Kạhri* may be a name, in which case *siri* (*i.e.*, *Sri*) belongs to this. The Santals apparently do not know any person or godling having such a name, but those from whom the *ojha* has originally got this word may 'know' such a person. A Maṛ *ojha* (a man belonging to the local Pahaṛia tribe) has told that *Kạhri* is the name of a godling residing in Hades, something akin to *Jọm raj*, the king of Hades; it might be added that Santal *ojhas* have learnt also from Pahaṛia confrères. Another possible explanation might be to connect it with Urdu (Arabic) *qahr*, force, power; this, however, seems to be a little too far-fetched. Some Santals try to connect the word with Hindi *kahna*, to

The following is another formula:

Akhṛa khoḷe, piṛ khoḷe, khuṭi khoḷe, rola khoḷe, bata khoḷe, cal khoḷe, caḷin khoḷe, mudhaini khoḷe; ke khoḷe? Guru khoḷe, guru gean; mae khoḷe, khoḷae siri Kạhri gean, Kạmru guru dohae.

That is, He sets (or possibly, I set) the place of performance free; he sets free the stools to sit on; he sets free the poles, he sets free the rafters; he sets free the laths, he sets free the roof, he sets free the thatch, he sets free the roof-ridge. Who sets free? The *guru* sets free, by the *guru's* knowledge; the Mother sets free; he causes to be set free by knowing the propitious wording (or as above); by the grace of Kamru *guru*.

When the opening ceremonies have been gone through, as stated, all is ready for the commencement of the teaching.

The teaching of this course comprehends the following:—

(1) *Mantar*, rigmaroles to drive away disease, or the supposed supernatural cause of any disease, the *mantars* being different for the different diseases. See previous paper, Sec. IX, and below.

(2) *Jhaṛni*, also different for the different cases, and used only in connection with certain complaints; the *jhaṛni* is sung or chanted to a special melody that differs somewhat according to the words; the disciple has to learn the words, the melody and the manner of application. See previous paper, Sec. IX, and below.

(3) The songs to be used at the *Dasãe daṛan*, the dancing and begging wandering, when the course is finished off at the time mentioned above.

(4) The special dances and play acting, and how to be possessed (*rum*).

(5) Medicines to be used when *mantar* or *jhaṛni*, or both, are ineffective.

Details will be given further on.

When the evening's lesson is done (the *guru* sits with his disciples in his court-yard for an hour, more or less, at a time), the *celas* start for their respective homes.

The writer has naturally never been present at any such occasion; but from the experience he has had of *ojhas*, it seems natural to draw the conclusion that it must take a fairly long time to teach anybody a short *mantar*. Cf. footnote, p. 18.

Before the disciples go away, the *guru* 'closes' the business of the evening; he first mutters a special *mantar* or charm, the object of this being to close the *akhṛa*, so that persons not concerned may not vitiate the proceedings; the court-yard, momentarily 'consecrated' for the purpose, is made an ordinary court-yard again. Thereupon he mutters another *mantar* to ensure the safety of the disciples when

---

say, tell, etc.; from the same root they have a couple of words *kạhni*, a folktale, *kạhtuk*, a proverb. How the word should have got this form, is outside their thoughts. These people give the word the meaning of 'saying,' 'wording' or 'formula.' In this case the words would mean 'by the fortunate, propitious wording,' *i.e.* the *mantar* proper. This gives some sense to the *ojha*, one might think. The following renderings may thus be attempted: 'for luck (or, by fortune, luck), by the knowledge (or, command) of Kahri,' or 'by the knowledge of the fortunate (luck-bringing, propitious) wording,' or 'by the knowledge (or command) of *Sri Kạhri*.' Whilst 'by knowing the fortunate, lucky, propitious wording' is the meaning attached to the expression by most *ojhas*, the most probable translation is "by the knowledge of *Sri Kạhri*"; *Kạhri* is then taken as the name of a now entirely forgotten *guru* who taught the old *ojhas* and in this way made himself remembered.

going home. These *mantars* are called *bandhọn mantar*, a *mantar* to tie up by a charm.

The first is as follows:—

Akhṛa bandhọn, kẹ bandhẹ? Guru bandhẹ; pịṛ bandhẹ, cal bandhọn, cạlin bandhọn. kẹ bandhẹ? Guru bandhẹ, guru gean, Kạmru guru dohae bandhọn.

Translated it means: To close up the place of performance; who closes up? The *guru* closes up; he closes up the stools to sit on, to close up the roof, to close up the thatch. Who closes up? The *guru* closes up, by the *guru*'s knowledge. Close up by the grace of Kamru *guru*.

The charm to protect the disciples runs as follows:—

Kulhi jaete kulhi bandhọn, chatka jaete chatka bandhọn, aṅgna jaete aṅgna bandhọn, duạr jaete duạr bandhọn, ghọr jaete ghọr bandhọn, khạṭi jaete khạṭi bandhọn, pạṛ jaete pạṛ bandhọn, rola bandhọn, khẹṛ bandhọn; kẹ bandhẹ? Guru bandhẹ, guru giã; mại bandhẹ, bandhẹ siri Kạhri giã, Kạmru dohae bandhẹ.

The meaning is somewhat as follows:

"When going through the village street, the village street to be closed (to evil influence); when entering the door to the court-yard, the door to be closed (to evil influence); when entering the court-yard, the court-yard to be closed (to evil); when entering the door, the door to be closed (to evil); when entering the house, the house to be closed (to evil); when going between the poles of the house, the poles to be closed (to evil); when going under the beams, the beams to be closed (to evil); when going under the rafters, the rafters to be closed (to evil); the thatching grass to be closed (to evil influence). Who closes (to evil influence)? The *guru* closes by the *guru's* knowledge; the Mother closes (to evil influence); closes knowing the fortunate wording (or as above), closes (to evil influence) by the grace of *Kamru*."

When above-mentioned *bandhọn* has been executed, the young men are free to go home, without fear. They return next evening at the same time. The first thing then to be done is to 'release' this *bandhọn*; it is done in the same way as the first evening, by the *guru* pronouncing the *Akhṛa khollom*, etc. whereupon they proceed with the *mantar*, etc., as the first day. Before separating they go through the same *bandhọn*.

The same routine is gone through every evening, so long as the course lasts.

2.

Parts of the course specially concerned with the Dasãe daṛan. *Final touches.*

Up to about the beginning of the month of Bhador (Aug.–Sept.) they continue learning *mantars* and *jhaṛnis* and nothing else. The *guru* makes the *celas* repeat before him what they have learnt and he corrects them. How much of a precaution this may be, may be judged from what has been stated previously. By this time the *guru* will also have gained some insight into the qualities of his disciples, especially will he know whether any of them takes sufficient interest in the real *ojha* work, or whether they have come to his course mostly to be coached for the *Dasãe daṛan*.

From this time on, the *guru* will pay attention, on the one hand, to make his disciples fit to participate in the *Dasãe daṛan* fun, and on the other hand, to give those of his disciples whose interests are of a more serious character, the final touches before he gives them the *sid* or initiation.

They now pass through what is called *pạisạri*.[1] The *guru* collects some five or six fowls or pigeons from his disciples, or money with which to buy these. It is said that not all give, but only the most proficient ones among the disciples, especially the so-called *paṭ cela*, who intend to receive *sid* ultimately. The *guru* takes his disciples out somewhere away from the village houses and there sacrifices these fowls or pigeons to the *guru boṅga* and other *boṅgas* of the *ojha*. One object of these sacrifices is to secure the disciples who are now soon ready to act their part, against the enmity of malevolent powers. They are performed in the afternoon.

The following is a sample of the invocation offered on this occasion:—

Johar tọbẹ, Kạmru guru (or *Lọhbọr guru*, or *Buạṅ guru*, etc.) *cela cạtiạṅ duṛuṕ akat'koa ; tọbẹ onko ṅutumteṅ emape kana, bes baṛẹko cel idi ma, ar teheṅ khọnko ḍakaopea : khusite kusạlte hijukpe ; arko ẹnẹca, jãhãe bạdi bạiri jinthi pạthri lagao alo bajao alo hoyok̕ ma. Judi jãhãe menae khan sẹ gun pạthri emanteak̕ jọtọge pe sahaṛ giḍia, cela cetanre alo baṛe bajaok̕ ma.*

That is, Be greeted then, Kamru guru (or Lohbor guru or Buaṅ guru etc.). I have made the disciples and pupils sit down (to learn); then on their behalf I am giving you this; may they continue to learn well, and from to-day they will commence to call you: with pleasure, with enjoyment come; they will dance and play: let no spell or evil charm of any enemy or adversary be thrown or hit. If there is any such, or any magic or evil charm, or the like, you will move all such away; may nothing fall on the disciples!

Thereupon the *guru* applies *sindur* to the peacock feathers of the disciples, and also to their cymbals.

When this is done, the disciples commence to learn to dance *Dasãe* fashion; this will be described later on; most of them will know the proper way of *Dasãe* dancing from before, as it is to be seen every year in the villages. They further learn the songs sung at the same occasion; these will be found in a separate section below.

They are also taught to 'call' the *boṅgas* and to become *rum* (see p. 34, footnote). This, of course, refers to *boṅgas* whose names are not kept strictly secret, anyhow not to the disciples, more specially to the *guru boṅgas* and some others, nameless ones, called, according to the actions of those 'possessed' by these, 'cow' *boṅga*, 'cowherd' *boṅga*, 'tiger' *boṅga*, and so on, as will be presently told.

---

[1] The word *pạisạri* is used, so far as I know, in Santali only about what is here mentioned. Some Santals apparently connect the word with Hindi *pai* and say it really means to stand straight on one leg and worship or implore; others have offered the explanation that the word is derived from *paesa* (or *poesa*), pice, because the *guru* collects pice to buy fowls for the purpose here mentioned. The two explanations are mentioned as an example of popular etymology. I suppose one might compare the Hindi *paisar* which means 'access, entrance, admission, ability, power' (Platts' Dictionary). No *ojha* has been able to give a satisfactory explanation; but I suppose, one will not be much mistaken, if one takes it to mean to be given preliminary admission to the *ojha* craft, a kind of certificate that one has been through a course, giving them the right to call on certain *boṅgas*.

To call the *boṅga* they clash cymbals and beat brass-cups, and sing the following gibberish:

Kasa ṭhọklẹ kạsim rāwāe, kọn kọn debla yawaere?
Yawae sẹ ho, Kạmru guru (Gaṇḍo guru, Lọhbọr guru, etc.).
Hạṛū boṅga (Jugi boṅga, etc.).

That is:

They beat the brass, how it is sounding! Which godlings are coming?
Come then, Kamru guru (Gando guru, Lohbor guru, etc.).
Hanuman bonga (Jugi bonga, etc.).

Naturally only one *guru*, or one *boṅga*, is mentioned at the time. During this singing and cymbal beating one after the other of the disciples becomes *rum*, that is, possessed by one or the other of the *boṅgas* mentioned (they are also possessed by the former, now dead *gurus*).

What here follows is a description of 'possession' by the above-mentioned 'nameless' *boṅgas*; they go through regular rehearsals of the plays they are to act in the villages during the *Dasāe daṛan* (also acted at the *chata* festival). The order in which these *boṅgas* are made to appear may vary; only some of them have to come in groups. I shall mention the plays in the order in which they are said to be mostly gone through. The different songs are recorded exactly as heard; some of them are in Santali, generally far from perfect as to form; others are in a rustic kind of Bengali or Bihari, also far from correct; on the one hand there is the 'licentia poetica,' on the other, a very curious negligence of the Bengali conjugational forms, the form of the third pers. sing. being, *e.g.*, used for the 1st pers., according to what Santals explain. There are also some 'songs' in a mixture of Santali and Bengali, Bihari or Hindi; it is very common for them to use Bengali and Hindi nouns with Santali verbal suffixes; here the opposite is done.

First of all the *hạṛū boṅga*, the Hanuman *boṅga*, is mentioned.

The *guru* and *cela* sing:

Kal Bhaerọ, Masaṅ Kal,
Gaṅga Gạuṛạ, sạṛimrẹ
Huluman bir ya Loṅkac ḍahaoket.

That is: Kal Bhaero, Masaṅ Kal, Ganga Gaura—the mighty Hanuman is on the roof, he burnt up Lanka.

The first three names are names of *boṅgas* who are addressed.

According to Santal traditions, the ancestors of the present people went along with Rama to Lanka. The song is in Santali.

When this is sung, two or three of the disciples become 'possessed' and act like monkeys, mount to the roof of the house, etc. It is said that this 'possession' is resorted to at the *Dasāe daṛan*, when they see pumpkins on the roof of a house visited, and want to get these. When they have been 'possessed,' the others sing:

Lut, puṭạ, Hạluman Loṅka jabe,
Loṅka jabe, puṭạ, Phọloṅka jabe.

That is (according to Santals): Jump, my boy; Hanuman is going to Lanka; he is going to Lanka, my boy; he is going to Phalanka.

Lut is said to be pronounced also *lup*, equal to Beng. *lapha*.

Next they will call for the *jugi boṅga*. In Santali *jugi* means a wandering Hindu ascetic. They sing:

Jugit gosãe, Sirạm Parbạti,
Ram Ram Hạrit bọlọ he!

That is, O Jugi Gosãe, say 'Sri Ram Parbati, Ram Ram Hari'! (The *t* at the end of *jugi* and *Hari* is 'poetical.')

Generally two are then possessed, and the others sing:

Jugikin, jugikin, sat jugikin na, naego, kọemar jugikin.
Toka disomem dāṛālela? sat jugikin na, naego, kọemar jugikin.
Turuk disomem dāṛālela? sat jugikin na, naego, kọemar jugikin.

That is:

The two jugis, the two jugis, the trustworthy two jugis, girl (*na*); o mother, the two begging jugis.
What country dids't thou wander to? the two trustworthy jugis, girl; o mother, the two begging jugis.
Dids't thou wander to the Mogul (Turk) country? the two trustworthy jugis, girl; o mother, the two begging jugis.

(The language of this gibberish is Santali, but not as it is spoken at present in these parts.)

The two 'possessed' ones sit down on their haunches and say: *ḍirrr bul bul bul bul, roṅga lạṭi dao, sili dao, tumbạ dao, tilok dao, ḍirrrr bul bul bul bul, gañja dao!* The first words are only meant to draw attention; next they order (using a Hindi verb, but otherwise mostly Santali names for the things wanted) a knotted stick, a hair rope (twisted of a cow's tail hair, supposed to be effective in driving away the *boṅgas*), a gourd (*tumbạ*, the hard shell of Cucurbita lagenaria, used by the Santals for water bottles, when out on tour, and as receptacles for small things), a mark on the forehead (the Hindu *tilak*, not otherwise used by the Santals), and finally ganja, the Indian hemp. It might be remarked that some of the pice collected (as referred to above) are spent to buy ganja, which is only exceptionally used by the Santals. The two *boṅgas* are supplied with all this and play their rôle, until the audience is tired and somebody gives them a thump in the back, whereupon they come to.

Next comes a call for the *gại* (cow) *boṅga*. One is possessed as a cow, another as her calf. They walk on all fours; the one possessed by the 'cow' *boṅga* makes a sound like a lowing cow, saying *bẹ̄ẹ̄ẹ̄ẹ̄* (the sounds represented as repeated are meant to express only one long sound; they are otherwise written as pronounced by the Santals).

The others sing:

Yo goal goalrẹ! Yọ goal kāhārẹ?
Bạchurẹ tọ baghe mare!

That is:

O goala, goala! where are you, o goala?
The calf—the tiger is killing!

Or else they sing:

Bagalrẹ bagal! kãhã roilorẹ?
Sugi gại baghe mar dilorẹ!
Jãnde tãnde bạchur bãndhẹ.
Sugi gại baghe mar dile!

That is:

O cowherd, cowherd! where are you?
The tiger has killed the Sugi cow.
Somewhere the calf is tied up,
The tiger has killed the Sugi cow!

Immediately another is 'possessed,' this time the *mahra boṅga*, the goala *boṅga*. This one walks upright and says *iạạạ iohẹl iohẹl!* according to the manner of the goalas, when calling to their cattle. The cow *boṅga* follows after him, and a stick is given into his hand. He pats the calf *boṅga* on the back, and this one answers, emitting a sound like a calf's. The others again sing:

Lakwalaṅ icạk hạiạr, họbọrwalaṅ nule ḍhạurạk'.
Gateṅ ho delaṅ calak ran gola dọ!
Gateṅ ho delaṅ calak muṅge darere saṅga!

That is,

We two shall pare the *icạk*[1] bar, we two shall take the mango branch in our arms;
Come along, my companion, to go to the medicine store-house[2];
Come along, my companion, let us go, there is a beam in the *muṅgạ* tree.[3]

Now the *bạghut* (that is, tiger or leopard) *boṅga* appears a little distance away from the others, moving on all fours and saying *hmmmm* or *ũũũ*, imitating the call of a tiger or a leopard. The *mahra boṅga* naturally has to take action to save the 'cow' and the calf; he attacks the 'tiger' and beats him with his stick. It is, of course, only fun, but they may handle each other rather roughly, so the others try to prevent the 'goala' hitting with his stick, and the *guru* and *cela* blow into the ears of both to hinder them from fighting.

The others also sing:

Dạu ma ḍạu mar mar ḍạu!
Taramre ma timạre tamare,
Sulạṅre ma limạṅe lamaṅ.

---

[1] *Icạk* is the Santal name for Woodfordia floribunda, Salib., a common jungle bush, small bars of which are often used for digging up wild roots in the forest.

[2] *Gola* is the name for round grain granaries; here naturally the forest is meant, where the *ojha* has his 'stores.'

[3] *Muṅgạ* is the Santal name for Moringa pterygosperma, Gärtn. The tree is commonly planted. The leaves are much used for curry; the flowers and fruit are also eaten. The tree or rather its products are made use of in several ways; the wood is, however, unsuitable for carpentry of any kind. The Santals believe that the odour of the wood will drive snakes away, specially when put in their holes.

That is,

It is flaring up, at it! at it! it is flaring up!
Walking it is flowing down,
Joyfully playing it is trailing along.[1]

When all is finished, the 'possessed' ones come to.

Next they sing:

Sat dhubin kapọṛ kacae, caudạ sẹ porilọ dhubi tọ;
Na bọlọ yọlọṅka tọlọṅka, dhubi tọ Hori bọlọ he.

That is,

Seven *dhubi* (washerman) women are washing dumping cloth; the *dhubi* is down giddy and prostrate;[2]
Don't say ornaments tornaments, the *dhubi* is saying *Hori.*[3]

Immediately one is 'possessed' by the *dhubi* (washerman) *boṅga*. He moves in a bent position and calls out *kapọṛ kacẹ, kapọṛ kacẹ*, several times (that is, according to Santal explanation, not *he*, but *I* am dumping cloth; see remark above). He takes his own cloth, if he has any suitable on; otherwise, and preferably, he catches hold of the clothes of somebody present and commences, dhubi fashion, to beat the ground with this, at the same time emitting sounds like those emitted by the dhubi, when dumping cloth.

Now they sing:

Jal pkẹkọ, kẹ̃oṭa guru ho!
Kẹ̃oṭa guru ka biṭi ya suru suṭạ kaṭe, goi;
Nana suṭạ jhimri bonae dẹ!

That is,

Cast the net, o fisherman *guru!*
The fisherman *guru*'s daughter is spinning fine thread, hey!
Make a fish-trap of thin thread (slips) and give here!

A man is 'possessed'; he stands or kneels and says *bọṛọ mãc, bọṛọ mãc* (big fish, big fish) again and again. The *dhubi boṅga* goes up to this one, takes him by the throat, scolds him that he is making muddy the water in which he washes clothes and they have a great quarrel, until the others separate them.

Then they sing:

Leṅgaka hate raja yayela debta;
Ghurạ ho ghurạ, sạki,[4] ghurạ ho Leṅga ghurại;
Ghurạ ho saṭọr bhạiạ, ghurạ ho cãware ḍolae!

---

[1] The words are in Santali, with some of the additions often used to make the words fit in with the tune. What this and the preceding 'song' have to do with the 'tiger' *boṅga*, is difficult to say. They may possibly be something formerly found in some other connection, and then kept on here. It would be a misunderstanding to think that these 'songs' always convey any special sense to the public or the actors.

[2] The word translated 'giddy and prostrate' means 'fourteen,' his head feels like turning round to fourteen sides.

[3] That is, being on the point of dying he calls out to Hari, Krishna.

[4] *Sạki* is a female friend, a mendicant dressed as a female, it is the same as Hindi *sakhi*.

That is,

In the hand of the Lenga (*boṅga*),[1] o king, the godling has come;
Turn round, o turn round, friends, turn round, o Lenga, cause to turn round!
Turn round, o seventy brothers, turn round, o, swinging the hair-wisp!

During this singing a couple of the young men are 'possessed' by the *caṛ cạṛi boṅga*, the scourge *boṅga*.[2]

The 'possessed' ones call out *lele lele, caṛ cạṛi ho* (bring the scourge!); they clap their hands and wheel their right arm round.

The others sing:

Kās tọrẹ tọrẹ, raja ho yayela;
Duio bohin sọnẹ kiri tạḍ.

That is,

Brass-cups rows rows, the king has come;
Both sisters (have) *tạḍ* made of gold.[3]

When they call out *lele lele caṛ cạṛi*, they put their hands and feet out to be struck; they do so, at the same time facing towards the east.

Sometimes one is possessed by the *bindi* (spider) *boṅga*. They sing:

Bindigọr bindi rạimạt lẹndọṅ,
Taṛamre ma timạre tamare;
Sulạṅre ma limạṅe lamaṅ.
Sạrukiạri noṛak laṅ-,
Bindi raṛore laṅ-.

That is,

Spider's spider, rạimạt centipede,
Walking it is trailling along,
Joyfully playing it is flowing along.
Sarukiari's[4] house we two shall—,
At the spider rock-rapids we two shall—.

The spider *boṅgas* mount the roofs and move on all fours there.

Sometimes they are 'possessed' by the *raekakaṛbak* (chameleon) *boṅga*. Those 'possessed' move on all fours with the peculiar backward and forward swaying motion of the chameleon, and say *hoooo*.

---

[1] I have not heard any Santal understanding the real meaning; they have learnt it and repeat it, mostly only part of it, leaving out the last line. *Leṅga* is here said to be the name of a *boṅga*; the word otherwise means 'left.' This *boṅga* is in the hand, it is said.

[2] *Caṛ cạṛi* is the name of a kind of rope's end, made for the purpose, of *bachọm* (Pollinia eriopoda, Hance.), the sabai grass. They take as much as can be held in the grip of one hand and tie this together at the root end. The grass is then divided into three parts; the first two of these parts are twined together, then the third is wound round the other two, the whole being again tied at the top end. They strike with this first at the wrists and then at the ankles.

[3] The translation is as the words are understood by Santals. The 'king' is the *boṅga*. *Tạḍ* is an ornament worn on the upper arm by women; it is large and hollow; it is not seen now in common use, only very exceptionally. I have heard it said that Santal women at the time of the Santal rebellion (in 1855) carried money hidden inside these ornaments.

[4] The translation is doubtful; no Santal has been able to explain to me the real meaning, if there is any *Sạrukiạri* is supposed to be the name of a *boṅga*. The text probably refers to the way in which some spiders move.

Some also are possessed by the *hạti* (elephant) *boṅga*. They sing:

Hạtigọr cạṛi, rạigọr ṭạṇḍi,
Taṛamre ma dhamase dhumus,
Sulạṅre ma riọle rọyọl.

That is,

The elephant shed, the mustard field;
When walking it is heavily,
When joyfully playing it is high stepping.

The elephant *boṅga* moves slowly and heavily along on all fours; when he puts one hand down, he puts the other up on his back; the hand on the back is perhaps meant to show the trunk's motion.

Then there is the *bạckạr boṅga* (*bạckạr* is a juggler or conjurer). One is 'possessed' by this *boṅga*, saying *bạji dek, bạji dek!* (summersault, look!) and turning summersaults.

The others sing:

Bạji bạjilo, bạckạr?
Kạti lọbẹ bạjilo, bạckạr?

That is,

Did you turn summersault, o juggler?
What is your profit turning summersaults, o juggler?

They also call out singing:

Dudu ḍuḍu bajilom, bạckạr, ḍuḍu.

That is, Drumming, drumming, I turned summersault, o juggler, drumming. (The word *bạji* is here taken in the meaning it has in Santali.)

When they have seen enough they give him a thump in the back, and he comes to.

Sometimes the *bir sindič boṅga* also will take possession of someone. I have not heard any song in connection with this one, nor anything about how he is acting. *Bir sindič* is a name the Santals have for a kind of monkey; this monkey is not, however, found in the forests where the Santals now live. I have heard Santals visiting the Calcutta Zoo wondering whether the orang-utan seen there might not be the *bir sindič*.

We shall now return to the *ojha's* course of instruction. He teaches his disciples, so far as he knows, the songs, etc., mentioned, and also how to act the respective rôles, so far as this might be thought necessary. The acting is otherwise left to the sense and ability of the actors who have personal knowledge of most of the animals or persons they are to represent.

During the *Dasãe daṛan* the whole string of *boṅgas* are naturally not shown at every place they visit, but some here and some there. As already remarked, some of these 'boṅgas' are always shown in groups, thus the 'cow,' the 'cowherd' and the 'tiger' *boṅgas*, and the 'washerman' and the 'fisherman' *boṅgas* together.

These proceedings throw some light on the real conception of *rum* among the Santals. Those who are 'possessed' for this play act, to start with, just like one 'possessed' by an ordinary *boṅga*, that is, one of those ordinarily worshipped by the Santals. The *boṅgas* here acting are, however, never otherwise represented as such among the Santals, and, of course, never worshipped. The idea seems to be, that in order to be able to play a rôle properly, one has to be 'possessed' by the spirit of the part acted. The same as with us, only otherwise expressed; something concrete is wanted by the Santals.

As already remarked, possession is brought to an end in every case when the action has been going on sufficiently long, generally by a sharp reminder in the back of the actor.

In connection with the preparation for the *Dasãe daṛan* there are one or two matters more to be mentioned. The disciples have to learn to use one or the other of two kinds of stringed 'musical' instruments. One is called *kab kubi*. It is a hollow cylinder, generally of wood, but may also occasionally be seen made of a hollow gourd. One end is covered with skin (generally of a goat or a sheep, occasionally also of a kind of large lizard or of a large snake). This skin is pierced and a double string of catgut is run through, a small bit of wood or anything suitable being put in the string loop, to prevent it from slipping through the skin. When playing, the cylinder is kept in the left armpit, the covered end towards the back. The double string, coming through the cylinder, is often (not always) run through a small 'pipe' (mostly the narrow end of the hard shell of a gourd, Cucurbita lagenaria) and tied together, a small bit of wood or gourd stalk being used as a kind of handle to keep the strings taut. Keeping the strings in his left hand the player strikes them with a tiny stick; whilst doing this he alternately tightens and slackens the strings. The sound produced is remarkable.

Another instrument is the *buạṅ*. This consists of a bow with two strings of catgut, fixed like the string of an ordinary bow; the bow has a hollow gourd fixed to its middle. When playing the gourd is kept against the player's stomach; he strikes the strings with a small stick, alternatively pressing the gourd hard against his body and loosening it. The sound produced is very much like that of the *kab kubi*. Any one hearing it must needs think that the players must suffer from hunger.

The two instruments mentioned are used only during the *Dasãe daṛan*, not otherwise; they are, as will be understood, neither elaborate nor expensive. They sometimes last from one year to the next; they will in any case have to be repaired. This and the making of new ones must, as a matter of course, be done during daylight, and does not come into the business of the evening 'sessions.'

The other instruments used during the begging are not peculiar to this occasion and need no special mention here.

What has been described above concerns, as will have been seen, matters specially concerned with the *Dasãe daṛan*. The *ojha guru* does not, however, neglect his serious disciples. These, of course, also participate in the fun, but they receive instruction in genuine *ojha* practices at this stage. They are thus taught, how to perform *sunum boṅga* (see Sect. X., p. 16, where the proceedings are described) and other matters.

Previous to the last named instruction in play-acting the more proficient *celas* go through certain exercises, the only object of which seems to be to assist them in their future professional work. It belongs to the course, but is not practised outside.

To assist a *cela* to become proficient in being 'possessed' (*rum*) the following is done: The *guru* makes the *cela* sit down on a *guṛgu*, the cylindrical stone used in a Santal household for crushing spices; the *cela* sits on his haunches with his feet on this stone; in order not to tumble down he supports himself with his two hands on the ground spread out. He now commences to turn round (apparently always to the right) having the *guṛgu* as a pivot. After some turns round he becomes giddy and falls down 'possessed'. If any one has any difficulty in becoming *rum*, the *guru* ties the *cela*'s hair in knots; this is supposed to produce the desired effect; the *cela* is in this way given into the charge of the *boṅga*, and the *boṅga* is egged on. The man is supposed to be literally taken by the hair by the *boṅga*.

By this time the *paṭ cela*, the principal disciple (there may, of course, be more than one) asks the *guru* to be made *kaṭ khuṛạ*.[1]

He wants to go through a ceremony that makes him a recognized candidate for receiving the final *sid*. The *ojha* does not object, but orders the *celạ* to bring the required *samagiri*, the things necessary for the performance, viz. a *guṛgu*, a new *haṭak* (winnowing fan), a *chiṛ sakọm* (a kind of wristlet, of iron, now not in use among the Santals), and a *jọnọk* (a broom made of *sirom*, Andropogon muricatus, Retz.).

When these things are brought, the function is gone through. The *cela* sits down on his haunches; the *guru* hands him the *haṭak* which he keeps in his lap, the rimmed bottom-end outwards, and the other end close to his body. When the *cela* is sitting properly, with his left hand holding the *haṭak*, the *guru* puts a small handful of *adwa* (sundried) rice in the *haṭak*. The *cela* commences to rub out this rice heap, moving his hand round and round.

During this the *cela* becomes possessed, whereupon the *ojha* addresses him as follows: *Dewa jạnu sewa jạnu raja jạnu math, Gosãe! Raj dọ muṇḍạ dọ sadọman catọmanteko ñir hẹc họjọr hijuka; inạtele baḍaea oroma, ni raj ni muṇḍạ kanae mẹnte. Boṅga dọ buru dọ celate cạtiạte duṛupen betharen, buru maṫ mahle haṭak sapkel tọhọpkel khan, sok caole bagaṛ caole ghasaokel suturkelkhan dhiṛu gạí dhinuạr gạí leka ñir hẹc họjọr hẹcenkhan sirạ gaṇḍo pạta gaṇḍo belket aṭetket khan sewakak maswarkakale.*

That is: To worship, you see, to adore, you see, a king, you see, a head, my Lord! Kings, Muṇḍas with horses, with umbrellas they come running, come hurrying; thereby we know, understand, this one is a king, this one a Muṇḍa. A *boṅga*, a spirit, through a disciple, a pupil has sat down, has taken a seat, when a winnowing fan made by a Mahle of hill bamboo is held, taken hold of, when clean rice, impure rice has been rubbed out, rubbed down, when like a cow in milk, like a cow with calf he came run-

[1] So far as the writer knows, the expression is not otherwise used in Santali: I shall not here make any attempt at finding out the original meaning. Possibly this expression and *pạisạri* both refer to some specific action, now quite forgotten. The word is in Santali used about what is here described. Popular Santal etymology connects the word with *gọkhuṛ*, proficient.

ning, came hurrying, when the principal stool, the solid stool has been placed, been put, we shall make worship, pay homage.[1]

The possessed one grunts and is further addressed: *Dẹ dẹkhọn Gosāe, ọkọeṭak em tićen, em bọṛena, hesak latar baṛẹ latar siṛạ gaṇḍo paṭa gaṇḍo belkeṭ aṭelkeṭ, jạṭak janamak lạilem, tọbẹ nạ̃hĩ ale kā̃ṛā̃ andhra manwale baḍaea oromale, nui boṅga nui buru kanac mẹnte; tọbẹ nạ̃hĩle sewakak maswarkakale.*

That is: Please let us see, my Lord, who thou art who art stretched like a string, like a straw rope; under the pipol tree, under the banyan tree the principal stool, the solid stool has been placed, been put; tell first (thy) race (thy) birth, then we blind sightless human beings shall know, shall understand, that it is this *boṅga*, this spirit[2]; then only we shall make worship, pay homage.

Then the '*boṅga*' (that is, the possessed man) replies: *Sạ hạ̃ hạ̃ hạ̃k! Dek tọbẹkhan iń dọ khọjkidiń tạpuskidińkhan dhĩrũ gạị dhinuạṛ gạị lekań ńir hẹć họjọr hẹćenań. Hesak latar baṛe latar sıṛạ gaṇḍo paṭa gaṇḍo belkeṭ aṭelkeṭkhan duṛupenań beṭharenań. Tọbẹ iń dọ Lọhbọr guru kanań; tọbẹ cele mẹnte jạṭak janamak dọń oko dọhọea, rẹbeṭ dọhọea. Porasale bańkhan ũhũk! Dek ja bhọ̃ṛọ̃ bhọć!*

That is: Yes, yes, yes! Look, since you asked for me, enquired for me, like a cow in milk, a cow with calf I came running, came hurrying. As under the pipol tree, under the banyan tree the principal stool, the solid stool has been placed, been put, I sat down, I took my seat. So then, I am Lohbor guru (this name as an example); now then for what purpose shall I keep hidden, keep back what is (my) race, (my) birth. That is all and true, else nothing here, no! Look out, you bulky bumpkin![3]

---

[1] The translation is in a couple of places only tentative. The words are as uttered by Santals; but the language is faulty, and according to ordinary usage, in several places ungrammatical, the subject pronouns being mostly omitted. I have not heard of any Santal understanding all of it. The thrice repeated *jạnu* is not Santali; it may possibly be the same as Hindi *janno*. *Muṇḍạ* means here, not the Muṇḍas of Choṭa Nagpur, but the Pahaṛias of the northern parts of the Santal Parganas. The Pahaṛias were the zemindars or landowners in former days.

[2] *Buru* in Santali means 'mountain, hill'. Some have tried to make out that 'spirit' is the original meaning of the word, but they are very likely mistaken. *Buru* is the general name the Santali language has for mountains and hills; there are a number of other words also, but these refer to some particular form of hills and could not be used about mountains in general. According to Santal traditions, when the *godets* of Ṭhạkur, the Supreme Being (*godet* is the village headman's messenger), once rebelled, saying that as they were doing all the work they should also have the power, they were driven away from the presence of Ṭhạkur and came and settled down on the earth, on hills, in streams and pools, rocks and crevices, etc. (it is a very curious tradition resembling what has been told from the Hawaian islands, and the biblical narrative of the fall of the angels; it would be intensely interesting to find out the origin of this tradition among the Santals). It is Santal belief that all hills have resident spirits. It is against all analogy that a name for spirits (for which moreover the Santals have other words) should be employed as a name for a natural object. On the other hand we find all over the world, both at the present time and in former ages, that the name of a place or of the abode of a king or some power is used for the resident. It is unnecessary to give examples, such as Pharaoh, Mikado, the Sublime Porte, Rome, the Holy See, Downing Street, Quai d'Orsay, etc. *Boṅga* is the common name for spirit, whatever its derivation may be; *buru* is a mountain, and a spirit that resides on a mountain. *Bonga buru* is a general name for spirits and mountain spirits, a kind of collective to include all sorts; *buru boṅga*, a very common expression, means literally a hill or mountain spirit. Etymologically possibly near related words in other languages mean 'mountain'

[3] The first words *sạ hạ̃ hạ̃ hạ̃k* (there may be as many *hạ̃* as one likes) are interjectional and used to signify that the *boṅga* is present, in accordance with expectation. They are always used in similar circumstances. *Porasale*, at the end, is not understood by the Santals, the commonly offered explanation being that it stands for *purạ* and *sạı*, that is, that the rigmarole is finished and true. It may possibly be some corrupt word or other, meaning that the 'exhibition' is at an and. The last word is mostly used in jest about very stout people.

The *ojha* has rehearsed the whole with the man beforehand and taught him his answer.

The invocations quoted are samples; there are several variants, but what has been cited will be sufficient to show the nature of these proceedings.

The *cela* who has been made *kaṭ khuṛạ*, as described, is henceforth given special treatment. The *ojha* takes him along when he goes on professional visits, shows him how to feel the pulse, to understand the different symptoms, etc., teaches him to prepare the medicines, and where to find them, in short, does what he can to qualify him to become an *ojha*.

There are one or two matters more that should be mentioned. The *ojha* instructs his disciples, besides in what has already been told, also in some specific kind of divination. They are to learn how to foretell what kind of a calf a cow will bring forth, sex and colour, whether a woman will give birth to a boy or a girl, how to tell what kind of food people eat, and so on. It is done very much in the same way as when divining by oil-leaf. The disciple takes a *sal* leaf, marks it with oil in several places, *e.g.*, one mark for a bull calf, one for a female calf, one for a red, one for a white calf, and so on, one mark for every possibility. Uttering an appropriate *mantar* (the same as in the ordinary divination, only omitting the unsuitable parts, and adding what is thought necessary) he puts a covering leaf on, places the whole on the ground, takes it up, salutes the leaf, takes the covering off and sees what the 'oracle' tells. Time will show whether the disciple has been successful or not; one for whom the oracle shows what proves to be correct is deemed lucky; he has the favour of the powers behind. It is perhaps also to find this out that this kind of divination is practised by the *celas*; one hears otherwise very little of it in the villages.

Only those who take a sufficient interest in *ojha* science among the *celas* will attempt these matters; the others may be more or less interested onlookers.

3.

The sid *or initiation.*

To become a full-fledged *ojha* it is necessary to receive what is called *sid*.[1] The *ojha* gives this to a *cela*, who asks for it and who is deemed fit for it.

The course of instruction described is, as mentioned, brought to its conclusion shortly before the *Dasãe daṛan*. All *celas* are supposed to become *pạisạri*, that is, in reality a person who has been through a course; one or two may be made *kaṭ khuṛạ*, and such a one is supposed to be fit for receiving the *sid*. One who is made *kaṭ khuṛạ* has generally attended two or three years' courses.

As already touched on, only a very few of the disciples receive *sid*, or care to go

[1] *Sid* is a word come from Hindi (originally Sanskrit *siddhi*); in Hindi it means 'accomplishment, perfection, proof, final emancipation, etc.; also the acquisition of supernatural powers by magical means or through the performance of certain mystical or alchymical rites or processes, and the supernatural faculty so acquired' (Platts, Dictionary giving practically the same meanings as in Sanskrit). In Santali the word is used exclusively for a ceremony initiating in anything more or less occult, more especially for the final function making anybody an *ojha*, and the initiation of a *ḍạn*, making a woman a witch.

so far; those who receive *sid* may do so on the morning of the day of *belbọrọn* (as understood by the Santal *ojha* and his disciples); often, perhaps generally, it is given at some other time; there is no rule as to time, provided the recipient is a finished *cela*.

It might be noted that it is not the *ojha* who declares that a *cela* is now ripe for receiving the initiation. It is the disciple who takes the initiative, asking the *ojha* to give him the final touch. He has been following the old *ojha* some time, has learnt his practice and thinks that he may now be able to work independently. The *ojha* will not refuse, he only demands the necessaries for the function. These are the following: A new loin-cloth, a goat, one pair of pigeons and some fowls (these are all to be sacrificed; the number of fowls varies, but is generally five; and all *ojhas* do not want pigeons), one rupee (some *ojhas* demand five rupees) and one 'pot' of beer.

On the *cela* agreeing to this, the *ojha guru* will, as soon as the *cela* has collected the necessaries, go to the house of the disciple, alone or accompanied by his wife, and give the *sid* there. It is not done in the *guru*'s house. It is done in the following way:—

The two concerned first go and bathe, such being a necessary preliminary to a sacrificial performance. Having returned, they 'clean' a small place in the court-yard with cowdung, and the *ojha* here puts down a few small handfuls of *adwa* rice and makes some *sindur* marks at each small heap, the number of heaps, and consequently also of *sindur* marks, varying according to the number of sacrifices to be made. The *cela* provides the rice and the *sindur*, handing it to the *guru* in leaf-cups, according to custom.

Sitting down on the new loin-cloth, spread in the court-yard for the occasion, the *ojha* performs the sacrifices; the *cela* holds the goat, the fowls and the pigeons whilst the *guru* beheads them. In one corner of the cloth the money to be given to the *guru* is tied up, and when the sacrifices are performed, he takes cloth and money.

The head of the sacrificed goat is cooked with rice, and the brain is made into 'cakes'; this is all eaten by the two principals.

In addition to the goat mentioned, the *ojha* will sacrifice a pair of pigeons, or a fowl to some special *boṅga* of his. This is done in the following way:—The *cela* holds the fowl and lets it feed on the rice put down. The *ojha* thereupon utters the following or some similar invocation:—

Mẹn tọbẹ, phalna, phalnae celjoṅ kana, uni ṭheniṅ jimạ kam kana: uni hatte atanme; uni ṭheniṅ soprotkam kana; jāhāre ojhakae, jāhā hilokre ame ṭikạwam khan ar ame ṅumlem khan, rugiye bogelen khan dāṛẽm ṅamkoa; bac bogelen khan bam ṅama.

Translated, this 'invocation' (which is in Santali) means: "Beware then, thou so-and-so (name of *boṅga* is mentioned), so-and-so (name of disciple) is learning; I am giving thee into his charge, receive by his hand; I am handing thee to him; somewhere or other he will do *ojha*-work; when he some day or other makes a mark for thee and he names thee, then if the patient gets well, thou wilt receive sacrificial animals; if he does not recover, thou wilt receive nothing."

At this time the *guru* tells his *cela* the names of the different *ojha boṅgas* to be invoked.

The two men are not alone; any one may be a spectator. When the flesh of the sacrificed animals is ready prepared for cooking, the *ojha* will instruct the father of the *cela* to call the headman of the village and some of the more important villagers. At the same time, he gives instructions with reference to the above mentioned 'cakes,' and also that the flesh of the two pigeons (if such are sacrificed) is to be kept separate and made into cakes.'

Whilst the flesh of the goat and the fowls is cooked as curry and eaten by all present, the 'cakes' mentioned are reserved for the two *ojhas*; the cake prepared from the pigeons (or if pigeons are not sacrificed, then from a fowl) the *cela* is instructed to divide into two. The *guru* and *cela* are now covered by a cloth, so they cannot be seen; they sit in the middle of the court-yard. The *guru* instructs his disciple to take forcibly away from him the part of the 'cake' that he first takes to eat; even if he has got it into his mouth and is chewing it, he is to pick it out and eat it. If he is not able to do this, the *ojha* says, he will not be able to take up the work like his master; his inability is a sign that he has not learnt.

This is gone through whilst they are hidden by the cloth; likely Santals seeing them doing this would feel disgusted. It is probably meant as a symbolic act; the *guru* gives his disciple of his very own, and the *cela* shows his power.

The *sid* has now been given; it is consequently the revealing of the names of certain *boṅgas*, combined with sacrifices and the symbolic 'cake' eating, as described. From now on the disciple is through the action of the *guru* brought into direct contact with the supernatural powers invoked by *ojhas*.

After all formalities have been gone through, the people collected commence to drink the beer. The *guru* announces, that he has given the young man the *sid*. The beer is to celebrate the occasion, and they are witnesses.

When they have eaten and finished the beer, they separate.

The *cela* is now a full-blown *ojha*. It will, however, be easily understood, that the course described is not sufficient to teach a man what an *ojha* is supposed to know or to be able to do. He may possibly be able to pick up a sufficiency of *mantars*, etc., to be able to perform this part of an *ojha*'s work. So far as the other part of his work is concerned, the real treatment of disease, according to their lights, he will have to seek knowledge and experience wherever it is to be found.

Remembering the nature of his 'knowledge' and 'science,' it is obvious that his success as an *ojha* must to a very large extent depend on his personal ability to make people believe in him. Cf. the preceding paper Sect. VIII. On the whole I should say, that taking all into consideration it is difficult for a working *ojha* to avoid becoming an utter humbug and a cheat. There may be some who believe in their 'art'; but there are just as many who only practise because they earn money and good food. I have heard several *ojhas* confess that it is all humbug, so far as the 'spiritual' side of their work is concerned.

What an *ojha* is expected to know and be able to do has been described in detail in the body of this paper; his medical knowledge and practices have been described in the Santal Medicine, to which the reader is referred.

4.

The boṅgas *invoked by the* ojhas.

Besides the five *boṅgas* mentioned above the *ojhas* have quite a number of others that may be invoked. Some have a predilection for one, others for another, and certain *boṅgas* are invoked in certain diseases only.

The names of these *boṅgas*, so far as the writer has been able to ascertain, are the following:—

Sib Ṭhạkur (probably a form for Shiva).

Bolman Ṭhạkur (lit. the powerful *Thạkur*).

Dhạrti muni mãi (or *mae*, a female *boṅga*, possibly another name for one of the Hindu goddesses; *muni* is undoubtedly Hindi, but may in Santal pronunciation be the same as either *muni*, or *mani*).

Dhạrti ṁae, probably the same as *Dhạrti muni mae*; it might be noted that this female *boṅga* sometimes seems to be taken as the complement or necessary adjunct to the *Serma Siṅ Ṭhạkur*.

Jitu siṅ (invoked at the time of the Jitiya festival).

Ma Monsa (invoked at the Monsa festival; these last ones are females).

Gaṅga gạuṛạ.

Parbạti.

Pirthi kũãr.

Baset kũãr.

Bãs bir, probably the name of a bamboo-clad hill.

Mahabir, the same as Hindi *mahavira*, whether it is meant to represent Vishnu, or the Jain teacher; possibly the *ojha* does not know; it is sufficient that there is a *boṅga* so named.

Maha parasnat, the *boṅga* supposed to reside on the Paresnath hill in the Hazaribagh district to the west of the Santal Parganas.

Miluṅcu, or *Maloṅca*, the spirit supposed to reside on the Maloncha hill in the southern part of the Jamtara Sub-division of the Santal Parganas; this spirit is much feared and believed to be very powerful; ordinary people make vows to him, and it is reported that human sacrifices have been offered to him formerly.

Siṅ bạhni (also *Siṅ bạhni*), a *boṅga* supposed to reside on the Kaṛakaṭa hill in the Santal Parganas; supposed to be a very powerful spirit; Santals passing the hill when on their way, *e.g.*, to a tea garden, make vows to this spirit to offer a sacrifice when they return. The name is very likely a corruption of Skr. *Sinha vahini*, borne on a lion, an epithet of Durga; the *boṅga* is, however, supposed to be male.

Bãs pahaṛ, lit. bamboo hill or mountain, a hill *boṅga* of a hill so named. The *oṛak boṅga* or house-god of the Santal Hãsdak̔ tribe has the same name.

Raṅga pahaṛ, a hill *boṅga*, male.

Boka pạhṛi, a female hill *boṅga*, residing at a hill so called.

Pāċbạhni, a hill *boṅga*, residing on a hill so called, female.

Pahaṛ dana, a hill *boṅga*, said also to be the name of an *abge boṅga*.

Dhan ghara, the same is the *abge boṅga* of the Santal Marṇḍi and Ṭuḍu septs; also said to be the name of a *kisāṛ boṅga*.

Nạrsiṅ, a hill *boṅga*.

Lilạ bạti, a female *boṅga* supposed to reside on a hill in the district of Manbhum, said to be the greatest *boṅga* of the witches.

Maraṅ buru, lit. the great mountain, the principal national godling of the Santals; he has a peculiar double position, as he is also worshipped (specially libated to) together with the Ancestors.

Mạñjhi haṛam, the village-headman *boṅga*, by many counted to be identical with *Pilcu Haṛam*, the first man; supposed to reside in every village, where there is a *Mạñjhi than*, a small structure in the village street just outside the entrance to the headman's house.

Pargana, the overchief *boṅga*, a rather feared spirit.

Dẹs mạñjhi, a *boṅga* supposed to be a departed sub-overchief, so called. This last mentioned *boṅga* is not commonly worshipped by others than the *ojhas*, like the three others just mentioned.

Gosãe era, a lady of the holy grove, national godling, invoked against sores (*uri*).

Jaher era, also a national godling, female, invoked in cattle disease.

Kạuạ cọndọn.

Sikrạ bạṛi.

Mae sạhri.

Sirkạuk.

Nag nạgin (or *Lag lạgin*), likely not different from the well-known godlings, but adapted to *ojha* ideas, supposed to be able to prevent epidemics, also to end such; invoked also in cattle disease.

Lilạ cạṇḍi, female, also the *abge boṅga* of the Santal Hembrom sept.

Gaṛ dana, also an *abge boṅga* of the Santal Besra sept.

Karhaṛ dana.

Gaṛ siṅkạ, also an *abge boṅga* of the Santal Hembrom sept, said to be residing on some hill or other.

Siṅghạsor nat.

Siṅsor ẹkọṭ.

Bhạnsiṅ, a *jatra boṅga* with *Dulạr siṅ*, his wife.

Sagram Siṅ, also a *jatra boṅga*.

Gurạiạ, also the *oṛak boṅga*, house or family god of the following Santal septs, *viz*., the Hembrom, Marṇḍi and Soren. *Guraia* is a well-known godling of the lower strata of Hindus (cp. Crooke, Popular Religion).

Ṭhuṇṭạ tursạ, also the *oṛak boṅga* of the Santal Ṭuḍu sept.

Gurạiạ cãora, also an *oṛak boṅga*.

Cor dana, lit. theft giver, said to be the *boṅga* specially invoked by thieves; this is, however, quite outside the Santal pale; they have no professional thieves.

Jaṭa cãora.

Dhara cãora (has *cãora* any connection with Hindi *caura*, the funeral pile on which *sati* is performed ?).

Roṅgo ruji, a *bonga* to whom worship is made the night before the men start for the annual tribal hunt, with utterly obscene songs and practices.

Kal cãora.

Lilạ cãora (should *lilạ* have anything to do with Malto *lila*, a tortoise? The writer has, some years ago, seen a place of worship called *lila than*; in the vicinity there is a stone tortoise; the place has been a Pahaṛia one.)

Luri lora, invoked in small-pox.

Ghaṭ cãora.

Gaṛ cãora.

Jog dana.

Sara dana.

Caṇḍi dana.

Lilạ dana.

Band kũãṛ.

Jolon kũãṛ.

Koelo kũãṛ.

Ṭak biraḷ.

Kal bisạ.

Duriạ barḍo, invoked in madness.

Kudrạ caṇḍi, female.

Kal caṇḍi, female.

Dhana caṇḍi, female.

Dhara caṇḍi, female.

Sara caṇḍi, female.

Bisạ caṇḍi, female (also named *Besa caṇḍi*), invoked when there is poison.

Risạ caṇḍi, female.

Nason caṇḍi, invoked in madness.

Ban ḍuri, female, said to be identical with *Sara caṇḍi*.

Bhelwa raṅgi, female.

Raṭni raṅgi, female.

Kuṇḍli pukhri, the *boṅga* of the tank so named; *see* p. 7, footnote.

Kapaṭ darha, the *boṅga* of a waterpool so named, said to be on the south side of the Brahmini river, not far from the Haripur Inspection Bungalow in the Dumka Sub-division, S.P.

Naṅgin koilo (or *Nagin koelo*), female.

Leloṛi, female.

Gohal ghurạ.

Āk duạra.

Āk deora, female.

Kal deora, female.

Dhaṛap kiạri.

Bisạ rạṅgi, female.

Koelo rạṅgi, female.

Bạrchi rạṅgi, female.

Rạṅgin cạṅgin, female.

Sǫlma Sę̃ṛę̃, female (also Sǫlma Sę̃ṛę̃.)

Hisi, female.

Dumni, female.

Ulumpạikạ.

Julumpạikạ, this and the preceding one are *boṅgas* whom the traditions tell the Santals' ancestors invoked to find their way when they were running away out of fear for Mandhǫ Siṅ.

Kạpi Karan, lit. battle-axe Karan.

Bhạluạ Bijại, lit. swallow Bijai; *bhạluạ* is likely short for *bhạluạ kạpi*, the name of a common form of their battle-axes. The two last named are personages from the same event or period as *Ulumpạikạ*; all these last named four are seldom invoked; they are said to be specially invoked when labour is protracted.

Pat cirạ, female.

Kal Bhaerǫ.

Masaṅ Kal.

Rǫkǫt Kũạri, female.

Most of the *boṅgas* mentioned are worshipped by sacrificing animals, pigeons or fowls to them, mostly as a result of a vow in case of recovery. This has been described in the previous part of the paper. To some of them *bul māyām* is offered, viz., to those who are supposed to have come out when the oil-oracle was consulted; the operations have been fully described previously (see p. 22 ss.).

In addition to the *boṅgas* also the *ojha gurus* are invoked, more especially in the *mantars*. Every *ojha* is supposed to invoke his own *guru* from whom he has learnt and received his *sid*; it is not, however, always, or even commonly practised, anyhow not so long as the *guru* is alive. When a *guru* is dead, he becomes, according to Santal belief, a *boṅga*.

Among the *gurus* the following are specially remembered and invoked: First of all the reputed original teacher, *Kạmru* (or, *Kạmbru*) *guru* who is mentioned in the great majority of *mantars*. Further, *Gaṇḍo guru, Sidhạ guru, Bir hǫṛ guru, Kẹoṭa guru, Ḍaṇḍo guru, Rohṛa guru, Bhaerǫ guru, Mạnsiṅ guru, Ṭirom guru, Buạṅ guru, Poṭa guru, Lǫhbǫr guru, Jitu guru, Keṛha guru, Būhǫṛ guru.*

All the names mentioned, both of *boṅgas* and of *gurus* (and I have no doubt they might be considerably added to), are of very little interest to the ordinary reader. They have, however, for several reasons been recorded here.

They may be of some slight assistance towards tracing the connection between the Santal people and part of the religious worship found among the lower strata of the inhabitants of northern (and north-eastern) India. The writer is under the impression that there is considerably more of this kind of interaction or dependence than is generally thought.

When it is remembered that the Santals believe that the hills and rivers, etc., are the residence of some *boṅga* or other who may get his name from such a hill or river or pool, these very names may, if it is possible to locate them, possibly show a connection between such localities and the ancestors of the present people, or, anyhow, that these ancestors have had some connection with people who have been living near, or have known such places. The wanderings of the Santals are so little known that one likes to press into service anything available to try to find out a little. A few of the names recorded above are easy of identification.

The names may, in their Santali garb, have some small philological interest.[1]

5.

The Dasãe daṛan, *the September wandering.*

The course of instruction is, as mentioned, finished for the year a few days before the *Dasãe pọrọb*, the festival of the *Dasãe*, or Aświn, month. This is the common name among the Santals for the *Durga puja*. This is naturally not a Santal festival; it is celebrated by the many Bengalis living in the country, the Santals participating as active spectators. The festival plays some rôle in the life of the Santal villagers, a large number of people, especially young men and girls, going *ńẹńẹl*, looking, as it is called. They go and view the image prepared for the festival, and sometimes even bow to it. At the final act, when the image is immersed, Santals are often hired to carry it, and the din and noise always accompanying this last act in these parts is to a large extent due to the drumming and shouting and hubbub of the Santal spectators. Incidentally it might be remarked that the *Dasãe pọrọb* is one of their time-markers. The Santals do not worship Durga.

When the *guru* and his disciples have held their final function, the *belbọrọn* (as described here below, and generally a few days before the Hindu *belbọrọn*), they are ready to commence the *Dasãe daṛan*, lit. Dasãe wandering about.

Those who may participate are, as remarked, the *ojha* and his disciples; besides

---

[1] It has previously been stated (see p. 1) that the Santals consider all *boṅgas* to be malevolent and inimical, the only exception being *Cando boṅga*; but he is confused with the Supreme Being who is good.

As regards the *ojha boṅgas* there is likely little difference in the *ojha*'s and the ordinary Santal opinion, as to the nature of *boṅgas*. The *ojhas* may have adopted some ideas concerning them from the Hindus; specially may this be the case with the most known and publicly worshipped members of the Hindu pantheon adopted by them.

There is one idea concerning the *boṅgas*, borrowed from Hinduism, and foreign to the ordinary Santal mind, *viz.*, that the *boṅgas* may be obliged to obey a *mantar*. It does not, however, seem to be the *mantar* knowing *ojha* whom they must obey, but the *ojha* acting as the representative of certain gods.

This shows from where the *ojha* must have received his 'science,' and at the same time, that the Santal *ojha* has adapted the 'doctrine' to serve his own ideas. It might be interesting to discuss these matters.

those of the current year, also any of previous years' courses who may remember enough of the songs, etc., and who may wish to participate in the fun, and even the disciples of other *ojhas*, provided they live in the village.

The raison d'être of the *Dasãe daṛan* is on the one hand the fun and merry-making and the showing off of the 'scholars;' on the other hand there seems to be some sense of appreciation that these young men have gone through a course of instruction in fighting the foes of man.

Those who participate have to dress in a special manner. Instead of the ordinary *ḍeṅganak*, or loincloth, such as worn by the Santals, they wear what is called *kạcni*. This is a bit of cloth some three to four yards long, taken plaited round the waist and fixed by being turned in over the *ḍora* (this is the string worn by all male Santals round the waist). The *kạcni* is consequently a kind of skirt; over the *kạcni* they have a narrow bit of cloth tied round the waist. Inside they have a *bhagwa*, a narrow strip of cloth passed between the legs and fastened in the *ḍora* in front and behind. I have been told, that formerly it was not the custom to use *kạcni*; they had ordinary *ḍeṅganak* or *dhuti* on.

To cover the breast they may use anything, even a coat at the present day, often a small bit of cloth just thrown round the shoulders and breast. On the head they have a kind of turban, never anything very elaborate.

They may, or may not, according to ability or wish and predilection, have one or more of the following: *Pạingạn*, hollow anklets, with small pebbles or bits of iron inside, making a sound at the least motion; *lipur*, an anklet of leather with small *jhuṅkạ*, globe-shaped metal bells, fixed on, and *urmạl*, a loin belt, of the same stuff and make as that of the *lipur*, also with *jhuṅkạ*. All these make a tinkling sound. They may also put on what is called a *kọmọr piṭi*, a broad waist belt, of skin with red cloth and mica, etc., sown on; sometimes also what is called *kọmọr kạṭhi*, a kind of loin ornament, made with shells and tied round the waist so that part of it stands out behind like a kind of short tail. None of these ornaments is obligatory.

All have peacock feathers; during their dancing these are kept in the right hand high up, and the hand is twisted in time with the dancing steps, giving the feathers a peculiar roundabout swing. Formerly they were in the habit of having the *ṭạini theṅga*, the *ṭạini* stick. This is a stick, from five to six or even more feet long, and one to two inches thick, of bamboo or other suitable wood. At the top it has a peculiar 'crown' of iron. A bit of iron is divided into three or four 'branches'; these are twisted (to the left) and a few small iron rings (often also twisted) are slipped in on the 'branches' (one I have before me has six small twisted rings). The 'branches' are joined together and the whole driven like a nail into the top end of the stick. The iron 'crown' is some three inches high more or less. When this stick is stamped on the ground the rings tinkle.

The *ṭạini* is now very seldom seen, and is practically not used any more by the *Dasãe koṛa*; but the *ojha* himself may carry one along during the *daṛan*. When a *ṭạini* is carried they use *ḍeṅganak* and not *kạcni* for loincloth, I am told.

Formerly, it is said, every disciple had a *ṭạini theṅga*, and this was the only thing they had when going begging: their dancing was simply to walk round and round in the court-yard, constantly stamping the *ṭaini* stick end down on the ground.

It is said, that formerly the *ojhas* were in the habit of carrying such a stick when going on professional visits. When in Japan some years ago, the writer saw at Nagasaki in a temple yard a Shinto priest walking with a stick that to me looked just like a *ṭaini*; it was, of course, not possible to examine the thing more closely. In connection with this *ṭaini* stick it is of interest to note that several of the Santal subsepts are by custom not permitted to make use of it.

The *Dasãe koṛa* (lit. *Dasãe* boys, September boys) as they are called at the time, have a number of 'musical' instruments. The *kab kubi* and the *buạṅ* have already been described; they further carry cymbals and brass cups (used as bells), some small bells, a *ḍẹḍgẹr* (a small kettle-drum), a *ḍhulki* (a small drum of wood, both ends covered) and Santal flutes. They also carry the common Santal *banam* (a one-stringed violin, played with a bow) with them, both *banam* and bow being for the occasion furnished with tassels and feathers.

It will be seen the *Dasãe koṛa* are fairly well furnished with instruments, anyhow for making noise.[1]

The begging party consists of some twenty to thirty young men, according to the size of the village and its number of young men. As previously remarked, former *celas* will join, and also other youngsters go along, even if they have learnt nothing; such, however, only to swell the crowd. One such party will carry with them some four to five pairs of cymbals, one or two brass cups, four to five *kab kubi*, a couple of *buạṅ* (the carriers of this are always placed at the end of a row because the *buạṅ* would otherwise interfere with the movements of the other dancers), one *ḍẹḍgẹr*, one *ḍhulki*, three to four small bells (*ghaṇṭi*), a couple of *banam* and one pair of flutes (these last ones, in Santali called *tirio*, are always made in pairs tuned together).

We shall then hear how the actual *Dasãe daṛan* is gone through. On the morning of the *ojha belbọrọn* day (as already remarked this does not generally fall on the same day as the *belbọrọn* of the Durga puja, but is taken one or a couple of days earlier) the *guru* and *celas* start for some place at a distance away from the village, preferably close to a forest. They are all on an empty stomach. They have some rice and flour with them, *sindur* and *aenọm*, cooking pots, fire and fowls (and pigeons) for sacrifices. When they have found a suitable spot, preferably at the foot of a tree, a fairly large *kọ̃ṇḍ* is made and plastered with cowdung; small handfuls of rice are put down here, *sindur* is applied (five streaks for each *boṅga* or *guru*); the *aenọm*

[1] It might be mentioned that this *Dasãe daṛan* is imitated by others who have nothing to do with the *ojhas*, but make use of the occasion to go round and beg Indian corn on their own hook. These competitors generally operate in couples; they nearly always use the *buạṅ*, and frequently carry with them what is called *ṭap* and *cadọr badọni*, puppets worked with the fingers, sometimes quite a show with a number of figures, mostly, however, only one figure put on one finger and two wooden hands put on two other fingers of the same hand. The hands are clapped before the puppet, and songs are sung. The *Dasãe koṛa* and these others should not be mixed up together; they have nothing to do with each other; only they operate at the same time. Incidentally it might be remarked that, otherwise, clapping hands is the opposite of applause with the Santals: it means derision, a fairly sure sign, if needed, that this puppet show is not original with them.

(black eye paint) is also applied. The disciples sit in a row, whilst the *guru* sacrifices the fowls, one after the other in the ordinary way, first letting the fowl feed on the rice. When sacrificing the *ojha* mutters an invocation of which the following is a sample:

Johar tọbẹ, Kạmru guru (or, *Lọhbọr guru*, or *Gaṇḍo guru*, etc.) *teheṅ dọle belbọrọnok̄ kana, disom belbọrọn ṅutumtele belbọrọnok̄ kana: ona ṅutumtele emape kana. Disomle daṛana ṅindạ ṅutạ, ṭaṭka biṛki alo hoyok̄ ma; jāhāe guniye baḍaekhan, ban pạthriye calaokhan, alo lagao bajaoale ma; ape dohaete disomle dāṛā ạgui ma. Hoṛhọ akale, jaṅge akale tahẹnpe!*

That is: Be greeted then, Kamru guru (or Lohbor guru, etc.), to-day we are performing the *belbọrọn*; we are performing this on account of the *belbọrọn* of the country; in the name of this we are giving you. We shall wander about in the country at night in darkness, may there be nothing to frighten, to suddenly scare; if any one knows sorcery, if any one works black magic, may it not have effect or hit us! Let us by thy grace wander through the country and come back. Keep watch over us, be our constant guard!

These invocations vary according to the knowledge of the *guru*. At this time the *ojha* applies *sindur* to the peacock-feathers of the disciples, viz., to those they are to carry along, during the *Dasãe daṛan*.

When the sacrifices have been performed, the ojha party is joined by the village people, any man who cares. The fowls (and pigeons, if such have been sacrificed; some say that pigeons are not taken, others assert the opposite) are then singed and all what is not eatable destroyed, whereupon they cook the fowls with the rice to a kind of hash.

Whilst this is being cooked, the disciples pass the time calling up the *boṅgas*, specially those 'nameless' ones mentioned in the previous chapter, and are 'possessed' by one or the other of these.

At this time one revolting thing happens. One young man has been 'possessed' by the *bạghut boṅga*, the tiger spirit. The other disciples are sitting round him, singing; a white fowl is then let loose there, and the *boṅga* pounces on the fowl and bites through its neck.[1] When the play is over, the young man who acted as 'tiger' *boṅga* makes 'cakes' of this fowl and eats these himself alone.

When they have all eaten, the *kọṇḍ* is destroyed and they start on their way back. As many as are going to be dancers change their clothes at this stage.

It will be understood that there is very little more than the name in common between the Durga Puja *belbọrọn* and that of the *ojha*'s, except the particular time observed.

---

1 One would not think of meeting anything of this kind with the Santals. They explain it themselves by saying that at the moment they are *rum*, they are *boṅga*, and not man. It might be remarked, that at one of their festivals (the *baha*, flower, festival, in the spring when the *sal* trees stand in blossom) some men who have been 'possessed' by certain *boṅgas* and act as such, suck up blood of fowls that have been sacrificed to them (viz., the *boṅgas* they represent). It is significant that a man 'possessed' can get himself to do such a thing: a Santal in his senses would abhor the thing just as much as anybody else.

The *ojha guru* does not go straight home. Now comes what is called *ran jagao*, a kind of blessing' of the medicinal roots, etc., used by the *ojha*. Followed by his *paṭ cela* and a few others who carry a wooden bar(*khonta*) or something to dig with, he goes round in the forest. In his hand he has a leaf-cup, in which he has flour kneaded out with a little water. When they pass a tree or a bush that is considered to have medicinal value, the *ojha* takes a little of the kneaded flour and sprinkles this on the ground, telling that this is medicine against such and such a disease. The *celas* who follow then dig out a bit of the roots and take this along.

From these performances they all return to the *ojha guru*'s house. In some cases they are reported to come so late, that there is time for nothing more that day; in such cases they go from the *guru*'s house to their respective homes and return to the *guru* next morning, to start from there. As a rule they will be back during the afternoon. They first dance in the *guru*'s court-yard; here also some of them are 'possessed,' and they act as described. In the meantime, the *ojha guru* crushes the medicinal roots, etc., brought, mixes the stuff with rice-flour and water in a leaf-cup (*bhãutić*, a small cup made of one leaf, this being plaited and stitched with a straw in four corner places), and taking this cup and his *ṭaini* stick he and his followers commence the *daṛan*, their wandering to beg. Whilst walking along the village street, they sing the following over and over again:

Jagao guru ho, jagao cela, aṭharo goṇḍa mantar jagao
Solo goṇḍa biru,
Jagao jagao ho, Ṭhạkin Ṭhạkrạn,
Jagao jagao ho, sara des jagao!

That is:

Make efficient, o *guru*, make efficient, o disciples, seventy-two mantars make efficient,
Sixty-four forest-roots,
Make efficient, o, make efficient, Thakin Thakran,
Make efficient, o, make efficient, the whole country make efficient![1]

As is proper the first object of their walk is the house of the *ato mạñjhi*, the village headman. When they reach this place, they enter the court-yard in Indian file style, the *paṭ cela* leading, all keeping their peacock feathers high, jerking them at each step, as they enter and walk round the court yard some three to four times. When entering they sing the following (or some variant; there are several, different according to different *gurus*):

Dasãea ka jhala mala, Dibire Durgạ,
Nayaka jhala mala, keo ho, jhalaelọma, jhalaelọm?
Jhala mala Kạmru des ho.

---

[1] *Jagao* is used for making efficient; we might perhaps often translate it 'bless.' In Hindi it means to awaken; here to awaken the inherent properties or power of what is mentioned. During the Sohrae festival the cattle are similarly made *jagao*.

Aṭharo goṇḍa, lit. eighteen sets of four, a very common way of counting. *Solo goṇḍa*, lit. sixteen sets of four. These numbers may possibly have some reference to the numbers of mantars and medicines taught. *Ṭhạkin Ṭhạkrạn* refers to Durga.

Hate lela silia, desere jugia yeho yarwa cala,
Desere jugia, yeho kańca dudą pąire ma pąikate,
Maha gąrurą bunąloma sar khelaere.
Hate lela silia, kande lela ḍuriạ,
Mae tọ yaelọm, des desi jugia,
Mae tọ yaelọm nańgare bulạị.
Hạri Hạri, kal baje kãsã baje,
Mahakaete sirạ sindur,
Dibire Durgạ sar khelaelọm.
(or,—*telek sindur, Tinik debta sar khelaere.*)

Translated (it is a rather mixed language, just a little Santali with partly quite misunderstood and not correct Hindi-Bihari) it is something like this (I might again remark that I translate in accordance with what the Santals believe to understand to be the meaning):

The resplendence of the *Dasãe* festival, o Dibi Durga,
Is there no resplendence?[1] Who then? I made it resplendent, I made it resplendent,
Resplendent, the country of Kamru.
With the *sili* (hair) rope in their hand the jugis give them this sundried rice;
Give the jugis this fresh milk, *pại* (pint) by *pại*;
I have become a great Adjutant bird,[2] the play is true!
With the *sili* (hair) rope in the hand, with a tassel on the shoulder,
O mother, I have come, jugis from all countries (are there),
O mother, I have come, to walk about in the town.
Time after time they call out Hari, Hari! time after time they sound the brass (cymbals),
Making it smell sweetly the finest sindur,
O Dibi Durga, I have made play the real thing.
(or,—marking sindur, A number of godlings, the play is true, or real, or in straight rows. The words are differently understood).

Whilst the dancers walk round and round the court-yard, the *guru* goes with his leaf-cup and sprinkles a little of its contents on the waterpot stand and a little over the entrance door (on the eaves). The lady of the house or some other female (daughter or daughter-in-law of the headman) brings a stool for the *guru* to sit down on.

Now the dancers form up in lines of eight to ten and commence to dance; one with a *buạń* is, as already remarked, always the last of a line, the others place themselves as

---

[1] This is how the Santals understand it, or rather guess at its meaning. As is known *Nayaka* is one of the *taktis* of Durga's. Such a misunderstanding is instructive.

[2] The Adjutant bir: (Ardea argala) plays a certain rôle in the superstitions of the Santals. A feather is thought to be efficacious against snake bite, even only the mentioning of its name. It is told and believed that if the shadow of an Adjutant bird sweeping past falls on a snake on the ground the snake dies. The Hindu origin of this belief in the magical powers of the bird is obvious. *Gạruṛ* is borrowed from Hindi where the word is the common form for Skr. *garuḍa*.

they please. The 'dance' is of a very simple kind. The dancers take a few steps with a swaying motion forwards, and the same steps backwards, drumming and playing anything they have, holding their peacock feathers up as described and jerking them, all singing one or the other of the *Dasãe* songs (these will be mentioned further on). When they have made these steps backwards and forwards a few times, the dancing 'master' says *ḍirrrr ḍirrrr*, and the whole company turns round, at the same time making a kind of cringing bow. Thus they continue, playing, dancing, singing, until the headman's wife or some other lady of the house comes out with some Indian corn in a winnowing fan. She lets the Indian corn fall into a basket which the *Dasãe koṛa* have brought along. They expect to get a quantity, so they always take along a man with a shoulder-stick or banghy-pole and slings (*bhaṛia̤ marãṛ* and *sikuạr*) and baskets, to take the Indian corn. This is for the *Dasãe koṛa*, the performing young men.

The *guru* also gets a share, generally the same quantity as that given to the boys. In his case the Indian corn is put on the ground in front of him and he has to pick it up himself; he twines a piece of string and puts the cobs on this, carrying the whole on a stick over his shoulder.

When they have got the Indian corn, they stop dancing (it is understood that the people are satisfied with what they have seen and heard) and go away in Indian file, singing the above quoted *Jagao guru ho, jagao cela, etc.* After this visit to the headman's house they proceed to visit the other houses of their village, taking all in succession, until they reach the end of the village street, when they go back and visit the houses on the other side of the headman's house. The homesteads of a Santal village lie on both sides of the village street, ordinarily well away from each other (that is, where outside influence has not made the Santals alter their own comparatively sanitary way of building). When 'taking' the street they do not work one side first and the other side coming back, but take both sides at once. They do not visit only the Santals, but if people of other races are living in their village, they will also visit them and beg, even Mohammedans. Brahmins, they tell, may ask them to become *rum* and act before them.

As soon as they get out into the street, they walk along two, three or four abreast; they sing again, as they walk, *Jagao guru ho, etc.*

When they enter any court-yard, they act in the same way as they did entering the headman's house, sing the same, dance and drum, etc. The *guru* in every house sprinkles his medicinal rice-water on the waterpots or their stand and over the entrance door. When they have received the Indian corn, they start for the next house.

The same is repeated in every house with only few variations. When they on entering a court-yard see that an *ojha* lives here (that is, see an *ojha*'s *than*, cf. above p. 46), or know that such a one is living there (there may be several in a fairly large village), they go through the same performance as in other houses, but here in addition the following: a couple of the young men become *rum*, possessed by some *guru boṅga* or other, and also (but not always) by some of the 'play' *boṅgas*. The house-wife, or, if she is not there, or is incapacitated, another grown-up female, brings some *sindur* mixed with oil in a *bhąutič* (see above p. 72) leaf-cup and gives this to the *guru* who proceeds to make *sindur* marks in five places, beside the *than* or somewhere in the court-yard; he also smears *sindur* on the foreheads of the *rum* young men and on their backs (it should be remarked that this is always done when anyone is possessed by a *bonga*). When all is done and they have received what they want, they walk out, one after the other saluting the housewife who stands at the entrance door with her hands kept turned upwards and together, as a woman does when receiving a salute. The *guru* takes the unused *sindur* along with him; it is his.

There is one other variation, referred to previously. If they, on entering a court-yard, see a number of pumpkins on the roof, presently one of the *Dasãe kora* becomes 'possessed' by the *hąrũ bonga*, climbs up on the roof and takes a pumpkin.

In the evening they return with their spoils to the *guru's* house, where they finish the day, dancing, singing, becoming 'possessed' and the like. They do not stay long, and return to their respective houses for the night.

The next morning they return to the *guru's* house, clothe themselves according to custom, dance a little, and start to finish the village.

When there is no house left to beg in, they again go to the *guru's* house, and make ready to visit some other village. The object is the same, to beg and to have some fun.

Before they start they dance a little, whereupon they sing:

:/: *Delabon guru ho* :/:
Disomte dǫ ho, guru ho, disomte dǫ ho!
:/: *Delabon guru ho* :/:
Deste dǫ ho, guru ho, deste dǫ!
Disomre dǫ ho, guru ho,
Celko ńamoka, guru ho? celko ńamoka?
Desre dǫ ho, guru ho,
Celko ńamoka, guru ho? Celko ńamoka?
Disomre dǫ ho, guru ho,
Sunume sindur ho, guru ho, sunume sindur;
Desre dǫ ho, guru ho,
Naenǫm kajar ho, guru ho, naenǫm kajar.
Sunume sindur dǫ, guru ho,
Cekae anečem, guru ho, cekae aneč?
Naenǫm kajar dǫ, guru ho,
Cekae anečem, guru ho, cekae aneč?
Sunume sindur dǫ, guru hoń
Sindur lągil ho, guru hoń sindur lągil.
Naenǫm kajar dǫ, guru hoń
Kajar lągil, guru hoń kajar lągil.

That is,

Come let us go, o *guru*,
Out in the country, o guru, out in the country!
Come, let us go, o guru,
Out in the land, o guru, out in the land!
In the country, o guru,
What things are to be had, o guru? What things are to be had?
In the land, o guru,
What things are to be had, o guru? What things are to be had?
In the country, o guru,
Oil and sindur, o guru, oil and sindur,
In the land, o guru,
Eye-paint and lamp-black, o guru, eye-paint and lamp-black.

Oil and sindur, o guru;
What are you going to do with that, o guru, what are you going to do with that?
Eye-paint and lamp-black, o guru,
What are you going to do with that, o guru, what are you going to do with that?

Oil and sindur, o guru,
Oil and sindur, o guru, I am going to apply, going to apply;
Eye-paint and lamp-black, o guru,
Eye-paint and lamp-black, o guru, I am going to apply, going to apply.[1]

Having finished this song they start, walking across the field to the village they intend to visit. On their way they stop at some suitable place to arrange their clothes, specially to take on the loin cloth *kạcni* fashion (if they start in the morning without previous dancing anywhere, they go dressed as usual). When they reach the end of the village street, they march along to the first house (here not to the headman's house first), singing as they pass along the street the following:—

Kulhi jagao naṭ bạṭi, raja ho,
Nakhṛa jagao naṭ bạṭi, raja ho,
Raja puṭạ dhọrọme duạr,
(or, *raja puṭạ, dara mạñjur ae*)
Hạri, Hạri raja ho,
Raja puṭạ dhọrọme duạr.

---

1 The here cited song is, as will be seen, really an alternating song between *guru* and disciples. It is, however, sung by all. The language is genuine Santali with a couple of 'poetical' peculiarities, and one form that is often heard with certain individuals, but is not otherwise ordinary language, *viz.*, *neč*, or fully, *aneč*, added to the finite verb instead of simply *a*. There are some individuals who have got into the habit of nearly always using this.

Sunum sindur is the *sindur* with the oil that is necessary to prepare the 'paint' used. *Aenọm* (*naenọm* is the poetical form with prefixed *n*) *kajar* are two words for the same thing. The first word is "eye-paint,' the second is their name for lamp-black that is used as eye-paint. They paint this on the eye lids. They also use the same stuff in certain sacrificial performances, that is to say not the ordinary sacrificer, but the *ojha*. (Cf. p. 31.)

That is,

The village street make efficient, the brass-cup of the dance, o king,
The place of dancing make efficient, the brass-cup of the dance, o king,
The king's son, at the sacred entrance.
(or, The king's son, coming along the road like a peacock,—according to Santal translation).
Hari, Hari, o king,
The king's son at the sacred entrance.

Whenever they pass along the street of a village not their own they sing the above gibberish.

When they enter the court-yard of a house they sing *Dasãea ka jhala mala, etc.*, and otherwise act just as in their own village. Here, however, the *guru* does not bring any medicine-water with him to sprinkle on the water pots. When they enter the court-yard of an *ojha*, they go through the same as in their own village. Whilst in their own village everybody is supposed to give some Indian corn, many in 'foreign' villages are not inclined to give. When they enter a house of such people they are at once informed that they have no one there who could give. No woman shows herself, and the *Dasãe koṛa* naturally do not stop, but go to the next house.

During their wandering about they will frequently meet a party from some other village out on the same business; in such cases they get some extra fun. This will be described in a chapter below.

According to the size of the villages visited and the number of houses where they are received, they manage to 'do' two or three (not more) villages in one day. Every evening, often long after sun-set, they return to their own village and deposit the results of their begging in the *guru*'s house, and again start from there the next morning.

As a rule they go begging up to three days, the last day in any case being the *bas..n hilok*, the day of immersion or dismissal, as the Santals call it. On this day they may attempt some begging in the forenoon, but will not get much. They all march with their *guru* to the *dibi ṭaṇḍi*, lit. the goddess plain, the open place near the house where the Durga image has been standing, and where generally crowds of people come together, in these parts also very large numbers of Santals. Here they dance and sing, drum and play; here they are one after the other 'possessed' by the different *bongas* mentioned and perform their various plays. *Sindur* is not used here, and there is no begging.

When all is over they march to their *guru*'s house and have some final dancing and other performances, whereupon they go to their respective homes.

The Indian corn collected remains in the meantime in the charge of the *guru*. The amount collected varies. In each house visited they receive, I am told, from one to four *jhumbli*. One *jhumbli* is four cobs of Indian corn, tied together by the covering leaves of the cobs that are pulled back. The amount of maize given may consequently turn out to be anything from half a seer to two seers in each house. In this is not included what is given to the *guru*. He receives his corn separately and keeps all for himself; it is his due, a kind of payment for all the trouble he has taken.

The *celas* go to the *guru* every evening, now not for instruction or anything similar, but to separate the Indian corn from the cobs. The maize must first be properly dry; it generally takes a couple of weeks to get this done. They may ultimately have a couple of maunds of Indian corn. They will now do one of two things; they may sell the maize and for the money buy a *khạsi* or a *bạdhią*; or they have a festival called *cela karam*.

A *khạsi* is a castrated he-goat, a *bạdhią* a castrated pig. The animal is killed and divided between those who have participated, besides which every household in their village gets a share; they are particular that none shall be left out.[1] They do not have a public feast, eating together; each takes his share home, where it is prepared as curry (*utu*, as they call it) and eaten with their rice.

When they have done as described some years in succession, the *guru* who, as a matter of course, still leads them, proposes to them that they should have the *karam* festival. He supports his proposal by saying that they have now so many times given their own village people food; now they ought to do something for the whole country-side, and let them taste their Indian corn.

Agreeing to this they measure what they have of Indian corn and possibly *janhe* (Paspalum scrobiculatum, L., a millet grown by the Santals and said to give intoxicating beer. Where people have no Indian corn they may give some *janhe* instead, I am told), to find out how much beer (*hạṇḍi*) they may be able to manufacture. They may brew from the maize and the *janhe*; sometimes they exchange the Indian corn for rice or *janhe*. The stuff is portioned out to the different households in the village, and the people are requested to brew. In consultation with the village headman, his deputy and other village people, a day is fixed for the celebration, and those who have received the Indian corn, etc., for brewing are requested to have the beer ready on the day notified, adding that on that day they are all to come together at the *guru*'s house. The intended celebration is announced in the neighbouring villages and all are invited to come.

In the morning of the day appointed all the beer is brought to the *guru*'s house, and one pot is drunk at once; this is called *jan hạṇḍi*, the beer of knowing, or intimation. In the evening people come together. During daylight they have looked out a *karam* tree in the forest; after sunset a dozen or so start with drums to fetch a branch (*karam* is the Adina cordifolia, H.f. & B., a large forest tree). A small branch is cut and brought by two unmarried young men, and by the same two planted in the village street just outside the entrance to the *guru*'s house. Now the actual festival commences.

A little beer is libated beside the planted branch, some for *Pilcu haṛam* and

---

[1] When the Santals club together to buy an animal for food, they are anxious that all may get equal and just shares according to their contributions. All eatable parts are cut up into small bits and divided into as many portions as there are 'shares' (one such portion is called *joṛo*), every portion getting the same amount of each kind of meat, fat, intestines, etc. It is quite a serious business with them.

Pilcu buḍhi (the first man and woman), some for *Mạṅjhi haṛam* (the spirit of the original village chief, by many Santals considered identical with the first man) and some to *Maraṅ buru* (the principal national godling). The libation to *Mạṅjhi haṛam* may be omitted. Some one recites the *binti* for the occasion.[1]

Now the beer drinking and dancing commences. First the village people drink in the *ojha guru*'s house and go out to dance. They dance some four *akhaṛ* (rounds). When they have done they call the people of some village or other whom they have seen present. These come in, get each two leaf-cups of beer and commence to dance. When these have had two *akhaṛ* of dancing, the people of another village are called and treated in the same way, and so on, until all villages present have had their turn. According to the number of villages represented this dancing may go on until cock-crow or even longer. Up to this time they dance in the street round the planted *karam* branch a certain kind of dance, called *karam ẹnẹc*, or also *riṅjạ* (*ẹnẹc* means dance or play). There are songs sung to a special melody, the dancing drum is beaten to a special time. No one commences dancing before he is called with his village; but as soon as they have commenced, they may continue as much as they like, only not too close to the *karam* branch, in order not to hamper those 'legitimately' there.

When all have been called, the dance is changed to what is called *bhinsạr*, that has other dancing steps, other drumming and songs with other melodies. At sunrise the two young men who brought and planted the *karam* branch go and pluck it up. The one who takes hold of it runs round with it a couple of times, keeping it high up. The girls present jump up and try to pluck a leaf of the branch. If there are girls present wishing to pledge themselves to special friendship, they put the leaf they have taken in each other's hair; from this time on these pairs are connected in special intimate friendship; they call each other *karam ḍạr* (*karam* branch) and do not use their names.

The two young men thereupon run with the branch to a tank or other fairly deep water, enter the water until they are sufficiently in to be able to immerse themselves. The one who has the branch lets it go whilst under water.[2] Hereupon they return to the others, after having bathed. Then the dancing ceases and all visitors return to their respective villages. Those of the village continue drinking what beer may be left and dance (now *lagṛẽ*, the most common Santal dance) until noon. Then all is over.

No sacrifices are offered, only beer libated as described.

There are a couple of things that should be mentioned. The Santals have a large number of different dances, with corresponding different songs and different drum beating. The dance used at the *Dasãe daṛan* is called *Dasãe* or *lọbọe*; the

---

1 A *binti* is a recitation of appropriate tradition and precepts, statements, often in figurative language, of what they are at the particular occasion occupied with. The *binti* varies; at certain occasions it is a long story, reciting the traditions from the very commencement of the world, literally *ab ovo*, down to the moment of recitation. So here, there are not many who know the *binti* properly; one who is known to know is therefore generally called in to recite.

2 Very much the same kind of diving is gone through when they go to the Damuda river with the bones of dead people. The bones are let go by the man carrying them whilst he is immersed in the water.

songs and melodies have the same name; of the last named there are several different ones.

6.

When Dasãe *begging parties meet.*

The *Dasãe daṛan* is not restricted to begging in one's own village; as a matter of fact they do more begging in other villages than in their own, although they, of course will receive more liberal gifts at home than abroad. As every village is supposed to have a *guru* and every year to have a course of instruction as described. and as they all end their courses at the same time and in the same manner, it will naturally happen that the begging parties meet.

When meeting they have some wrangling, one party trying to outdo the other and to show themselves superior in power. It may to an outsider sound rather harsh; the fact that they have learnt these songs and questions and answers at their course shows that it is not to be taken at its face value.

As soon as they see one another, they both sing:

Jhạri loṭa cepel cepel, horlo lolo; tọkọe guru dọe lẹvẹr sẹtẹren?
Horlo lolo, tọkọe cela dọe lẹvẹr sẹtẹren?

That is:

A lota with a spout, brimful, swaying, lulling, which guru has come swaying here?
Swaying, lulling, which disciple has come swaying here?

Yọrẹ tạpuạ, hamar sọṅge lạgis kẹnẹrẹ?
Bãwẹ̃ bãwẹ̃ ban calabo, tọlẹ tọlẹ pạthri yuṛabo.

That is:

Hey, you dunce, why will you pit yourself against me?
High through the air I shall set magic in motion, deep below I shall cause the (opposite) sorcery to disappear.

Dabha lad bad, ḍabha pạki gel,
Tomara biconme khae jaga, amar sọtẹ juạn ke?

That is:

The orange is soft, the orange is ripe;
I shall eat your seed; who is stronger than myself?

Thereupon the answer comes:

Gun calare gunia,
Hae, hae! guru gunia,
Hae hae! guru na gunia

That is:

Work your magic, sorcerer!
Alas, alas! the *guru* sorcerer,
Alas, alas! the *guru* is no sorcerer.

Gun menaktam khan mar ge calaome!
Pạthri menaktam khan mar ge ñedeñme!

Gunem sambṛaotiṅkhan marge teṅgonme!
Pạthrim daramtiṅ khan mar ge hijukme!

That is:

If you have any magic power, do work it!
If you have any sorcery, do hit me fatally!
If you can restrain my magic, do stand up!
If you can meet my sorcery, do come here!

After this braggadocio they come nearer and commence a more friendly intercourse. They ask each other (using a Bihari dialect): *Suluk jaebe na guru, bạdi jaebe?* Will the *guru* not go in peace, will he go with ill-will? They answer: *Suluk jaebo*, we shall go in peace. Hereupon they sing:

Johari guru ho, dẹbo johara;
Johari guru ho, dẹbo beohara.

Johar, johar, guru ho, cete johar?
Beohar, beohar, guru ho, cete beohar?

Cela celakin dọ balaea johar,
Guru gurukin dọ so johar.

That is:

Be greeted, o *guru*, come let us greet each other;
Be greeted, o *guru*, come let us show courtesy to each other.

Greeting, greeting, o *guru*, what greeting?
Courtesy, courtesy, o *guru*, what courtesy?

The disciples between themselves the greeting of men whose children are married;
The *gurus* between themselves the 'equal' greeting.[1]

There is then some greeting gone through. Next they ask each other for lime and tobacco. The most common way of using tobacco among the Santals is to chew tobacco leaf pounded and mixed with unslaked lime of mussels in the hollow of one's hand; this tobacco chewing is in use among men (formerly never among women) and is a very common way of commencing a talk with other people. Strangers (provided they are Santals) will ask each other for lime and tobacco; if the party addressed is unwilling it means either great hurry or non-acceptance of the invitation to talk. The *Dasãe* boys may ask for tobacco in the ordinary way; but they have also some songs, used at this occasion. The following is one of these.

They sing:

Thamakur, thamakur; gosãe, maṇḍa thamakur,
Baha leka daka, sẹṅgẹl leka pạurạ,

[1] The greeting or salutation performed between two men whose children are married is a very elaborate and rather curious acting: it is the finest form of salutation between equals known to Santals. The *so johar*, lit. equal greeting, is a form used by persons who are unrelated and do not know their respective ages. They both 'receive' each other's salutation. See the writer's paper on the different kinds of salutation used by the Santals, J.A.S.B., Vol. LXVII, Part III, (1898), where a full description is found.

Buṛhi chagol mare cọbọr rase,
Ạṇḍiạ mạṅjhi, mạṇḍiạ paranik.
Den bạbu, cun thamakur ẹmọk talaṅme.
Mil din laṅ jọma, juger jug ṅutum tahẹn talaṅa.
Dẹn ho peṛa naṅcarretam ghẹ̃ṭ thamakur,
Ḍanḍaretam rẹbẹl cun;
Hẹ̃ṭ guru bhẹ̃ṭ celalaṅ jọmletamge.
Makṛe sutạm, makṛe jhilmil,
Kẹ judi belware mala gathe pare,
Se am khaete pare.

That is:

Tobacco, tobacco, my lord, pounded tobacco,
Cooked rice like flowers, liquor like fire,
Old juice of an aged she-goat, just sufficient,
A powerful headman, a vigorous deputy headman.
Do, young man, give us two lime and tobacco,
It is one day we two eat; age upon age a name will remain for us two.
Give, o friend, the tobacco tied up in the edge of your cloth,
The lime stuck in your waist;
The outdone *guru*, the visiting *cela*, we two shall first eat what you have.
Twisted thread, twisted shutter;
If any one can string the bael necklace,
He will be able to eat the mango.

The language is a curious mixture.

Whilst sitting together to chew tobacco, they attempt to try each other's knowledge, and to show their superiority, if they have any, something like the rivalry between the disciples of different schools. They ask questions and expect answers, all stereotype, and strangely enough, generally in a foreign, mixed and incorrect language. The following are examples.

Bin bhiṭuạk phule jo hilạì lagae,
Bin baklak kaṭher nam jo kạhi dẹhọre, guru ho.

That is,

The stalkless flower waving,
The barkless tree's name, please, *guru*, tell.

The answer is:

Tumi ho guru, ami ho guru,
Bin bhiṭuạk phule jo hilạì lagae,
Bin baklak kaṭher nam jo kạhi dẹhọ re, guru ho.

That is,

You are a *guru*, I am also a *guru*, that is, the stalkless, etc.

Kọn kọn bin rọkọt kaṭ, babaji?
Uhi je bajae lakta he,
Uhi je bin rọkọt kaṭ, babaji.

That is,

What can you cut without shedding blood, o babaji?
Why, listen, it is sounding,
Why, that is cutting without shedding blood, o babaji.

The following is an answer to a scolding:

Are, sala sala bolis na, sal gac tọ moṭa hoilo,
Huluk na buluk na, marte marte camme chaṛega;
Ḍẹdgẹr daṗkate lagṛẽ salre huḍuk ḍubuk karta he re.

That is,

You fellow, don't say *sala* (brother-in-law), the *sal* tree has become thick;
Don't loaf about; thrashing you I shall flay your skin off;
Covering a kettle-drum with it I shall make it sound lustily at the lagṛẽ dancing place (*sal*).

The play on *sala*, the *sal* stick that may be used, and the dancing *sal*, might be noted.

Hal bhaṅglo, pal bhaṅglo, jual bhaṅglo, des jae.
Kọn des? Des jae, Kạmru des.

That is,

The plough broke, the ploughshare broke, the yoke broke; I have started for the country.
Which country? I have started for the country, Kamru's country.

The samples given must suffice; most, if any, of the conundrums with their answers have nothing to do with *ojha* 'science' and are of very little interest, except it should be from a linguistic point of view, as they show, how a foreign language can be 'murdered' by those who do not know anything of it. One is often reminded of the Latin of the Epistolae obscurorum virorum.

7.

The Dasãe *songs.*

When the *Dasãe koṛa*, the 'September boys,' dance in the court-yards they have as mentioned, a number of special songs sung to special melodies that fit in with their dancing steps. These are, as mentioned above, called *Dasãe sereń*, also *lọbọe sereń*; *sereń* is the Santali name for a song; *lọbọe* refers to the steps of the dancing.

The *Dasãe* songs are practically all in Santali, with many poetical peculiarities, as to the form of words and also as to the grammatical construction.

Bindire sutạmteben ṭuṇḍạń kan dọ,
Bindire tọṛẹteben gẹmẹń kan dọ;
Bindire Siń bir dọ lọk kan dọ,
Bindire Man bir dọ hasa ḍigiren.

That is,

O spider, you two are moving along the thread (web),
O spider, you two are climbing slowly up the gossamer;

O spider, the *Siń* forest is burning,
O spider, the *Man* forest has become dust and ashes.[1]

Ọt ma lọlọ, Kạmru guru, serma setoń, Buạń guru,
Yọ haere, cela dọlań lalaokelko.
Sui sutạm gutukate sẹnẹrre lań galańkako,
Reaṛ kaṇḍa, sitạ nala latarrelań dọhọkako.

That is,

The earth is hot, o Kamru guru, the sky is fierce sunshine, o Buan guru;
Alas, alas, we two have tantalized the disciples;
We two shall thread a needle and weave them on the rafter,
In a cool waterpot, below the Sita valley we two shall put them.

Cetan khọn cọń latar khọn coń koemar jugi darao kan,
Kọemar jugi cetete lań bidạye?
Kọemar jugi toatelań bidạye,
Kọemar jugi dahetelań bidạ bahere.

That is,

Whether from up-country or from the low country a jugi is coming,
Wherewith are we two to send the begging jugi off?
We two shall send the begging jugi off with milk,
We two shall send the begging jugi off and away with curds.

Siṅgi siń siṅgi ńindạ hãs hạsil cẹ̃ṛẽ, dại, kin rọdọn akada;
Do sẹ, do sẹ lạiaepe,
Jaher ɛra lạiaepe,
Bareakin manewakin nupel akana.

That is,

All day and all night the swan pair, o elder sister, have been bothering,
Do, do, tell her,
Tell the Lady of the holy grove,[2]
Two human beings have appeared.

Tọkọe guru nurạlte pohoko dọko nãṛgolen?
Tọkọe cela baherte pakaṛeko ṭuṇḍạń kan?
Kạmru guru nurạlte pohoko dọko nãṛgolen,
Kạmru cela baherte dọ pakaṛeko ṭuṇḍạn kan.

That is,

Through which guru's incitement did the locusts come down?
Through which disciples' calling out are the larvæ moving about?

---

[1] *Tọṛẹ* is a fabulous thread mentioned in the traditional account of the creation of the world, as going between heaven and earth. Gossamer thread floating in the air is called *tọṛẹ*: apparently they are not quite certain whether it is gossamer. *Siń bir* and *Man bir* are forests mentioned in the Santal traditions.

[2] According to Santal traditions the first human pair came out of two eggs of a pair of swans. When the Creator first made a human pair from earth, the Day horse came and kicked them to pieces just as he was going to give them souls. So he made a pair of swans from what he plucked off his breast, and these two got two eggs from which the first human pair came out. The introduction of *Jaher ɛra* is entirely unknown in the traditions.

Through the incitement of Kamru guru the locusts came down.
Kamru's disciples calling them out the larvæ are moving about.

Naire ma naigor hako biolę boyolę;
Hae, hae! gadare ma tayan biolę boyolę;
Hae hae! natore ma nato kurikin bilit balan.

That is,

In the big river the river fish are swimming about;
Alas, alas! in the big river the crocodile is swimming about;
Alas, alas, in the village the two village girls go glittering about.

Horre hesak sakam hipire hipire,
Hoete hesak sakam hipir hipir;
Daharre bare sakam ńohore ńohore.

That is,

On the road is the trembling pipol leaf,
The wind makes the pipol leaves tremble;
On the cart-track is the glossy banyan leaf.

Horre kasmar kulai bir ma tilai lo,
Kulai pedel pedel, gate, kulai homor homor,
Marna lagae kulai do,
Kulai pedel pedel, gate, kulai homor homor.

That is,

On the road a kasmar tree, a hare, in the forest the tilai bush is burnt,
The hare is jumping about, the hare is mourning, o companion,
The hare is going to die,
The hare is jumping about, o companion, the hare is mourning.

Logo burure, guru ho, kadlak matkom ho, guru ho, kadlak matkom ho,
Hae hae! ghanta barire, guru ho, caole sarjom ho, guru ho, caole sarjom ho!
Hae hae! halan hapatin ho, guru ho, kadlak matkom, guru ho, kadlak matkom ho,
Boeha boehakin, guru ho, halan hapatin ho, guru ho, halan hapatin,
Ńatea ńateakin, guru ho, cepeč hapatin, guru ho, cepeč hapatin.

That is,

On the Logo hill, o guru, there is a middle sized mahua tree, o guru, a middle sized mahua tree,
O dear, dear! on the Ghanta bari, o guru, there is sal grain, o guru, sal grain;
O dear, dear! to pluck and divide, o guru, the middle sized mahua tree, o guru, the middle sized mahua tree.
The two brothers, o guru, will pluck and divide, o guru, will pluck and divide;
The two wives of the two brothers will, o guru, suck between them, o guru, will suck and divide.[1]

[1] *Matkom*, the mahua, Bassia latifolia, Roxb.
Ghanta bari, lit. the stir about field (or homestead) may possibly refer to the Mandar hill (in the south of the Bhagalpur district) where the gods churned the ocean.

Cetane disom dọ, guru hoe dakkeḷa ho, guru hoe dakkeḷa ho;
Latare disom dọ, guru hoe jạrikeḷa ho, guru hoe jạrikeḷa ho.
Gaṅ nại dọ, guru ho, pẹrẹčena ho, guru ho, pẹrẹčena ho,
Soṛa nại dọ, guru ho, coṛaṅenare, guru ho, coṛaṅenare.
Cekate, cekate, guru holaṅ parọm calak ho, guru laṅ parọm calaka?
Miḷ sutạm dọ, guru ho, cọtẹ lọbẹre, hae hae!
Bar sutạm dọ, guru ho, buạṅe ḍạṇḍire, guru ho, buạṅe ḍạṇḍire;
Miḷ jaṅga dọ, guru ho, tọrẹ sutạmre, guru ho, tọrẹ sutạmre, hae hae!
Miḷ jaṅga dọ, guru ho, buạṅe ḍạṇḍire, guru ho, buạṅe ḍạṇḍire.

That is,

In the up-country, o guru, it rained, o guru, it rained;
In the low-country, o guru, it poured, o guru, it poured.
The Ganges river, o guru, was filled, o guru, was filled,
The Sora river, o guru, ran overflowing, o guru, ran overflowing.
How, how, o guru, will we two get across, o, guru, we two get across?
One thread, o guru, high above, o dear, dear!
Two threads, o guru, in the buaṅ stick, o guru, in the buaṅ stick;
One foot, o guru, in the gossamer thread, o guru, in the gossamer thread, o dear, dear!
One foot, o guru, on the buaṅ stick, o guru, on the buaṅ stick.

Tọkọe gururen cela dọko noḍoṅen dahades dọ, guru ho, dahades?
Tọkọe-gururen cela dọko noḍoṅen? sarag ḍihạn bharṇḍo leka dhuṛiko noṭaṅeḷ.
Kạmru gururen cela dọko noḍoṅena, dahades dọ, guru ho, dahades dọ, hae hae!
Kạmru gururen cela dọko noḍoṅena, sarag ḍihạn dhuṛiko noṭaṅeḷ.

That is,

Which guru's disciples have come out over the country, o guru, over the country?
Which guru's disciples have come out? right up to heaven like a whirlwind they spread the dust.
Kamru guru's disciples have come out over the country, o guru, over the country; alas, alas!
Kamru guru's disciples have come out, right up to heaven they spread the dust.

Hako hako, guru ho, ḍaṇḍa ḍaṇḍa, hae!
Dhiri cetan, guru ho, hako bele, hae hae!
Cạuṛạ cetan, guru ho, hakoe bubrum kan.

That is,

Fish, fish, o guru, fins, fins, o dear, dear!
Upon the stone, o guru, the fish egg, o dear, dear!
Upon the rock, o guru, the fish is sitting on eggs!

Kuṛikin na tọrẹteben tuṇḍaṅ kana, hae hae!
Kuṛikin na tọrẹteben gẹmẹñ kana, hae hae!

Kuṛikin na naben nasul sangarte, nisi sermań tetańena ;
Nardo kuṛikin tohoń nasulleben,
Nardo kuṛikin tohoń sańgarleben!

That is,

You two girls, you are moving along the gossamer, o dear, dear,
You two girls, you are crawling along the gossamer, o dear, dear!
You two girls, supporting and taking about you two for twenty years I became utterly destitute;
Any more, you two girls, I shall certainly not support you two,
Any more, you two girls, I shall certainly not take you two about with me!

Toķoe gururen cela doko noḍońena lale lal do, guru ho, lale lal do?
Toķoe gururen cela doko baherena, maṭ barahe, guru ho, caṛhi barahe?
Kamru gururen cela doko noḍońena lale lal do, guru ho, lale lal do, hae hae!
Kamru gururen cela doko baherena, maṭ barahe, guru ho, caṛhi barahe!

That is,

Which guru's disciples have come out so red, o guru, so red?
Which guru's disciples have come out in the country, with a rope of bamboo, o guru, with a three-stranded rope?
Kamru guru's disciples have come out so red, o guru, so red, o dear, dear!
Kamru guru's disciples have come out in the country, with a rope of bamboo, o guru, with a three-stranded rope!

Kuṛikin na, ḍhińki lebedben na, kuṛikin,
Numul noyońben, hae hae! kuṛikin!
Caole sokojben na, kuṛikin, sańkha natenben!

That is,

You two girls, tread the dhinki, you two girls,
Look down where the shade is, o dear, dear! you two girls!
Toss up the rice, you two girls, listen to the sound the shell wristlets are making!

Toķoe guru racare hesaķ beleķ kan, guru ho,
Hesaķ beleķ kan, hae hae?
Toķoe guru baṭere baṛe beleķ kan, guru ho,
Baṛe beleķ kan, hae hae?
Care kisnikin cero beroķ kan.
Mane huhāṛ do gurukin kena kiniķ kan,
Gurukin kena kiniķ kan.

That is,

In which guru's court-yard is the pipol ripening, o guru,
The pipol ripening, o dear, dear?
In which guru's property is the banyan ripening, o guru,
The banyan ripening, o dear, dear?
The two pied-starlings are twittering,

The two fine green doves, o guru, are chattering,
O guru, the two are chattering.

Tọkọe guru racare divhe jolok kan, guru ho,
Hae hae, divhe bamberok?
Kạmru guru racare divhe jolok kan, guru ho,
Hae hae, divhe bamberok.

That is,

In which guru's court-yard is the lamp burning, o guru,
O dear, dear, the lamp shining?
In Kamru guru's court-yard the lamp is burning, o guru,
O dear, dear, the lamp is shining.

Tọkọe guru ho, guru hoe akhṛaleta ho,
Guru hoe akhṛaleta ho, hae hae?
Kạmru guru hoe akhṛaleta ho,
Guru hoe akhṛaleta ho, hae hae!

That is,

Which guru, o guru, provided the place for performance,
O guru provided the place for performance? O dear, dear!
Kamru guru provided the place for performance,
O guru, he provided the place for performance, o dear, dear!

Hae hae, Kạmru cela dọ cela dọe pinḍleta ho;
Cete lạgit ho guru hoe akhṛaleta ho,
Guru hoe akhṛaleta ho?
Sunume sindur lạgit guru hoe akhṛaleta;
Naenọm kajar lạgit cela hoe pinḍleta dọ.

That is,

O dear, dear! Kamru's disciple, the disciple made an altar;
For what purpose did the guru provide a place for performance,
O guru, did he provide a place for performance?
To use oil and sindur, o guru, he provided a place for performance,
To use eye-paint and lamp-black the disciple made an altar.

Hae hae! sedae Siaṛsiń kumạṅ
Kọdẹ piṭhạ silpińteko sińlede,
Janhẹ ḍombok dakateko lebdaledea.

That is,

O dear, dear! in the old days father's sister's husband Siaṛ Siń
They shut up with a door of kode millet bread,
With a ball of cooked janhe millet they threw him down.

Tokare dọ ho, guru ho, ḍhak saḍe kan, guru ho, hae hae?
Tokare dọ ho, guru ho, rạnkhi rāwāok kan, hae hae?
O̱t ma patalre, guru ho, ḍhak saḍe kan, hae hae;
S̱erma cọtẹre dọ, guru, rạṅkhi rāwāok kan, guru ho.

That is,

Where, o guru, is the kettle drum sounding, o guru, o dear, dear?
Where, o guru, are the brass cymbals chiming, o dear, dear?
The earth, in the world below, o guru, the kettle drum is sounding, o dear, dear;
In the sky above, o guru, the brass cymbals are chiming, o guru.

Hae hae! dur dese yạile, buhin, jhaṭkạite bidại de!
Hae hae! jạite jạite bạḍi dur jhaṭka, buhin, bidại de!

That is,

O dear, dear! I have come to a country far away, o sister, be quick to send me off!
O dear, dear! walking, walking I have come very far, be quick, o sister, and send me off!

Hae hae! kisãṛ nera mẹc gando mạcire goe duṛup̄ akan,
Hae hae! ḍạṅguạ kuṛi satere goe racak̄ kan.
Hae hae! kọcẹ kọcẹteye bẹṅgẹladiń,
Hae hae! kokombeye landawadiń.

That is,

O dear, dear! the master's wife is sitting on the chairs, planks and stools, o brother-in-law,
O dear, dear! the maiden is standing pulling the straw of the eaves, o brother-in-law.
O dear, dear! she looked at me sideways,
O dear, dear! she turned her head aslant and laughed to me.

Hae hae! Sarag ḍihọn patalreko ẹnec̓ kana,
Hae hae! guru dọ, guru dọe nẹmok̄ kan dọ sunume sindur,
Hae hae! cela dọ, cela dọe nẹmok̄ kan dọ naenọm kajar.

That is,

O dear, dear! right to heaven and in the netherworld they are dancing,
O dear, dear! the guru, the guru is giving oil and sindur,
O dear, dear! the disciple, the disciple is giving eye-paint and lamp-black.

Hae hae! dẹ gọ yayọ bhik yayọ,
Arwa cạl, eka ḍạli ḍar lạgil,
Hae hae! eka kodar mạṭi lạgil;
Yuhi dẹkhọ mora saṅgare bhại yayọ.

That is,

O dear, dear! do, o mother, o mother, give what I beg, o mother,
Sun-dried rice, one basket for the branches.
O dear, dear! one hoe for the earth;
See him, my dead brother-in law, o mother.

Hae hae! kuli kuli sunte jabọ ghọrẹ ghọrẹ;
Hae hae! khelte jabọ, hae hae! na hạmi jabọ, go,
Sẹbọkẹrọ bạṛi duạre.

That is,

O dear, dear! I shall go through the street to listen from house to house;
O dear, dear! I shall go to dance, o dear, dear! No, I am not going
To the door of the worshippers' house.

Hae hae! nape dọ, gọ nayọ, noṛak duạrre,
Hae hae! nale dọ, gọ nayọ, serma setoṅre;
Hae hae! kọe dọ, gọ nayo, nemalepe,
Hae hae! kọe dọ, gọ nayọ, bidạkalepe!

That is,

O dear, dear! You, o mother, o mother, are in your house and home,
O dear, dear! we, o mother, o mother, are in the heat of the sun in the sky
O dear, dear! what we beg, o mother, o mother, give us,
O dear, dear! what we beg, o mother, o mother, send us off with that!

Hae hae! nẹtọm ḍaṅgra dọ, guru ho, kọṅẹrekade,
Hae hae! kọṅẹ ḍaṅgra dọ guru hoe ẹtọmrekade;
Hae hae! guru hoe burumen dọ, guru hoe burumen dọ;
Kuyạ lekan kuṛi, guru hoe lại baṛae kan, guru hoe katha baṛae kan.

That is,

O dear, dear! The right side bullock, o guru, he has put on the left side,
O dear, dear! The left side bullock he has, o guru, put on the right side.
O dear, dear! o guru, he lay down, o guru, he lay down;
A girl black like a wild dog, o guru, is telling it, o guru, she is spreading a report of it.

Hae hae! dẹs lọbẹ disom cayayen,
Hae hae! guru ho, delabon dẹste,
Hae hae! guru ho, delabon disomte;
Hae hae! dẹs lọbẹ disom baheren,
Hae hae! guru ho, delabon dẹste,
Hae hae! guru ho, delabon disomte!

That is,

O dear, dear! the desirable country, the land has become stinking,
O dear, dear! o guru, come let us go out into the country,
O dear, dear! o guru, come let us go out into the land;
O dear, dear! the desirable country has become defiled,
O dear, dear! o guru, come let us go out into the country,
O dear, dear! o guru, come let us go out into the land!

Hae hae! tọkọekoren piạri ghuṛi
Likide likide, guru ho?
Hae hae! tọkọekoren poṇḍko sadọm
Dọmọgẹ, guru ho, dọmọgẹ dọmọgẹ?
Hae hae! Kạmru gururen piạri ghuṛi
Likide likide, guru ho.

Hae hae! Kạmru celaren pọṇḍko sadọm
Dọmọgẹ dọmọgẹ, guru ho, dọmọgẹ.

That is,

O dear, dear! whose lovely mare
Is gracefully galloping, o guru?
O dear, dear! whose white horses
Are jumping, o guru, jumping and plunging?
O dear, dear! Kamru guru's lovely mare
Is gracefully galloping, o guru.
O dear, dear! Kamru's disciple's white horses.
Are jumping, o guru, jumping and plunging.

Hae hae! siṅgi siṅ siṅgi ṅindạ
Hãs hạsil cẹṛẹ gurukin rọdọn akada re.
Hae hae! cete lạgit, gurukin rọdọnkeda re?
Hae hae! manwa lạgit, gurukin rọdọnkeda re.
Hae hae! dal cetanre, gurukin cipiạ kan, gurukin cipiạ kan;
Hae hae! dal cetanre, gurukin tupukạ kan, gurukin tupukạ kan.
Hae hae! dal cetanre, gurukin beble kan, gurukin beble kan,
Hae hae! dal cetanre, guru ho, manwa jọnọm dọ, guru họ, manwa jọnọm dọ;
Hae hae! tokare dọ, guru ho, gạiko jọnọmlen, guru ho, gạiko jọnọmlen?
Hae hae! tokare dọ ho, guru ho, gạiko busạ̃ṛlen, guru ho, gạiko busạ̃ṛlen?
Hae hae! kạsi ṭạṇḍire, guru ho, gạiko jọnọmlen, guru ho, gạiko jọnọmlen;
Hae hae! kạsi ṭạṇḍire, guru ho, gạiko busạ̃ṛlen, guru ho, gạiko busạ̃ṛlen.

That is,

O dear, dear! All day and all night
The swan pair, o guru, have been bothering.
O dear, dear! for what, o guru, did they bother?
O dear, dear! for the human being, o guru, they bothered.
O dear, dear! on the water-dal, o guru, they are searching for each other, o guru, they are searching for each other.
O dear, dear! on the water-dal, o guru, they are making a nest for themselves, o guru, they are making a nest for themselves.
O dear, dear! on the water-dal, o guru, they are laying eggs, o guru, they are laying eggs.
O dear, dear! on the water-dal, o guru, was the birth of man, o guru, was the birth of man.
O dear, dear! where, o guru, were the cows born, o guru, were the cows born?
O dear, dear! where, o guru, were the cows brought forth, o guru, were the cows brought forth?
O dear, dear! in the kasi grass field, o guru, the cows were born, o guru, the cows were born;

O dear, dear! in the kasi grass field, o guru, the cows were brought forth, o guru, the cows were brought forth.

Hae hae! Tuṛi Pukhuri, guru ho, naṭal baha dọ, guru ho, naṭal baha dọ;
Hae hae! Baha Bandela, guru ho, toa baha ho, guru ho, toa baha ho.

That is,

O dear, dear! at Toṛe Pokhore[1], o guru, is the aṭal flower, o guru, is the aṭal flower;

O dear, dear! at Baha Bandela, o guru, is the milk flower, o guru, is the milk flower.

Hae hae! kạsi ṭạṇḍire kạkiye janamlena re, kạkiye janamlenare;
Hae hae! celem cedaere mãi nam ńẹlledea?
Hae hae! celem cedaere mãi nam cịạledea?
Hae hae! raca jọjọkreń ńẹlledea, guru hoń ńẹlledea;
Hae hae! gurić giḍireń cịạledea, guru hoń cịạledea.

That is,

O dear, dear! in the kasi grass field aunt was born, aunt was born (or, bore);

O dear, dear! what were you doing, o girl, when you saw her?

O dear, dear! what were you doing, o girl, when you discovered her?

O dear, dear! whilst I was sweeping the court-yard, o guru, I saw her, o guru, I saw her;

O dear, dear! whilst I was throwing the cow-dung away I discovered her, o guru, I discovered her.

Hae hae! haṭ bajarre, guru ho, ḍạṅguạ kuṛi, guru ho, ḍạṅguạ kuṛi;
Hae hae! lilạm bajarre, guru ho, chạḍui kuṛi, guru ho, chạḍui kuṛi.
Hae hae! chạḍui kuṛi dọ, guru ho, lumạm lugṛi, guru ho, lumạm lugṛi;
Hae hae! ḍạṅguạ kuṛi dọ, guru ho, lumạm sạṛi ho, guru ho, lumạm sạṛi ho.

That is,

O dear, dear! in the market town, o guru, a maiden, o guru, a maiden;

O dear, dear! in the auction town, o guru, a divorced girl, o guru, a divorced girl.

O dear, dear! the divorced girl, o guru, in silken cloth, o guru, in silken cloth;

O dear, dear! the maiden, o guru, in a silken sari, o guru, in a silken sari.

Dẹntiń, gọ, jạṛi jote! dẹntiń, gọ, kindiri banam!
Hae hae! tọkọe gururen cela dọko nodọńena, lale lal dọ, guru ho, lale lal?
Hae hae! Kạmru gururen cela dọko baherena lale lal dọ, guru ho, lale lal.

That is,

Give me, o mother, the fibre yoke-rope! give me, o mother, the stringed fiddle!

---

[1] Tore Pokhore Baba Bandela is a place mentioned in the Santal traditions, where the ancestors deliberately gave up some old customs and adopted new ones.

O dear, dear! which guru's disciples have come out so red, o guru, so red?
O dear, dear! Kamru guru's disciples have come out in the land so red, o guru, so red.

Hae hae! guru dọ, guru dọ, gẹl bar guru dọko nạcurenare;
Hae hae! cela dọ, cela dọ, gẹl bar cela dọko baherena.
Hae hae! nọdọṅako guru nera basna dak dọ;
Hae hae! belako guru nera pạṭa gaṇḍo dọ.

That is,

O dear, dear! gurus, gurus, twelve gurus turned round;
O dear, dear! disciples, twelve disciples came out.
O dear, dear! the guru's wife will bring a cup of water,
O dear, dear! the guru's wife will place solid stools for them to sit on.

Hae hae! toka disom dāṛākeda, guru ho?
Hae hae! toka disom saṅgarkeda, guru ho?
Hae hae! bhāṇḍ disom dāṛākedaṅ, cela ho,
Hae hae! Tuṛuk disom saṅgarkedaṅ, cela ho.
Hae hae! bhāṇḍ disom dọ, cela ho, bhọ̃ṇḍgea,
Hae hae! cela ho, Tuṛuk disom dọ baṅ bogea.

That is,

O dear, dear! which country did you travel in, o guru?
O dear, dear! which country did you go about in, o guru?
O dear, dear! I travelled in the defiled country, o disciple;
O dear, dear! I went about in the Mogul country, o disciple.
O dear, dear! the defiled country, o disciple, is unclean?
O dear, dear! o disciple, the Mogul country is not good.

Hae hae! toka disomben dāṛākeda,
Jugikin, jugikin na, sat jugikin?
Hae hae! bhāṇḍ disom dāṛākeda,
Jugikin, jugikin na, sat jugikin.
Hae hae! Tuṛuk disomben saṅgarkeda,
Jugikin, jugikin na bunum baraṛiṅ.

That is,

O dear, dear! where did you travel,
You two jugis, two jugis, two trustworthy jugis?
O dear, dear! in the defiled country you travelled
You two jugis, two jugis, two trustworthy jugis.
O dear, dear! in the Mogul country you went about
You two jugis, two jugis, o girl, the giant wasp.

Hae hae! kạsi ṭaṇḍire kạsim gẹlẹlenare, kạsim gẹlẹlenare.
Hae hae! goṛa mutulre bajgọr bahalenare, bajgọr bahalenare.
Hae hae! cetem cekaere kạsim ṅẹlledare, mại na?
Hae hae! raca jọjọkre kạsiṅ ṅẹlledare, kạsiṅ ṅẹlledare.

Hae hae! guric gidire bajgor cialedanre, bajgor cialedanre.
Hae hae! pachia hoeye hoekeda, kasi gele notanenare, guru ho, notanenare;
Hae hae! purua bharndo rakapena, bajgor baha livelenare, guru ho, livelenare.

That is,

O dear, dear! in the kasi grass field you formed ears, o kasi grass, you formed ears, o kasi grass.
O dear, dear! at the cattle-shed gable the bajgor bush blossomed, the bajgor bush blossomed.
O dear, dear! what were you doing when you saw the kasi grass?
O dear, dear! whilst I was sweeping the court-yard I saw the kasi grass, I saw the kasi grass.
O dear, dear! whilst I was throwing the cowdung out I discovered the bajgor, I discovered the bajgor.
O dear, dear! the west wind was blowing, the kasi grass ears were blown away, o guru, were blown away;
O dear, dear! a whirlwind from the east came up, the bajgor blossom drooped, o guru, it drooped.

Purua dak do poroye poroye, pachia dak do halaye halaye,
Gada mundu dak, dai na, hudure hudure.
Hae hae! Logma buru, Ghanta bari cetante
Talse rakapen, guru ho, talse rakapen.

That is,

Rain from the east is drizzling, rain from the west is storming and pouring,
Rivers and jungle full of water, o elder sister, thundering, thundering.
O dear, dear! Over the Logma mountain, the Ghanta bari hill
(The water) dashed up, o guru, dashed up.

Hae hae! delabon, delabon ho jhimbri,
Deste do re, jhimbri, disomte do re!
Hae hae! cete lagil do jhimbri,
Deste do re, jhimbri, deste do re?
Hae hae! cete lagil do jhimbri,
Disomte do, jhimbri, disomte do?
Hae hae! sunume sindur lagit jhimbri
Deste do re, jhimbri, deste do re.
Hae hae! yaenom kajar lagil jhimbri,
Disomte do re, jhimbri, disomte do re.

That is,

O dear, dear! come along, come along, o fish-trap,
Out in the land, o fish-trap, out in the country!
O dear, dear! for what purpose, o fish-trap,
Out in the land, o fish-trap, out in the land?

O dear, dear! for what purpose, o fish-trap,
Out in the country, o fish-trap, out in the country?
O dear, dear! to catch oil and sindur, o fish-trap,
Out in the land, o fish-trap, out in the land.
O dear, dear! to catch eye-paint and lamp-black, o fish-trap,
Out in the country, o fish-trap, out in the country.

Dara hara catọm noṛak kuṛikin na,
Dela sẹ, dela sẹ noḍoṅlenben!
Hae hae! naṭal goṇḍal nataṅ piṇḍạ kuṛikin na,
Dela sẹ, dela sẹ baherlenben!
Hae hae! sona chatar chatarkate
Rupegọr badha, badhakate kuṛikin na,
Dela sẹ, dela sẹ noṇḍoṅlenben,
Dela sẹ, dela sẹ baherlenben!
Hae hae! toka họeye họekeda, sona chatar notaṅenare!
Hae hae! toka bharṇḍoe bharṇḍokeda, rupegọr badha nạpirenare!

That is,

You two girls in the splendid hip-roofed house,
Please come, please come, come out at once!
O dear, dear! you two girls in the large and glorious receiving veranda,
Please come, please come, step out at once!
O dear, dear! shading yourselves with an umbrella of gold,
You two girls with sandals of silver on,
Please come, please come, come out at once,
Please come, please come, step out at once!
O dear, dear! what wind came blowing, the gold umbrella was blown away!
O dear, dear! what whirlwind came whirling, the silver sandals were swooped away!

Siṅ bir dọ lọk kan, Man bir dọ hasa ḍigiren,
Do sẹ, Chitạ, ṅẹl nạgui kũi dak̕ dọ!
Do sẹ, Chitạ, ciạ nạgui ḍạḍi dak̕ dọ!
Ciạ hõṅ ciạkeda kũi dak̕ dọ,
Ṅẹl hõṅ ṅẹlkeda ḍạḍi dak̕ dọ.
Kũi dak̕ dọ pẹrẹć akan, ḍạḍi dak̕ dọ talse rakapen.
Do sẹ, Chitạ, lo nạgui kũi dak̕ dọ,
Do sẹ, Chitạ, bhurạk nạgui ḍạḍi dak̕ dọ,
Siṅ bir laṅ dulak̕, Man bir laṅ nirci nĩṛĩja.

That is,

The Siṅ forest is burning, the Man forest has become dust and ashes,
Do, Chita, go and see what water there is in the well!
Do, Chita, go and find out what water there is in the spring!
I have been and found out about the water in the well,
I have been and seen what water there is in the spring.

The well is full of water, the spring is brimming over with water.
Do, Chita, draw water and fetch it from the well,
Do, Chita, dip your vessel and bring water from the spring,
We two shall pour water on the Siń forest; we two shall sprinkle on the Man forest and extinguish the fire.

Toka birko sendera kan? sisạ ṭamak saḍe kan,
Sakewa dọ huḍure huḍure.
Toka birko kareka kan? sisạ ṭamak saḍe kan,
Sakewa dọ huḍure huḍure.
Siń birko sendera kan, sisạ ṭamak saḍe kan,
Sakewa dọ huḍure huḍure.
Man birko kareka kan, sisạ ṭamak saḍe kan,
Sakewa dọ huḍure huḍure.
Tọkọekoko sendera kan? sisạ ṭamak saḍe kan,
Sakewa dọ huḍure huḍure.
Tọkọekoko kareka kan? sisạ ṭamak saḍe kan,
Sakewa dọ huḍure huḍure.
Mọ̃ṛẽkoko sendera kan, sisạ ṭamak saḍe kan,
Sakewa dọ huḍure huḍure.
Mọ̃ṛẽkoko kareka kan, sisạ ṭamak saḍe kan,
Sakewa dọ huḍure huḍure.

That is,

In which forest are they hunting? the leaden kettle-drum is sounding,
The horn is making a din.
In which forest are they following the chase? The leaden kettle-drum is sounding,
The horn is making a din.
In the Siń forest they are hunting, the leaden kettle-drum is sounding,
The horn is making a din.
In the Man forest they are following the chase, the leaden kettle-drum is sounding,
The horn is making a din.
Who are those who hunt? The leaden kettle-drum is sounding,
The horn is making a din.
Who are those who follow the chase? The leaden kettle-drum is sounding,
The horn is making a din.
The Five (the country side) are hunting, the leaden kettle-drum is sounding,
The horn is sounding.
The Five are following the chase, the leaden kettle-drum is sounding,
The horn is making a din.

Hae hae! nạire ma, guru ho, gãnḍ gạruṛ, guru ho, gãnḍ gạruṛ;
Hae hae! tala Gaṅgare, guru ho, sọnẹr gidi, guru ho, sọnẹr gidi.

Hae hae! nạguwalaṅ dọ, guru ho, sọnẹr gidi, guru ho, sọnẹr gidi;
Hae hae! sẹṭẹrwalaṅ dọ, guru ho, gãṇḍ gạruṛ, guru ho, gãṇḍ gạruṛ.

That is,

O dear, dear! in the river, o guru, is the Adjutant bird,[1] o guru, the Adjutant bird;
O dear, dear! in the middle of the Ganges, o guru, is the king-vulture, o guru, the king-vulture.
O dear, dear! we two, o guru, shall fetch the king-vulture, o guru, the king-vulture;
O dear, dear! we two, o guru, shall bring the Adjutant bird here, o guru, the Adjutant bird.

Nạire dak dọ, kuṛikin, ḍhipre hasa,
Numben na, kuṛikin, naṛkanben.
Kocare ḍubuạ sunum, pakhare kundạr nạkič,
Rọdọk̃ben na, kuṛikin, nạkijok̃ben.
Ḍaṅre cạuričtaben, kocare toa baha,
Suduk̃ben na, kuṛikin, bahak̃ben!

That is,

In the river there is water, you two girls, on the bank there is earth,
Bathe, you two girls, wash your hair.
In the corner there is bottle oil, in the niche there is a hair comb,
Tie up your hair, you two girls, comb yourselves.
On the pole are your plaits of cow's tail hair, in the corner is the milk flower,
Tie your hair in a knot, you two girls, fix a flower there!

Hae hae! dẹsre dọ ho, guru ho, juri jugi dọ, guru ho, juri jugi dọ;
Hae hae! disomre dọ, guru ho, juri banam dọ, guru ho, juri banam dọ.
Hae hae! celem cekaere dọ, juri banam, guru hom ńẹleda ho?
Hae hae! celem cekaere dọ juri jugi, guru hom ciạlelkin?
Hae hae! disom daṛanre dọ, guru hoń ńẹlleda juri banam dọ,
Hae hae! disom saṅgarre dọ guru hoń ciạlelkin juri jugi dọ, guru ho, juri jugi dọ.

That is,

O dear, dear! in the land, o guru, a pair of jugis, o guru, a pair of jugis,
O dear, dear! in the country, o guru, a double fiddle, o guru, a double fiddle.
O dear, dear! what were you doing when you, o guru, saw the double fiddle?
O dear, dear! what were you doing when you, o guru, discovered the pair of jugis?
O dear, dear! whilst going round in the country, o guru, I saw the double fiddle,
O dear, dear! whilst travelling about in the country, o guru, I discovered the pair of jugis, o guru, the pair of jugis.

---

[1] *Gãṇḍ gạruṛ* in Santali generally means rhinoceros; here it is said to be used for the Adjutant bird.

Hae hae! tokare dọ, guru ho, gạiko janamlen, guru ho, gạiko janamlen?
Hae hae! tokare dọ, guru ho, boṅgae nupellen, guru ho, boṅgae nupellen?
Hae hae! kạsi ṭaṇḍire, guru ho, gạiko janamlen, guru ho, gạiko janamlen.
Hae hae! kạsi ṭaṇḍire, guru ho, boṅgae nupellen, guru ho, boṅgae nupellen.
Hae hae! cete lạgit, guru ho, boṅgae nupellen, guru ho?
Hae hae! cete lạgit, guru ho, gạiko janamlen?
Hae hae! sunume sindur lạgit, guru ho, gạiko janamlen, guru ho, gạiko janamlen,
Hae hae! naenọm kajar lạgit, guru ho, boṅgae nupellen, guru ho, boṅgae nupellen

That is,

O dear, dear! where, o guru, were the cows born, o guru, the cows born?
O dear, dear! where, o guru, did the bonga appear, o guru, did the bonga appear?
O dear, dear! in the kasi grass field, o guru, were the cows born, o guru, were the cows born.
O dear, dear! in the kasi grass field, o guru, the bonga showed himself, o guru, the bonga showed himself.
O dear, dear! for what purpose, o guru, did the bonga appear, o guru?
O dear, dear! for what purpose, o guru, were the cows born?
O dear, dear! to get oil and sindur, o guru, the cows were born, o guru, the cows were born,
O dear, dear! to get eye-paint and lamp-black, o guru, the bonga appeared, o guru, the bonga appeared.

Disom daṛanre dọ, Kạmru guru, nam baṛẹ lahakme,
Nale dọ họe jivi, hasa họṛmọ hoetele bindạṛok, nam baṛẹ bereťkalem!

That is,

When we walk about in the country, o Kamru guru, please you go in front.
We are souls of air, when our body of earth will by the air fall to the ground, you please put us on our feet.

Nape purub khon, guru ho, nale pạchim khon, guru ho,
Maj kulire, gurulaṅ, gurulaṅ nāṛgo ńapamen.
Bọhọkretam, guru ho, ṭoya dhaca,
Tarenretam, guru ho, lal gamcha.
Johạri, guru ho, johạri,
Johạri, guru ho, dẹ laṅ johara.

That is,

You coming from the east, o guru, we coming from the west, o guru,
In the middle of the village street, we two, o guru, we two, o guru, came down and met.
On your head, o guru, you have a plume of blue jay feathers,
On your shoulder, o guru, a red strip of cloth.
Greeting, o guru, greeting,
Greeting, o guru, come let us salute each other!

Hae hae! cetane disom dọ, guru ho, nalom calak ho, guru ho; nalom calak;
Hae hae! latare disom dọ, guru ho, nalom sẹṭẹrok, guru ho, nalom sẹṭẹrok.
Hae hae! nạsul miru leka, guruko sikṛi dọhọkem,
Hae hae! nạsul kare leka, guruko biṛi dọhọkem.

That is,

O dear, dear! to the up-country, o guru, don't go, o guru, do not go;
O dear, dear! in the low-country, o guru, do not arrive, o guru, do not arrive.
O dear, dear! like a kept parakeet they might chain and keep you, o guru,
O dear, dear! like a kept maina, o guru, they might fetter and keep you.

Except in a very few places no remarks of any kind have been made to explain the above quoted songs; they must speak for themselves and show what is in the minds of the Santals when they are out for *Dasãe daṛan*. Some of the songs recorded show reference to countries in which the ancestors of the present-day Santals have, according to their own traditions, at some time been living, and to events that happened in those countries, now only indistinctly remembered, that may, or may not, have had some connection with the predecessors of the *ojhas*. It is with our present knowledge not possible to do more than guess at the possible time of the events referred to. Likely they are not less than three to four hundred years old, perhaps more.

Others of the songs refer to the present time, partly in veiled language, and others again to the doings of the *Dasãe koṛa* themselves. It might be noted, that there generally is no direct begging in any of the Santali songs. Most of the songs refer to matters that ordinarily seem to have a very small place in the Santal mind.

There are, of course, other *Dasãe* songs than those here cited. It will be observed, that the Santals do not make use of rhyme, and to make the words scan smoothly they very frequently introduce a vowel, not used in ordinary language, omit something, or add a *re* not otherwise heard. I have reproduced so many verses, because they are of some interest to the student of the language.

8.

Mantar *and* Jhaṛni.

The 'medicinal' side of the *ojha*'s work has been mentioned elsewhere. Previous to giving medicine the *ojha* will generally try the effect of his various *mantar* and *jhaṛni*, which are supposed to be able to drive all evils away by their inherent magic powers. That these never are efficacious apparently do not prevent their use. So long as they believe, or anyhow their patients have any belief in them, there is, to them, always the possibility of their working power. Even if they do not have any visible effect, it may be thought advisable to resort to them to keep on the safe side with the spirits.

Below will be given specimens of the different *mantar* and *jhaṛni*. As elsewhere mentioned the *jhaṛni* is not spoken, but sung to special melodies (see p. 14).

According to Santal ideas there is a natural enmity between an *ojha* and the witches. The *ojha* tries to undo the evil work of the witches, and these will naturally attempt to hinder the *ojha* in doing his work; he must consequently also guard himself against the possible sorceries of the witches, and naturally against all inimical and malevolent powers.

When the *ojha guru* opens his course of instruction one of his first acts is to secure his course and his disciples against the dangers mentioned (see p. 47) and to take measures to protect his disciples when they go and come (see p. 50).

Here is a *mantar* which the disciples are taught to use to protect themselves:

Tel tuṛi rại sursạ, cul culte cul bandhọn, mul multe mul bandhọn, ghicạ calte ghicạ bandhọn, chạti calte chạti bandhọn, pañjra calte pañjra bandhọn, ḍaṇḍa calte ḍaṇḍa bandhọn, cuke calte cuke bandhọn, jaṅgu calte jaṅga bandhọn, ṭhemna calte ṭhemna bandhọn, supti calte supti bandhọn; kẹ bandhẹ? Guru bandhẹ, guru gean, mae bandhẹ, bandhẹ siri Kạhri gean, Kạmru dohae bandhẹ.

That is translated something like this: Oil *tuṛi, rại, sursạ* (different kinds of mustard from which oil is pressed). When applied to the hair, the hairto be charmed; when applied to the head, the head to be charmed; when applied to the neck, the neck to be charmed; when applied to the chest, the chest to be charmed; when applied to the ribs, the ribs to be charmed; when applied to the loins, the loins to be charmed; when applied to the eyes, the eyes to be charmed; when applied to the thighs, the thighs to be charmed; when applied to the knees, the knees to be charmed; when applied to the feet, the feet to be charmed; who charms? The *guru* charms, by the *guru*'s knowledge; the Mother charms, charms by the knowledge of *Kạhri* (or: charms by knowing the propitious wording), charms by the grace of Kamru.

Any of the oils mentioned is supposed to be applied at the time.

When an *ojha* goes on a professional visit, he will to protect himself use the same *mantar* as that cited p. 50. When passing through a forest with dangerous animals he may use the following:

Hare bagha, muṛ cọlte muṛ bandhọn, dãt cọlte dãt bandhọn, gola cọlte gola bandhọn, chạti cọlte chạti bandhọn, dāṛā cọlte dāṛā bandhọn, jạṅghi cọlte jạṅghi bandhọn, guṇṭhi cọlte guṇṭhi bandhọn, ṭena cọlte ṭena bandhọn, suptiċ cọlte suptiċ bandhọn, roa cọlte roa bandhọn; kẹ bandhẹ? Guru bandhẹ, Kạmru guru dohae bandhẹ.

Translated: O tiger (or, leopard,) when moving the head, the head to be charmed; when moving the teeth, the teeth to be charmed; when moving the throat, the throat to be charmed; when moving the chest, the chest to be charmed; when moving the loins, the loins to be charmed; when moving the thighs, the thighs to be charmed; when moving the knees, the knees to be charmed; when moving the legs, the legs to be charmed; when moving the feet, the feet to be charmed; when the hair is moving, the hair to be charmed; who charms? The *guru* charms, by the grace of Kamru *guru* he charms.

When he has pronounced this *mantar*, the tiger will sit quiet without moving.

If he should meet any one who looks threatening, the following is effective; the *ojha* takes up some dust and scatters this in front of him towards the person coming; at the same time he says: *Are Hindu Musạlman, na kaṛes, amko dekhia, mukhe dekhia hạsi uthe!*

That is, O Hindu, Musalman, don't abuse, seeing me looking at my face may you feel inclined to laugh.

The witches are believed to be able to hit people in the following way: they take a small stone or (preferably) a small bit of charcoal and blow this out from the mouth towards the person to be hit; if nothing is done to counteract the 'shot', the person 'hit' in this way will fall down in a swoon, anyhow become suddenly ill (it is one form of what they call *ban pạthri*). The following *mantar* is used; *Dẹsẹ pọrọb dekhle jabe, ḍhelka mạṭi uṭhại libo, poṛhae dibo*; *kise libo? Kopale chạtiye ar guru gun cale, se gun kạṭia amar gun lạgiạ jae.*

Translated: She will go and see the festival of the country; I shall pick up a clot of earth; I shall 'read over' it and give it; what shall I receive it in? In the forehead, in the breast, another *guru* uses magic; doing away with that sorcery I shall use my own magic.

The above is supposed to be an effective guard.

If any one is supposed to have been 'hit' the following is used: *Pạthri ke pạthri udạilọm, band ke band udạilọm*; *kẹ udạilọm? Guru udạilọm, dohae Kạmru guru!*

That is, I sent spell after spell flying, I sent charm after charm flying; whom did I send flying? I sent the *guru* flying, grace, o Kamru *guru*!

Whereupon the *ojha* blows over the patient. Thereupon medicine.

When children are crying without apparent cause, or when they suffer from a peculiar form of vomiting and diarrhoea, they are supposed to have been exposed to what is called *aha*, the effect of the evil eye. The following *mantar* is used:

Kạndni gẹlọ, nidạni ạilo, kọtọ khọn kande he? Hạṭ kandoni, baṭ kandoni, chạlụ kandoni; i kandoni kẹ phukẹ? Guru phukẹ, guru gean, mae phukẹ, phukẹ siri Kạhri gean, Kạmru dohae phukẹ.

That is, Cryer went, sleepy came, how long is it crying? Market crying, road crying, child crying; this cryer who blows away? The *guru* blows away, by the *guru*'s knowledge; the Mother blows away, blows away by the knowledge of Sri Kahri, by the grace of Kamru he blows away.

Finished off with blowing.

Mantar against headache:

Matha piṛạ kẹ phukẹ? Guru gean, mae phukẹ, phukại, siri Kạhri gean, Kạmru dohae phukẹ, chuṭiạ ja.

That is, Headache who blows away? By the *guru*'s knowledge, the Mother blows away; causes to blow away by the knowledge of Sri Kahri, by the grace of Kamru he blows away, get away!

Finished with blowing.

Against *aha* (another):

Purub pạchim utọr dạkhin cạr kọ̃ṇḍ cạr poa mạṭi bandhọn; dọs bhại nọñjọr bandhọn, hã kọrile mukhe nakha, Dibi Durgạ Sitạ Bhọrọt dohae.

That is, East, West, North, South, the four corners, the four quarters, to be charmed; the ten brothers' view to be charmed; if you gape (I shall give it you) in your mouth, in your nose, by the grace of Dibi, Durga, Sita and Bhorot.

The *ojha* blows and performs *bulạu* (see, p. 26) with the kernel of *sọsọ* (Semecarpus anacardium) and a bit of a broom.

Against *mẽt haso* (lit. eye pain) the following is used: the patient is in the evening after dark taken out and told to look at the stars; the ojha takes a garlic in his mouth and blowing into the eyes of the patient three or five times he utters the following *mantar: Cọk uṭhe; i cọk kakhe uthe? phalna kẹ phạlni kẹ, i cọk kẹ phukẹ? Guru phukẹ, guru gean, mae phukẹ, phukại siri Kạhri gean, Kạmru dohae, siri dohae phukẹ.*

That is. The eye pains; who causes this eye-ache? So and so (man), so and so (woman), this eye-ache who blows away? The *guru* blows away by the *guru*'s knowledge, the Mother blows away, causes to blow away, by the knowledge of Sri Kahri, by the grace of Kamru, by luck, by grace, he blows away.

After having got his eyes blown into, the patient is to go straight in without looking anywhere.

The following is another against the same:

Cọk cọk, i cọk na dukhẹ, na phulẹ; kẹ phukẹ? Guru phukẹ, guru gean, mae phukẹ, phukại siri Kạhri gean, Kạmru dohae phukẹ.

That is, Eye, eye, this eye does not pain, does not swell; who blows away? The *guru* blows away, by the guru's knowledge; the Mother blows away, causes to blow away, etc. (as above.)

Against pain anywhere in the body (here called *betha*, a name ordinarily used about pneumonia, pleurisy and intercostal rheumatism) the following *mantar* is used: *Betha betha, muṇḍer betha. dãter betha, kokhar betha, pañjar betha, ḍaṇḍar betha, i·bethar bis kẹ jhaṛẹ? Guru jhaṛẹ, guru gean, mae jhaṛẹ, jhaṛae siri Kạhri gean, Kạmru dohae jhaṛẹ.*

That is, Pain pain, headache, toothache, pain in the side, pain in the ribs, pain in the loins, who lays this pain? The *guru* lays it by the *guru*'s knowledge, the Mother lays it, etc. (as above).

Then follows the *jhaṛ*, the laying or exorcising of the pain through passing the left hand, in which he has a peacock feather, as previously described, from the head downwards, and singing the following *jhạṛni: Bethagọr betha, muṇḍer betha, bethagọr betha, dãter betha, bethagọr betha, kokhar betha, bethagọr betha, ḍaṇḍar betha, bis jhaṛọñre; kọner guru hamar jhaṛae to jhaṛae? kọner cela hamar jhaṛa sere bis dọ? muṇḍer betha, dãter betha, kokhar betha, pañjar betha, ḍaṇḍar betha bis jhaṛọñre.*

That is, The pain causing pain, the headache, the pain causing pain, the toothache, the pain causing pain, the pain in the side, the pain causing pain, the pain in the lions, to stroke the poison; which *guru* by his stroking causes me to stroke? which disciple strokes the poison down in me? Headache, toothache, pain in the side, pain in the ribs, pain in the loins, the poison— stroke it out.

The above which is in a corrupt form of Bihari is immediately followed by the following in Santali: *Delañ betha; oḍokokme, delañ betha, baherokme, gọrọmlañ dọe okta kana, hiromlañ dọe cintạ kana; delañ betha, oḍokokme, delañ betha, baherokme!*

That is, Come, o pain, come out, come, o pain, get out, our (inclusive dual is used) namesake is speaking evil, our co-wife is backbiting; come, o pain, come out, come, o pain, get out!

If this does not help, medicine is to be applied invoking the boṅgas; *bul māyām* is to be resorted to.

The following is another *mantar* for the same: *Betha betha, golar betha, chạtir betha, pañjar betha, hũk betha, suk betha, bhitri betha, boṅga betha, i betha kẹ jhaṛẹ? Guru jhaṛẹ, guru gean, mae jhaṛẹ, jhaṛẹ siri Kạhri gean, Kạmru dohae jhaṛẹ.*

That is, Pain pain, throat pain, chest pain, rib pain, lumbago pain, gradually developed pain, inside pain, boṅga-pain, who is stroking this pain out? The *guru* is stroking it out, by the *guru*'s knowledge, the Mother is stroking it out, stroking, etc. (as previously).

The *jhaṛni* then follows: *Betha dọ jhaṛ se, Kạmru guru kera betha dọe jhaṛa, Kạmru cela kera betha dọe nija, betha dọ jhaṛ se, Ḍanḍo guru kera betha dọe jhaṛa, Ḍanḍo cela kera betha dọe nija se bis dọ.*

That is, The pain to be stroked out, Kamru *guru* will stroke the caused pain out, Kamru's disciple will take the caused pain; the pain to be stroked out; Ḍanḍo *guru* will stroke the caused pain out, Ḍanḍo's disciple will take the caused pain, the poison.

The following is a third *mantar*, showing what an *ojha* may include under the name of *betha: Betha betha, ceṅgha betha, ḍọṇḍ bại, palaniạ adgao, gola biṛhi sunorio, i betha kẹ jhaṛẹ? Guru jhaṛẹ, guru gean, dohae Kạmru guru!*

That is, Pain pain, colic convulsion, convulsion by strangulation of intestines, carbuncle on the back, sores in the throat, inflammation of the gums, who strokes this pain away? The *guru* strokes by the *guru*'s knowledge, by the grace of Kamru *guru*.

This is finished off with blowing over the patient and the following *jhaṛni*: *Yọrẹ yọrẹ betha, muṇḍạ jo betha jhaṛea nāṛgoea, sirome jọṅkte jhaṛea nāṛgoea, saparọm jọṅkte giragọr baher.*

That is, Hey there, hey there, o pain, where pain in the head it is stroked out, brought down, with a *sirom* broom it is stroked out, brought down, with a *saparọm* broom it is swept out and away.

Against colic the following *mantar* is used: *Nun nun, purub nun, pạchim nun, utọr nun, dạkhin nun, i nun kẹ poṛhae? Guru poṛhẹ, i nun kakhe dei? Phalnarẹ, phạlni; kẹ piṛạ pẹṭ tambhẹ? Jivi chaṭ paṭ jivi tambhẹ? Guru tambhẹ, tambhae siri Kạhri gean Kạmru dohae, guru dohae tambhẹ.*

That is, Salt salt, east salt, west salt, north salt, south salt, who causes to read over this salt? The *guru* reads; to whom shall I give this salt? So-and-so (man), so-and-so (female); who is making the stomach ache to cease? The soul is restless, who is making it quiet? The *guru* is making it quiet; causing it to be quiet, etc. (as previously).

This was a *mantar* to make the salt effective, in a corrupt and mixed form of Bihari. Then comes immediately another *mantar* to make the water in which the salt is dissolved safe. It runs thus: *Pạni pạni, purub pạni, pạchim pạni, utọr pạni, dakhin pạni, i pạni kẹ poṛhae? Guru poṛhẹ, guru gean, mae poṛhẹ, poṛhae siri Kạhri gean, Kạmru dohae pọṛhẹ.*

That is, Water water, east water, west water, north water, south water, who causes to read over this water? The *guru* reads by the *guru*'s knowledge; the Mother reads, causes to read, etc. (as previously).

The salt is during this dissolved in the water and the patient drinks it all without breathing.

When a woman's breast suppurates, the following is used: *Dud dud, i dud, ghoṛa aṅgarea goborea, i dud, kẹ jhaṛẹ? Guru jhaṛẹ, guru gean, mae jhaṛẹ, jhaṛẹ siri Kạhri gean, Kạmru guru dohae.*

That is, Milk milk, this milk, red and black, dark, this milk who strokes it away? The *guru* strokes, by the *guru*'s knowledge; the Mother strokes, strokes, etc. (as previously).

(The translation of three words is uncertain, *viz.*, *ghoṛa aṅgarea goborea*, not known to any Santal I have met; it is also a question whether the Santals do not here take *dud* to be equivalent to 'breast' like in their own language, where they have same word for milk and a woman's *mamma.*)

The *mantar* is followed by this *jhạṛni: Dudegọr dude, delaṅ, dude, oḍoṅokme; delaṅ, dude, baherokme. Dudegọr dude, sẹṅgẹl dude, rupegọr dude, gọṛọmlaṅ dọe okta kana, hiromlaṅ dọe cintạ kana; delaṅ, dude, oḍokokme, delaṅ, dude, baherokme, bis!*

That is, Milk of milk, come, o milk, come out; come, o milk, get out. Milk of milk, fire milk, silver milk, our (inclusive dual is used) namesake is speaking evil, our co-wife is backbiting; come, o milk, come out, come, o milk, get out, the poison!

They call a certain complaint *sagak* (the word really means the awned seed of certain grasses, very troublesome at the time of ripening, because they stick and prick the skin; as a name for a complaint it is used about fever supposed to be due to the presence in the body of any small foreign body); against this they use the following *mantar: Ạpcul karọn, kaṅgari karọn kẹ kukarẹ? Guru kukarẹ, kukạrlom ekṭhene guṭi ạilom, bạhrạre upọr ho.*

That is, What is caused by hair, what is caused by charcoal who rubs? The *guru* rubs; I rubbed it, I brought it together at one place, get up to the surface. (Above is a good specimen of how a foreign language may be made to serve, being misunderstood, the words being partly remoulded and given a meaning corresponding to the meaning of a Santali word similar in sound).

After the *mantar* comes a *jhạṛni: Lunḍano, lunḍano abe bisa lunḍ lalare.* (I rubbed, I rubbed, now the poison is brought here by rubbing.)

During the operation two *boṅgas* (*saket*) are also invoked. It might be mentioned, that what is translated 'rub' (in Santali *lunḍạn* or *lunḍạu*) is to rub gently with a circular motion, sometimes making use of a ball of rice, flour or other stuff to make the rubbing more effective.

Another *mantar* for the same complaint is the following: *Gaḍa gaḍa bag jae, nice nice siạl jae, se bag roa, se bhạluk roa, se bilar roa, se kukur roa, se mạnus roa, i roar bis kẹ jhaṛẹ? Guru jhaṛẹ, guru gean, mae jhaṛẹ, jhaṛac siri Kạhri gean, dohae guru jhaṛae.*

That is, The leopard (or tiger) is walking along in the river bed, below the jackal is going along, this leopard's hair, this bear's hair, this cat's hair, this dog's hair, this human hair,—the poison of that hair who strokes it away? The *guru* strokes, by the *guru*'s knowledge; the Mother strokes, causes to stroke by the knowledge of Sr Kahri, causes to stroke by the *guru*'s grace.

Then the *jhaṛni: Koṇeṛ raṇḍini, koṇeṛ pạpini, bisa tora dilạise? yabe bisạ bis jhaṛoṅre.*

That is, Which widow, which sinning woman caused to give you the poison ? now the poison, stroke the poison away.

The *jhaṛni* is continued in Santali: *Cetete dọ, gurulaṅ jhaṛe noḍoṅa? Cetete dọ, celalaṅ girom bahera? Saparọm jọnọkte, gurulaṅ jhaṛe noḍoṅa, lukui jọnọkte dọ, celalaṅ girom bahera.*

That is, Wherewith, o *guru*, shall we two stroke it away ? Wherewith, o disciple, shall we two sweep it out ? With a *sirom* broom, o *guru*, we two shall stroke it away; with a *lukui* broom, o disciple, we two shall sweep it out.

The following is a third specimen against the same: first the *mantar: Jạmbir jạmbir, sọnẹk jạmbir, rupẹk jạmbir, i jạmbir kẹ jhaṛẹ? Guru jhaṛẹ, Kạmru guru dohae.*

That is, Citron citron, golden citron, silver citron, this citron who strokes it away ? the *guru* strokes, by the grace of Kamru *guru*.

Whilst uttering this *mantar* the *ojha* strokes the patient, applying at the same time some oil, over which a *mantar* has been previously 'read.' It is the same as the '*tel tel, rae tel*', etc., (see p. 18) uttered when performing *sunum boṅga* (see also p. 16 ss.).

When the poison in this way has been gathered at one place, the *ojha* bites it out with his teeth; he draws blood; what he in this way gradually (biting several times) gets out he spits into a leaf-cup. Into this he pours a little water and takes it away some distance to see what has come out, whereupon he throws it away.

Against *hũk* (lumbago) and similar complaints they use this *mantar: Hũk, ḍanḍar hũk, kokhar hũk, paṅjar hũk, i hũk kẹ jhaṛẹ? Guru jhaṛẹ, guru gean, mae jhaṛẹ, jhaṛae siri Kạhri gean, Kạmru dohae jhaṛẹ.*

That is, Lumbago, pain in the loins, pain in the side, pain in the ribs, this lumbago who strokes away? The *guru* strokes, by the *guru*'s knowledge, the Mother strokes, causes to stroke, etc. (as previously).

And then the following *jhaṛni: Hũk jhaṛọṅ, betha jhaṛọṅ, kọnẹr guru hamar jhaṛae tho jhaṛae? kọnẹr cela hamar jhaṛae sẹrẹ bis dọ.*

That is, Stroking away the lumbago, stroking away the pain, which *guru* is causing to stroke away for me, causing to stroke away ? which disciple is causing to stroke the poison away for me ?

Against fever (malaria and others) the following *mantar* is used: *Lag jọr, pap jọr, i jọr kẹ phukẹ? Guru phukẹ, guru gean, mae phukẹ, phukẹ siri Kạhri gean, Kạmru dohae phukẹ.*

That is, Fever applied (*i.e.*, due to the action of witches or *boṅga*), fever due to sin (*i.e.*, venereal), this fever who is blowing off ? The *guru* blows it off, by the *guru*'s knowledge, the Mother blows it off, blows, etc. (as previously).

A variant of above is the following: *Lag jọr, pap jọr, amọl jọr, piti jọr, deṛ pọhọriạ jor, i jor kẹ* etc., as above. That is: Fever applied, fever due to sin, fever due to acidity of the stomach, fever due to gall, six hours' fever, this fever, etc., as above.

The following is a *mantar* against high fever: *Taṛka taṛka, kaṭ kaṭe, maṭ maṭe, akaṛ bindi, bhurme phuṭẹ, bap bir Nạrsiṅ guru dohạe; jhiṭi kuṭi ḍheba band, ạsia guru dhọrọmiạ kaj jug bijun nijhur, thak thak jib rak Kạmru guru dohae.*

That is, Quick, rat-tat, gnashing, crooked, piercing, giddy, broken, o father man of valour, Narsiṅ *guru*, grace! Taking all along, shutting up, having come, by the *guru*'s righteousness, doing work without hindrance, be quiet, keep the soul, by the grace of Kamru *guru*.

Finished off with blowing.

Language is corrupt and mixed.

A number of complaints are called *bại*; generally some kind of convulsions, loss of control of the body, fit, etc.

The following is a *mantar* against *bại*: *Bại bại, sonẹk bại, rupẹk bại, i bại kẹ jhaṛẹ? Guru jhaṛẹ, guru gean, mae jhaṛẹ, jhaṛẹ siri Kạhri gean, Kạmru dohae jhaṛẹ.*

That is, Convulsions convulsions, gold convulsions, silver convulsions, these convulsions who strokes away? The *guru* strokes, by the *guru*'s knowledge, the Mother strokes, strokes, etc. (as previously).

The following is another; the *ojha* first 'reads over' mustard, *Hal dhorlom tae bonlom sursạ, i sursạ kẹ pọṛhẹ? Guru pọṛhẹ, guru gean, mae pọṛhẹ, Isor Mahadeb dohae pọṛhẹ.*

That is, I caught hold of the plough, I sowed the mustard seed, who reads over this mustard seed? The *guru* reads, by the *guru*'s knowledge; the Mother reads, by the grace of the Lord Mahadeb he reads.

The *ojha* thereupon scatters the mustard seed over the patient, uttering the following *mantar*: *Sursạ sursạ siri sursạ, sursạ phule jabọ loṅka ghurbạ toke jhaṛ guru re bis.*

That is, Mustard mustard, fine mustard, I shall go to fetch the mustard flower very far away, I shall bring it back to you, o *guru*, stroke the poison away.

This is a third for the same (*mantar*): *Bại bại, rọs bại, amọl bại, kheptọ bại, i bại ke jhaṛẹ? Kạmru dohae jhaṛẹ.*

That is, Convulsions convulsions, convulsions due to the juices of the body, convulsions due to acidity, raging convulsions, these convulsions who strokes away? By the grace of Kamru he strokes away.

Whereupon the following *jhaṛni*: *Yọrẹ yọrẹ bại dọ munḍe jọ bại dọ sirome jọnọkte jhaṛea nāṛgoea, saparọm jọnọkte giṛạgọr bahera; Kạmru guru jhajaṛ kanae, Gaṇḍo guru dọe giṛạgọr baherela.*

That is, Hey, hey! o convulsions, what convulsions are in the head, with a *sirom* broom he is stroking and bringing it down, with a *saparọm* broom he is sweeping it out; Kamru *guru* is stroking, Gaṇḍo *guru* is sweeping it out.

Finished off by blowing over the patient.

Against *ḍọṇḍ bại* (strangulation of the intestines) the following *mantar* is used: *Ceṅgha jhaṛọṅ, paṭha jhaṛọṅ, i bis kẹ jhaṛẹ? Guru jhaṛẹ, guru gean, mae jhaṛẹ, jhaṛae siri Kạhri gean, Kạmru dohae jhaṛẹ.*

That is, Stroking the colic, stroking the swelling, who is stroking away this poison? The *guru* is stroking, by the *guru's* knowledge; the Mother is stroking, causes to stroke, etc. (as previously).

Followed by the following *jhaṛni: Hatkan jharoṅ, palania jharoṅ, ceṅgha jharoṅ, patha jharoṅ jharre bis.*

That is, *Hatkan* (a medicinal plant, Leea) stroking, stroking the sore on the back, stroking for colic, stroking for swelling, stroking stroke the poison out.

Against *gaṇḍ* (swelling of a gland, specially in the loins) the following *mantar* is used: *Kōṇḍ kōṇḍ, agil kōṇḍ, pachim kōṇḍ, i kōṇḍer bis kẹ jharẹ? Guru jharẹ, guru gean, mae jharẹ, jharae siri Kahri gean, Kamru dohae jharẹ.*

That is, Region region, front region, west region, who is stroking the poison of this region away? The *guru* strokes, by the *guru's* knowledge, the Mother strokes, causes to stroke, etc. (as previously).

Against a cut by a sickle the following *mantar* is used: *Hāsua katel ghao jiri hiri rokotẹ porẹ, jiri hiri pani porẹ, i rokot kẹ phukẹ? Guru phukẹ, guru gean, mae phukẹ, phukai siri Kahri gean, Kamru dohae phukẹ.*

That is, Wound by the cut of a sickle, blood is trickling flowing, water is trickling flowing, who is blowing at this blood? The *guru* blows, by the *guru's* knowledge, the Mother blows, causes to blow, etc. (as previously).

Against a wound caused by stumbling against anything they have the following *mantar*: *Pathol katlom, ghao jiri hiri rokot porẹ, i rokot kẹ phukẹ? Guru phukẹ, guru gean, mae phukẹ, phukai siri Kahri gean, Kamru dohae phukẹ.*

That is, Stumbling I cut myself and got a wound, the blood is trickling flowing; this blood who is blowing at it? The *guru* blows by the *guru's* knowledge, the Mother blows, causes to blow, etc. (as previously).

Then follows a *jhaṛni*: *Rokotẹ jhaṅja kal, rokotẹ bohae jhaṅja kal.*

That is, The blood is flowing the whole time, the blood is flowing the whole time gushing.

The following is a *mantar* against a cut by any kind of implement: *Taṅgate bajilom, jiri hiri rokot bohae, se rokot kẹ tambhẹ? Guru tambhẹ, guru gean, mae tambhẹ, tambhae siri Kahri gean, Kamru dohae tambhẹ.*

That is, I hurt myself on an axe (or, as the case may be, by a knife or any other instrument, which is named in the *mantar*), the blood is trickling flowing, who stops this blood? The *guru* stops by the *guru's* knowledge, the Mother stops, causes to stop, etc. (as previously).

Followed by this *jhaṛni*: *Taṅgate bajilom, jiri hiri rokotẹ bohae, phukite phukite yanda kale, Kamru guru, se rokot tambhiloma ṙe bis.*

That is, I hurt myself on an axe, the blood is trickling flowing, blowing blowing loudly, o Kamru *guru*, I stopped that blood, poison.

Against sores caused by *soso* (Semecarpus anacardium) they have also a *mantar*: *Bhel bhelwa bhelar mukhi se bhelwa porlo, i bhelwar ghao kẹ phukẹ? Guru phukẹ, guru gean, mae phukẹ, phukai siri Kahri gean, Kamru dohae phukẹ.*

That is, The marking nut, the opening of the marking nut, that marking nut touched, the sore of that marking nut who is blowing at it? The *guru* is blowing by the knowledge of the *guru*, the Mother blows, causes to blow knowing the fortunate wording (or as translated above), by the grace of Kamru he blows.

Against the bite of a mad dog or jackal they use the following *mantar*: *Kạri kukur kulu ḍulu, e kukur dãt, e kukur bis, e bis kẹ jhaṛẹ? Guru jhaṛẹ, guru gean, Mae jhaṛẹ, siri Kạhri gean, Kạmru dohae jhaṛẹ.*

That is, The black bitch hanging the head, the tooth of this bitch, the poison of this bitch who is stroking it away? The *guru* strokes by the *guru's* knowledge, the Mother strokes, causes to stroke, knowing the fortunate wording (or as translated above), by the grace of Kamru he strokes.

Followed by this *jhạṛni*: *Kukur kaṭa Maesa jhaṛọñ, jhaṛre bisại nindạñ jhaṛọñ.*

That is, The bite of the bitch Monsa is stroking, stroke away the poison, she is stroking the lying one.

If the poison has entered the body, that is, if rabies has developed, the following *mantar* is used: *Gaḍa gaḍa bag jae, nico nico suạr jae, i bag roa, bhạluk roa, i cul kẹ guṭại? Guru guṭại, guṭại siri Kạhri gean, Kạmru dohae guṭia.*

That is, In the river bed the tiger (or leopard) walks along, below the boar walks, this tiger-hair, this bear-hair, this hair who collects? The *guru* causes to collect (in one place), causes to collect knowing the fortunate wording (or as above translated), by the grace of Kamru he collects.

Against dog's bite the following is used: *Are kukur kara kara, tọkọr dãt, tọkọr bis kẹ jhaṛẹ? Guru jhaṛẹ, guru gean, mae jhaṛẹ, Isor Mahadeb dohae jhaṛẹ.*

That is, O thou black black dog, thy teeth, thy poison who strokes away? The *guru* strokes by the *guru*'s knowledge, the Mother strokes, by the grace of the Lord Mahadeb (Siva) he strokes away.

Followed by this *jhạṛni*: *Seta banaṛ se ho, seta banaṛ se ho ṭunḍạñ kan, bando banaṛ se ho, bando banaṛ seko gujuk kan. Tọkọe guru dọ rẹ jhaṛẹ nãṛgoea, tọkọe guru dọre jhạṛni bahera? Kạmru guru dọye jhaṛẹ nãṛgoea. Kạmru cela dọye jhạṛni bahera, kar dohae? Isor Mahadeb dohae!*

That is, The dog vermin (some ant-like insects or larvæ believed to come out after being bitten by a mad dog), the dog vermin moves about; the *bando*-flower like vermin, the *bando*-flower like vermin is dying. Which *guru* will stroke this down? Which *guru* will pass this out and away? Kamru *guru* will stroke it down, Kamru's disciple will pass it out and away, by whose grace? By the Lord Mahadeb (Siva's) grace.

Against the bite of a chameleon they have the following *mantar*: *Girgiṭi sãp, i bis kẹ jhaṛẹ? Guru jhaṛẹ, guru gean, mae jhaṛẹ, jhaṛẹ siri Kạhri gean, Kạmru dohae jhaṛẹ.*

That is, The chameleon (or, lizard) snake, this snake, this poison who strokes away? The *guru*, etc. (as above).

Followed by a *jhạṛni*: *Sirkuṭ khaele, girgiṭi gulman khaele, kal bisa, hạrio, dada, sọnẹrọ bis dọ hạru harare kãs piṭạrer bis.*

That is, The scolopender ate, the chameleon ate by mistake the poisonous vermin; take it away, o elder brother, the extremely dangerous poison, o Hari, the many coloured lizard's poison.

The following is a *mantar* against being hurt by the sting of a scorpion: *Bichi bichi, khulir bichi, ṛaṅglir bichi, e bicher bis kẹ jhaṛẹ? Guru jhaṛẹ, guru gean, mae jhaṛẹ, jhaṛae siri Kạhri gean, Kạmru dohae jhaṛẹ.*

That is, Scorpion scorpion, light coloured scorpion, reddish scorpion, this scorpion's poison who strokes away? The *guru*, etc., as above.

The following is a variant: *Bichi bichi, kuili bichi rạmbṛu bichi tọkọr dãt, tọkọr bis kẹ jhaṛẹ? Guru jhaṛẹ, guru gean, mae jhaṛẹ: kar dohae? Ma Monsa Dibir dohae.*

That is, Scorpion scorpion, black scorpion, brownish scorpion, this one's tooth, this one's poison who strokes away? The *guru* strokes, by the *guru's* knowledge, the Mother strokes, by whose grace? by the grace of the Mother Monsa Dibi.

Against the bite of *Kul sereñ*, a lizard so called, the following *mantar*: *Kul ḍạṇḍkạ dhuruṅ dhusuṅ, gache uṭhlo, sarage dhũã dekhele nam namre bis; e bis kẹ jhaṛẹ? Guru jhaṛẹ, guru gean, mae jhaṛẹ, jhaṛae siri Kạhri gean, Kạmru guru dohae jhaṛẹ.*

That is, Leopard mite, grey with dust, he mounted the tree; seeing the smoke in the sky come down, o poison; who strokes this poison? The *guru* strokes, etc., as previously.

We shall now hear some of their *mantars*, etc., against snake bite; it may be noted that the Santals believe practically all snakes to be poisonous. They believe that the bite of a good many lizards, of some frogs and similar animals is also poisonous; and less than a bite is enough to be hurt; being touched is often sufficient, according to their belief. I suppose much which is believed due to poison is really due to fear, although the Santals as a general rule take a sensible view of matters; I have, however, seen cases bordering on collapse that were entirely due to fear.

In connection with snake bite *mantars* are used, but more than *mantars* they use the *jhạṛni* combined with *jhaṛ*. The following are examples:

Mantar: *Ma Gạndhạri Gạuṛạ Rạti, ạmi jạni nare sãpa kọn kọn jạti cĩoti, cõuti, malonti, bhabona, pạṭhuṛạ surup sạ̃p, khuili sạ̃pin. Kar ghọrẹ khuili ki kar bape jại, tọkọr guṇạ mọṅgọl pan? kẹ jhaṛẹ? Guru jhaṛẹ, guru gean, mae jhaṛẹ, Isor Mahadeb dohae jhaṛẹ; kar dohae? Ma Monsa Dibir dohae.*

That is, Mother Gandhari Gaura Rati, I do not know what kind of snake, whether Russel's viper, the *couti*, the *malonti*, the *bhabona*, the *pạṭhuṛạ*, exactly what snake, black female snake. In whose house did you eat him or whose father will go, by whose virtue will he get felicity? who strokes? The *guru* strokes by the *guru's* knowledge, the Mother strokes, he strokes by the grace of the Lord Mahadeb (Siva); by whose grace? by the grace of the Mother Monsa Dibi.

Here is another: *Lilạ lilạ je khaner bis sei khaner mile jae, caṭ cuṭki cuṛạ mala, i bis kẹ jhaṛẹ? Guru jhaṛẹ, Kạmru guru dohae jhaṛẹ.*

That is, Play play, the poison of any place shall be collected at this place, in the very uppermost parts; that poison who is stroking? The *guru* strokes, by the grace of Kamru *guru* he strokes.

Followed by this *jhaṛni : Tọkọe biṅe jọjọm kana bis dọ? Jhaṛa se jhaṛ se guru bis dọ ; namase nạmi gelare bis. Nayaṅ biṅe jọjọm kana bis dọ ; gaṇḍet biṅe jọjọm kana bis dọ, etc.*

That is, Which snake is 'eating,' the poison? The *guru* will stroke, yes, stroke the poison ; come down, it came down the poison. The cobra snake is 'eating,' its poison ; the karait snake is 'eating', its poison, etc.

If the snake is known, only the name of this one is mentioned ; if it is unknown, the *ojha* will enumerate all the snakes he knows ; it is of importance that the name of the snake responsible should be mentioned.

The *ojha* who gave above *mantar* and *jhaṛni* is also responsible for the following in connection with treatment of snake-bite. The *ojha* first mutters the following : *Citi citi sãp citi, jọler citi, maha gaụṛa aṅkaṛe* (that is, Variegated, variegated, snake variegated, water variegated, in the grasp of the great adjutant bird), whereupon he proceeds to charm the patient (*bandhọn* it is called) to prevent the 'wick from falling,' as it is called, that is, to secure the bitten one against dying. He does this by blowing into the nose of the patient, whereupon he utters the following *mantar* : *Dãt bandhẹ, nak bandhẹ, jib bandhẹ, i bandhẹ ; kẹ bandhẹ? Guru bandhẹ, guru gean, Kam guru dohae bandhẹ.*

That is, He charms the teeth, he charms the nose, he charms the tongue, he charms this ; who charms? The *guru* charms by the *guru*'s knowledge, he charms by the grace of Kam (*i.e.* Kamru) *guru*. At the same time he ties the limb with a string, some hair, or whatever may be handy, if the bite is in a place where this is possible.

If blood comes out from the nose, this is taken to be a sure sign that the 'wick has fallen down', that the person is beyond help, and the *ojha* will declare his inability to do anything, saying that 'the eaters have prevailed ; he could not manage it.'

The following is a *mantar*, against snake bite : *Dhọnder bis niṅguṛ ke jae, mukhe dekhia loṛbi, ṭan bhelar mukhu sunbar kạhni sat sat ke bis kọrlọm ; i bis kẹ jhaṛẹ? Guru jhaṛẹ, guru gean, mae jhaṛẹ, jhaṛae siri Kạhri gean, Kạmru dohae jhae jhaṛẹ.*

That is, The poison of the *dhọnḍ* (a water snake, non-poisonous ; here mentioned as an example) will come down to the tail, seeing me you engaged to fight ; as soon as I heard the story, I at once ascertained the poison ; who is stroking this poison? The *guru* strokes, by the *guru*'s knowledge, the Mother strokes, causes to stroke knowing the fortunate wording (or as translated above), by the grace of Kamru he strokes.

Then comes the following *jhaṛni* :

Culer sọṅjọk namal bisạ matha bạrire bhelase bis dọ,
Mathar sọṅjọk namal bisạ daṭa bạrire bhelase bis dọ,
Dãter sọṅjọk namal bisạ jibạ bạrire bhelase bis dọ,
Jibạr sọṅjọk namal bisạ gola bạrire bhelase bis dọ,
Golar sọṅjọk namal bisạ chạli bạrire bhelase bis dọ,
Chạtir sọṅjọk namal bisạ pẹṭẹ bạrire bhelase bis dọ,
Pẹṭer sọṅjọk namal bisạ ḍaṇḍa bạrire bhelase bis dọ,

Dandar sonjok namal bisa gunthi barire bhelase bis do,
Gunthir sonjok namal bisa themna barire bhelase bis do,
Themna sonjok namal bisa thopa barire bhelase bis do,
Thopar sonjok namal bisa angur barire bhelase bis do,
Angur sonjok namal bisa gãwa barire bhelase bis do.

That is,

The poison that was in the hair has come down and is now on a level with the head, the poison,

The poison that was in the head has come down and is now on a level with the teeth, the poison,—

and so on, the poison is brought gradually down from the teeth to the tongue, from the tongue to the throat, from the throat to the breast, from the breast to the stomach, from the stomach to the loins, from the loins to the knees, from the knees to the legs, from the legs to the feet, from the feet to the toes, and from the toes to a level with the village (that is, down into the ground).

If possible, the *jhar* against snake bite is performed with a feather of the adjutant bird; if that is not available, a peacock's feather is used or, if nothing else part of a broom (*sirom* or *saparom*). See p. 73, footnote 3.

Mantar is used also against cattle disease. Here is one, used when a buffalo is troubled with a swollen neck, so that it cannot have the yoke on. A scorpion is found and put on the buffalo's neck to make it sting, and the following *mantar* is uttered: *Hadgar kur kuri hingur lore se bonhaete asite site seromre matha.*

What this really means it is difficult to make out; as the present text stands it is a mixture of Santali and Bihari. It may possibly be something like: 'Lean, in the gripes, reddish exudation, to charm this to come, coolness, a head on the neck.'

Even against a blight of the crops *mantar* is used; the following is one: *Gudi gudi, purub gudi, pachia gudi, utor gudi, dakhin gudi, amar khete yaela gudi, sat samud Lonka gar phukia uria jahre gudi.*

That is, Flying bug, flying bug, east bug, west bug, north bug, south bug, in my paddy field the flying bug came, past seven seas to the Lanka fortress be blown and fly away, flying bug.

I have more *mantars* and *jharnis*; the specimens quoted are sufficient to show their nature.

It might be remarked, that *jhar* may be performed without a sung *jharni;* the *ojha* may make the 'passes' simply reciting a *mantar*. The *jharni* is sung only once; but as elsewhere mentioned, the *ojha* will sometimes continue the *jhar*, whistling the *jharni* melody.

It will be observed there is a distinct difference between a *jharni* and a *mantar*. The *jharni* is more of a persuasive character; it seems to be an attempt to get the illness or its cause away by gentle means, and not by force. It is only exceptionally that the *guru* or a spirit is mentioned; where that is done it is perhaps not a *jharni* proper. The *mantar*, on the other hand, is a reference to higher powers, an attempt to remove disease or its cause by the force of spirit power, or even by a word alone, if one only has the proper word. It does not seem difficult to deduce from what source these *mantars* must have originally come, or in any case, the idea of the possibility of using them. The *ojha* takes care to state that he acts as the representative of and by the grace of some spirit or other.

A couple of things seem to be vital to success. The spirit at whose command the disease should disappear must be the proper spirit having the proper power; and the disease, or whatever it may be, must be named by its proper name.

A name is to a Santal something more than it generally is to us; it is not only a means of identification, it represents, is part of, somebody or something. If the proper name is not used, the person (or the disease) is not properly or effectually called. The connection between caller and called is not properly established.

This is a peculiar trait of the Santals; with the fear they have of the *boṅgas* they are quite unconcerned when speaking of them using general terms, even when using the vilest epithets. If the supposed real name is mentioned, all is altered. The 'owner' of the name is brought to one's presence.[1]

It will have been observed that when uttering a *mantar* a large number of names for different objects are used, the purpose apparently being to make sure, so far as possible, that the thing or disease or cause is mentioned and properly mentioned, partly on account of the belief just referred to, partly to ensure that nothing or no possibility is left out.

In support of this one may refer to the *mantars* used against snake-bite. When the snake is known, this snake alone is mentioned; if, as frequently happens, it is unknown what kind of snake has bitten, every known species is enumerated.

One may further refer to the *mantars* used when 'reading' over oil; all likely kinds of oil are mentioned to make sure that the oil present is not forgotten. In the same way, when the *ojha* charms his disciples to make their going and coming sure, every possible source of danger is enumerated.[2]

To be safe all and everything must be included.

9.

Special snake-bite mantars *in corrupt Bengali.*

In connection with snake-bite they have quite a number of *mantars*. Besides those quoted above I have a very long and curious one, or rather a string of *mantars*,

---

1 The following may show this. It happened many years ago; I had a Santal to pull the pankha for me. One day, I asked him who his *abge boṅga* was (the *abge* is a kind of tutelary *boṅga* whose name is not disclosed, specially not to women; it is said that when a man feels his end coming he will whisper the name into the ears of his eldest son). The man answered, that he did not know; when his father died, he had been quite a child; none had mentioned the name to him, and he had not had anything to do with *boṅga* worship. This was also likely true. I then asked him which sept he belonged to; on his telling this, I asked whether his sept's *abge* was not called so and so. I have seldom seen fear like in him. He commenced to tremble and to perspire profusely; ultimately he ran away and did not return until a couple of hours had elapsed. When I asked him, why he had bolted, he answered that he had heard that these *boṅgas* were very dangerous and powerful, and when they were mentioned by name, they might come, and he would not stay to be exposed to what might happen. He had no doubt as to the reality and nature of the spirits. But, as will be seen, the mentioning of the general term of *abge* did not affect him; as soon as the supposed real name was spoken, the fear of the presence came.

2 One is here reminded of the old Norse tale of the death of Balder. All creation had been made to swear that they would not hurt Balder; somehow the mistletoe had been forgotten or left out; and it was the mistletoe that killed him

giving charms, etc., for a good many matters connected with snake-bite and the call of the *ojha* and what he must do in self-protection (it seems) and to counteract the poison. It is of some interest to have all these in extenso; they number in all 66. A few are translated here below; the whole of them are printed without translation p. 116 ss.

They are in a very corrupt form of Bengali with here and there Hindi words and constructions interspersed, also in a couple of places Santali. I asked a Bengali friend to help me with it; he sent it back saying he could not understand it; there are so many strange words, not found in any dictionary and not known to an educated Bengali. Since I have tried to get through it myself, the whole is, however, so uncertain, that I do not think it would do to publish a translation. Incidentally it might be remarked that the *ojha* himself does not understand it; he has only a most vague idea of the contents. This does not, of course, spoil the magic, according to *ojha* ideas.

The *mantars* referred to in several respects show a decided difference from those previously given; one seems to be transferred to another sphere; I take it that the influence of Hinduism is much stronger here. *Kạmru guru* is only occasionally mentioned; strangely enough 'the grace of *Kạmru*'s country' is heard. The Hindu deities have a rather large place; Monsa, the snake-goddess is very often mentioned, generally coupled with Dibi (*i.e.*, Durga); Krishna is also often mentioned under different names; further Mahadeb (Siva) and possibly also Vishnu, and often Vishnu's bird, the *gạruṛ*. Also other deities are named, Saraswati and others. A few of the *mantars* are quoted:

Hukạ bọlẹ gaṛa guṛu, hulkạ bọlẹ cãe,
Hukạr pạni cahẹ guru, tar bis nae.

The huka says *gaṛa guṛu* (gurgles), the huka bowl gives up ashes,
The water of the huka the *guru* wants, there is no poison in that.

Dhulạ dhubli, dhulạte loṭae har har, bis uṛiạ palae.

White dust, I roll in dust again and again, the poison is evaporated.

Dhulạte luṭu puṭu, biser jala bạmi ache, mukher kotha;
Mae Monsa Hori bọlọ, Hori sọbdẹ nạire bis.

Roll in dust again and again, the pain of the poison is abated,—the word of (my) mouth;
Mother Monsa, say Hari, in the word Hari there is no poison.

Sọrọsạti, Sọrọsạti, lilọl bọrọnẹ, rọkọti Sọrọsạti
Kuntọl kọrọne ạgu jại, ma Monsa khae;
Pichu jại Mahadeb Dibi, as kọrẹ khas na;
Amake chuṛio na, amake chuṛis tọ,
Khại Isor Mahadeber matha.

Saraswati, Saraswati, blue coloured, saves Saraswati,
Hair on ear, goes ahead, Mother Monsa eats;
Behind go Mahadeb and Dibi, do not eat with hope;

Do not taunt me, if you taunt me,
I eat up the Lord Mahadeb's head.

(This last is used for self-protection by the *ojha* when going anywhere at night.)

Thak, sapına, nicole, tor mukh bandbo lohar sikolę,
Lor cor koris na; judi lor cor koris to khai Isor Mahadeber matha.

Stay, snake, in your cover, I shall tie thy mouth with an iron chain,
Don't move, if thou movest, I shall eat the head of the Lord Mahadeb.

Bati jagao, bati sar bati he,
Samdor pat bati jagao nathu dę.

Lamp (of life) burn, true lamp of life,
With a *samdor* leaf make the lamp burn, putting it in the nose.

The language is mixed; *bati*, in Santali, lamp or wick, is used about the principle of life; it is specially heard when people have been bitten by snakes; *e.g. bati ńūrena*, the lamp-wick has fallen, means, that there is no hope, life is extinct. *Jagao* is to awaken, make effective, keep alive.

Sat simoler asę bańka, tae bosi goruṛ pańkha,
Goruṛ pańkha jhāpę jhūpę, bolę Gopaler gha mukhe.

Twisted with the fibre of seven simols, hence the *garuṛ*'s, wings are closed,
Closing his wings *garuṛ* says, Gopal's sore is in his head.

Poddo pate jonmo hoilo, Manik ar Bisai Ṭhakur,
Tae sati jani; kon tolę agun hobę, kon tolę pani?
Kon tolę bis namhę? bhatis lani Mahadeb amar ma bap?
Goruṛ muher sis, ęk hatę bis jharbo dękho tohor this;
Arhai baihar jha, siaṛ condor mukhe ja.

On a lotus leaf they were born, Manik and Bisai Thakur;
This I know for certain; below what will it become fire, below what will it become water?
Below what will the poison go down, o light-bringer Mahadeb, my father and mother?
With the remedy in the mouth of the *garuṛ* I shall with one hand stroke the poison down, look, thy anger.
Away it go past two and a half low-lying fields, off to the mouth of the *siaṛ condo* snake.

(Translation somewhat uncertain; the Santals have a belief that there is a kind of small ball or tablet in the head of the *garuṛ* bird, supposed to be an infallible cure for snake-bite.)

Ban ban, sil ban, pathri ban, i ban kę mare? Guru mare, guru geane, mae mare; kar dohae? Mahadeb Gaurar dohae marę, raja Bhojke dohae.

Dart dart, stone dart, flint dart, who shoots this dart? The *guru* shoots by the *guru's* knowledge; the Mother shoots, by whose grace? by the grace of Mahadeb Gaura he shoots, by the grace of king Bhoj.

Sapi, sunu, sapina, Gokhuler kotha: pọ̃ńc tạri Kisun jọnmọ hoilo kotha? Jọnmọ hoilo Mạdhupure doibar ghọrẹ, bãsad tulạị dile Gokhule, nạị dhọrẹ Kisna hate mọhọn bãsi, matha campa phul; hạ̃site khelite gẹlọ Kạlidọhẹr kule sate, ẹki lagal dhum.

O snake, listen, o female snake, to the words of Gokhul: The rescuer of the five (*i.e* here, humanity), Kisun, where was he born? He was born in Madhupur in a cow-milking house, Gokhul gave him his caste; the midwife put a sweet sounding flute in Kisna's hand, the champaka flower on his head, laughing he went with Kalidoh's relatives to play; with them he started a noise.

Ọrẹ Nitạị dhubinir bis, kal kuṭir bis, gha mukhẹ jhaṛẹ; kar dohae? Ma Monsa Dibir dohae.

O Nitai, dhubi-woman's poison, mortal poison, the sore with my mouth I charm away; by whose grace? by the grace of Mother Monsa and Dibi (Durga).

Nitạị dhubin, Nitạị dhubin litui kapọṛ kacẹ he, chahọ dẹsẹ pọṛetọ, hae hae! libọ tọ libọ aṅger saj.

Nitai dhubi-woman, Nitai dhubi-woman every day dumps clothes, if it should fall to the country (*i.e.*, the owner die), alas, alas! I should acquire the ornaments of the body.

Yọrẹ yọrẹ kul sereń, yọrẹ yọrẹ girigiṭi, daretem dẹjok kan dọ, dela sẹ nãṛgolenme;
Nalaṅge bhạị, nalaṅge bundhu; cọlọ cọlọ kiser ḍakọn.
Yọhẹ baba he, sọroṅge ki sẹrọ dhũạ̃ je uṛiche?
I parẹ Gaṅ nadi, u parẹ Jabo hoyeche, baba he,
Saraṅge kiser dhũạ̃ je uṛiche?

Oh oh 'tiger-song' lizard, oh oh brown lizard, thou art mounting the tree, please come down at once;

Thou and I are brothers, thou and I are friends; come quickly, there is a call cf something or other.

O father, in the heavens the smoke of what is drifting?

On this side is the Ganges river, on that side the Jabo is, oh father, the smoke of what is drifting?

(Above is at first Santali; refers possibly to the near approach of death and cremation.)

Sat sae simol gachẹ bose achẹ gạruṛa, sat sae simol gachẹ bose ache gạruṛa, Kạnạị bhọire, Kạnạị bhạị!

In seven hundred simol trees *gạruṛ* are sitting, in seven hundred simol trees *gạruṛ* are sitting, o Kanai brother, Kanai brother.

Asọn gachẹ Maniạra kaṛ, sat sae kạṭ bhaṅgia, siạṛ cand dhọrọm tuṛia, kaha so sọroṅge dhũạ̃? Kạrinạṅgin dohae, dohaere dohae nomou.

In the ason trees on the one side of the Maniara country having broken seven hundred pieces of wood the *siạṛ cand* snake, having broken righteousness—wherefrom is the smoke in the heavens? O *Kạrınạṅgin* (the king cobra), grace, oh grace, grace, come down.

From the specimens quoted the difference from the commonly used Santal *ojha-mantars* will be apparent. These are likely quite recently borrowed from Hindu sources. They are interesting from a linguistic point of view, showing how a language may be ill-treated by those who do not understand it. In order to put on permanent record a specimen, which otherwise might be lost, I add below the full text of the lengthy *mantar* alluded to in the beginning of this paragraph.

1. *Hukạ bọlẹ gạṛa guṛu, kulkạ bọlẹ cãe,*
Hukạr pạni cahẹ guru, tar bis nại.

2. *Dhulạ dhubli, dhulạte loṭae*
Har har, bis uṛiạ palae.

3. *Dhulạte luṭu puṭu, biser jala*
Bạmi ache, mukher kotha;
Mae Monsa Hori bọlọ, Hori sọbdẹ nạire bis.

4. *Simol tọlẹ bicchạ uṛilọ, gayẹ pọrilọ;*
Gayẹ cọmkọre bis nại, bhọbọnẹ uṛilọ bis.

5. *Gamcha laṛọṅ, gamcha calọṅ;*
Gamcha caltẹ nạire bis.

6. *Gamcha laṛọṅ, gamcha calọṅ;*
I gamcha piṛhi marọ, bis kọrilam pạni.

7. *Sọrọsạti, Sọrọsạti, lilọl bọrọnẹ,*
Rọkọti Sọrọsạti kuntọl kọrọnẹ
Ạgu jại, ma Monsa khae; pichu jại Mahadeb
Dibi, as kọrẹ khas na; amake chuṛio na;
Amake chuṛis tọ, khại Isor Mañadeber matha.

8. *Thak, sạpina, nicole, tor mukh bandhọ lohar sikọlẹ;*
Lọṛ cọṛ koris na, judi lọṛ cọṛ koris tọ
Khại Isor Mahadeber matha.

9. *Jọl bandhọn, thọl bandhọn,*
Bandhọn apọn kaya, tin kọn pirthimi bandhọ; tin maha maya.

10. *Bạṛki gundhi ạsudhini,*
Bạti jogao nạthu dẹ.

11. *Bạti jogao, bạti sar bạti he,*
Samdọr pat, bạti jogao nạthu dẹ.

12. *Baṛa je badọl, jọl borsa par hũyạ̃?*

13. *Tumi katlẹ asẹ, ạmi puchạlam ghãsẹ.*

14. *Mae Gandhari gaura rati ami.*
Ami jani nare, sãpa kon kon jati?
Chĩuti, cõuti, malonti.

15. *Soronge garura, patalahĩ garura ;*
Garura jo sobde, bis je uri gelo.

16. *Sat simoler ase banka,*
Tae bosi gorur pankha ;
Gorur pankha jhãpe jhũpe, bole Gopaler gha mukhe.

17. *Kaliyare kaliya!*
Kotha jas palayẽ?
Tor bis marbo, calane caline, akase concol ;
Patale ghor, Kaliyare kalkoti.

18. *Bhel bhelae mukhe, lag bhelake sobae mukhe.*
Sat din sat rat, i bis bojor hũyã thak.

19. *Gat bhangom, gatri bhangom ;*
Bhangom lohar sikol.
Tin tuhri dar samne, namre bis ;
Dorhor bis patalke jai.

20. *Car ganda car sãpa,*
Aru lag, pãru lag, celia phat liya, andi cihar candor,
Kon sãpa khailen bapa?
Ami jani na, jani to Isor Mahadeb bapa.

21. *Poddo pate jonmo hoilo, Manik ar Bisai Thakur,*
Tae sati jani ; kon tole agun hobe, kon tole pani?
Kon tole bis namhe?
Bhatis lani Mahadeb amar ma bap?
Gorur muher sis, ek hate bis jharbo, dekho tohor this ;
Arhai baihar jha, siar condor mukhe ja.

22. *Bis bis, i bis, kal kotir bis gha mukhe jhare.*

23. *Ban ban, sil ban, pathri ban, i ban ke mare?*
Guru mare, guru geane, mae mare : kar dohac?
Mahadeb Gaurar dohae mare, raja Bhojke dohae.

24. *Ore! sapinar bis, kal kotir bis, gha mukhe jhare.*

25. *Sapi, sunu, sapina, Gokhuler kotha :*
Põnc tari Kisun jonmo hoilo kotha?
Jonmo hoilo Madhupure doibar ghore ;
Bãsad tulai dile Gokhule, nai dhore
Kisna hate mohon bãsi, matha campu phul ;
Hãsite khelite gelo Kalidoher kule sate, eki lagal dhum.

26. *Kon mọntọr jhạṛni pọkkhẹ?*
Pọbọn cọltẹ ban sidhọrni, i dhọrni lọṛẹ cọṛẹ,
Isor Mahadeber piṛi.

27. *Dhọrọm cintạ bạnsi dhọrni,*
I dhọrni na pại bat.
Amar gurur nam Ram tạri;
Sikkhot bạnsi dhọrni; i dhọrni lọṛẹ cọṛẹ,
Gọrdọn kạtia rọktọ khại, dhọbar pạt mathae lẹ.

28. *Sọt guru bandhọ, i nọt bandhọ;*
Sọ ạsi hajar phirbi kundọr bandhọ,
Ḍẹli sọrdar ghọṛẹ, achẹ du biddạ;
Bạpu mae pọkhẹr beṭa, pọkhẹ achẹ.
Nọkhẹ khiciạ sọt bọl, phuṭbẹ bọṛna guni huyạ chi.
Sãp khelibar ạmi, ạmi boṭi Laler sik;
Bisnu kisnu lilạ jạni, sapinar bisak kọrẹchẹ.
Gunạgara pạni, Bọl dẹkh murmuk cũạ?
Aṛek kiạ, ẹk jiạ, nana sãpẹr bis mal s̃aṭẹ jhaṛẹ.

29. *Goruṛ ban ọka sọka, Pọrọmẹsọrẹr sẹk sọn manpur;*
Rukhiạ kọṛọ bạṛi cọndọn, kãhã jae?
Purub jae, purub bandhọ.
Pạchim jae, pạchim bandhọ.
Utọr jae, utọr bandhọ, dạkhin jae, dạkhin bandhọ.
Kẹ bandhẹ? Guru bandhẹ, guru chaṛe mae bandhẹ,
Bandhẹ sẹrẹ bandhẹsẹ Kạhri gia Kạmru dohae.

30. *Tilhạr mạṭi, didir haṛ;*
Sọb sapinake aṭhẹ kuṭhẹ amakẹ dekhẹ baṛhabẹ.
Tuṇḍ Isor Mahadeber mathae khas.

31. *Kon ḍọlẹr kon ḍọlẹr mọñjọr?*
Sọb sapina aṭhe kuṭhe, kon ḍọlẹr sọrbọ ma sapinake?
Dhọrọm duṭi pa, i kon ḍọlẹ harabitọ.

32. *Ḍạn gun aṭ caṭo, carkha carhae kẹ kaṭẹ?*
Guru kaṭẹ, guru chaṛẹ mae kaṭẹ;
Kaṭẹ sẹrẹ? Kaṭẹchi, Kahari gia Kạmru dohae kaṭẹ.

33. *Choṭẹ moṭẹ nạriya kera singhạ.*
Bạṭular pat, hạru har uṭ, Mahadeber jaṭ sumbhạr,
Hạru har, nại nụi jogin, Kạmru kamechake dohae.

34. *Choṭẹ moṭẹ bilạti ciñcir, rọktọ bharlo kẹs.*
Je gun gun calaeo, sẹ gunkẹ kaṭẹ;
Kẹ kaṭẹ? Mahabeb kaṭẹ.
Mahadeb geane guru kaṭẹ;
Nại nại jugin, Kạmru kamecchakẹ dohae.

35. *Amar ban rage jae,*
Ramer ban aṛe jae;
Se ban sil pathor bojor hũyą thak!
Kar dohae? Isor gaura.
Nae nae jogin, Kamru kamecchake dohae.

36. *Kari kurthi, Monsa jati.*
Jaore ban phalnake khate!
Harda khão, hardi khão, muṛi mocrike karji khão;
Jaore raṅga dhori, dhori bis;
Usike satme jao!
Kar dohae? Ma Monsa Dibir dohae.

37. *Jol bhaṅgo, jolom bhaṅgo, jolate pa bhaṅgo,*
Osṭi noṅgor mathae baṛ, dhãe dhũi;
Tulsir mala ulią dego, ulią de morite khai;
Jole morite khai. dharę bhorsate ḍhumor bhase;
Sam sun sundori, kal bhuṛ bhuṛ koreche;
Kal koṭir biske unotriske uṛailam.
Kar dohae? Ma Monsa Dibir dohae.

38. *Ore sapinar bis!*
Kal koṭir bis gha mukhe jhaṛe.

39. *Kopale kopale betola;*
Ciron ciron tur dãte lagilo he.
Je bate ailere sapinar bis;
Sei bate jaibere sapinar bis.

40. *Ore raj saper bis!*
Kal koṭir gha mukhe jhaṛe.
Kar dohae?
Ma Monsa Dibir dohae.

41. *Dhulą yache luṭur puṭor, biser jala;*
Ogo hebai! E mukhe raj saper biser jala.

42. *Ore, mora saper bis!*
Kal kuṭir bis gha mukhe jhaṛe.

43. *Cho mase culą jhare punir sãp;*
Cho mase culą jhare punir sãp;
Jhaṛase guru mae, nami gelare bis;
Nijase guru mae, nami gelare bis.

44. *Ore, baro rupą sãp!*
Tomar bis jobore jolon.
Kal kuṭir bis gha mukhe jhaṛe.
Kar dohae?
Ma Monsa Dibir dohae.

45. *Jahorẹ, jahorẹ bisọñjọr molae;*
Hạigo, khuler nit̤hurẹ kạnu murmur sãp.

46. *Ọrẹ Nitại dhubinir bis,*
Kal kuṭir bis, gha mukhẹ jhaṛẹ.
Kar dohae?
Ma Monsa Dibir dohae.

47. *Nitại dhubin, Nitại dhubin*
Litui kapọṛ kacẹ he,
Chahọ dẹsẹ pọṛẹtọ, hae hae!
Libọ tọ libọ añger saj.

48. *Hạliạṛẹ, haler mạṭi kal poṛaetẹ bis nại.*
Gayẹ bis nại, payẹ bis nại.
Bisna bhại, bistum! sobae Hori bọlọ, bhại;
Hori bol!
Hori sọbdẹ bis uṛẹ jae.
Kar dohae?
Ma Monsa Dibir dohae.

49. *Hẽṭẹka khijurika piṛia, upọr pạnir ghạilạ.*
Hẽṭẹka khijurika piṛia, upọr pạnir ghạilạ.
Ogo, cuḍur cuḍur sapini!
Jọ jaebe, guni morarẹ paelam.

50. *Bọsọ, hẹrọ, bọsọ capẹ simoler tọlẹ.*
Bicchạ bhọbọnẹ uṛilọ, bis pọri gayẹ comkorẹ.
Bis nại, Bisṭum bir sọn, mọn mọn mọt nại.
Pọbọnke uṛẹ jae, kar dohae?
Ma Monsa Dibir dohae.

51. *Sat sae simol gachẹ bose achẹ gạruṛa,*
Sat sae simol gachẹ bose achẹ gạruṛa,
Kạnại bhạire, Kạnại bhại!

52. *Asọn gachẹ Mạniạṛa kaṛ,*
Sat sae kaṭ bhañgia, siạṛ cand dhọrọm tuṛia,
Kaha so sọrọṅgẹ dhũạ̃?
Kạrinạṅgin dohae, dohaere dohae nomou.

53. *Yọrẹ yọrẹ kul sereñ, yọrẹ yọrẹ girigiṭi,*
Daretem dẹjoḱ kan dọ, dela sẹ nãṛgolẹnme;
Nalañge bhại, nalañge bundhu;
Cọlọ cọlọ kiser ḍakọn.
Yọhẹ baba he, sọrọṅgẹ ki sẹrọ dhũạ̃ je uṛiche?
I parẹ Gañ nạdi, u parẹ Jabo hoyeche,
Baba he, sọrọṅgẹ kiser dhũạ̃ je uṛiche?

54. *Sãp kore ke jore bhai, rokol pore cim cim,*
Ure apone nir bis. Kar dohae?
Ma Monsa Dibir dohae.

55. *Chani, chani, chani, biser nam jani;*
Rokolei tubu tubu, rokoter jani.
Añk loker pani gha mukhe jhare.
Kar dohae?
Ma Monsa Dibir dohae!

56. *Rokolei tubu tubu;*
Pabone kãye kamore khailen sãpa.
Caporei nai. Kar dohae?
Ma Monsa Dibir dohae.

57. *Sãp cahe kor sãp, pitme raho?*
Sahe dhula ale uli mare thopi bis.
Utorke jabo ba patalke puri.
Kar dohae?
Ma Monsa Dibir dohae.

58. *Sit gaga lil boron, sãk cil lil boron.*
Urao bis tin bhobon, Su campa satek bakor
Ur jao bis tũi hatek capor.
Kar dohae?
Ma Monsa Dibir dohae.

59. *Ek jhal jhalea dhuduame;*
Hua jagia to jagia, mitri jagia.
Na dise kotri samudor sikkha;
Nam, namre bis tajia, Halumanke dohae.

60. *Sapi, sunu, sapinar jonmo hoilo kotha?*
Jonmo hoilo jotha totha Doibikir ghore.
Basudebe tule dile Gokkhula nai ghore.
Hate tule dilen mohon nistu kistore bhai;
Mathae campa phul, ki korile pare re bhai?
Sei mayer baper sapiner soron kore;
Garur mohabir, garur moha birore bhai;
Ponkhe boro jor, ponkhe kore cechan.
Guru Kalidoher jol, hete to Kalidoh, upore to sei ghor;
Sei ghor bhangia to harre bis!
Kar dohae? Ma Monsa Dibir dohae.

61. *Naire, naire bisor gaye kio bis naire naire.*
Rombha khola phutaye biske diske korilam pani.
Naire nai solo soi gopini tare ondo nond pran.
Hori bol, bhai, Hori bol.

62. *Dhut cun cuni musri basę, kaha jae?*
Gogon gorasi, hẽ yã, hẽ põa, hẽ candrae!
Amka oṅger biskę, unotiskę uṛailam.
Kar dohae? Ma Monsa Dibir dohae.

63. *Mahadeber pusbo ḍāṛi saji noyę khola;*
Bọri rekha tolę poddo pale, poddo patę jonmo hoilo;
Kũāri jonmo, paola bhaṅgia gelo patal bhobonę.
Kõa deber ma nae khe, monę lagi betha:
Saka sunu sapinar sundorer kotha.
Upolęka lęka hori, orę biskę liliję.
Ekhonę ki achore bis?
Kar dohae? Ma Monsa Dibir dohae.

64. *Khotok ḍumurer trisuk, mal chaṛa bis;*
Tũi borom kopalę, borom kopalę diyẽ tali.
Jarę bis tũi kuli kuli.
Kar dohae? Ma Monsa Dibir dohae.

65. *Bond kor kor Indujir namę;*
Meghlal megher arę bosę bond koręchę.
Kęu na kęu dękhę, lag sopi bondi korę;
Du bhaike rakhę, jokhon baron gel chilo;
Basupiri ṭhãyę sat hajar kolsir bis pãyachilen dan.
Se bis rakho rakho, thoro thoro.
Araiṭikurer bis mal satę jhaṛę.
Kar dohae? Mai Monsa Dibir dohae

66. *Khoṭ khoṭon to gaṛuṛ bapa,*
Gaṛuṛ nijer ghorę hamasa jachen.
Ki korichen? Ghurę mon pabo na.
Goruṛti golae roth katę, bahũrẽ bahũrẽ;
Bis tũi jao soron batę.
Biyae gelo sapina, rowã gelo kola kola.
Sotalę porbote bis namchę.
Sonar tola, arek kia, nana sãper bismal satę jhaṛę.
Kar dohae?
Ma Monsa Dibir dohae.[1]

---

1 The transliteration of above is as written by a Santal, only here and there made conform with the style of writing use of Santali.

APPENDIX II.

Kạmru guru.

The personage venerated above all other *gurus*, invoked in the majority of *mantars*, and also regularly worshipped by the Santal *ojhạ*, is *Kạmru guru*. He is, as stated, their reputed first teacher. He is also, by some, said to be the first teacher of *jan* science (see p. 41), and also to be the one who first instructed the witches. All agree as to his being the first teacher of *ojhaism*; but some deny his being the originator of witchcraft. In any case he plays a large rôle within the range of Santal ideas and life; his influence has made itself felt, and even now, is felt in a marked degree; how, may be gathered from the previous pages.

On account of the place he holds in Santal medical practice and superstition it may be of interest to know what ideas the Santals have formed concerning him. They have several stories about him; these belong, as they are at present told, decidedly to the realm of fairy-tales; but a few grains of historical fact may possibly be extracted from them, and some facts may be gleaned concerning the development of the Santals and their connection with peoples other than themselves. The reader may himself judge from what is told here below.

First a few words regarding his name. This is supposed to be *Kạmru* or *Kạmbru* (the *b* being probably inserted in pronouncing the word; Santali has several analogous words, as *mamla* and *mambla*, *ramṛa* and *rambṛa*). I have heard a variant *Kamruk*; the word is by *ojhas* often pronounced *Kamru*, with stress on the first syllable, and without resultant vowel; now and then I have only been able to hear *Kam* (in *mantars*). The word is not of Santali origin; this does not, however, prove much, as the majority of the Santal proper names are of Aryan origin. It seems natural to connect the word with Skr. *kama*, and *kamarupa*, whether in its original meaning of 'taking any shape at will, beautiful, pleasing,' or as the name of a country, the western portion of Assam. This makes it possible to take it either as the name of a person so called, or as the name of a person from Kamrup.

A tradition that the Santals learnt witchcraft from a blackmith whilst they were living in *Kamruk* seems to have its origin in a popular derivation of the name from the word *kamar*, a blacksmith.

The Santal traditions as told by the old Kolean *guru* expressly state, that their ancestors have learnt *ojha* 'science' from Kamru, and this authority adds, 'in very old times his country and our country were close to each other' (the word does not mean bordering on each other).

The question then arises: have the Santals ever been in the east during their wanderings? Their traditions, as they are recounted at the present day, speak about wanderings in one main direction, viz., towards the east; it is not possible to deduce anything else. On the other hand, I have heard Santals giving expression to a vague idea, that their ancestors have once been in the east. It is just possible that the name of Kamru may have given rise to such tales, combined with the knowledge the present people have of Kamrup and Assam.

Incidentally it might be noted that this question touches a problem that is coming to the front at present, the problem of the linguistic connection between a large number of races living in India and in the countries to the east, north-east and south-east of India.

If the ancestors of the Santals have ever been in the east, in the present Assam, it must have been in a very remote antiquity previous to any time about which we have any reports. It is certain, that the ancestors of the Santals lived on the Chota Nagpur plateau some four to five hundred years ago, and it is probable that they had then been living in those parts of the country for centuries.

The Santal traditions tell that their ancestors helped king Ram against Ravana on Lanka; strangely enough one school of the traditions expressly deny that they went there. Taking it for granted that the story of the Ramayana has some foundation in fact, further that the monkey-king stands for the chief of the aboriginal assistants, this would all go to make it probable that part of the ancestors of the Santals some two thousand years ago or more were living in the vicinity of the present Oudh, if not actually there. The Santal traditions and what may be deduced from them, practically all seem to point to the west.

The language found in the *mantars* and *jhaṛnis* does not point towards any very remote antiquity and certainly not to the east.

The following is heard among the Santals about Kamru :—

Kamru's birth is said to have taken place on the water under a lotus leaf, and he is said to be of the race of godlings or *boṅgas*; therefore he is invoked up to this day. It is also told that *Monsa* (as the Santals call the snake goddess Manasa) was born at the same time; Kamru is, however, a little younger. According to the Santali story *Monsa* was the daughter of *Sib Ṭhakur*; he had been sitting on the lotus leaves; when he returned to heaven and looked down, he to his great astonishment saw a girl (*Monsa*) sitting where he had just been. (It is a separate story and shall not be repeated here; it is just mentioned to show where there may be some connection between the two tales.)

They were two brothers, of whom Kamru was the younger one; the elder one of whom nothing is told, died leaving two sons who stayed with Kamru. Kamru was married, but his wife was a witch.

Kamru apparently was a great medicine-man, although nothing is told in the tales about his knowledge and doings. Then it happened when Kamru was old that he was bitten by a snake. He called his two nephews and told them to go to some hill and fetch from there a certain medicine; they were to recognize the medicine by seeing that it (it is not stated whether it was the tree or the ground or anything) was shining like fire. The two nephews at once went, found the tree, dug out and took with them a part of the root, and were on their way back when they were met by Kamru's wife.

She had heard her husband instructing the two young men and had followed after them. When she met them, she said: "What are you going to do with that medicine? Your uncle is dead." When they heard this they became very grieved and said: "What is then the use of this dirty medicine?" whereupon they threw it away and went home empty-handed.

When they reached there they saw that their uncle was alive. He at once asked them for the medicine, and they explained that their aunt had met them and told them that he was dead, wherefore they had thrown away the medicine. "Then I am going to die," Kamru said to them; "now then remember, when I have been burnt, you two must pour water over the place; then you will find two small pieces (of flesh); eat them, then you will acquire my *bidią* (science); otherwise you will be quite unable to acquire it."

Now Kamru really died, and people came together to take the body away and burn it. They built the funeral pyre, placed the body there and put fire to it, and it was burnt. The two nephews then went to pour water on the place, whilst the other people were there in the vicinity.

Just as Kamru had told them, the two young men really found two small bits of flesh; they looked at each other, whispered and asked each other: "Look here, shall we two eat this?" Both of them urged the other one to be the first to eat; the result of this contention was that they said: "By no manner of means, we shall not eat it; for if we eat it now, will not people see us?" And saying so they threw the two bits into the water and let it flow away. Consequently they did not acquire the 'science' of their uncle.

The one who did was their aunt. She had observed it, got hold of the two bits and ate them, and acquired her late husband's 'science.' But so it always is when you have to do with women; a man is unable to cope with them. And now, the story ends, there are only women in Kamru land.

It is difficult to decide what science' the story really refers to, whether it is witchcraft or magic. The Santals have several stories telling how women learnt witchcraft; these have one point in common with what has been related above, viz., that the women outwitted the men and by deception acquired knowledge or power really intended for the men. One variant of the story referred to tells how the women by subterfuge learnt witchcraft from *Cando boṅga*, the same story being otherwise told about *Marań buru* and *Kąmru guru*, who apparently is supposed also to have known witchcraft.

We shall not enter into any discussion of these matters here. We shall only just hear a few words about the ideas of the present day Santals regarding *Kąmru* or *Kamrup* country, to see whether this can give us any assistance in deciding the question raised.

Many now living Santals have been in Assam as labourers in tea-gardens and otherwise; they have also been in, or passed through, the district of Kamrup. Even if they do not mix up the present district of Kamrup with the traditional Kamru country, the similarity of the names is sufficient to make them think that the traditional Kamru country is in the east. Now people who have come back from there have told some very tall stories, after the fashion of some travellers, the stories generally going towards confirming the tales current about the Kamru country, e.g., telling how they have been caught and kept for years by women who during daytime have kept them hidden or made them into rams or the like and let them out at night, who have taught them sorcery, and so on, and from whom they have only escaped with the greatest difficulty, risking their lives.

The contents of the folk-tales amount to the following: There is really a country called Kamru; it is in a direction southwards from where the Santals are now living; to reach there one has to cross the sea (this would not take one to the present Kamrup, but more towards the Chittagong and Burma side). The country is very rich and fertile, and there are only women living there, or else the women predominate, and no one is able to go there and stay. Another report is that there are men also, but they are not liked by the women (definite reasons that cannot be recorded are given). Once a Santal had gone there and was at once caught by a woman. He told that he had come to learn their 'science,' and was kept for five years by the Kamru woman who during daytime had him covered by a *diṛmi*, a large bamboo basket, and instructed him during the night. At last he got *sid*; the woman turned him into a kite and he flew back to his own country.

Another story tells of a Santal child who was caught by a vulture and carried to Kamru country; here he grew up and ultimately married. He wanted to get back to his own country and with much difficulty persuaded some one to help him. But every time having started to go in the morning, when it became evening he found himself coming back to the place he started from. At last a woman told him, that he must leave every thing behind, not take anything of that country along; else he would never succeed. On doing this he got away.

And so on. The traditional Kamru country is a country of strange people with strange powers; the inhabitants can at will turn a man into a dog or any other animal. In those parts of the world the fabulous *ekaguḍia* and *ghoṛmũha* are found, with one leg and heads like that of horses, otherwise like human beings, who buy and eat people.

All in all, Kamru country is a land full of magic and witchcraft; but the stories told seem to imply that it is the women who are so dangerous and powerful.

It is difficult to deduct anything from the stories told by the present day Santals. It is possible that the ancestors of the people have in some remote time been in some touch with eastern people, so different from themselves that they have attributed what they have not understood to magic and sorcery

It is possible that Santals of this and the nearest previous generations, who have been in Assam and have brought back with them tales of strange peoples, and also the name of Kamrup, may have been the real originators of the idea that Kamru's 'science' has come from this part of the world. It would be only natural, if they were inclined to seek the origin of a matter like magic in a part of the world that they do not really know, where there is room for mysticism and what is not understood; the unexplored and unknown has many possibilities other than what is known and seen every day.

I am most inclined to think that the present-day *ojha* 'science' among the Santals has been taught them, in the first instance, not in the eastern parts of India, but somewhere in the western forests by a Hindu *ojha*, by the Santals called Kamru, now an entirely mythical personage, probably a western man, possibly an eastern man emigrated to the west, the name being either a *n. pr.* or an appellative, in this case denoting a man from Kamrup or a man with Kamrup 'science.'

APPENDIX III.

Santali Tunes.

With reference to the tunes here recorded, I have to acknowledge the assistance rendered by Mr. Jakob Soren, a Santal bandmaster and singing master in the Santal Mission's Boarding School for boys at Kaerabani. Two of the Dasãe tunes and three of the Buaṅ tunes are as they were recorded, by the late Mr. Skrefsrud some forty years ago; these are easily recognized by the tremolants inserted; these are very common in genuine Santal song, not affected by Western ideas of music. Jakob has not recorded these.

The Santals have songs in both the major and the minor key, the last one predominating in their music.

The specimens here recorded are only examples; there is not a large difference between the tunes to which one class of songs are sung; but they have a fairly large number of different classes and a large number of songs for each class. They apparently have no difficulty in producing verses to be sung.

In the specimens recorded, the theme is easily recognized, also how it is worked.

Jhapni tunes.

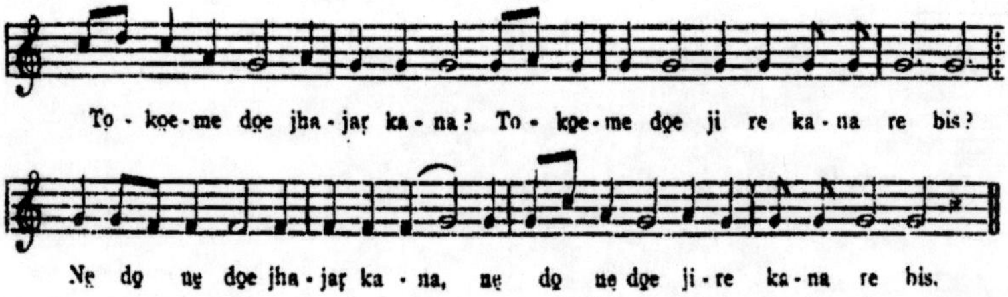

To - koe-me doe jha - jaṛ ka - na? To - koe-me doe ji re ka - na re bis?
Nẹ dọ nẹ doe jha - jaṛ ka - na, nẹ dọ nẹ doe ji - re ka - na re bis.

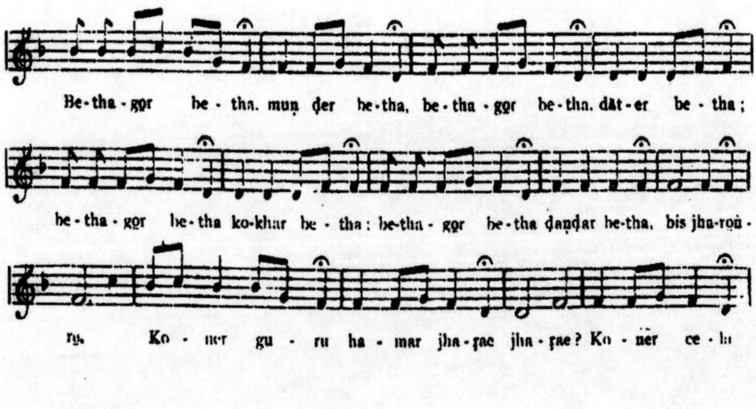

Be-tha - gor be - tha. muṇ ḍer be-tha, be - tha - gor be-tha. dāt-er be - tha;
be-tha - gor be-tha ko-khar be - tha: be-tha - gor be-tha ḍanḍar be-tha, bis jha-roṅ-
ṅg. Ko - ner gu - ru ha - mar jha-ṛae jha-ṛae? Ko - ner ce - lu

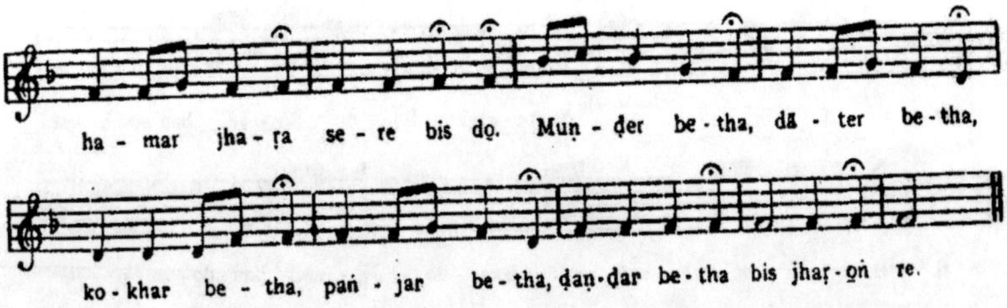
ha - mar jha - ṛa se - re bis dọ. Muṇ - ḍer be - tha, dā - ter be - tha,
ko - khar be - tha, paṅ - jar be - tha, ḍaṇ - ḍar be - tha bis jhaṛ - ọṅ re.

Dasāe tunes.

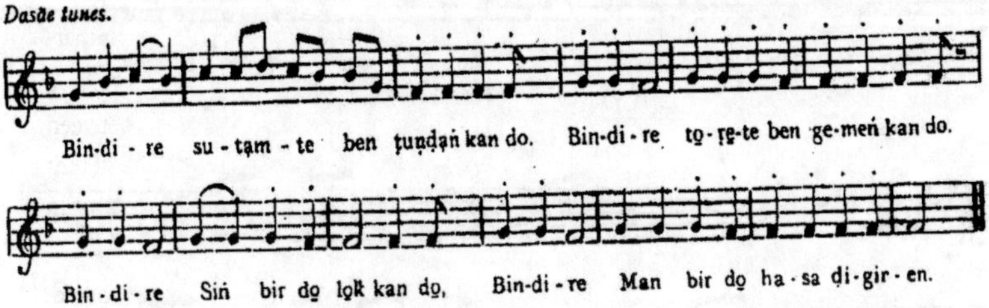
Bin-di - re su - tạm - te ben ṭuṇḍạṅ kan do. Bin-di - re tọ - ṛẹ-te ben ge-meṅ kan do.
Bin - di - re Siṅ bir dọ lọk kan dọ, Bin-di - re Man bir dọ ha - sa ḍi - gir - en.

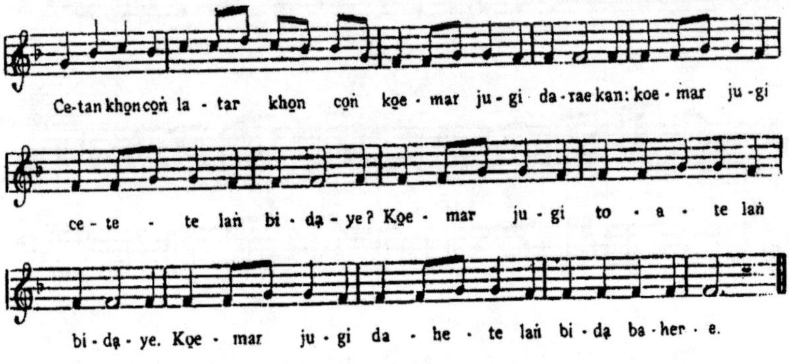
Ce-tan khọn cọṅ la - tar khọn cọṅ kọe - mar ju - gi da - rae kan: koe - mar ju - gi
ce - te - te laṅ bi - dạ - ye? Kọe - mar ju - gi to - a - te laṅ
bi - dạ - ye. Kọe - mar ju - gi da - he - te laṅ bi - dạ ba - her - e.

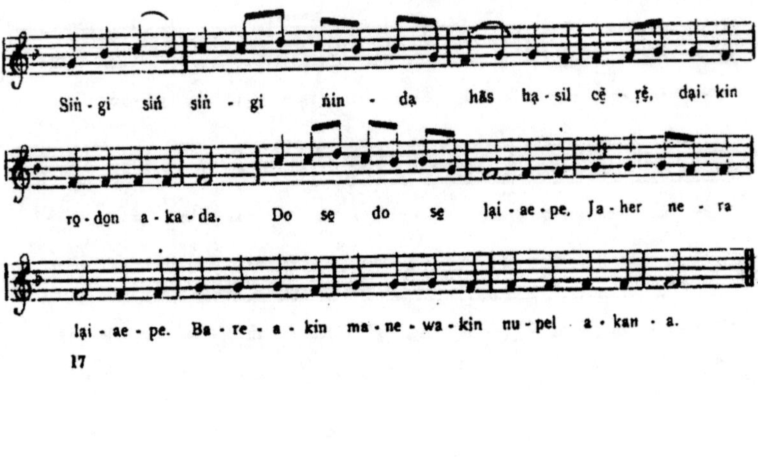
Siṅ - gi siṅ siṅ - gi ṅin - dạ hās hạ - sil cẹ̄ - ṛẹ̄, dại. kin
rọ - dọn a - ka - da. Do sẹ do sẹ lại - ae - pe, Ja - her ne - ra
lại - ae - pe. Ba - re - a - kin ma - ne - wa - kin nu - pel a - kan - a.

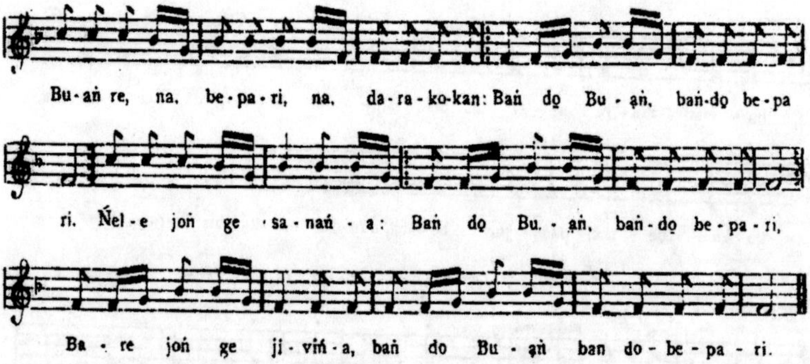
Bu-aṅ re, na, be-pa-ri, na, da-ra-ko-kan: Baṅ dọ Bu-ạṅ, baṅ-dọ be-pa
ri. Ńel-e joṅ ge sa-naṅ-a: Baṅ dọ Bu-ạṅ, baṅ-dọ be-pa-ri,
Ba-re joṅ ge ji-viṅ-a, baṅ do Bu-ạṅ ban do-be-pa-ri.

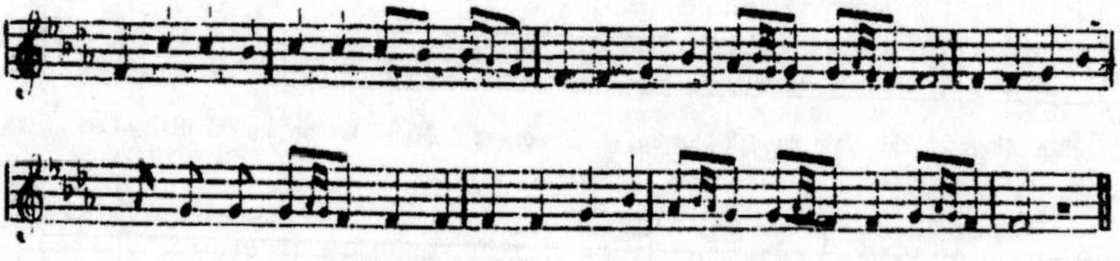

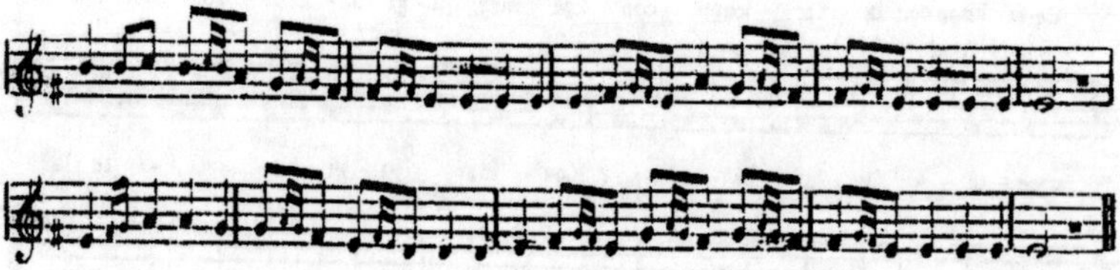

Buạṅ tunes.

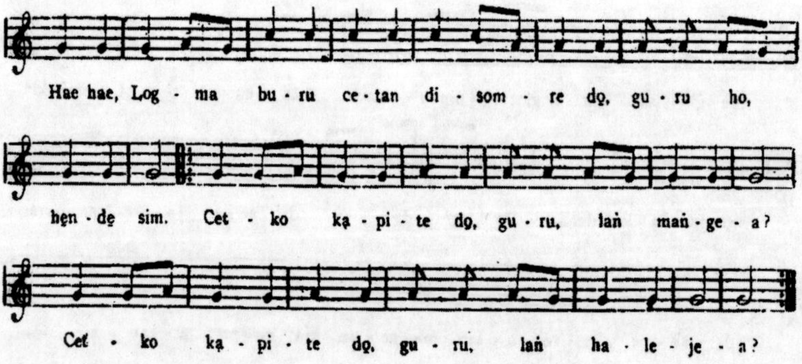
Hae hae, Log-ma bu-ru ce-tan di-som-re dọ, gu-ru ho,
hẹn-dẹ sim. Cet-ko kạ-pi-te dọ, gu-ru, laṅ maṅ-ge-a?
Cet-ko kạ-pi-te dọ, gu-ru, laṅ ha-le-je-a?

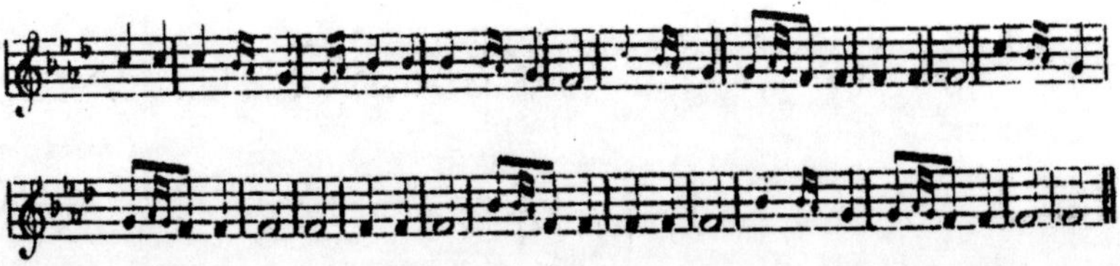

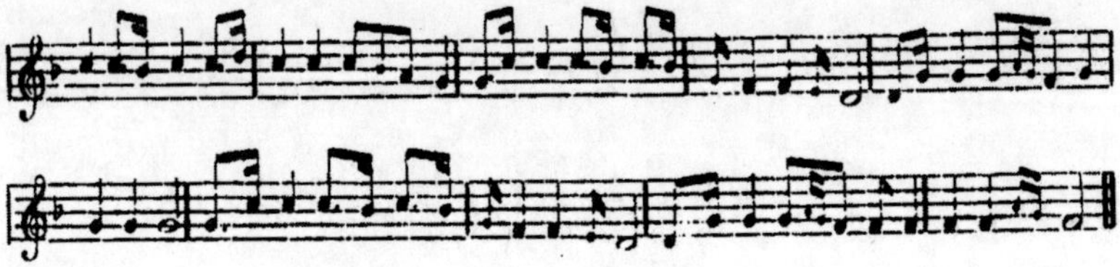

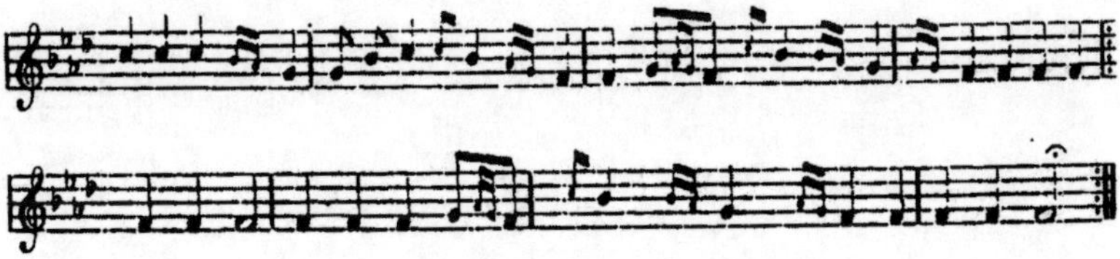

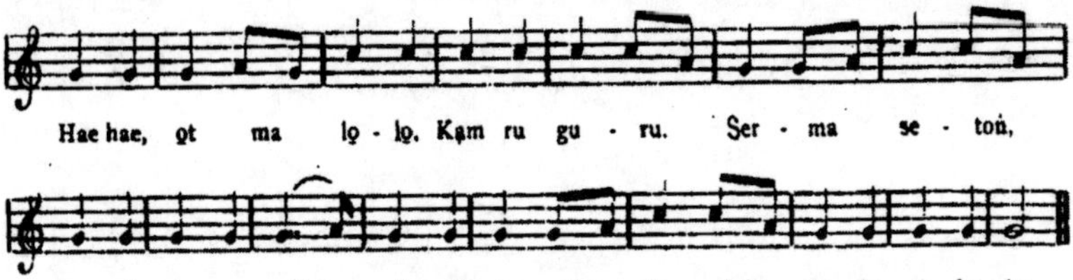
Hae hae, ọt ma lọ - lọ. Kạm ru gu - ru. Ṣer - ma se - toṅ,
Bu - ạṅ gu - ru, Nu - mi - naṅ ce - la dọ laṅ to - ka - re - ka - ko;

PART II

SANTAL MEDICINE

SANTAL MEDICINE.

By THE REV. P. O. BODDING, *Mohulpahari, Santal Parganas.*

Introductory Remarks.

I.

In the paper called The Santals and Disease, the general ideas of the Santals as regards the nature and causation of disease, their superstitions, and their general attitude in connection with disease and death have been stated. The doings of their medicine-men and *ojhas* have also been told, samples of their *mantars* and invocations have been given, and so on. For all such matters the reader is referred to the paper mentioned. Practically nothing has been mentioned in that paper concerning what corresponds to what we understand by medicine. This will be given in the here following pages. Before entering on details some remarks may be called for, as regards the origin of this work and as regards certain sides of the Santal way of practising medicine, and other matters that have not found a place elsewhere.

The writer's interest in the matters here treated of is of a double nature, partly and principally ethnological, and partly 'medicinal.' It should, however, be added that the writer is not a medical man, perhaps the very reason why he has taken up a work like the present one, and he hopes, it will be found that he has nowhere attempted to intrude into the domain of the profession.

To know how an uncivilized people tries to face and fight disease and everything connected therewith, is to know how they try to tackle, or evade tackling, some of life's great problems. Facing disease man often reveals what is otherwise only seldom seen.

As regards their medical practice, the attitude of the Santals may be summed up as being, according to their lights, practical treatment, combined with superstition, resulting in, sometimes, a quite sensible attitude, and sometimes in absurd attempts to gain the victory over the enemy.

Knowledge of their medicine will, within certain limits, show their knowledge of nature, and how they use this knowledge.

It is also of some interest to know what diseases a people like the Santals has, or knows of, and to ascertain their amount of knowledge in this respect. In this respect I have had assistance from properly qualified doctors (from Mrs. Bodding, M.B. & Ch. B. (Edin.) and, at one time, from Dr. B. B. Bögh).

There is just a possibility that in the very large heap of medicinal ingredients made use of by the Santals there may be one or two, the qualities of which it might be advantageous to find out and to test.

When the writer in January, 1890 came out to the Santals, he was from the very first brought into contact with their medicine. It did not take long to be made aware of the Santals having medical treatment and medicines of their own, and of their belief in this. They might doubt the efficacy of certain medicines; but many were affirmed to be 'proved,' as they called it.

It was not seldom to hear them profess to be able to cure what European doctors consider hopeless. In some cases (not hopeless ones) that came to the writer's notice it also seemed to be a fact that they had applied remedies of an efficacious nature.

This possibility that something of value might be found, in connection with ethnological curiosity, made me commence taking down 'prescriptions' of theirs that I happened to come across. I think the first I ever wrote down was one of their remedies for rabies. One of our workers had a large scar at the pit of the stomach. Being asked how he had got this, he told he had once been badly bitten by a mad dog. His grandfather had given him some medicine, and nothing had happened to him, whilst others that had been bitten by the same dog and had got no medicine, all died. Then came a remedy for gravel, another for dysentery, and so on, to be followed by 'medicines' to prevent a wife from running away, and remedies of a similar nature. As will be understood, I got from the very first into the middle of it and was met with examples of what might be sensible, and with examples of rank humbug and superstition.

There is scarcely a grown up Santal man who has not some knowledge of the kind of medicine treated of here, as is only natural considering the lack of real professional help amongst the people; every one has to rely to some extent on himself. One man knows, *e.g.*, a remedy for cough, another for diarrhœa, a third for snake bite, and so on. It is reported to have helped some, then why not others? Some are regular specialists in the treatment of, *e.g.*, tuberculosis or venereal disease, charging specialists' fees. Some persons may have established quite a reputation and are sought by patients from far away.

It might also be mentioned that the Santal young men are supposed to go through a kind of course in *mantars* and medicine among other matters. This has been fully described in the paper entitled The Santals and Disease.

Some know remedies for several diseases, and a few have taken up seriously "medicine" as a profession and are all round medicine-men who try to, or profess, to cure all diseases and ills not caused by supernatural agencies, *i.e.*, by *boṅgas* (evil spirits of sorts) or by witches.

It should be mentioned, that there are very few Santals, if any at all, who have "medicine" for their only means of subsistence. For most it is a mode of earning just a little outside the ordinary, a means of getting good food and a drink now and then. For some few it may mean a good income in addition to their agricultural earnings.

It is generally only men who practise. Women may sometimes be found assisting their husbands when they give certain medicines, *e.g.*, to females.

A practising woman would undoubtedly be suspected of being something more than a "doctor"; she would be taken to be a witch very likely. It may, however, happen that a woman "knows" some remedy or other and may make use of such knowledge. I have heard of a very few women practising, all considered 'doubtful,' but also clever "doctors."

As mentioned above, the writer commenced taking down "prescriptions" and other matters connected with Santal medicine some thirty-four years ago, and continued doing so occasionally, so long as people were found who could be "tapped." How many such sources there have been, it might be difficult to say. I shall mention a few of my sources as examples.

At Mohulpahari where the writer has spent most of his time in India and has his home, a Santal, living in the village of the same name was regularly practising. He was one of the most sensible of his class that I have come across. His remedies were all herbs, roots, barks and fruits of sorts, never a large conglomeration of all kinds of stuff (some of them next to impossible to procure, a method offering an easy expedient, although perhaps not often resorted to, of putting the blame for failure on the absence of some of the stuff enumerated). I also saw this man setting a fractured bone very nicely and doing other things which one would not think an uncivilized Santal capable of, and which they, for the matter of that, also generally are unable to do properly.

I prevailed upon this man to sell me his knowledge. He came when he "remembered" something, and some three scores of the "prescriptions" recorded are due to him. He made me promise, that so long as he lived I should not divulge his mode of treatment or any of his secrets to any one here in these parts, in order not to give him competitors and deprive him of certain means of income. He is dead now many years ago. This man did not believe in *ojhaism,* but I have been told, that in order not to lose his practice, and to please his patients he had to affect appeasing the *boṅgas* by offering sacrifices to them, a significant feature both as regards himself and as regards his patients.

Another Santal from whom I have got a large number of prescriptions is one of our mission-workers now in the Dinajpur district. He had been practising both in this district and in Dinajpur long before he became a Christian, and has continued, although perhaps not to such an extent as formerly. Having heard of his reputation I asked him to write down his "knowledge." Not being much of a calligrapher himself he dictated what he had to tell to a schoolmaster. In many cases he has given also some of the symptoms of the diseases. He apparently has a very strong belief in the efficacy of his medicines. This man is the most "learned" Santal 'physician' I have come across. He has collected "prescriptions" from all sides, according to his lights not uncritically, as I have understood him to know of much that he has not put down, because he did not believe in it. Most he has got from other Santals, a few he must have got from Bengali sources.

A third "authority" who might be mentioned is now an old man who has been with the writer for more than thirty years, as a literary helper and ethnological collector.

When he heard about this matter being looked into he became quite excited and forthwith commenced to go round collecting stuff from all he could get hold of. Many "remedies" the essential part of which is based on superstition and belief in magic have been collected by him.

Other people showed a similar interest, when they heard about the prospect of something being published on their own medicine. Several persons came and offered their "knowledge," sometimes for a consideration, but just as often out of interest in the fact that their own medicines were to be brought to the knowledge of others. The large number of contributors made it possible to follow several of these remedies to some common source. There may also be some common forms of treatment, presupposing a kind of 'school,' if such an expression is permitted.

I have to thank my old friend and colleague, the late Mr. H. J. Muston, for having relieved me of the drudgery of transcribing and translating most of the Santali original manuscripts. Wherever possible it has been thought to be of interest to have a literal translation. When there seems to be no doubt on the subject, our names of diseases have been given.

I am sorry I have not been able to get the botanical names of all the plants used in Santal medicine, and I am not quite certain as to the correctness of all the botanical names given. The Santali names are there, and if any one should wish to investigate the nature of the stuffs used it will always be possible to procure the genuine article itself. I have, as to botanical names, drawn freely on Dr. Campbell's dictionary.

It would have been easy to cut the whole down so as to leave only the botanical ingredients of the different "prescriptions." Doing this would, however, have made the present work serve only one of the purposes for which it is written, and that not the essential one, *viz.*, to be of some possible service to medicine. When so much more has been recorded and a literal translation has been given, the great ethnological interest attached to the subject must serve as an explanation and excuse.

II.

As to the original sources of these 'prescriptions' it is difficult to say anything with certainty; it seems that the bulk of them is indigenous. The ingredients are mostly what is to be found in the forests of the Santal country; the names are mostly Santali ones.

So far as I remember only two are of clear European origin, that of Cod-liver-oil for night-blindness, quite recently received through missionaries, and carbolic acid used against syphilis. This last one they have very likely received from some compounder or other. The use of hot tea for dysuria and constipation is likely a 'discovery' of their own.

A few are easily traced to Indian bazar medicine, *viz.*, those that for ingredients have stuffs bought in the bazars, all having Bengali or Hindi names.

Some may possibly have originally come from one of the Hindu systems of medicine. Those who have studied these will be able to tell whether this is so or not. I have understood that some Santal *ojhas* have learnt from non-Santal *ojhas*, from some belonging to the *kamar* (blacksmith), *ḍọm* and other castes, also (very rarely) from Paharias and even Jolhas. All this will, however, amount to very little.

It may in this connection not be out of the way to mention, that the traditions of the Santals state, that their ancestors have learnt *ojha* 'science' from *Kamru guru* undoubtedly a non-Santal, very likely a Hindu. With regard to this person the reader is referred to the paper The Santals and Disease. One gets, however, the impression that what the Santal *ojha* has learnt from *Kamru guru*, whoever he may be, is not so much medicine as magic, *mantars*, charms, etc., with which to subdue or drive away the supposed malevolent spirits.

Kamru guru has in any case been a teacher of more than medicine. It might be remarked, that his followers, the *ojhas* of the present day, base their reputation as 'doctors' just as much, or perhaps even more, on their supposed ability to deal with the supernatural powers, as on their knowledge of medicine.

The *ojhas* guard their professional secrets with great jealousy.

Whatever there may be of foreign origin, the medicines are now generally 'santalized.'

There are no invocations or *mantars* connected with the collection and preparation of the medicines. The only thing of a similar nature is the *ran jagao,* the 'awakening' or blessing of medicine, at the time of the Santal *Dasãe pọrọb* when the year's course in *ojha* 'science' is finished (see paper The Santals and Disease, where all this has been described); this does not, however, refer to any special ingredient, but to the effectiveness of medicine in general. There are, as will be seen, certain instructions given as to time and mode of collection of certain ingredients; but this is all, so far as I have noticed, and the medicine-men deny the use of invocations. This does not, as is mentioned elsewhere, exclude that *mantars* and invocations, partly combined with sacrifices or sacrificial acts or promises of such, are resorted to by the *ojha* and the patient's relatives. This is part of the *ojha*'s business. All this does not, however, seem to have anything to do with the application of the remedies as such; it is resorted to, not to make the stuff itself efficacious, but as a safeguard, by excluding or preventing the influence of malevolent spirits. The *mantars* muttered when using the oil-oracle, also the 'reading' over oil, salt and such things, might be mentioned; but it is not the efficacy of the remedies that is the primary object.

As to the age of the 'prescriptions' here recorded it is with our present knowledge not possible to say anything. Some of the remedies are of quite recent date, others may be followed back for some generations. They are also very likely adapted to time and locality, 'improved' or otherwise.

How they have got some of their remedies a couple of examples will show.

The writer had many years ago a dog famed for his exploits as a snake-killer. Once during my absence from home this dog was badly bitten by a poisonous snake. His neck, I was afterwards told, swelled up to a large size and all were sure the dog would succumb. Then the dog was seen to go to a place in the compound and there ate some herb or other, whereupon he recovered. A servant had followed the dog and saw what he did. He and the others were sure the dog had shown an infallible remedy for snake-bite.

Santals are reported to have watched the common lizard or the mongoose and to have seen what these have used for sting of scorpions and scolopenders and for snake-bite. During such encounters lizards and mongooses, it is told, have been seen to eat certain plants or the bark of certain trees, and also to rub themselves against the same trees or plants.

I have heard a story of a couple of men watching an old hanuman monkey treating and curing a couple of young monkeys bitten by a cobra. The old hanuman was acting like a regular doctor, feeling the hands, *i.e.*, the pulse, of the patients. Having in this way ascertained what was the matter he had bitten off the bark of a certain tree, had chewed this, and spitting it into their mouth he had made them eat this whilst he also applied some of the same stuff on the spot bitten. The young monkeys recovered very quickly, whilst before treatment they had been very low.

Now this story is a rather tall one and likely invented to make people believe. But even so, such stories show that the Santals believe in, and are not unwilling to make use of the animal instinct. It should, however, be added that all stories of this kind that I have heard are restricted to the class mentioned, to find an antidote against poison, as is quite natural.

Another remedy was got in the following way: One night a man dreamed that a dead relative of his came and told him about an infallible medicine for *puni*, atrophy in babes. The remedy was the egg of the humming bird, to be eaten. This is just mentioned because it may be of some psychological interest.

In this connection it may be noted that the Santals have also a belief that a disease may be either caused or cured by some stuff the name of which sounds similar to the name of a disease, or the shape of which may in some way remind one of some of the symptoms.

They say that eating *mandargọm* (Anona squamosa) will cause *manda*, a cold. They do not, however, seem to heed this much; they are fond of *mandargọm*.

The roots of a shrub they call *pẹṭ cambṛa* (Helicteres Isora), the fruit of which has a peculiar twisted shape, is believed to be a remedy for colic.

Among the ingredients used for small-pox are the conical prickles of the simol tree (Bombax malabaricum, DC.) and the 'warts' found on the leaves of the Ficus glomerata, Roxb., both likely reminding a Santal of the small-pox eruptions.

The remedies just mentioned may be classified as belonging to what is called homœopathic magic. They have a fair number of these, especially for the many kinds of what is called *bạị*, convulsions, cramps, an involuntary state or movement of the body, or any part of the body, over which one has no control. They distinguish a large number of *bạị* according to the symptoms.

For what they call *dhinuk bạị*, bow-cramp (something like the convulsions in tetanus), one remedy is the dirt scraped off a bow.

For what is called *halman bai*, monkey cramp, one remedy is to get the head of a monkey and rub this against a stone and smear on the stuff thus procured.

For *harna bai*, deer cramp, so called because the patient is in trepidation, grinds the teeth and moves the upper lip like a deer when eating, a deer's horn is rubbed against a stone; part is smeared on his forehead, and the patient is to lick it.

For icterus one remedy is as follows: A bit of the bark of the mango tree with a little lime smeared on is given to the patient who is to stand turned towards the sun, when it is rising, with the bark in his hand. The medicine-man then takes a cup of water and pours the water on the patient's hand, whilst somebody else rubs him. In this way all yellowness is supposed to be washed away.

For what is called *jhapni bai*, when the patient is unable to open his eyes, as in coma, they use a remedy consisting of a small plant called *jhapni* by them (the leaves close up at night), and the 'eye' of a peacock's feather; these are ground together, plastered over the whole body, and also licked.

For what is called *kandon bai*, continual crying, especially in children, they use the dirt from a cart axle; the more the cart was squeaking the better; the dirt from a *carkhi*, a machine used to separate the seeds from the cotton, also squeaking, has the same effect.

For other examples of the same kind the reader is, among several, referred to Nos. 130, 134, 135, 140, 141, 143 and 148, in the work itself.

The last one mentioned treats of what is called *suar bai*, pig cramp; the patient foams at the mouth like a pig; he makes a sound like a pig smacking when eating. Here one ingredient is the jaw-bone or the skull of a pig, to be ground together with certain other stuffs, part to be plastered all over the body, part to be eaten. It is 'prescribed' that the pig whose bones are to be used should have been killed by a tiger or leopard; if such is not available the bones of a healthy pig may be substituted. That the bones of a pig killed by a tiger should be more efficacious than those of a pig killed in an ordinary manner touches another Santal belief, that qualities in an agent may be passed on to what has been acted on; in a similar way an implement used with success may be supposed to get special inherent qualities. We shall not follow up these superstitions here; traces are found elsewhere among the Santal remedies.

A couple of other examples of the above mentioned superstition may be referred to.

In diseases in which blood is seen, something of a red colour may be found among some of the remedies. Thus for spitting of blood in phthisis the red Nymphæa rubra is used, also a bit of a red woollen blanket (preferably of European make). In menorrhagia similar red-coloured ingredients are applied.

For male impotency one of the ingredients is a male sparrow to be eaten together with certain other stuffs. The sparrow is by the Santals considered to be especially strong in what is here desired, so much so, that 'like a sparrow' may be heard used as an opprobrium.

The remedies resorted to in supposed female barrenness might also be mentioned (see No. 261). Among the stuffs used is the dried umbilical cord; some midwives will secure a bit of this, dry it and keep it to be able to give to barren women.

One of the remedies for *aha*, vomiting with diarrhœa, especially in children, believed due to the evil eye, also belongs here. One is to take the kernel or stone of the fruit of Spondias mangifera, Pers., that has been sucked and thrown away; this is to be ground and given to be drunk in water.

For *ṭaru lạndup̣*, perforating ulcer of the palate, one remedy consists of a hare's excrement, hare's hair, and the stomach or quills of a porcupine. Likely the peculiar movement observed in the nose of the hare has been the origin of this remedy.

To cause mother's milk to dry up, a little milk is buried in a plough-furrow.

For a suppurating breast earth heaped in front of a plough when ploughing is moistened with water and applied.

A number of other 'homœopathic' remedies may be found; but the reader must be referred to the work itself.

To sum up: As regards the origin of the great bulk of the medicines practically nothing is known; but one may be justified in supposing that what has been the case with others has also happened with the Santals. They have hit upon something in some way or other and may have thought it efficacious; they may then have tried the same for other complaints than the one it was originally used for, have found it useless or possible, and have in this way been guided by experience according to their lights.

Sometimes one wonders whether people like the Santals have not more of the primitive instinct left than we have. Certain phenomena of a psychological nature might seem to point this way (so to say 'standard' dreams of theirs are curious, *e.g.*, about coming rain). Any number of vegetable poisons may be found in their forests, but it is very seldom indeed that one hears of a Santal having suffered by mistaking these for something else. To mention a concrete example of something similar: the Santals are very fond of eating some of the edible mushrooms. As is well known, some of the poisonous mushrooms may look very similar to certain edible ones. In Europe mistakes are sometimes heard of; among the Santals they are very seldom indeed. The writer has never heard of such cases; but as they have medicines to be used in such cases, they must be happening.

III.

As may be expected, the diagnosis of disease is a great difficulty with them, as soon as they are confronted with anything different from the common diseases of every day occurrence.

There are few grown up Santals who have not killed or assisted in killing animals and cutting them to pieces; they have also frequent occasion to see something, *e.g.*, when a dead body is burnt, although their natural feelings will keep them at some distance; they consequently must have some vague or general idea of the anatomy of their own bodies. They might be thought to get some assistance from this, but apparently do not get much. Bearing in mind how observant of details a Santal generally is, it is strange that they do not know more of their own bodies and the nature of their ills than they seem to do. Likely their superstitious fears that disease is frequently due to the malevolent influence of evil spirits may have something to do with this.

In this connection attention might be drawn to their names for diseases. Most of these are symptomatic, as will be observed. Exceptions are names borrowed from other races, however, also often symptomatic, and the names of a few diseases of a well known and easily recognized character, or of diseases attributed to some specific action of the spirits or the witches. The name is generally taken from some easily recognized, striking symptom observed. But as several diseases have symptoms in common the same name may be used for different diseases. On the other hand some diseases will show different symptoms at their different stages of development. The same disease may therefore be known by several names.

A few examples will show the position. Take tuberculosis of the lungs. As may be expected, they do not recognize the nature of the disease in its first stages. It is then called cough of some sort, generally getting a name according to the peculiar sound of the coughing or the amount of phlegm expectorated. In its more advanced stages it is mostly called *dhọk;* this name is also used for some form of bronchitis. As soon as haemoptysis sets in, all other names are discarded, and it is called *raj rọg*, the king-disease, that is, not the disease of kings, but the sovereign disease. I have an impression that the ordinary Santal often thinks that an entirely new disease has taken possession of the patient, when the spitting of blood commences. Tuberculosis in other parts of the body than in the lungs is naturally not recognized as such.

Or take syphilis. To start with, any venereal disease may be called *gurmi*, a name meaning heat and also used for some other quite different ailment. During the later stages when sores break out, these sores have different names according to site and appearance, and are generally considered to be due to different diseases.

A disease like cholera has many names. Their regular name for this is *hawa duk*, lit. air affliction,[1] a name that points to the supposed origin or spreading of the disease. The most common name is, however, *marañ laċ oḍok*, the great stomach outcoming, any abnormal evacuation being called *laċ oḍok*, stomach outcoming. Another name is *aṛhạia*, lit. two and a half, *viz.*, *pọhọr*, periods of four hours each, "the ten hours." This name refers to the rapid course of fatal cholera.

Murhuċ jọm, leprosy, is often called *marañ rọg*, the great disease. *Guṭi*, small-pox, is frequently referred to as *lạṭu kasra*, large scabies.

The use of names like these last ones is due to a peculiarity of the Santals: they do not like to name a thing by its proper name, especially if it is something of

[1] It might be noted that the name used by the Santals for an epidemic is *disom duk*. This may be literally translated "country affliction" or "grief." *Duk* means affliction, sorrow, grief. *Duk* alone is often used for separate instances of death, through a fatal disease or otherwise. *Disom duk* is used for what we call an epidemic, provided it is something with a high mortality. Their point of view is the way in which the whole land is affected.

a serious nature or something to be feared. To be bitten by a snake is thus generally referred to as being "hurt by a twig."

IV.

The work here published will give some idea as to the occurrence of disease among the Santals. They have at the present day generally speaking the same diseases as are found in the tropics among other races. They tell that they did not have syphilis, tuberculosis and leprosy until after the Santal rebellion, really an attempt to rid themselves of the foreign money-lender, in 1855. This is very probably a too sweeping statement; but this rebellion marks the end of an epoch in the life of the Santal people. Up to that time they were living much more by themselves, in the forests, fairly unexposed to infection from other races, and leading so strenuous a life that likely only the strongest survived, persons who had the power of resistance. In any case the state is now quite different. Venereal disease is fairly common, although not at all to such an extent as it is reported to be found among the surrounding Bengalis and Biharis from whom they have likely acquired the contagion. Tuberculosis is becoming fearfully prevalent among them, in spite of their out-door life. Their lack of understanding the nature and the infectiousness of this disease makes them careless. When the disease has entered a family it generally reaps a fearful harvest. Leprosy was not common among the Santals formerly; during the last generation it has become alarmingly so.

My wife who is a qualified doctor tells me that in her experience malaria is, as to prevalence, far ahead of all other diseases, also among the Santals. Next come skin diseases, such as scabies, eczema, ringworm, etc, and then bowel complaints. Dysentery is very common and often fatal.

Eye diseases are very frequent, and many have lost their sight through sheer ignorance and want of timely treatment. It might be noted that the Santals generally have splendid eyesight; cataract is very common and often seems to afflict people at an earlier age than is usual in our countries.

Pneumonia and pleurisy are of much more frequent occurrence than one would expect in a hot climate; the same may be said of rheumatic complaints; their exposed life and carelessness as to exposure explains this.

Tumours, malignant or otherwise, are not rare. Some of the horrible diseases caused by Filaria, so commonly met with in other parts of India, and also fairly frequently seen amongst Hindus living in the same country, are very rare among the Santals.

As a curiosity it may be mentioned that I have not heard that appendicitis has been met with among the Santals, only one suspected case has come to notice.

Among the so-called infectious diseases common in Europe most occur also among the Santals, with a couple of exceptions. Scarlet fever I have never heard of among them, and so far as I have been able to find out, diphtheria is practically unknown.

Among epidemic diseases the Santals recognize four or five, *viz.*, cholera, small-pox, measles, plague and chicken-pox. As regards the plague (with a borrowed name called *maha mạri*) they have fortunately not had it among themselves and consequently have only vague ideas regarding it; it has, however, been near enough to them to let them know its deadliness.

As regards chicken-pox, it is fairly common among them; this is not, however, classified as *disom duk* on account of its mild character, and medicines are scarcely used. If any one should become very ill or even die from this, it will be thought to be real small-pox with which this disease is often confused by them, and it is then treated accordingly.

Measles are of yearly occurrence and also feared; it is a fact that many children die from the after-effects of this disease, mostly on account of their ignorance of its nature.

Their ideas about cholera have been mentioned elsewhere; they know its dangerous character and are very much afraid of it. It will be found among the 'prescriptions' that some medicine-men warn against in any way touching the patient and against taking food or drinking water in their houses, and the person who takes the medicine to the house is advised to have a quid of ginger and some other stuff in his mouth as a prophylactic. With regard to small-pox they know the seriousness of the disease, its common course and symptoms and they are very much afraid of it.

In this connection some 'prophylactic' measures of theirs might be mentioned, as they specially aim at guarding against small-pox and cholera. Prophylactic must, however, here be taken in a sense different from what is the common meaning of the word with us.

These precautionary measures are of a double nature, on the one hand invocation of the spirits and sacrifices, on the other hand medicines.

In the month of *Magh* (Jan.-Febr., the month when the Santals change from the old into the new year; some customary remnants show that this month must have been the first of their year; now they follow the Bengali or the Christian year) the entire male population of the village, at a day fixed and after the usual preparations and abstinence, at the end of the village street sacrifice a black female kid and a black pullet and bury them there. At the same time they make vows to the spirits of the village boundaries that they will give them certain sacrifices next year, if they remain free from disease during the whole year. This 'precaution' refers to all kinds of disease, both among men and beasts, also against misfortunes and accidents, but especially also to small-pox and cholera. The sacrifices are followed up by giving some pills to every person found in the village. These pills are made by grinding some 46 different kinds of medicinal stuff and

[1] It might be mentioned that what they call *bobṛẽ ṭikạ*, lit. brahmin vaccination, inoculation with small-pox virus, has now and then been practised by them. I have not heard that it is being done at the present time; but I have met old people who have been through the treatment and even have been practising it themselves in their younger days, now some sixty and more years ago. This inoculation was naturally dangerous, and people died from the thus acquired small-pox. Since the introduction of calf-lymph vaccination this inoculation has gone out of vogue. The name used shows that the Santals have got this vaccination from others. It is not an original practice of theirs.

mixing them with country liquor. Where the sacrifices are performed they are divided into as many portions as there are house-holds in the village, whereupon the *ojha* prepares some rice-water in a leaf-cup. With the whole in a winnowing fan the whole assembly starts for the village, and entering every courtyard, beginning from the village street end, the *ojha* sprinkles the waterpots with the rice-water, whereupon the pills are given. This is thought to secure the inhabitants for the coming year. A full description will be found in No. 244. It may be resorted to even now; but I have no concrete example to refer to. Cp. the *ran jagao* described in The Santals and Disease, p. 72.

A similar proceeding is described in No. 243.

Precautionary measures taken against small-pox alone are of a similar kind. The male members of the village prepare themselves for a sacrificial performance, and a brown female kid is brought. The *ojha* engaged for the specific performance comes with a stick and the bark of Oroxylon indicum (called 'bear's winnowing fan' by the Santals) and a stick and the bark of Callotropis gigantea. At the entrance to the village street the *ojha* divides the barks into two portions, calling on *Siń boṅga* (the sun god) and *Dhạrti mae* (mother earth), and orders the village men to bury portions of the bark here and there at the end of the village street, whereupon they walk through the village street with the two sticks. Next they take the kid mentioned to the eastern boundary of the village and here let her graze in the name of *Nag Nạgin*; when the kid has grazed they walk round the village boundary with the two sticks and the kid; returning to the place where she grazed, she is sacrificed. The decapitated kid and the two sticks are left here. If they escape an epidemic, sacrifices are offered next year. If small-pox should appear in the village, some prophylactic medicines are taken by all. A detailed description will be found under No. 191.

It might also be mentioned that the Santals make frequent use of several kinds of amulets, worn in a string round the neck, the waist or at the elbow. The most frequently used form is a *mandoli*, a small hollow metal receptacle; medicines are put into the receptacle. Another form is what is called *amsam dhiri*, lit. dysentery stone, really ancient stone-beads found buried here and there, believed to act as a charm to keep dysentery away; these beads are of various colours, some resembling the evacuations of dysentery, and believed, when used as an amulet, to be a charm against the form of the disease, the evacuations of which correspond to the colour. A third form is a bit of a root or a bark tied up with hair (a bear's hair should be there) and kept on the body somewhere. These amulets are intended to keep away disease, and in some cases to keep attacks of a disease at bay (as, e.g., in epilepsy and bronchitis, cough, etc.). They are very commonly used and often tied by mothers on some part of the body of their children.

Going through the list of diseases will show what the Santals have, or rather what they think they have; but the above-mentioned symptomatic nomenclature with the possibility of wrong diagnosis must be borne in mind, also that they necessarily have diseases not recognized by them, counting them as forms of something else than what they really are.

V.

There is one matter that might be mentioned in this connection. The Santals have splendid teeth. It is not only that their food is likely less destructive to the teeth than what many other races eat; it has become a habit with them to keep their mouth clean. They brush and clean their teeth at least once daily. It is the first thing they do in the morning, many refusing even to drink water, until they have had a general teeth and mouth cleaning. It is performed with the help of a short twig of a *sal* branch.

This is chewed at one end, until it becomes something like a brush, and is then vigorously used, whereupon the mouth is rinsed with water. The *sal* contains some resin or juice that may likely be of some assistance in preserving, in any case in cleaning the teeth. The Santal children get accustomed to this mouth cleaning from their infancy, and all look upon it as an absolute necessity. This habit of theirs must to some extent influence their health; if they did not take such care of their teeth, one would likely hear a good deal more than one does of bowel complaints, remembering what they are treating themselves to in the way of food.

When Santals living in this district go to visit friends settled where *sal* trees are not found, they will always take along with them a good supply of *daṭaụni* (as they call these toothbrush twigs) for their own use and to give to their friends who have difficulty in procuring them; they know that such gifts are much appreciated. What has been told will show what the Santals think of the preservation of their teeth. Inflammation of the gums is not frequent. Caries of the teeth is, of course, met with; they believe this to be due to some *tejo*, worms or larvæ, that eat the teeth.

A few words on the sanitary conditions of the people may also find a place here.

The Santals are a jungly people; they have to be classified as agriculturists; but they have even now a good deal of the roaming nature of their ancestors in them. They like an open air life, sleep outside, and live more in the open than inside their houses. Their villages are much more sanitary than what one generally sees among the neighbouring races. They are, wherever possible, built on fairly high land, the homesteads lying well apart from each other, on both sides of a fairly broad street. The houses are put up round a courtyard, into which all doors lead. No door leads from the street directly into any house. There is one house for the family, until the sons grow up, when these will generally start a new household in separate houses, often on a separate plot of land. There may be two or three houses for human habitation on the same courtyard, I do not think I have ever seen more. Then there is a cowshed and a shed for goats or sheep. There will thus in time be four houses round the yard, one on each side of it. It is seldom really crowded. The sheds for the cattle are generally open and people often take there their bedsteads to lie on during daytime when the cattle are out. People who are ill are often put there during daytime.

The Santal houses are not sanitary. They have only one door and no windows. They are consequently dark. The roof may permit of some ventilation, but much is left to be desired here. As a rule they cook their food outside but always have a fireplace inside. During the cold season they generally, and also sometimes at other seasons, cook their food inside, the result being that the house, especially at night, is suffocatingly full of smoke. This does not, however, seem to affect the Santals much. In the house they store their rice and all other things for which they can find a place. Here the fowls also live at night. It is, of course, not possible to keep such a house clean, even if they tried. They have a regular housecleaning, generally once yearly, all being swept and the whole inside sprinkled with a special kind of clay-earth. It is considered the duty of the housewife or whomever she may put to do it, to sweep the floor and also the courtyard every morning before sunrise or just after, and once weekly, if so often, a Santal wife will clean the floor and often part of the yard with cowdung. This cowdung cleaning seems strange to others, and it may be thought to be a hot-bed for germs, but the Santals feel a house properly plastered in this way to be eminently clean. It keeps down the dust, whatever else it may do.

The Santals have practically no furniture. They have some pieces of wood to sit on and also some low stools, always without a back, and they have bedsteads, a frame on four legs with a woven bottom of string, always their own manufacture. They are never large, generally much too short according to our ideas, but properly made, they are comfortable to lie on. They use them as beds at night, and as seats during daytime; when not in actual use they are raised on one side and put out of the way. They are light and carried without difficulty by one person from one place to another. They may be said to be sanitary, really in this respect as good as any beds. In case of need they also sleep on mats, on straw or on anything.

The above is a very incomplete description of the daily environment of the Santals, but will be sufficient to give an idea of how they are situated. In certain respects the circumstances are good enough, in others they leave much to be desired.

They are fairly clean with their bodies, some scrupulously so, others rather the opposite. Generally speaking, there is room for improvements in this respect. They wash hands and feet whenever there is a need for it, and use oil of sorts to keep their skin soft and cool. Their own women wash their clothes, boiling them with ashes.

As regards food they are scrupulously clean, both when preparing it and when eating. They wash and scour their plates and cups; if they use leaf-cups, and leaf-plates, these are thrown away after use and never used twice. They will not eat what has been touched by others, except by certain near relatives. A wife may eat what has been left by her husband, but not *vice versa*. They may eat what has been touched by their children. Except certain near relatives they will not drink water from the same cup, until it has been thoroughly scoured and washed. They wash their hands and rinse their mouth before eating and always use their right hand to eat with, the left hand being used for certain ablutions, etc., and never for food or the like. What may be said on this point is that they are in ignorance of the necessity of having a 'clean' watersupply, and that they, as a matter of course, do not know what is essential, and what not, to avoid contamination. When they see that the water is clear, they think it is good.

They may be said to be less careful with what they buy of foodstuffs in the bazars. And they are not careful enough when they handle things. It is strange, they are sensible and careful with their own, but much less so, if at all, careful with things bought in the shops.

It should further be mentioned that they have a good deal of vermin, especially bugs, in their houses.

Whilst the Santals are very careful to go far away from their houses to pay their debt to the old usurer, as they sometimes style it, they are not so careful with passing water, and when anybody suffers from some bowel complaint, they do not always take the proper precautions, especially not with children. They do not know the need of being careful when spitting.

It should be mentioned that the Santal houses as a general rule are cheap structures, built by themselves. When a person has died in a house, especially when death is due to some dreaded infectious disease, it often happens that they let that house stand unused and build a new one, often some distance off. In this way the whole village is sometimes moved to a new site.

VI.

Apart from the ingredients which are bought in the bazars or from "medicine"-vendors and which are easily spotted by their foreign names, practically all the stuffs used by the Santal medicine-men are such as may be procured in their own villages, or found in their forests.

So far as the writer has been able to judge, the genuine Santal remedies do not consist of a composition of a large number of ingredients. They have in each case one or two that are considered to be the essential ones; one may hear the medicine-men mention these as such; then they have one or more which are considered necessary to bring out the proper qualities of the essential ingredients, or to make it possible to take the medicine. This, of course, refers to internal medicines. Externally applied medicines may need to be mixed with something, but may also be applied pure.

Santal medicine thus also makes use of what is called vehicles. Most of these will not call for any remarks. They represent what they have or use to make a stuff possible of being administered. It is perhaps more the last mentioned consideration than anything else that operates. The Santals do not object to their medicines being bitter or the like to taste; they rather expect it to be "tasty" in this way; then they will more readily believe that it is efficacious. It is not rare to hear them criticize European medicines as only tasteless water and consequently ineffective.

Some ingredients used are of a disgusting nature. I remember an old very respectable Santal who told me in confidence that some medicines of his had helped a large number of people against certain diseases. I do not remember what it was, and somehow none of this man's remedies have been recorded; but his great secret was that he in preparing certain medicines made use of *gẹl bar serma reak ič*, human excrements twelve years old.

There is one household medicinal stuff of the Santals which may be mentioned here; it is what they call *kạṅji dak*, lit. sour water, stale ricewater. When they have emptied the earthenware pots in which they have boiled their rice, they pour in a small quantity of water and let this stand in the pot until just before it is to be used for boiling rice next day. Then the pot is "washed" with this water which is thereupon poured out into a separate pot reserved for the purpose. When they boil their rice, the superfluous water after boiling, a quart or so, is drained off and also poured into the pot mentioned. In a couple of days the stuff will turn sour, if it is not poured into already sour old *kạṅji*.

This *kạṅji dak* is used as food for pigs and cattle which are said to like it. It is further used to exhibit other medicines and also as a medicine in itself, both for human beings and for cattle. Especially when intended for medicine it may be kept for a long time. The writer has seen some *kạṅji dak* which he was informed was five years old, an awfully horrid smelling stuff. It is kept separate in a covered pot, some new *kạṅji* being added occasionally to replenish what has evaporated.

VII.

As regards the collection of Santal medicines the following may be noted:

As mentioned above there are no special ceremonies or religious observances connected with the collecting of the different ingredients, so far as the work of the ordinary medicine-men is concerned. *Ojhas* might be thought to try to copy Hindu medicine-men; but it is explicitly denied that they use *mantars* or invocations. The 'religious' side of their work comes in, when they are going to apply their remedies. This has been described in detail in the paper The Santals and Disease.

Some special precautions taken will be mentioned below (see Sec. IX).

If some of the ingredients are commonly known and no mistake is possible, or they are of the kind that has to be bought in the bazar, the medicine-man may ask those who have called him in, to fetch, or, as the case may be, to buy the stuff wanted. As a rule he will bring all himself; as might be expected, he will not give much concrete information regarding the stuff he uses, or concerning his way of finding it. It is unnecessary to say more on this point.

An *ojha* or medicine-man will generally procure and keep with him a supply of ingredients that are not easily procurable. Thus, if he happens to come across a rare medicinal tree, shrub or plant he will take some of the bark, or whatever may be used, home with him, and in any case keep in remembrance the exact spot where he has seen it. A Santal is naturally observant of details; they do not soon forget what they have seen with their own eyes.

The bulk of the Santals has up to the present time been living in parts of the country more or less covered by jungle or forest; they have generally not far to go to find what they want. With some ingredients there will, of course, be difficulties.

It may be impossible to find the exact stuff. In such cases one ingredient may have to be left out, or something similar substituted. I understand that this is often done. The patient naturally has to pay the cost of the medicines, besides the fee.

The medicines employed are mostly part of trees, shrubs or plants. Sometimes the leaves or the fruits are used; frequently it is the bark; or the roots, or the bark of the roots. This last is so much the case that a common name of theirs for their own medicines, as distinguished from other, *e.g.*, European medicines, is *ręhęl ran*, lit. root medicine. They have an idea, that the roots of a tree, or what is underground, will preserve the inherent qualities better than what is above ground, exposed to all kinds of influences.

The medicine-man who goes to find medicines will carry along a *khonta*, the instrument always used for digging for medicines. A *khonta* is a wooden bar with a flat bit of iron fixed in one end, or it may be simply a bar of hard wood (so was the custom in former times, it is said). In such cases the wood is either *hesel* (Anogeissus latifolia, Wall.), reputed to be the hardest wood they have, or *icąk* (Woodfordia floribunda, Salisb.). This last is common in the forests and often used by the *ojha*, *e.g.*, at the time of *ran jagao*, when the *ojha* shows his disciples some of the most common root medicines (see the paper The Santals and Disease, Appendix I).

VIII.

As regards the preparation and administration of the medicines the following may be mentioned:

Some stuff may be given in its natural form without any special preparation, outside what may be done with foodstuffs or drinks, but will in such cases, if taken in, scarcely be classified as medicine, any more with the Santals than with others. An example of this is the use of *sińjo̜*, the bael fruit (Aegle Marmelos, Correa.)

Some stuffs are macerated in *go̜to̜m*, the Santal name for what in North India is generally known as *ghi*, clarified unsalted butter, specially in *go̜to̜m* prepared from the milk of cows, not so often from the milk of buffalo cows which is in many cases considered unsuitable for medicinal purposes by the Santals, or even what doctors call contra-indicated. Some stuffs are soaked in mustard oil, others again soaked in water or some other fluid and then strained. Some medicines are boiled, and even boiled down, *e.g.*, to the consistency of molasses. Some are prepared by infusion or by decoction.

Only in chronic cases, or in diseases that are recognized and known to take some time to run their natural course, will they resort to a mode of preparation that requires any length of time. The general custom is to prepare the medicine on the spot for immediate use.

The most common way of preparing medicines is to grind the ingredients on a flat stone with the help of a cylindrical stone called *guṛgu*, both found in every Santal household as indispensable utensils, and used for domestic purposes every day, specially to grind turmeric and spices. These two stone implements are, as a matter of course, well cleaned both before and after being used for preparing medicines, before, to be sure that no foreign particle shall vitiate the medicine, and after the operation to ensure clean food.

The proceedings when using the *guṛgu* are so characteristic, that a description may be of interest. When the stones have been properly cleaned, the medicine-man calls for a cup of water and some *sarjọm* leaves (*sarjọm* is the Santali name for the tree generally known as *sal*, Shorea robusta, Gärtn.; the leaves are fairly large and strong, and otherwise used by the people for making leaf-cups of sorts and plates). He thereupon takes the medicinal ingredients, roots, bark, leaves, or whatever they may be, one by one, and carefully washes them to remove all traces of earth or dirt.

The man takes his first ingredient, washes and crushes the stuff, using one end of the *guṛgu* as a hammer, and grinds it by rolling the *guṛgu* a sufficient number of times over it. He then adds his next ingredient, treating it in the same way, and so on, until the whole is crushed, ground and mixed. As the process goes on, a little water is sprinkled on by hand.

The medicine-man now takes a small leaf-cup made of one *sarjọm* leaf, and squeezing the prepared ingredients in his right hand he lets the water trickle down into the leaf-cup; one to two ounces of fluid extract will be the result. If a larger dose is wanted, the ingredients may be ground once more with water added and then squeezed anew.

The thus prepared medicine is thereupon taken in the leaf-cup to the patient who drinks the stuff,being instructed to lie quietly down for a while after taking the dose, to prevent vomiting, if there should be any such tendency.

Most internal medicines are administered as described. In some cases the stuff is warmed a little, and if anything else than a cold extract, prepared as described, is wanted, the medicine is boiled, as mentioned above, in water, in mustard oil or in *ghi*.

Internal medicine is preferably given on an empty stomach in the morning, repeated at noon and again in the evening, if deemed necessary.

When there is no immediate danger, consequently no great hurry, and it is understood from the known or supposed nature of the disease that it will take time to run its course, the medicine may be made up into pills and left with the patient with instructions to take them at certain stated times. The same may be done with liquid stuff, specially when the vehicle is some kind of oil, *ghi* or spirits. Some of the medicine-men seem to have a predilection for using this last stuff, something called *pạurạ*, spirits distilled from the dried *mahua* blossoms. In all such cases the personal presence of the medicine-man is not deemed essential.

It is in this connection of interest to observe, how instructions are given as to dosage. With freshly prepared liquid medicine the amount given is the contents of a one leaf leaf-cup, anything from one to two ounces.

With some preparations the patient is instructed to take as much as will go in a mussel shell, of which they generally distinguish three sizes, a small, a middle-

[1] This cup is made in the following way: a *sal* leaf is taken, the tip is just nipped off, whereupon the two ends of the leaf are folded doubly, a bit of stiff straw being pierced through the folds to keep the ends in position.

sized and a large one, in size equal to a small tea-spoon, a small desert spoon, or a small table spoon, respectively. If larger quantities are to be given at a time, they use either their own different kinds of leaf-cups, made of more than one leaf, as standards, or the common Indian measures for liquids. In the "prescriptions," when measures are specially given, they have generally been reduced to their English equivalents.

When the medicine is given in the form of pills, the size of these vary considerably. The size is given by reference to some well-known natural object of a fairly constant size. It may be a fly's head, a mustard seed, a pea, the excrement of a hare, of a goat or of some other animal, a cross-bow ball, and so on.

It will be observed that the dosage varies considerably. In some cases, perhaps generally, it is not really large; in others it must be called heroic. In such cases, knowing what they are about, they will watch developments and, when necessary, administer counteracting medicines.

If the remedy is for external use, an extract is not considered sufficient; something stronger is wanted. The ingredients are crushed and ground as described, then mixed with a little water as necessary, and placed in a potsherd which is put over some burning charcoal until the whole is sufficiently heated, that is to say, made just warm enough not to burn. The medicine-man then applies the medicine with his left hand.[1]

The plastering on of medicines is sometimes carried to extremes by ignorant persons and may become the cause of serious inconvenience.

When necessary or desirable the plaster or embrocation may be covered by a plantain leaf tied on. Bandages, as we understand the term, are, of course, unknown; rags and strips of old cloth, washed or dirty, have to do service. The plantain leaf is really a good substitute for an oilcloth or the like, and has the advantage of costing them nothing.

In connection with external remedies the following further methods may be noted.

The medicine is sometimes burnt to ashes and then sprinkled on. It may be rubbed on mixed with one's own saliva. Cuts may be first treated by passing water on them and then covering them with lime burnt from mussels.

In certain cases it will be observed that the medicine-man chews the stuff and thereupon spits it out, either in a bit of cloth to be used for the application, or directly on the affected part (such as the eye or the ear). Sometimes a fowl's feather is used for the application of the medicine.

---

[1] The right hand is not considered proper or felicitous. The left hand is constantly used in their medical practice. Why this should be so, is not so difficult to understand. When they say that it is infelicitous to use the right hand, it may possibly be to have an excuse for obviating the use of this hand. The left hand is otherwise the hand of dishonour, very much more so with the Santals than with us, because it, as remarked above, is used for certain undignified purposes, especially for certain ablutions. To use the left hand for any ceremonial purpose, for handling food, for greeting, or for handing anything to anybody, would be considered grossly insulting in a person who is supposed to know the proprieties. Why the left hand with all this against it, should be propitious for applying external medicine, for this I have never heard an explanation offered.

To reduce *prolapsus recti* they use the foot.

When bandaging bone-fractures splints are used made of cut pieces of *sar* (Saccharum Sara, L.), tied together at the ends so as to become stiff lengthways and flexible the other way. They are not unserviceable.

For certain maladies they resort to a kind of medicinal steam-bath. A simple steam-bath seems to be unknown. The ground, or otherwise prepared, ingredients are put in a generally new earthenware pot, the mouth of which is tied over with a leaf-plate. The contents are brought to boiling point, the leaf-plate is pierced to let the steam escape, and the pot is put under a bedstead (with a string bottom), on which the patient lies down covered with cloth that reaches down to the ground all round. The purpose is to make the patient perspire profusely with the help of "medicated" steam.

Another "medicated" steam-bath is given in the following manner: Some medicinal ingredients are ground and mixed with *ghi*. A bit of a shoot of a certain tree (Zizyphus Jujuba, Lam.), about six inches long, is covered three fourths of its length with the medicine. This "candle" is stuck in a ball of cowdung, the uncovered bit in the cowdung, the medicine-covered part standing out. The patient is made to sit on a low stool and is covered up with a sheet. The "candle" is lighted and kept under the cloth, until it is burnt down. The patient must not look at the "candle" during the whole operation; otherwise it will not be effective. This steaming is repeated several times, the object being to remove œdema.

In certain cases they make use of a proceeding, the idea of which seems to be to smoke out the *tejos* (worms) that are supposed to be the cause of the malady. It is a ludicrous sight to see when used, *e.g.*, for *reṅgol*, as the worms are called that are supposed to cause caries of the teeth, 'eat' the teeth, as they express themselves.

A kind of cupping is sometimes, but very seldom resorted to. My impression is, that very few Santals know anything about this practice; it is used by non-Santal medicine-men.

Surgery is practically unknown among them. They have no implements. They may lance a boil with a red hot iron, or make a puncture with a long thorn. Thorns, or now-a-days mostly needles, are used for puncturing some peculiar nose-trouble, called *simbṛa* by the Santals, and very common with them, whatever it may be. Strangely enough it is often women who perform this operation.

The disastrous way of trying to cure cataract by pushing down the lense with a needle I have not heard of any Santal doing; but I have met several Santals who have lost their sight utterly by having this done to them by persons of other races.

As a curiosity it may be mentioned that the writer has heard it told, that they have resorted to making a person dead drunk in order to make him insensible to pain when they have been forced to handle painful accidents.

They may be able to stand pain, but perhaps not more than other people belonging to the same stage. As an example of what they are able to do, the following may serve. Some people were out watching silkworms; then one man was bitten in the foot by a poisonous snake. They had a fire burning, and they took at once a firebrand and applied it, burning the whole out. The man did it himself.

IX.

What has been stated above is a description of the way in which medicines are ordinarily collected, prepared and administered. There will always be room for departure from the commonly accepted or practised course. In connection with disease many considerations of a personal nature will make themselves felt, combined with the feeling of difficulties caused by their lack of ability and knowledge, by fear and superstition, both with the patient and with the medicine-man. Religion will naturally come in, not to appeal to the goodness or mercy of the spirit world, but to attempt to appease or satisfy the supposed enemies, and to induce some special spirit-powers to keep the supposed acting inimical powers away, or to drive these away, if they are at all able to effect this; also these spirits have to be 'paid' for their services. This matter has been dealt with in the paper The Santals and Disease, to which the reader must be referred.

Some of the departures from the ordinary may be of interest ethnologically, and also of interest to the student of human nature.

A fairly large number of remedies are ordered to be given on certain days to be efficacious, especially on a Sunday morning, the very first thing, even before they pay their 'dues' to nature. Sunday is considered a felicitous day, not only for administering medicine, but also for a good many other things.

In some 'prescriptions' instructions are given, that the water to be used for the preparation of the medicine has to be dew. The dew is collected in the following way: a clean piece of cloth is taken out and dragged over the grass in the morning and then squeezed out. The dew is supposed to have certain qualities due to its mysterious appearance.

Similar qualities are attributed to hail-water. Hail stones are sometimes collected and kept in a bottle for future possible medicinal use. That the hail immediately melts does not matter; the supposed quality remains, as the propelling force is supposed to remain in a spent bullet or in a supposed 'thunderbolt'. I cannot remember having heard that rainwater is especially used, as might have been expected.

Considerations of a similar nature are probably underlying certain specific instructions given in connection with some remedies. Certain qualities of purity, that is to say, of being untouched, or unused, or of being unexposed to extraneous influence, are supposed to be necessary for, and to give efficiency, to the medicine. Foreign influence is in certain cases supposed to hinder or vitiate the action of the remedies.

The simplest form this takes is the employment of a new, unused earthenware pot for preparing or administering a remedy. It has likely also something to do with the idea of cleanliness, as we understand it. The idea especially to be compared is, however, that of religious or social contamination. Dirt is objectionable, but may be removed. When a vessel has been handled by anybody for use some undefinable matter or quality or influence of this somebody is supposed to stick to the vessel; it becomes polluted for others, whilst it is quite good for those who have it in use.

When girls who have not been married are mentioned now and then in connection with certain ingredients, it is probably not so much the idea of virginity that is thought of, as the fact that such a girl has not been exposed to, or is not under the influence of other people than her own family, and perhaps specially of *bongas* worshipped by the members of another family than that of her father. To understand this it should be remembered that a Santal woman has no religion of her own: all her regular relations with the supernatural have to go through her male relatives, father, brother, husband, or son, as the case may be. A woman has to keep away from participation in sacrifices. When married she is supposed to be under the influence, or within the sphere, of her husband's *bongas*.[1]

The above statement should not be taken as implying that the Santals disregard morality. There is much to be desired in this respect among them: but they really prize chastity in their woman-kind. An unmarried loose character would not in any way be thought proper for the herein mentioned cases.

It will be observed that chastity is expressly demanded in many 'prescriptions'; see remarks at the end of this section. In one 'prescription' it is said: 'You, the medicine-applier, must be chaste and have no intercourse with women, and the patient must remain so also until he is cured' (see No. 90.). Even when applying medicines to cattle this is mentioned (see Vet. No. 2, c.).

Some similar vague idea seems to be underlying the application of the warm dung of a heifer which has not calved (see No. 156, c.).

In one case (for Tinea tonsurans) instructions are given that the maternal uncle of a child suffering from this should bathe on a Sunday morning, then come and after wiping his feet wring out the water from his wet towel on the head of his nephew or niece. These relatives (maternal uncle and nephews or nieces) are supposed to show each other particular respect and honour, honour each other like honouring the sun (or Supreme Being), as they express themselves.

In some of the 'prescriptions' it is said that a potsherd of a pot broken by falling down from (the head of) an unmarried girl will be efficacious for certain sores, when rubbed in water and applied. The same is, however, also said about a potsherd that has been turned out of its hole by a certain snake, called *tutri* (Eryx conicus) by the Santals.

One medicine for puerperal fever is to take some leaves of one tree and the roots of another, grind these and mix them with the urine of the woman's husband who is to apply the remedy to her abdomen; he himself must do it, no one else.

In one case it is ordered that the medicine-man must not see the patient for two weeks, but must send the medicine by someone else. The reason for this is not obvious. In another class of 'prescriptions' the applier is warned to keep his breath during the operation. It has to be done *mil satahẹlte*, in one breathing, the object apparently being to prevent contamination, and thereby

[1] To avoid misunderstanding it might be noted that it is the *bongas* a Santal woman is kept away from, that is to say, from all acts through which relations or connection with any *bonga* are supposed to be established. A woman is free to invoke the Supreme Being: she could not be prevented. If she tried to establish any connection with a *bonga* through a sacrifice, she would, if discovered, be treated as a witch.

lack of efficiency, by the remedy being exposed to the breath of the person acting. Strangely enough, this applies only during the operation itself, not at any other time.

In connection with this the reader may be referred to what is said about certain proceedings during protracted labour; it is instructive (see No. 270).

In certain cases the patient is instructed to walk home, or to go inside his house, after the application of the remedy, without looking back or anywhere. This is probably something of the same nature as that mentioned above; the patient is to be guarded against extraneous influence, only that it seems as if the object in view here is to prevent the patient from, in some way or other, becoming unsuitable for the effects of the medicine, more than to secure the efficiency of the remedy itself.

Something of the same kind also applies to the *ojha*; in certain circumstances he has to walk away from where the patient is, without looking backwards or to any side. He is taking something dangerous along with him, and this must not get an opportunity of slipping back to the patient. See The Santals and Disease, p. 26 s.

There is one more matter to be mentioned in this connection. It will be observed that in some cases it is ordained that those to be treated are to practise what is called *nẹo dhọrọm*. It has been translated 'become priests,' an expression that will need some explanation. The Santals have a custom (also met with among other races) strictly adhered to: during the night previous to the performance of any sacrifice all concerned, but especially the sacrificer, sleep on a mat, or on straw, on the floor, and not on a bed, and keep themselves away from women in order not to be polluted. This is what they call *nẹo dhọrọm*. As elsewhere remarked the women are kept away from religious observances; they are not fit for them and would pollute. It might also be noted that the Santals speak of sexual intercourse, even between married couples, as *bạṛič kạmi*, a bad act, an evil doing, that pollutes, the purification from which comes when a child is born. It is unnecessary here further to point out what may be implied by the demand of this precaution. The same is to be observed previous to 'medicine' being administered to cure barrenness in a woman.

X.

In connection with Santal medicine a few household remedies of theirs are to be mentioned that have not found a place among the prescriptions, or have not been properly described. A medicine-man or an *ojha* may make use of these, or order them to be used; but they are not considered as being inside the special domain of the profession, more than, *e.g.*, a hot-water bottle would be with us.

The household remedies to be mentioned here are four.

In cases of local pain, also when this is combined with some swelling, they resort to what by them is called *tobak*. The point of a sickle (often more than one is heated, so as to enable the operator to work quickly) is made red hot, and the painful or inflamed spot is pricked with this, that is, just touched, the distance between each prick being anything from half an inch to one inch. Before pricking the exact spots are marked with ashes, just a little. The operation is said to be not very painful. It is often resorted to as a cure for a kind of headache. I remember when I first saw the marks of this on the forehead of a Santal, I thought it must be some kind of tattoo, the marks being quite artistically arranged.

If an infant child is to be treated in this way, a needle is used instead of the sickle. The operation is meant to be what is called a counter-irritant, and is aseptic.

Another counter-irritant of theirs is what they call *sǫsǫ*. *Sǫsǫ* is the Santal name for the well-known marking-nut tree (Semecarpus Anacardium, L.), very common in their part of the country.[1]

The pericarp contains a juice which the Santals make constant use of for several purposes, especially for blistering. When a blister is wanted, they take the pericarp and cut a small hole in it so as to be able to get at the juice that is found inside. Having wound a little thread or the like round a small bit of wood they insert this into the pericarp and let it be saturated with the juice. With the 'brush' thus prepared the skin is marked where, and to such an extent as, wanted. In a few hours a blister will commence to develop with gradual accumulation of fluid. After a couple of days this is punctured. If careful, there is no suppuration. It is painless. It is extensively used both on human beings and cattle.

It might also be mentioned that the Santals "distil" an oil of the pericarp. This is placed in a small earthenware pot with a small hole in the bottom. The pot is exposed to heat whereby the oil exudes; dropping through the hole mentioned, it is collected in a "bottle". The oil is generally stored in a receptacle which is a buffalo's scrotum. The oil is used medicinally, mostly, however, for lubricating purposes.

The other household remedies referred to are *sekao* and *iskir*, both most excellent when properly applied.

Sekao is a kind of fomentation, given in the following way: a large potsherd with live charcoal (what in Santali is called *bursi seṅgel*) is put on the floor close to the person who is to be treated. The part of the body to be fomented is smeared with *ghi*; the hand of the operator is kept over the live coals, till it is as hot as can be borne and thereupon pressed gently down on the affected part and kept there for a short while, until the heat is used up. The operation is then repeated and continued for a shorter or longer period; it is frequently combined with more or less massage.

Sometimes a knot of the leaves of the Ricinus plant is used instead of the hand; the leaves are so tied together that they form a kind of ball with a narrow neck, used as a handle. This may be more pleasant for the operator, but may become too hot for the patient.

Sekao is very commonly used and resorted to for all kinds of painful swellings and internal pain. Combined with *iskir* it is what they at once apply when something occurs, before they call in the "doctor".

---

[1] The flesh (hypocarp) of the fruit is commonly eaten, especially by children, often with disastrous results: if all parts of the pericarp have not been removed from the flesh of the fruit, the result to the eater is extensive blisters and sores round the mouth and in the face generally.

Iskir is massage and is given for what is called *haḍi* and other complaints of a similar nature. It is very commonly resorted to in order to counteract muscular pain due to over-exertion, rheumatic pains, fatigue, or anything of a similar nature.

To be able to give *sekao* and *iskir* is considered to be a necessary part of a Santal woman's education; a woman unable to give this would not be considered desirable as a wife. Men also know the art. All are naturally not equally expert; some are really excellent and have a natural aptitude, the proper touch; most will be able to do it somehow.

XI.

For reasons that need not be enumerated the arrangement of the herein following subjects is rather arbitrary. To start with, the sequence followed by a Santal, *viz.*, from the head to the foot-sole, was followed; later on some grouping seemed natural. On account of the uncertainty of the proper equivalents for the Santal names of diseases no attempt has been made of preparing an index of these. The sketchy table of contents given here below will enable anyone interested to find what is wanted. The numbers refer to the sections, not to the pages.

Some veterinary medicines used by the Santals have been recorded at the end of the work. Last of all will be found an Index containing in alphabetical order the Santali names of all ingredients used, so far as possible with the botanical or other equivalents, and in a third column, the numbers referring to the sections where the stuff has been recorded. There are also a very few names of ingredients, known to be used by the Santals, but not recorded in the work itself; such have no numbers. If there should be any disagreement between what is found in the text and in this index, this last one should be taken as what is believed to be correct.

LIST OF SANTAL "PRESCRIPTIONS."

LIST OF SANTAL "PRESCRIPTIONS."

1. *Up hende ocoe.* To darken grey hair.

Medicines: *Bana ic'*, bears' excrement.

Mithi, Trigonella Fœnum Græcum, Willd.

Mix and grind these together and rub the mixture into the head on three successive Sundays, and the hair will become black again.

N.B.—This is only applicable for young people prematurely grey, not for old people.

2. *Caḍrak* (*Ṭak*). Baldness.

Symptoms: This may attack everyone, both children and adults; the hair falls off entirely.

Medicines: (*a*) *Muṅga chal*, the bark of Moringa pterygosperma, Gärtn.

Grind and smear on daily.

(*b*) *Bhelãoṅja*, Cæsulia axillaris, Roxb.

Ekasira dare chal, the bark of Cratæva religiosa, Forst.

Caili chal, „ „ „ Morinda exserta, Roxb. or, M. tinctoria, Roxb.

Grind, cook in mustard oil and smear on.

(*c*) Anoint the head with *sukri itil*, pigs' fat.

(*d*) *Seṅgel siṅ jo*, the fruit of Tragia involucrata, Willd.

First rub this on the bald place some three or four days, then mix this fruit with *mithi*, Trigonella Fœnum Græcum, and after grinding both together cook in *gai gotom*, melted butter of cow's milk, and apply this oil to the bald spot, when the hair will grow again.

Only applicable for young people, not old ones.

3. *Ruate potorlen khan.* When the hair falls off owing to fever.

Medicines: *Boṅga sarjom rehet' chal*, the bark of the roots of Ventilago calyculata, Tulasne.

Gabla darereko tolok tejo, the insects found on the leaves of Acacia arabica, Willd., including their chrysalis.

Grind these together, take a little *gotom*, melted butter, and an equal quantity of oil made from *bagluca*, Martynia diandra, Gloxin. and after mixing both heat and boil them, and then apply; the hair will grow again.

4. *Bhãuri.* Vertigo.

Medicines: (*a*) *Bhãuri mala*, a vertigo necklace, is worn on the neck, and they touch with the point of a redhot sickle along the edge of the eyebrows; this is enough to effect a cure.

When this malady attacks cattle

(*b*) Make a mark like a cross on the forehead, or the sign of multiplication, heat some *utiń sunum*, mustard oil, and pour it on the back of the neck, which will prove efficacious.

(*c*) *Gại ghuṛạ*, Polygala chinensis, L.

Bhā̃uri mala, a vertigo necklace.

Grind these together and make to drink.

5. *Bọhọk̄ khub lọlọlen khan, ona reaṛ ocoe.* To make the head cool when it feels very hot.

Medicines: (*a*) First of all twist the arms and legs vigorously and rub the soles of the feet with *etko hasa*, the burnt clay from inside the fireplace; then

(*b*) *Bharbhạri sakam*, the leaves of Ocimum basilicum, L. or O. canum, Sims. Grind these, tie them in a knot in a corner of a garment and give him to smell; then

Tale bạgṛạ, the stem of the leaves of Borassus flabelliformis, L.

Pound this to shreds, heat at the fire and wring out the juice, then add about the same quantity of *utiń sunum*, mustard oil, as you have juice, mix both well together, pour on the head and rub it well in. Do this two or three times and the head will become cool.

6. *Goṭa bọhọk̄ tugum tugum haso.* When the whole head feels heavy.

Medicines: (*a*) *Kohṇḍa jọ reak̄ bõk̄*, the stalk of the fruit of Cucurbita moscheta, Duchesne.

Dhubi ghā̃s, Cynodon dactylon, Pers.

11 *gol mạric*, 11 black pepper corns.

Grind these three, mix with water, and smear over the whole head.

(*b*) *Caole mạric rẹhẹt*, the roots of a kind of capsicum with seed like grains of rice.

Thoṛa goṭẹ rẹhẹt, a little of the roots of Croton oblongifolius, Roxb.

Thoṛa jạnum rẹhẹt, „ „ „ „ „ Zizyphus Jujuba, Lam.

Grind these three together and rub on the fontanel.

(*c*) *Jọjọ sakam*, the leaves of Tamarindus indica, L.

Mihndi sakam, „ „ „ Lawsonia alba, Lam.

Dạtrạ sakam, „ „ „ Datura alba, Nees. or D. fastuosa, Willd.

Thoṛa buluṅ, a little salt.

Grind together, make a thin mixture with water, warm in a large potsherd and apply as a plaster along the whole length of the spine; recovery will follow.

hok haso. Headache.

Medicines: (*a*) *Kahu botke da*, the bulb of Bryonia lacinosa, L.
Karla da, " " " Momordica dioica, Roxb.

Grind these and apply as a plaster to the painful part.

(*b*) *Tale bagra dak*, the juice of the stem of the leaves of Borassus flabelliformis, L.

Squeeze this out, smear some on and give some to drink.

(*c*) *Chatni chal*, the bark of Alstonia scholaris, R. Br.

Grind and apply warm as a plaster, and bandage it tightly.

(*d*) When the pain begins smear on to the painful part the juice of *peaj*, onions, or *rasun*, garlic.

(*e*) *Sengel siṅ rehet*, the roots of Tragia involucrata, Willd.

Grind and apply as a plaster, and touch the nerve with a red hot iron.

If the patient has *simbra*, a collection of blood inside the nose, prick it, and take

(*f*) *Mõrẽ gotaṅ gol maric*, 5 black pepper corns.
Jhal maric rehet, the roots of long capsicum.
Lonphul, cloves.

Grind these, strain through a cloth and drop 3 or 4 drops into the nose at whatever time of the day he has the headache.

(*g*) *Lilkathi rehet*, the roots of Polygala crotalarioides, Buch and Ham.
Gol maric, black pepper.

Grind and squeeze a little into the nose.

(*h*) *Latha cip cirip rehet*, the roots of a species of Achyranthes.
Lendet, an earthworm.
Bharbhari jaṅ, the seed of Ocimum basilicum, L., or O. canum, Sims.

Grind and smear or plaster on.

(*i*) *Sinduari*, Vitex Negundo, L.
Seta kata reak jaṅtet, the seed of Grewia polygama, Roxb.

Warm and smear on.

(*j*) *Sanci maric*, black pepper.
Andia dhurup, Leucas cephalotes, Spreng.
Pond rasun, white garlic.

Grind and drop the juice so obtained into the nose.

(*k*) *Dhubi ghās*, Cynodon dactylon, Pers.
Pond rasun, white garlic.
Adwa caole, rice that has been husked without boiling.
Taher sakam, the leaves of Cucumis sativus, L.

Plaster on the forehead.

(*l*) *Tale dandil*, the leaf stem of Borassus flabeliformis, L.

Roast this and take the liquid that exudes, add a little salt, and rub the entire head therewith.

(*m*) *Adwa caole*, rice made from sundried, not boiled paddy.
Jeleń mạric, a long Capsicum frutescens, Willd.
Dhubi ghãs, Cynodon dactylon, Pers.

Grind these together and plaster on the forehead.

(*n*) *Huṛhuṛạ sakam*, the leaves of Cleome viscosa, Willd.

Grind and plaster on the forehead along the edge of the eyebrows.

8. *Kaparjạdi bọhọk haso*. Neuralgia.

Medicines: *Lil kạthi rẹhẹt*, the roots of Polygala crotalarioides, Buch and Ham.
Pẹ gan gol mạric, some 3 black pepper corns.

Grind together, squeeze out and drop into the nose.

9. *Bọhọk mõk*. Swellings of the head.

Medicines: (*a*) *Choṛa lạdạuṛi rẹhẹt*, the roots of Vitis tomentosa, Heyne.
Sinduạri rẹhẹt, the roots of Vitex Negundo, L.

Grind together, warm slightly and plaster over the whole head.

(*b*) *Dhurup aṛak*, Leucas cephalotes, Spreng., or, Leucas Clarkei Hook.

Get and dry this, grind it to powder, and putting it into a leaf like a cigarette let him inhale the smoke through the nostril on the side that pains.

(*c*) *Karla sakam*, the leaves ot Momordica dioica, Roxb.

Rub these into shreds like tobacco, wrap them in a rag and go off to a deep pool, smelling them as you go; on reaching the water immerse yourself or dive in and at the same time throw away the rag and its contents. On coming to the surface go straight home, do not look back or speak to any one till you enter the house, and the pain will cease.

(*d*) *Caole mạric rẹhẹt*, the roots of capsicum with fruit like grains of rice.

Grind and apply as a plaster over the part of the forehead where the pain is.

10. *Mẹndok'*. Opthalmia, generally conjunctivitis.

Symptoms. There is considerable pain with a gritty feeling in the eyes night and day, and a quantity of matter is discharged.

It generally commences in this way:—when rain first falls people wash their face in muddy water or bathe in the same; then they get this disease. Sometimes it commences without any apparent cause. It may become so bad, that the inside of the eye peels off. Some people have become quite blind from this disease. They do not know any medicine, and so on account of the pain they apply the first best root, and so they become blind.

Medicines: When the eyes burn much.

(*a*) *Lọṅphul* 1 *gọṭẹć*, one clove.
Baṛe loṛe, the sticky juice of the banyan tree, Ficus bengalensis, L.

Grind these two together very fine, and wrapping it in a small piece of cloth, squeeze the juice out into the eyes, when the matter will come out profusely. If the matter has already been discharged, then apply the sticky juice only, and the burning sensation will cease.

(b) The leaves or roots of *piṭuạ aṛak*, Spermacoce hispida, L.

To be ground fine, put in a piece of cloth and the liquid squeezed into the eyes for about five days.

(c) *Dak̄ catọm aṛak*, Marsilia quadrifolia, L.

To be ground and applied as in (b).

(d) *Tạṇḍi catọm aṛak*, Desmodium triflorum, DC.

Rọkọc̆ dak, the water of small molluscs or periwinkles.

To be mixed and dropped into the eyes.

(e) *Sahraj bele*, the egg of the Indian crane.

Batapi sindur, a preparation of red lead.

Gọtọm, clarified or melted butter.

Grind the first two ingredients together, mix them in the third and anoint the eyes with the mixture.

(f) *Rạsun*, garlic.

Tạṇḍi catọm aṛak reak̄ sakam, the leaves of Desmodium triflorum, DC.

Grind the garlic and apply as a plaster above the eye-brows; grind the leaves, wrap them in a cloth and squeeze and drop the liquid into the eyes.

(g) *Nanha pusi toa*, Euphorbia thymifolia, Burm.

Ambṛa chal, the bark of Spondias mangifera, Pers.

Cun, shell lime.

Grind all together and apply as a plaster to the eye-brows.

(h) *Poṇḍ rạsun*, white garlic.

Sarjọm bhiṭuạk̄, leaf stem of the *sal*, Shorea robusta, Gärtn.

Chew both together and blow on to the eyes of the patient.

(i) *Piṭuạ aṛak̄*, Spermacoce hispida, L.

Grind and squeeze into the eyes and they will become cool.

(j) *Baṛe loṛe*, the exudation from Ficus bengalensis, L.

3 *gan lọṅphul*, about 3 cloves.

Grind, wrap in a piece of cloth and squeeze into the eyes.

(k) *Bir poraeni rẹhẹl*, the roots of

5 *gaṇḍa gol mạric*, 20 black peppercorns.

Raepan rẹhẹl, the roots of Smilax ovalifolia, Roxb.

Grind together, wrap in a piece of cloth and with some lukewarm water squeeze into the eyes. If the third ingredient is not obtainable, do without it. A cure will follow in ten minutes.

(l) First put 5 *chimbṛi rạsun*, 5 clusters garlic, into your mouth and keep them there, chewing a little. Then make the patient look up at the stars (for this must be done in the evening), address him by name and blow on him three times. Then he must go straight into the house without looking back. If in the course of that night he does not get well, then next day get

(*m*) *Nanha pusi toa*, Euphorbia thymifolia, Burm.

Grind this and smear on his eyebrows, and drop into his eyes the honey of the *luti* or *dumur*, two kinds of small honey bees.

(*n*) Rub some *phiṭkiri*, alum, on a stone and drop 2 or 3 drops of it into his eyes once in the morning and again once in the evening.

(*o*) Wait 2 or 3 days and if not recovered get

Bir poraeni rẹhẹl, the roots of

Grind and make into pills the size of a grain of Indian corn, adding to the roots 1½ black pepper corns ground, put into an iron spoonful of hot water; then wrap in a piece of cloth and squeeze it by drops into his eyes.

For opthalmia in babies.

(*p*) Let the mother squeeze a little of her milk into a mussel shell, add a trifle of *phiṭkiri*, alum, and drop a couple of drops at a time into the child's eyes; this is enough to effect a cure. Give no other medicine, or you will make the child blind for life.

11. *Rọn kana.* Hazy vision.

Symptoms: In this complaint people see dimly in the daytime and are unable to see far.

Medicines: (*a*) *Toyo caṇḍbọl rẹhẹt'*, the roots of Desmodium gangeticum, DC.

Utiń sunum, mustard oil.

Cook the former in the latter and squeeze and drop it into the eyes.

(*b*) *Gạruṇḍi ạṛak rẹhẹl*, the roots of Acternanthera sessilis, R. Br.

Grind fine, strain through a cloth and drop the liquid daily into the eyes till they become bloodshot and painful, when the treatment should cease.

(*c*) First rub the eye for 3 days with *kuclạ jań*, the seed of Strychnos potatorum, Linn. fil.

Then *rọkọć dak thoṛa*, a little of the water of small molluscs or periwinkles.

Bẹrẹl sasań thoṛa, a little raw turmeric, Curcuma longa, Roxb.

Bilạti thamakur thoṛa, a little imported tobacco.

Grind these together and for three days drop one drop daily into the eyes. Afterwards eat the meat of a *karanat sim*, a fowl whose feathers, bones and skin are black, as a curry or made into hand bread, and in 3 or 4 days clear vision will return.

12. *Tirsuṛ* or *Chạni.* Inflammation of the eye.

Symptoms: In this complaint the eye runs at first and is at the same time very painful; no matter exudes. It may be present with headache or fever.

In the beginning the eye feels gritty as if a particle of dust were in it and waters freely and continuously. The eye will gradually get quite red and the entire eyelid become bare; and if no medicine is applied the eye will turn white, and when the pupil is destroyed, there you are, blind.

Medicines: (*a*) *Rọl jọ*, the fruit of Terminalia Chebula, Retz.

This fruit to be rubbed and the eyebrows anointed therewith. The patient is sure to get well in 3 or 4 days.

(*b*) The ears or fruit of *hạti suṇḍạ*, Heliotropium indicum, Willd., to be ground, wrapped in a piece of cloth and the juice squeezed out into the eye. A cure will follow in some 5 days.

(*c*) *Peaj*, onions,
to be slightly roasted and the juice to be squeezed into the eye, then it will get well.

(*d*) Leaves of *piṭuạ aṛak*, Spermacoce hispida, Linn.
Bark of *dare piṇḍạ*, Randia uliginosa, DC.

Mix and grind these, wrap in a piece of cloth and squeeze out the juice into the eye. Also mix above leaves with genuine pure red lead, grind the mixture and smear it on the eyebrows.

(*e*) *Hạti suṇḍạ aṛak sakam*, the leaves of Heliotropium indicum, Willd.

Squeeze out their juice into the eyes.

(*f*) *Suruj mukhi ghãs aṛak rẹhẹt*, the roots of Helianthus annuus, L.
Ṭạṇḍi catọm aṛak rẹhẹt, the roots of Desmodium triflorum, DC.
Dak catọm aṛak, Marsilia quadrifolia, L.

Mix these three and squeeze the juice from them into the eye; a certain cure.

(*g*) *Mahadeb jaṭa rẹhẹt*, the roots of a certain variety of the rice plant, or of a small shrub so called.

Chew this well and spit on a piece of cloth and then apply to the eye. The real medicine is mingled with the saliva. Do this in the morning, and in the evening drop in some *tẹrọm rasa*, honey of *Apis florea*; the white on the eye will disappear.

(*h*) *Sinduạri sakam*, the leaves of Vitex Negundo, L.
Bẹrẹl sasaṅ, raw turmeric, Curcuma longa, Roxb.

Grind together and apply from the middle of the head down to the forehead covering with a leaf of the plantain. Do so daily for 3 or 4 days. Cover the eye too with a cloth dipped and wetted in the turmeric water. Apply also some *mare jọjọ amṭha*, old inspissated juice of the tamarind, Tamarindus indicus, L. to the eyebrows, and drop *baṛe loṛe*, the exudation from Ficus bengalensis, L., both of which will cool the eye.

(*i*) *Piṭuạ ghãs rẹhẹt*, the roots of Spermacoce hispida, L.

Grind, wrap in the hem end of a cloth, add a little water, and squeeze it out into the eye. Do this for a couple of days.

(*j*) *Khandadhar ręhęt*, the roots of.

Cook this in *gǫtǫm sunum*, melted butter, and let him drop it into the eye from time to time as well as foment the eye with it.

13. *Mẹ̆t dak jǫrǫk.* Watering of the eyes.

Medicines: *Dare bạṅki sakam*, the leaves of the large Vanda Roxburghii, R. Br.

Rạngu,

Grind and drop into the eye, the watering and pain will both cease.

14. *Tǫkę.* Sty in the eye. Chalazion, Hordeolum.

Symptoms. This begins with a small pimple on the eyelid that itches and grows in size from day to day, so that if you do not apply medicine quickly it will increase to such a size as to put the eye out of action.

Medicines: (*a*) *Ul chal sę bhiṭuạk rasa*, the juice of the bark or leaf stem of Mangifera indica, L.

To be applied on the sty.

(*b*) Rub the finger on the hand till it is warm and apply to the sty, which will cure it.

(*c*) Point at the highest hill near you and as you do so say three times, "You, such and such a hill, my sty is higher than you," and then pretend to pinch or nip. Do this early in the morning and you will come home all right.

15. *Ṭesra.* Leucoma. White spot on the eye.

Symptoms: This complaint results from disease of the eye or watering of the eye and so it becomes white.

Medicines: (*a*) *Saṅkha rạput*, fragment of a shell bracelet.

Sim ič, hendę lęhęrak rokawak, the fresh black thin excrement of a fowl

Lạli guṛ, refuse of molasses.

Rub the fragment of a shell bracelet, and mix what comes off with the other two ingredients, and apply daily to the eye, inside as well; he will get well. This is efficacious with cattle also.

(*b*) *Capot*, Desmodium cephalotes (?).

Chew the leaves or roots of this very small and spit into the eye. He will certainly be all right in three or four days.

Applicable also to cattle.

16. *Joka rǫg.* Pterygium.

Symptoms. Some people call this *mẹ̆t pilạ* or eye spleen. Spreading somewhat like the moving of a leech (*jǫ̆k*); something grows out of the corner of the eye and spreads over the middle and covers the whole eye.

Medicines: There is a small nerve extending from the corner of the eye to the ear. You can see this when one is eating food that it pulsates from the cheek bone below the the ear up to the corner of the eye. Follow this nerve accurately and apply in little spots the fruit of *sǫsǫ*, Semecarpus Anacardium, L. The patient will certainly get well.

17. *Jharao jharaote mẹ̃t kāṛālenre.* Blindness resulting from the watering of the eye.

Symptoms: The eye turns white from continued watering. This we call *chạni* (see No. 12). Many people become perfectly blind from this complaint, and unless medicine is applied the eye will be entirely ruined.

Medicines: (*a*) *Tẹrǫm rasa*, the honey of the *Apis florea*.
Nanha toyo caṇḍbǫl, or *Mahadeb jaṭa*.

Apply the honey in the morning, and in the evening, chew the roots of one of the two others to fragments, and after spitting in a piece of clean cloth put in these fragments and squeeze the juice into the eye. This treatment daily will remove the white.

(*b*) *Baṛe loṛe*, the sticky juice of the banyan tree, Ficus bengalensis, L.
Lǫṅphul, cloves.
Kǫrpur, camphor.
Suruj mukhi aṛak rẹhẹt, roots of Helianthus annuus, L.

Grind the cloves and roots together, then mix the sticky juice and camphor and squeeze into the eye, i.e., the drops; or, the application of the sticky juice and camphor only will have the same effect.

(*c*) The root of *piṭuą aṛak*, Spermacoce hispida, L. may also be applied.

(*d*) If above are unsuccessful, then on a Saturday evening procure the roots of *toyo sagak* grass and soak them in water in a brass plate or such. Very early on Sunday morning before going outside, moisten with your saliva the vein of the neck where it meets the end of the shoulder on the same side as the affected eye, or spit on the medicine and rub; then the white will disappear.

18. *Kāṛā mẹ̃t'*. Blindness.

Medicines: *Bir poraeni rẹhẹt*, the roots of
Kulạị tarǫp rẹhẹt', ,, ,, ,,

Grind together, wrap in a clean cloth and squeeze into the eye daily.

19. *Mẹ̃t' poṇḍlen khan*. When the eye turns white.

Symptoms: This is the result of protracted fever or ophthalmia, and if the pupil becomes white, blindness follows.

Medicines: (*a*) *Lẹhẹr sim ič*, the thin excrement of a fowl.

Apply a little at a time to the eye daily and the white will gradually disappear.

(*b*) *Mahadeb jaṭa*

Chew this throughly and after putting it into a cloth and spitting on it squeeze the juice into the eye; in the evening when retiring drop into the eye *tẹrọm rasa*, the honey of *Apis florea*.

(*c*) *Nanha catọm aṛak rẹhẹl*, the roots of Desmodium triflorum, DC.

Seta kaṭa rẹhẹl, the roots of Gynandropsia pentaphylla, L.

Seta aṇḍga rẹhẹl, „ „ „ Grewia polygama, Roxb.

Grind these two together and squeeze out about 2 or 3 drops into the eye and then

Dhurup aṛak rẹhẹl ar sakam, the roots and leaves of Leucas cephalotes, Spreng.

Grind both these together and drop two drops at a time into the eye.

20. *Mẽt ṭhu tolak bạisạu.* To set an eye which has "burst out."

Medicines: *Baṛe loṛe*, the exudation from Ficus bengalensis, L.

Nanha pusi toa rẹhẹl, the roots of Euphorbia thymifolia, Burm.

Grind and squeeze out the latter into a leaf cup, pour in and mix the former, and wrapping it in a piece of cloth squeeze into the eye, and in the evening foment it with *gọtọm sunum*, melted butter.

21. *Ạndhuạ* or *Rạt kana.* Night blindness.

Symptoms: People are unable to see at all at night, but in the day time can do so perfectly well.

One 'authority' says: This may begin of its own accord, i.e., without any known reason, sometimes it is due to the head being heated, and sometimes it follows the eating of rice or curry cooked in an iron vessel.

Medicines: (*a*) *Nanha dudhi loṭa rẹhẹl*, the roots of Ichnocarpus frutescens, R. Br.

Grind these fine, wrap in a cloth, squeeze and drop the liquid into the eyes.

(*b*) *Karanat sim*, a fowl whose feathers, bone and skin are black.

Let the patient eat the meat of such a fowl as curry or fried with flour and he will assuredly get well.

The gall of a black goat, fowl or buffalo or such animal should be roasted and eaten by the patient and from that very night he will be able to see. This has been proved to be efficacious.

(*c*) *Bẹrẹl sasaṅ*, raw turmeric, Curcuma longa. L.

Thamakur, tobacco.

Rọkọč dak, the water of small molluscs or periwinkles.

Grind the turmeric and tobacco together, wrap in a cloth and drop the liquid into the eyes. Afterwards pour in above water and he will recover.

(*d*) *Raṅgạini jạnum rẹhẹl*, the roots of Solanum Jacquini, Willd.

Mẹrọm reak haṛhaṭ sisir, the gall of a goat.

Grind the first fine, mix with the second, and after roasting let the patient eat it.

(e) *Rańgạini jạnum rẹhẹt* the roots of Solanum Jacquini, Willd.

Gạrunḍi rẹhẹt, the roots of Acternanthera sessilis, R. Br.

Gạì ghuṛạ rẹhẹt, the roots of Polygala chinensis, L.

Mạric rẹhẹt, the roots of Capsicum frutescens, Willd.

Mare malhan rẹhẹt, the roots of an old Dolichos Lablab, L., a little.

Mẹrọm sẹ gạì reak̕ haṛhat sisir, the gall of a goat or cow.

Thoṛa im, a little liver.

Cook all well together, and let the patient eat it one day in the evening.

(f) 3 *gan bher bherko ạcurok̕ dak̕ uru*, some 3 water beetles that revolve.

Grind, mix with his curry and let him eat for about three days.

Grind *kawet rẹhẹt*, the roots of Abrus precatorius, L. and make into pills which cover with *guṛ*, molasses, and give to eat; he will surely get well.

(g) *Hako itil sunum*, cod liver oil; sufferers for 10 years have been cured.

(h) Take the *haṛhat̕ sisir*, gall, of any animal and some meat, wrapt in leaves, and roast in the fire, then add bits of the meat raw and let him eat the whole after dark; an immediate cure will follow.

(i) *Tạnḍi catọm aṛak̕ rẹhẹt*, the roots of Desmodium triflorum, DC.

Barańgọm rẹhẹt, the roots of Vernonia cineria, Less., or Glossogyne pinnatifida, DC.

Caole mạric rẹhẹt, the roots of a kind of capsicum, fruit resembling grains of rice.

Haṛhat sisir, gall.

Mix all together, cook and give to eat or drink.

(j) *Pusi awar*, a cat's afterbirth.

Bir poraeni rẹhẹt, the roots of

Grind, wrap in a piece of cloth and squeeze drops into the eyes.

(k) *Karanat sim reak̕ im*, the liver of a fowl with black feathers, bones and skin, extracted before singing the feathers.

Karam pẹpṛẹt, the tips of the leaves of Adina cordifolia, H. F. and B.

Gọ̃ṛẹ̃ pẹpṛẹt, the tips of Stephegyne parviflora, Korth.

Bońga sarjọm chal, the bark of Ventilago calyculata, Tulasne.

Icạk̕ darereko tọlọk̕ tejo, the caterpillars found on Woodfordia floribunda, Salib.

Grind the last four together and thoroughly mix the first therewith, make the whole into a ball, wrap up in leaves and roast in the fire. Then in the evening take the patient, and also a cup of water, along with you to the gate leading from the courtyard of his house into the street, and there make him eat up all the mixture of medicine and liver that you have cooked, looking up at the stars all the time. Then make him wash his face in the cup of water, and after turning him round three or four times tell him, "Now go straight into the house and don't look round, otherwise your complaint will return." If he does this he will be completely cured. If this remedy should be inefficacious, then,

(*m*) after three days drop *sisir dak*, dew, into the eyes, make him rub them well and wash the face again in water and then in the evening he will see. If not, then the next day administer as above again and he will be cured entirely at once.

22. *Lutur kalak.* Deafness.

Medicines: (*a*) *Biṅ ḍimbu.*

Pound and crush some of the roots and leaves of this, squeeze the fluid out into a leaf cup or something similar, warm this on the fire and drop into the ear.

(*b*) *Ẹtkẹč sakam*, the leaves of Euphorbia antiquorum, Linn.

Warm these at a fire, squeeze out the fluid that exudes and drop this daily into the ear.

(*c*) *Hanḍi kunḍi rẹhẹl*, the roots of Physalis minima, Linn.

Grind these, warm them and drop the liquid in the ear.

23. *Lutur belek.* Otitis media suppurativa.

Medicines: (*a*) *Boṅga sarjom nạṛī*, a tendril of Ventilago calyculata, Tulasne.

Cut off about a span length of this, blow out the water from it and pour it into the ear.

(*b*) *Hesak sakam*, the leaves of Ficus religiosa, Willd.

Pound these, warm the resultant juice, and pour into the ear.

(*c*) *Arak sindur*, genuine red lead.

Mix with oil and pour into the ear.

(*d*) *Phuṭiạ kạuḍi cun*, the lime obtained from the small shells used in India as money.

Oṛak sạṛimre janamok kana aṛak, Commelyna bengalensis, L., that grows on the roofs of houses.

Grind these two with water, wrap in a piece of cloth and squeeze into the ear.

(*e*) *Kulại lutur*, Emilia sonchifolia, DC.

Dạtrạ sakam, the leaves of Datura alba, Willd., or D. fastuosa, Willd.

Grind and squeeze out into the ear.

(*f*) *Pitua ạrak rẹhẹl*, the roots of Spermacoce hispida, L.
Qhọc ạrak rẹhẹl, the roots of Boerhaavia repens, L.
Dare pinḍạ chal, the bark of Randia uliginosa, DC.
Biṅ kạṅcur, the slough of a snake.

Collect these and cook them in pure mustard oil, which should be dropped into the ear and is sure to cure.

(*g*) Grind the mushroom that grows on a bullock's horn and squeeze it into the ear.

(*h*) *Hoṛ rapak munḍhạlre arakge janamok ot*, grind the red mushroom that grows on a log that has been used for cremating a corpse, and squeeze it into the ear.

(*i*) *Rohoe kundri sakam sẹ rẹhẹl*, the leaves or roots of the cultivated Zehneria umbellata, Thew.

Cook in *utiṅ sunum*, mustard oil, and when cooled down pour into the ear.

(*j*) *Hoṛ rapak munḍhạlre janamok ot*, a mushroom that has grown on a log left after cremating a human being.

Cook this in *utiṅ sunum* mustard oil, and while the oil is hot throw in a live *kidiṅ kaṭkom*, scorpion, and when this is cooked take it out, and then pour the oil into the ear, and a cure will follow.

24. *Toa jorote lutur belė.* Ear suppuration from the entry of milk.

This arises from the carelessness of the mother while suckling the baby; some suckle while lying down and the milk dripping into the ear causes the mischief.

Medicines: (*a*) Make a leaf cup of the leaves of a shrub growing by the wayside, on which dogs have urinated. Let the milk drip into that cup and then pour it into the ear.

(*b*) *Ato kundri rẹhẹl*, the roots of a cultivated Zehneria umbellata, Thew.

Grind and without cooking pour into the ear.

25. *Lutur haso.* Ear-aehe.

Medicines: (*a*) Squeeze the juice out of *ḍimbu baha sakam*, the leaves of Ocimum Bascilicum, var. thyrsiflorum, L. into the ear.

(*b*) Roast *dare bạṅki*, Vanda Roxburghii, R. Br., squeeze out the juice, and after drawing this off pour into the ear.

(*c*) Proceed in the same way with *tale bạgṛạ*, the crushed leaf stems of Borassus flabelliformis, L.

(*d*) Grind and pour in *caole mạric*, capsicum resembling grains of rice.

(*e*) If there is pus take *dhãi aṛak rẹhẹl*, the roots of Grislea tomentosa, Willd., cook in mustard oil and pour into the ear.

(*f*) Grind *alo pinḍa*, Amorphophallus campanulatus, Blume, and pour into the ear.

(*g*) *Kidiń katkọm*, a scorpion.
Munḍhạl ol, a certain mushroom.

Cook in mustard oil and pour the oil into the ear.

(*h*) *Piṭuạ ghạ̃s aṛak*, Spermacoce hispida, L.

Grind small, put in a piece of cloth, squeeze and drop into the ear.

(*i*) *Tale ḍạr*, a leaf-stem of Borassus flabelliformis, L.

Pound and fry, foment and drop into the ear.

(*j*) *Kaṭ ot'*, an edible fungus that grows on wood.
Tale sakam reak' rọs, the juice of the leaves of Borassus flabelliformis, L.

Pour into the ear.

(*k*) *Malhan sakam*, the leaves of Dolichos Lablab, L.
Piṭuạ rẹhẹt', the roots of Spermacoce hispida, L.
Kaskọm rẹhẹt', „ „ „ Gossypium arboreum, L.

Grind these together and squeeze the juice into the ear.

(*l*) *Kundri sakam*, the leaves of the Zehneria umbellata, Thew.
Batapi sindur, a preparation of red lead.

Sprinkle the latter thinly on the former and half roast them, or wrap them in a leaf and roast them, and then squeezing out the juice into a leaf cup, pour this warm into the ear.

26. *Kanoaṛe lutur ghao.* Ear sore.

Medicines: Get a caterpillar found on either *gabla dare*, Acacia arabica, Willd. or *icạk goṭe dare.*

Grind and cook in *utiń sunum*, mustard oil, and let him apply this oil daily with a feather.

N.B.—This remedy is also good for *Uru ghao.*

27. *Kankoṭra.* (To extract) an earwig.

Medicines: *Gạrunḍi aṛak*, Acternanthera sessilis, R. Br.
Muć aṛak, Polygonum plebejum, Br.

Grind and pour into the ear.

28. *Simbṛạ bọhọk haso.* Headache caused by blood congestion in the nasal concha.

Symptoms. As in *Kaparjạḍi* there is pain on one side of the head, which occurs either in the forenoon or afternoon, and by this it may be known.

Medicines: When the pain is on, look inside the nose and you will see something like a blister. Prick and burst this and blood will at once come away. Then apply the seed of *sọsọ*, Semecarpus Anacardium, *L.* in two places under the eyebrows, in one place on the nose, in one place on the cheek bone and in two places on the nerve (*sir*) of the nape of the neck, and do nothing more that day. Then next day repeat the whole operation and he will recover.

29. *Mũ mãyãmok.* Bleeding of the nose.

Medicines: (*a*) Get quickly some *kaḍa guric̆*, buffalo dung, make it into a ball and give him to smell, when the bleeding will soon stop.

(*b*) *Hoṛo bohok*, the head of a tortoise.

Roast to burning point, mix in mustard oil and let him sniff it up the nose when the bleeding will stop.

(*c*) *Naksuri baha*, the flower of
Bonkapsi jañ, the seed of Thespesia Lampas, Benth. & Hook. f.
Suruj mukhi aṛak ṛehel, the roots of Helianthus annuus, Willd.

Boil these together in mustard oil, let him sniff some up the nose and smear some on the head.

(*d*) *Khet pipra aṛak ṛehel*, the roots of Urtica pentandra, Roxb. (?), growing in rice-fields.

Boil in water and drop a little on the head; also grind, squeeze out the juice and pour a little into the nose.

This is efficacious in bleeding of the nose in both human beings and cattle.

30. *Dãtrisi.* Bleeding of the gums.

Medicines: (*a*) *Kulai ic̆*, hares' excrement.
Sekra chal, the bark of Zizyphus rugosa, Lamk.
Edel roṅga, the knots on Bombax malabaricum, DC.
Nanha dudhi loṭa, Ichnocarpus frutescens, R. Br.

Cook in mustard oil and give to eat.

(*b*) *Terel cete*, the thin skin on the bark of Diospyros tomentosa, Roxb.

Grind small and cook in *gai gotom*, melted butter of cows' milk, and let him rub the gums with this for three days.

(*c*) *Loṅphul*, cloves.
Kalia jira, Nigella indica, Roxb.

Grind these to a powder, and some to be eaten daily.

31. *Reṅgol jom.* Caries of the teeth with toothache.

Symptoms. A kind of worms develop at the neck of the teeth which they eat, and if medicine is not given all the teeth will fall out. When they are at work the teeth ache intensely, and the whole cheek may swell up.

Medicines: (*a*) *Soso sunum*, the oil obtained by distilling the seeds of Semecarpus Anacardium, L. var. cuneifolia.

Heat this and drop it into the cavity; it will burn, but effect a cure.

(*b*) *Kanṭhaṛ dare kaṭic̆ ḍhompo*, little lumps on the Artocarpus integrifolia, L.

Bring these on a Sunday morning, pound slightly and tie them on to the patient's ear.

(c) *Man sạru*, a certain variety of Lasia.

Grind this fine, cook in mustard oil and apply to the affected parts.

(d) *Hẹsẹl rẹhẹl*, the roots of Anogeissus latifolia, Wall.

Heat in mustard oil and apply.

(e) *Akaona loṛe*, the milky exudation of Calotropis gigantea, R. Br.

Smear a piece of cotton with this and insert in the cavity.

(f) *Lilkạthi rẹhẹl*, the roots of Polygala crotolarioides, Buch. and Ham.

Grind, extract the juice and drop this into the ear on the effected side.

(g) *Ẹdẹl roṅgatẹt*, the knots on Bombax malabaricum, DC.

Tie on his ear on a Sunday morning before you go to relieve nature in any way.

(h) *Beṅgaṛ bet̤ahel jọ*, the fruit of Solanum stramonifolium, Jacq.

Grind, wrap in a piece of cloth, dip in oil and tie on to a piece of stick. Set fire to it and let the patient keep the smoke in his mouth, or make a leaf into a funnel and blow the smoke through this.

(i) *Hẹhẹl rẹhẹl*, the roots of Millettia auriculata, Baker.

Chew small, dip into hot mustard oil, and putting it into the tooth set fire to it.

(j) *Cip ciṛip rẹhẹl*, the roots of Achyranthes aspera, L.
Sạuṛi ghās rẹhẹl, " " Heteropogon contortus, R. & S.

Apply to the cavity on Sunday.

(k) *Meral dareren tejo*, the insect or caterpillar found on Phyllanthus Emblica, L.

Find and bring this secretly; then go to the patient on Sunday, ask him for some *utiṅ sunum*, mustard oil, in a leaf cup, and after putting the caterpillar quietly into it pour it quickly into the ear on the side where the pain is, and catching the oil again into the cup as it comes out of the ear show him the caterpillar. If on seeing it he is astonished the pain will cease there and then, and next day the swelling will subside. If he is not astonished or does not believe, then this means will not cure him and something else is necessary.

(l) *Rạṅgạini jạnum rẹhẹl*, the roots of Solanum Jacquini, Willd.

Dry these and grind to a powder, and putting it into the bowl of a leaf pipe let him draw the smoke in to the painful spot and he will be cured.

(m) Saturate a bit of cloth in oil and wrap it round a bit of stick and plaster on it *rạṅgạini jạnum jaṅ*, the seed of Solanum Jacquini, Willd.; then resting it on a leaf pottle and applying the flame of a lamp blow the smoke in; let the caterpillars fall into a cup of water and show them to him saying, 'Look at them.' And if he believes it he will be all right.

The whole thing depends on the credulity of the patient.

Another way of "smoking the worms out" is, as follows: The medicine man finds a fairly large potsherd; on this is placed dried cowdung which is set fire to. This produces a good deal of smoke. To guide the smoke a kind of leaf-chimney is put on the smoking cow-dung, a large leaf being twisted into a conical shape, wide at the bottom with only a small opening at top. The patient is made to sit down and to keep the potsherd in his hands. The operator sits in front, orders the sufferer to gape as much as he can, and using the hollow stem of a plant as a a blow-pipe he blows the smoke into the mouth of the poor fellow. It is a sight to see.

32. *Sọnpat.* Inflammation of the gums.

One "authority" says: The gums are painful and all the teeth get loosened. If you do not apply medicine quickly, all the teeth will fall out, and then it will be difficult to eat meat or anything parched. It is when you have teeth you can make a satisfactory meal, while if you have only the gums you turn the food from side to side and then swallow it. Therefore lose no time in applying medicine.

Medicines: (*a*) *Sondhaeni*, Tylophora longifolia, Wight.
Tọtnọpak chal, the bark of Eugenia operculata Roxb.

Cook in melted butter; to be kept in the mouth by the patient.

(*b*) *Dater mañjọn*, (tooth powder).

Rub the teeth with this, it is very advantageous.

(*c*) *Poṇḍ kawẹl rẹhẹl*, the roots of the white fruited Abrus precatorius, Willd.

Grind and apply as a plaster to the painful part and squeeze out a little into the ear.

(*d*) *Siñjọ banda*, the parasitical plant found on Ægle Marmelos, Correa.
Khijur rẹhẹl, the roots of Phœnix sylvestris, Roxb.

Grind, cook in mustard oil and pour into the ear. If the pain does not cease, then,

(*e*) *Ṭaṇḍi piṭuạ rẹhẹl*, the roots of Spermacoce hispida, L.

Grind with water and after warming slightly pour into the ear.

(*f*) *Bọkọm chal*, the bark of Melia Azaderach, L.
Matkọm chal, the bark of Bassia latifolia, Roxb.

Boil in water and with that let the patient wash out his mouth.

(*g*) *Tarọp chal*, the bark of Buchanania latifolia, Roxb.
Sekra chal, the bark of Zizyphus rugosa, Lamk.

To be pounded a little and kept in the mouth like a quid of tobacco.

(*h*) *Raj baha sakam*, the leaves of Nerium odorum, Soland.

Boil in a brass-cupful of water, then take the leaves out and throw them away, and boil the water down till there is only enough to fill a 4-anna brass cup; then take it off the fire, and with that water rub the teeth every night on going to bed by dipping the finger in it.

33. *Jaṛi phuṭauk.* Ulcerated tongue.

Symptoms. In this sores appear on the tongue of both children and adults.

Medicines: (*a*) *Baṛ chal*, the bark of Mimusops Elengi, L.

Boil in water and let him wash the mouth out with that water until recovery; no salt to be eaten for three days.

(*b*) *Aṭkir rẹhẹl*, the roots of Smilax ovalifolia, Roxb.
Kadar nāṛi rẹhẹl, the roots of Asparagus racemosus, Willd.
Bạrsạpakoṛ rẹhẹl, the roots of Grewia sapida, Roxb.

Mix and grind these and give to drink.

(*c*) *Campa rẹhẹl*, the roots of Michelia champaca, L.
Nanha dudhi loṭa rẹhẹl, the roots of Ichnocarpus frutescens, R. Br.

Grind these two with dust and after cooking in mustard oil give to eat.

(*d*) Grind fine a mushroom that is red like red lead and has grown on wood or something like that, and after cooking it in melted butter give to eat.

(*e*) *Sekra chal*, the bark of Zizyphus rugosa, Lamk.
Ul chal, the bark of Mangifera indica, L.
Nanha dudhi loṭa rẹhẹl, the roots of Ichnocarpus frutescens, R. Br.
Turạm da, the bulb of

Grind together, cook in mustard oil and give to eat.

(*f*) *Bhiḍi toa*, sheeps' milk.

To be drunk and smeared on the tongue.

(*g*) *Sẹrwaṅ rẹhẹl*, the roots of Vigna vexillata, Benth.
Nanha dudhi loṭa rẹhẹl, the roots of Ichnocarpus frutescens, R. Br.

To be cooked in melted butter of cows' milk and then eaten.

34. *Alaṅ poṭagok̲ sẹ paṛagok̲.* Rhagades linguae.

Medicines: *Sekra chal*, the bark of Zizyphus rugosa, Lamk.

To be kept in the mouth like a quid of tobacco and given an occasional chew. Some more of it to be boiled in water and every morning the mouth to be rinsed out with this water until cured.

35. *Moca ghao.* Sores in the mouth

Medicines: (*a*) *Nanha dudhi loṭa rẹhẹl*, the roots of Ichnocarpus frutescens, R. Br.
Kujri rẹhẹl, the roots of Celastrus paniculatus, Willd.

Grind these together, cook in mustard oil and apply to the affected part.

(*b*) *Kọnḍẹṅ da*, the bulb of Eriosema chinensis, Voq.
Sekra chal, the bark of Zizyphus rugosa, Lamk.
Utri dudhi loṭa rẹhẹl, the roots of Cryptolepis Buchanani, R. & S.

Grind these fine, cook in melted butter and smear on the sores.

(c) *Sekra chal*, the bark of Zizyphus rugosa, Lamk.
Khayar chal „ „ „ Acacia Catechu, L.

Let him chew either of these.

(d) Let him keep *bhiḍi toa*, sheep's milk, in the mouth: he will soon get well.

(e) *Sekra chal*, the bark of Zizyphus rugosa, Lamk.
Sẹkrẹč chal, „ „ „ Lagerstroemia parviflora, Roxb.
Dạtrạ rẹhẹl sẹ jọ, the roots or fruit of Datura alba, Willd. or D. fastuosa, Willd.
Rọl chal, the bark of Terminalia Chebula, Retz.
Atnak chal, the bark of Terminalia tomentosa, W. and A.

Grind together and apply both inside and outside the teeth.

Take *ẹdẹl roṅga*, the knots on Bombax malabaricum, DC. and after rubbing off the thorns, make a hole and hang on to the ear of the side that pains him, on Sunday.

(f) *Sirom rẹhẹl*, the roots of Andropogon muricatus, Retz.
Nanha dudhi loṭa rẹhẹl, the roots of Ichnocarpus frutescens, R. Br.

Grind these, cook in melted butter of cows' milk and give to eat and he will get well at once. Also smear on the lips the milky exudation of *bir sạru*, Lasia heterophylla, Schott. which will heal the sores on the lips.

(g) *Baṛe chal*, the bark of Ficus bengalensis, L.
Hesak chal, „ „ „ Ficus religiosa, Willd.
Pakaṛe chal, the bark of Ficus infectoria, Willd.
Nim chal, „ „ „ Melia Azadirachta, L.
Hạti ič, elephant's excrement.

Get all these, cook in mustard oil and apply.

(h) *Laṭha cip ciṛip jọ sẹ jaṅ*, the fruit or seed of
Mạṅjurjhuṭi rẹhẹl, the roots of

Grind these together and cook in *utiṅ sunum*, mustard oil, and apply daily with a feather.

(i) *Nanha dudhi loṭa rẹhẹl*, the roots of Ichnocarpus frutescens, R. Br.
Akaṛ baha, Limnophila Roxburghiana, G. Don.
Nanha catọm aṛak, Desmodium triflorum, DC.
Jhīk poṭa, a porcupine's stomach.
Bherṇḍa loṛe, the juice of Jatropha Curcas, L.

Grind these together, cook in *utiṅ sunum*, mustard oil, and apply with a feather. If the back of the mouth has sores:

(j) *Nanha dudhi loṭa rẹhẹl*, the roots of Ichnocarpus frutescens, R. Br.

Bạṛ baha chal, the bark of Mimusops Elengi, L.
Sirom rẹhẹl, the roots of Andropogon muricatus, Retz.

Grind these together, cook in *gại gọtọm*, melted butter of cows' milk ; to be eaten three times a day.

36. *Nulikor hoṛ.*

Symptoms. In this there are sores in the throat.

Medicines : *Sasaṅ baha*, the flower of Curcuma longa, Roxb.
Muṅgạ chal, the bark of Moringa pterygosperma, Gärtn.
Gol mạric, black pepper.
Piskạ da, the tuber of Dioscorea opposotifolia L.
Tumbạ ot', an edible form of mushroom.
Sukri ḍhumbạk', pig's excrement.

Grind these together and give to drink.

37. *Piṭkiri haso.* Angina.

Symptoms : There is pain in the neck under the jaw, and a choking sensation when swallowing the saliva.

Medicines : Every morning rub it with your own saliva, and then get a *rạnu guli*, ball of the ferment used in brewing rice beer, grind this, mix saliva with it and apply it over the painful spot. This to be done during the day time only after the morning rubbing.

38. *Gola kaṇṭa.*

Symptoms. This attacks the throat which swells up, so that if medicine is not applied it may stop the breathing and prove fatal.

Medicines : (*a*) *Gol mạric se caole maric*, black pepper or a kind of capsicum, resembling grains of rice.

Grind and give to drink.

(*b*) *Ato pinḍạ*, Amorphophallus campanulatus, Blume.

Grind and give to drink.

(*c*) *Kasmar chal*, the bark of Gmelina arborea, Roxb.
Rạsun, garlic.

Grind and give to drink, and foment externally with melted butter.

(*d*) *Caole mạric rẹhẹl*, the roots of a kind of capsicum resembling grains of rice.
Malhan sakam, the leaves of Dolichos Lablab, L.

Grind these together and give to drink ; and apply externally a mixture of
Phuṭiạ kạuḍi cun, lime made from the shells used as money in India.
Batapi sindur, a preparation of red lead.

39. *Kom kom.* Mumps.

Medicines: First of all foment the parts, and if this does not suffice, then

Dạtrạ jọ, the fruit of Datura alba, Willd. or D. fastuosa, Willd.

Rạṅgạini jạnum, Solanum Jacquini, Willd., leaves included.

Grind together and after warming in a leaf cup apply as a plaster over the swollen parts and recovery will follow in two or three days.

40. *Ạṅgur buḍhi.* Whitlow.

Symptoms. This may appear on any of the fingers or toes. At the commencement there is a pimple, reddish in appearance, that itches very much, and later on a burning pain.

Medicines: (*a*) *Turạm rẹhẹt*, the roots of

Suruj mukhi aṛak rẹhẹt sẹ jọtọge, the roots of, or the entire Helianthus annuus, L.

Grind and plaster on, wrapping a bandage over and then soaking the whole well in mustard oil; the pain will cease shortly.

(*b*) *Kolo da*, the bulb of Dioscorea daemonum, Roxb.

Rạṅgạini rẹhẹt, the roots of Solanum Jacquini, Willd.

Sarjọm chal thoṛa, a little of the bark of Shorea robusta, Gärtn.

Grind these together and apply, wrapping a bandage around.

When the sore breaks:

(*c*) *Maṭha aṛak rẹhẹt*, the roots of Antidesma diandrum, Tulas.

Turạm rẹhẹt, the roots of

Bhiḍi janaṭep rẹhẹt the roots of Urena sinuata, L. or Triumfetta rhomboidea, Jac.

Mix all these and apply.

At the very beginning, (*d*) if the milky juice of *bherṇḍa*, Jatropha Curcas, L., is applied the pain will cease.

(*e*) *Eṭkẹć dạr*, branch of Euphorbia antiquorum, L.

Hollow this out and put it on like a ring over the painful spot.

(*f*) *Eṭkẹć*, Euphorbia antiquorum, L.

Cut off a branch of this square and making a hole in it put it on the affected member. After being on for 24 hours take it off, get some *ṭạṇḍi catọm aṛak'*, Desmodium triflorum, DC., which grind and apply as a plaster.

(*g*) *Rạṅgạini rẹhẹt*, the roots of Solanum Jacquini, Willd.

Joka sakam, the leaves of Sida humilis, Willd.

Grind together and apply as a plaster.

(*h*) *Turạm rẹhẹt*, the roots of

Suruj mukhi rẹhẹt, the roots of Helianthus annuus, L.

Sim kaṭa aṛak rẹhẹt, the roots of Vitex peduncularis.

Grind these together and apply as an ointment; then wrap in a bandage and pour on mustard oil till it is saturated; immediate alleviation will follow.

(*i*) *Rangaini rehel*, the roots of Solanum Jacquini, Willd.
Bilati thamakur, imported tobacco.
Kolo da, the bulb of Dioscorea daemonum, Roxb.
Sarjom chal, the bark of Shorea robusta, Gärtn.

Grind these together fine and apply.

(*j*) At the commencement: *kada guric'*, buffalo dung.

Make this into a ball, burn it in the fire and stick it on like a thimble.

(*k*) If several days have clapsed, then
Latha cip cirip rehel, the roots of
Rangaini janum rehel, the roots of Solanum Jacquini, Willd.
Joka sakam, the leaves of Sida humilis, Willd.

Grind these fine and plaster on.

41. *Khẽrkhõc.*

Symptoms. This sore occurs on the palm or back of the hand or under the wrist. There are white pimples which ripen white and cause intense pain, and inside the sores there is a cup-like formation as in boils.

Medicines: (*a*) *Turam rehel*, the roots of
Suruj mukhi arak rehel, the roots of Helianthus annuus, L.
Bhidi janatep rehel, the roots of Urena sinuata, L. or Triumfetta rhomboidea, Jac.

Grind these three and apply.

(*b*) *Kolo da*, the bulb of Dioscorea daemonum, Roxb.
Matha arak rehel, the roots of Antidesma diandrum, Tulas.
Rangaini janum rehel, the roots of Solanum Jacquini, Willd.
Etka rehel, the roots of Mucuna pruriens, DC.
Sengel siń rehel, the roots of Tragia involucrata, Willd.

Grind these and apply.

42. *Hor khura.*

Symptoms. A "sore" appears on the sole of the foot as in *ras bat ghao.*

Medicines: (*a*) *Nanha jeleń rokoc*, a thin long mullusc or periwinkle.
Kauha chal, the bark of Terminalia Arjuna, Roxb.
Phutia kaudi, the small shell used in India as money.

Grind these together, boil in mustard oil and anoint the sore therewith.

(*b*) *Dare pinda jo*, the fruit of Randia uliginosa, DC.
Loto jo, the fruit of Randia dumetorum, Lam.

Grind together, boil in mustard oil and apply to the sore.

43. *Janga se idi paragok.* Rhagades.

This is something which affects only some people.

Medicines: Throw a nut of *Areca Catechu, L.* into *sasań dak*, turmeric (Curcuma longa, Roxb.) water, and on Saturday evening take it and put it down at the roots of a *telhec* (Sterculia urens, Roxb.) tree, and in doing so address it thus;

Make me a pair of shoes meanwhile; I shall come to-morrow morning. Having said this return home. On Sunday morning without relieving nature or passing urine go back there again and greet that tree; then sitting down kick it once with each foot and in doing so say: Here, take the worn out shoes, give me my good ones. Then go straight home without looking back, and from next year your feet will not crack.

44. *Janga kaṭuṗ ghao.* Sores on the toes.

Medicines: (*a*) *Icak̓ rẹhẹl*, the roots of Woodfordia floribunda, Salisb.

Mare nangle, an old leathern thong for fastening the yoke.

Take the first and chop them to the size of the stems of the tobacco plant; then boil them in about 2 or 3 pints of water, till their juice has been extracted; then take out and throw away the roots, and boil the water down to about 8 oz. Then roast the thong to burning point, grind it and strew it on the water, and mix well. Apply this mixture.

(*b*) *Joka sakam*, the leaves of Sida humilis, Willd.

Grind and apply of the consistency of porridge.

45. *Jan ruli.* (Osteo-myelitis.)

Symptoms. In this there is an intense aching and burning pain day and night all the way from the sole of the foot up the shin to the thigh bone.

Medicines: (*a*) *Bhuku chata*, a termites' nest.

Warm slightly and apply some three or four days.

(*b*) *Chạlni chal*, the bark of Alstonia scholaris, R. Br.

Warm and apply daily.

(*c*) *Akaona rẹhẹl*, the roots of Calotropis gigantea, R. Br.

Warm and apply daily.

(*d*) *Bir eraḍọm*, the wild Ricinus.

Apply daily without warming.

(*e*) *Bunum bhuku chata*, a termites' nest from the anthill.

Heat and apply; this is enough for a cure.

(*f*) *Dak̓ ghoṛa lada*, Vitis tomentosa, Heyne.

Kaḍa bhosam, the first stomach of a buffalo.

Kesari da, the tuber of Lathyrus sativus, L.

Mix and apply these warm.

(*g*) *Edẹl manj*, the heart of Bombax malabaricum, DC.

Bir họṛẹc̓, Atyllosia scarabædois, Benth.

Dare cetan reak̓ kaṭkọm janga, Viscum attenuatum, DC.

Grind all these together and after warming slightly plaster it over where it pains him and he will recover. If there is pus, *i.e.* if it is ripe, burn a hole with a red hot iron.

One "authority" says: This is the same as *uri*, commences like that and pains in the same way. This is said to burst from the bone and is therefore styled *ruli*. First apply what is prescribed for *uri*, and if inefficacious, then you know it is *ruli*. This complaint appears mostly on the thigh joint, thigh or knee, and therefore some people call it also *jaṅ uri*.

46. *Jaṅ rapudok*. Fractured bones.

Medicines: *Khode baha rehel*, the roots of
Bod laṛ rehel, the roots of Vitis adnata, Wall.
Kamraj rehel, „ „ „ Buettneria herbacea, Roxb.
Had joṛa nãṛiteḷ, the tendrils of Cissus quadrangularis, Willd.

Grind, apply as a plaster, and affix splints.

47. *Eklam seklam ruạ*. Ague.

Medicines: *Orsoreṅ rehel*, the roots of Zingiber Cassumunar, R. (?)
Kahu botke rehel, the roots of Bryonia lacinosa, L.

Grind and plaster the patient therewith.

48. *Ti jaṅga se jaṅ bhitri haso*. Pain in the limbs or bones.

Medicines: *Bonkapsi da*, the bulb of Thespesia Lampas, Benth. & Hook. f.
Kadar nãṛi rehel, the roots of Asparagus racemosus, Willd.
Atkir rehel, the roots of Smilax ovalifolia, Roxb.
Bir campa rehel, the roots of Ochna squarrosa, L.

Grind with water, and after squeezing the water out give about eight ounces of it to drink for three or four days.

49. *Ruạkateye kalhalenre*. Subnormal temperature after fever.

Medicines: *Paro da*, the tuber of Curcuma angustifolia, Roxb.
Berel sasaṅ, raw turmeric, Curcuma longa, Roxb.

Grind together and plaster the body therewith.

50. *Pali ruạ*. Intermittent fever (malaria).

Symptoms. In this the fever is not in evidence every day, but returns after an interval of one day or it may be two.

Medicines: (*a*) *Andia moron arak rehel*, the roots of Gymnema hirsutus, W. & A., var. Decaisneanum, Wight.
Nanha dudhi loṭa rehel, the roots of Ichnocarpus frutescens, R. Br.

Take a little of each of these and tie on the patient with thread.

(*b*) *Baṛe baha rehel*, the roots of Pentapetes phoenicia, L.
Datauni ger phodloteḷ, the frayed portion of a Santal tooth brush.
Pio il, the feathers of the Oriolus melanocephalus.
Sakri patṛa careć, pe senak, the leaf stem pins from three sides of a used leaf plate.
Bardũṛũć ulawak, the rejections from the mouth of a bat.
Bana up, a bear's hair.
Tarup up, a leopard's hair.

Tie these together and hang on to the patient's neck.

(c) *Ratcora*, Locusta viridissima.
Bare baha, Pentapetes phoenicia, L.
Suruj mukhi rehel, the roots of Helianthus annuus, L.
Catom arak rehel, „ „ „ Marsilia quadrifolia, L.
Sirom rehel, the roots of Andropogon muricatus, Retz.
Datauni reak togoc phodlotel, the chewed part of a Santal tooth brush.

Tie with a thread and hang on the neck. This must be done on a Sunday morning.

(d) *Tejo mala rehel*, the roots of Cissampelos Pareira, L.
Pound and give to drink; also
Dare cetanre omonok latha cip cirip rehel,
Arak garundi rehel, the roots of the red Acternanthera sessilis, R. Br.

Put a thread out in the dew on Saturday, then on Sunday morning tie these with that thread and then hang them on his neck. Or the following may be tied and hung on him in the same way:

(e) *Bana up*, a bear's hair.
Pio il, the feathers of the Oriolus melanocephalus, L.
Pitua ghãs, Spermacoce hispida, L.
Sirom rehel, the roots of Andropogon muricatus, Retz.
Bare baha rehel, the roots of Pentapetes phoenicia, L.

The leaf stem of Bassia latifolia, Roxb., that falls at night.

51. *Emne rua*. Various fevers.

Medicines: (a) At the commencement of fever, when it is uncertain of what kind it is:
Tejo mala rehel, the roots of Diospyros tomentosa, Roxb.

Grind and give to drink.

(b) *Caulia*, Ruellia suffruticosa, Roxb.
Damka dura,
Ranu ran, the ferment used to make rice beer.
Manjurjhuti rehel, the roots of
Kadar nãri rehel, the roots of Asparagus racemosus, Willd.
Atkir rehel, the roots of Smilax ovalifolia, Roxb.
Hund baha rehel, the roots of Jasminum arborescens, Roxb.

Grind these all together and give to drink.

(c) *Bonkapsi rehel*, the roots of Thespesia Lampas, Benth. and Hook. f.

Grind and give to drink.

(d) *Hat chal*, the bark of Holarrhena antidysenterica, Wall.
Latha cip cirip,

Grind together, strain and give to drink.

If the fever is persistent:

(*e*) *Akaṛ baha*, Limnophila Roxburghiana, G. Don.
Meral sakam, the leaves of Phyllanthus Emblica, L.
Hẹmsagọr, Cotyledon laciniata, Willd.

Grind the first two and give to drink, and plaster with the last.

(*f*) *Haṭ chal*, the bark of Holarrhena antidysenterica, Wall.
Lọpọṅ chal, the bark of Terminalia bellerica, Roxb.
Badgọcak, Lygodium flexuosum, Sw.
Bạru rẹhẹl, the roots of Schleichera trijuga, Willd.
Nãṛĩ gọd rẹhẹl, the roots of Aristolochia indica, Willd.

Grind and give to drink.

(*g*) *Mạṅjurjhuti rẹhẹl*, the roots of
Cero rẹhẹl, the roots of Imperata arundinacea, Cyr.
Ḍuṇḍukit rẹhẹl, the roots of Gardenia turgida, Roxb.
Sarjọm rẹhẹl, the roots of Shorea robusta, Gärtn.

Pound these and give to drink.

(*h*) *Goṭe rẹhẹl*, the roots of Croton oblongifolius, Roxb.
Nanha dudhi loṭa rẹhẹl, the roots of Ichnocarpus frutescens, R. Br.
Paṛọ, Curcuma angustifolia, Roxb.

Grind all these together and besmear therewith.

(*i*) *Lag jọṛ*,
Gõṛẽ chal, the bark of Stephegyne parvifolia, Korth.

Grind together and rub in, and give some also to drink.

(*j*) *Haṭ chal*, the bark of Holarrhena antidysenterica, Wall.
Adra cip ciṛip rẹhẹl, the roots of

Grind, strain through a cloth and give to drink.

(*k*) *Badgọcak*, Lygodium flexuosum, Sw.
Bọnkạpsi, Thespesia Lampas, Benth. & Hook. f.
Saram lutur rẹhẹl, the roots of Clerodendron serratum, Spreng.
Bir campa, Ochna squarrosa, Willd.
Lọpọṅ chal, the bark of Terminalia bellerica, Roxb.
Sarjọm chal, the bark of Shorea robusta, Gärtn.
Rạnu ran, the ferment used to make rice beer.

52. *Akal sakal rụạ.* Ardent fever.
Medicines: *Ọrsọreṅ rẹhẹl*, the roots of Zingiber Cassumunar, R. (?)
Kạhu botke rẹhẹl, the roots of Bryonia lacinosa, L.
Grind and plaster therewith.

53. *Gum gumi rụạ.* Low fever.
Medicines: *Patal kohṇḍa*, Pueraria tuberosa, DC.
Edẹl poha, a seedling of Bombax malabaricum, DC.
Tursi sakam thoṛa, a few leaves of Ocymum sanctum, Willd.

Mix and grind these and give to drink.

54. *Bhạlki ruạ.* High fever.

Medicines: (*a*) *Hẹmsagọr da*, the bulb of Cotyledon laciniata, Willd.

Grind and give to drink as well as plaster therewith.

(*b*) *Susurbaṅ chata*, a wasps' nest.

Bana up, bear's hair.

Ọkọe tejo kaḍẹčteko benao oṛak onko tejoak kaḍẹč, the sticks with which certain insects make their house.

Bardūṛūč phạkṛạk il, the 'feathers' of a bat's wing.

Dạtạuni kạṭič, a small tooth brush, *i.e.* a twig of Shorea robusta, Gärtn.

Baṛe jọrọ ḍọg ar rẹhẹt', the tip and root of the aerial root of Ficus bengalensis, L.

Pio il, the feathers of Oriolus melanocephalus.

Tie a little of each of these together and tie them on his neck.

(*c*) *Kadar nāṛī rẹhẹt'*, the roots of Asparagus racemosus, Willd.

Ṭạmpur cạili rẹhẹt, the roots of Morinda tinctoria, Roxb.

Badgọcak rẹhẹt, the roots of Lygodium flexuosum, Sw.

Sạuṛi rẹhẹt, the roots of Heteropogon contortus, R. and S.

Jọm jạnum rẹhẹt, the roots of Zizyphus Jujuba, Lamk.

Boṅga sarjọm rẹhẹt, the roots of Ventilago calyculata, Tulasne.

Bana haṭak chal, the bark of Oroxylon indicum, Benth.

Mix a little of these and give to drink.

(*d*) *Hoṛo rọṅgọ*, burnt paddy.

Hẹmsagọr da, the bulb of Cotyledon laciniata, Willd.

Grind together and smear over the whole body. Afterwards if he becomes cold, grind together *sunum muč*, a species of black ant, *bindi*, spiders, and smear on, when he will become warm again.

55. *Baṅ chuṭạuk ruạ.* Remittent or continued fever.

Medicines: (*a*) *Khẹt pipṛạ aṛak'*, Oldenlandia biflora, Roxb.

Grind and plaster over the whole body.

(*b*) *Orop' da*, the bulb of Costus speciosa, Sm.

Plaster the whole body with this and give some to drink.

(*c*) *Ul chal*, the bark of Mangifera indica, L.

Buc chal, „ „ „ Cordia Myxa, L.

Boil in water and wash the patient therewith from the elbows downwards and from the knees downwards; the fever will assuredly leave.

(*d*) *Gaḍa terel chal*, the bark of Diospyros montana, Roxb.

Hẹmsagọr da, the bulb of Cotyledon laciniata, Willd.

Grind these two together and besmear the body therewith.

(*e*) *Orop da*, the bulb of Costus speciosa, Sm.

Khẹt pipṛạ, Oldenlandia biflora, Roxb.

Grind these together and plaster over the whole body.

If the temperature is very high :—

(*f*) *Hẹmsagor*, Cotyledon laciniata, Willd.

Grind and apply a thin plaster of it over the whole body ; plastering thickly would be dangerous.

In high fever :—

(*g*) *Goṭe rẹhẹt*, the roots of Croton oblongifolius, Roxb.

Nanha dudhi loṭa rẹhẹt, the roots of Ichnocarpus frutescens, R. Br.

Hẹmsagọr rẹhẹt, the roots of Cotyledon laciniata, Willd.

Plaster with these for 3 or 4 days.

56. *Jarọ ruạ.*

Medicines : (*a*) *Etka rẹhẹt*, the roots of Mucuna pruriens, DC.

25—26 *gọṭẹć muthạ da*, 25 to 26 bulbs of Fimbristylis monostachya, Hassk.

Nańgrạuta rẹhẹt, the roots of Nardostachys jatamansi, DC.

Grind these together and smear on the head either so, or after cooking in mustard oil.

57. *Họrmọ jaljalaok*. Ardor of the body.

Symptoms : When there is some kind of fever, the body gets weak and the blood sluggish ; there is no thirst, but owing to great weakness the body dries up internally.

Medicines : (*a*) *Orop da*, the tuber of Costus speciosa, Sm.

Extract the juice of this and give the patient to drink with sugar three times or so, and the body will cool down at once.

(*b*) *Kadar rẹhẹt*, the roots of Asparagus racemosus, Willd.

Nanha dudhi loṭa rẹhẹt, the roots of Ichnocarpus frutescens, R. Br.

Soak both of these well and after mixing with sugar give the patient to drink daily until recovery.

(*c*) *Nanha pusi toa*, Euphorbia thymifolia, Burm.

Make a liquid preparation of this, keep it in a bottle and adding sugar let the patient drink of it daily fór about a fortnight, and he will get well.

58. *Koṛam jaljalaok*. Burning sensation in the chest.

Symptoms : When there is a burning sensation in the chest with intense thirst during fever apply this.

Medicines : *Korkoṭ rẹhẹt*, the roots of Dillenia indica, L.

Sarjọm dak sẹ chalge, the water or bark of Shorea robusta, Gärtn.

Bhorkọnḍ rẹhẹt, the roots of Hymenodictyon excelsum, Wall.

Grind all these together, mix thoroughly with *cini*, sugar, and give to drink. After that give some *dumur rasa*, honey of the small honey-bee, to drink, and after grinding *mẹrlẹc̓ sakam*, the leaves of Flacourtia Ramontchi, L. 'Herit. warm them slightly and plaster on the chest.

59. *Koṛam laṛao.* (lit. moving of the breast).

Medicines: (*a*) *Gạị ghuṛạ*, Polygala chinensis, L.
Kũs rẹhẹl, the roots of Themuda gigantea, Haskel.
Jhaṅkaṛe rẹhẹl, the roots of Thysanolaena acarifera, Nees.

Grind together and give to drink.

60. *Koṛam haso.* Pain in the chest.

Medicines: (*a*) First rub melted butter on and foment with hot sand.

(*b*) Grind *sekra chal*, the bark of Zizyphus rugosa, Lamk., warm it a little and apply as a plaster to the chest.

(*c*) Grind *kạuhạ chal*, the bark of Terminalia Arjuna, Bedd., warm it a little and plaster it on.

(*d*) Pound *dạtrạ rẹhẹl sẹ sakam*, the roots or leaves of Datura alba, Willd. or D. fastuosa, Willd., and extract 4 ounces of the juice, mix therewith 4 ounces *akaona loṛe*, the milky exudation of Calotropis gigantea, R. Br., and 4 annas (four pence) worth of *ạphim*, opium, stir all together and warm it somewhat in the sun, and then smear it over the seat of the pain.

(*e*) *Ghoṛa lạdạuṛi rẹhẹl*, the roots of Vitis tomentosa, Heyne.

Grind fine and apply to the place where the pain is.

(*f*) *Ḍhalka hạtkạn da*, the bulb of Leea macrophylla, Roxb.

Grind fine, warm slightly and apply.

(*g*) *Khayar chal*, the bark of Acacia Catechu, L.
Ruhen chal, the bark of Soymida febrifuga, Juss.

Grind and give some to drink and smear some on the chest.

61. *Ṭan ruạ.* Continuous fever.

Symptoms. If one walks about or works in the sun the limbs ache, the lower extremities are benumbed and locomotion unsteady, the body feels weak and tired and the urine is highly coloured.

Medicines: (*a*) *Kasmar chal*, the bark of Gmelina arborea, Roxb.
Mạhũt sẹ lạli guṛ, either of two kinds of molasses refuse.

Mix the juice extracted from the former with the latter and let the patient drink this for some five days; he will assuredly recover.

(*b*) *Sega rẹhẹl*, the roots of Mimosa rubicaulis, Lamk.
Badgọcak̓ rẹhẹl, the roots of Lygodium flexuosum, Sw.
Nanha dudhi loṭa rẹhẹl, the roots of Ichnocarpus frutescens, R. Br.

Soak all these together and let the patient drink it daily.

(*c*) *Bọnkạpsi rẹhẹl*, the roots of Thespesia Lampas, Benth. & Hook. f.

Grind these fresh daily and give the patient to drink, and he will recover. Tested and used.

(*d*) *Lopoṅ chal*, the bark of Terminalia bellerica, Roxb.
Mạhũt guṛ, molasses refuse.

Take the juice of the former, mix it with the latter and make the patient drink it, and he will certainly get well.

(*e*) *Tarop chal ros*, the juice of the bark of Buchanania latifolia, Roxb.

The patient to drink this for about five days and the aching of the limbs will cease.

(*f*) *Matkom chal*, the bark of Bassia latifolia, Roxb.
Adwa caole, rice made from sun-dried, not boiled paddy.

Mix these, soak them and let the patient drink the infusion daily; he will get well.

(*g*) *Nim sakam*, the leaves of Melia Azadirachta, Linn.
Mạhũt guṛ, molasses refuse.

Boil the former well, drain the water off and let the patient drink it hot mixed with the latter.

(*h*) *Kaḍa beṅjak rẹhẹl*, the roots of
Nanha cạuliạ rẹhẹl, the fine big and little roots of Ruellia suffruticosa, Roxb.
Mạṅjurjhuṭi rẹhẹl, the roots of

Grind all these together, boil them and let the patient drink it mixed with sugar.

When the fever is somewhat reduced:

(*i*) *Bonkạpsi rẹhẹl*, the roots of Thespesia Lampas, Benth. & Hook. f.
Mạhũt guṛ, molasses refuse.

Mix these two and give the patient to drink.

(*j*) *Kadam chal*, the bark of Anthocephalus Cadamba, Benth. & Hook. f.
Bạru chal, „ „ „ Schleichera trijuga, Willd.
Sarjom chal, „ „ „ Shorea robusta, Gärtn.
Hesak chal, „ „ „ Ficus religiosa, Willd.
Tejo mala rẹhẹl, the roots of Cissampelos Pareira, Linn.
Saram lutur rẹhẹl, „ „ „ Clerodendron serratum, Spreng.

Grind whichever of these you please and give him to drink.

(*k*) *Kadar rẹhẹl*, the roots of Asparagus racemosus, Willd.
Mạhũt guṛ, molasses refuse.

Mix the two and give him to drink.

(*l*) *Tejo mala rẹhẹl*, the roots of Cissampelos Pareira, Linn.
Nanha dudhi loṭa rẹhẹl, the roots of Ichnocarpus frutescens, R. Br.

Grind these together and let him drink it with *mạhũt guṛ*, molasses refuse.

(*m*) *Kadar rẹhẹl*, the roots of Asparagus racemosus, Willd.

Ạtkir rẹhẹl, „ „ „ Smilax ovalifolia, Roxb.

Ẹdẹl poha, seedling of Bombax malabaricum, DC.

The first two to be ground, the last cut into round slices, and the whole to be drunk with sugar.

(*n*) *Ul chal*, the bark of Mangifera indica, L.

Kadam chal, „ „ „ Anthocephalus Cadamba, Benth. & Hook. f.

Corco chal, „ „ „ Casearea tomentosa, Roxb.

Grind these together and give the patient to drink with *mạhũt guṛ*, molasses refuse.

(*o*) *Bọnkạpsi rẹhẹl*, the roots of Thespesia Lampas, Benth. & Hook. f.

To be drunk daily.

When there is fever at night:

(*p*) *Bọnkạpsi rẹhẹl*, the roots of Thespesia Lampas, Benth. & Hook. f.

Ạtkir rẹhẹl, the roots of Smilax ovalifolia, Roxb.

Badgọcak̕ rẹhẹl, the roots of Lygodium flexuosum, Sw.

Matkọm chal, the bark of Bassia latifolia, Roxb.

Grind a little of these together and let the patient drink about a tumbler full.

(*q*) *Campa rẹhẹl*, the roots of Michelia champaca, L.

To be ground and drunk.

(*r*) *Badgọcak̕ rẹhẹl*, the roots of Lygodium flexuosum, Sw.

Ạtkir rẹhẹl, the roots of Smilax ovalifolia, Roxb.

Ṅindạ ńũrok̕ matkọm chal, the bark of Bassia latifolia, Roxb. whose flowers fall at night.

Bharbhạri rẹhẹl, the roots of Ocimum basilicum, Linn. or Ocimum canum, Sims.

A little of these to be ground and drunk.

(*s*) *Kasmar chal*, the bark of Gmelina arborea, Roxb.

To be ground and drunk.

(*t*) *Ṭan dare rẹhẹl*, the roots of

Sarjọm dak̕, the water of Shorea robusta, Gärtn.

Atnak̕ chal, the bark of Terminalia tomentosa, W. and A.

Bọnkạpsi rẹhẹl, the roots of Thespesia Lampas, Benth. & Hook. f.

Saram lutur rẹhẹl, the roots of Clerodendron serratum, Spreng.

Sikuạr rẹhẹl, the roots of

Pound all together and give to drink for three days.

(*u*) *Kadam chal*, the bark of Anthocephalus Cadamba, Benth. & Hook. f.

Ambṛa chal, „ „ „ Spondias mangifera, Pers.

Ul chal, the bark of Mangifera indica, L.
Pańjọt sakam, the leaves of Clerodendron phlomoides, Willd.
Siṅjọ sakam, the leaves of Aegle Marmelos, Correa.
Gol mạric, black pepper.
Kạliạ jirạ, Nigella indica, Roxb.
Mẹrlẹć sakam, the leaves of Flacourtia Ramontchi, L' Herit.

Grind together, stir in water and give to drink.

(*v*) *Nanha dudhi loṭa rẹhẹt*, the roots of Ichnocarpus frutescens, R. Br.
Kadar rẹhẹt, the roots of Bonnaya veronicaefolia, Spreng.

Grind together and give to drink.

(*w*) *Bir campa rẹhẹt se baha*, the roots or flower of Ochna squarrosa, Willd.
Sarjọm chal, the bark of Shorea robusta, Gärtn.
Goṭe rẹhẹt, the roots of Croton oblongifolius, Roxb.
Bọnkạpsi rẹhẹt, the roots of Thespesia Lampas, Benth. & Hook. f.
Matkọm ḍạr reak bhitri gabeṭẹt, the pith of a branch of Bassia latifolia, Roxb.

Grind with water, squeeze out the water and give 6 to 8 ounces to drink for three or four days.

(*x*) *Sarjọm chal*, the bark of Shorea robusta, Gärtn.
Ul chal, the bark of Mangifera indica, L.
Kadam chal, the bark of Anthocephalus Cadamba, Benth. & Hook. f.
Corco chal, the bark of Casearea tomentosa, Roxb.
Hesak chal, the bark of Ficus religiosa, Willd.

Pound all, steep in water and give to drink.

(*y*) *Bir hoṛẹć*, Atyllosia scarabaedois, Benth.

Boil and give to drink with sugar.

(*z*) *Kaḍa beṅjak rẹhẹt*, the roots of
Mạṅjurjhuṭi rẹhẹt, the roots of
Cạuliạ rẹhẹt, the roots of Ruellia suffruticosa, Roxb.
Ḍamka ḍurạ rẹhẹt, the roots of
Kadar rẹhẹt, the roots of Bonnaya veronicaefolia, Spreng.
Ạṭkir rẹhẹt, the roots of Smilax ovalifolia, Roxb.

Steep all together in water, boil and give to drink with *mạhũt guṛ*, molasses refuse.

(*aa*) *Tejo mala rẹhẹt*, the roots of Cissampelos Pareira, L.
Nanha dudhi loṭa rẹhẹt, the roots of Ichnocarpus frutescens, R. Br.
Campa rẹhẹt, the roots of Michelia champaca, L.
Lọpọṅ chal, the bark of Terminalia bellerica, Roxb.

Grind all these together, soak in water and give to drink daily.

(bb) *Bonkapsi rehel*, the roots of Thespesia Lampas, Benth. & Hook. f.

Terel chal, the bark of Diospyros tomentosa, Roxb.

Mix and extract the juice, which give to drink daily.

(cc) *Baru chal*, the bark of Schleichera trijuga, Willd.

Matkom chal, the bark of Bassia latifolia, Roxb.

Caole ata rongo, rice fried to burning point.

Soak in water and give to drink morning and evening.

(dd) *Bonga sarjom chal*, the bark of Ventilago calyculata, Tulasne

Gote chal, the bark of Croton oblongifolius, Roxb.

Nāṛī murup chal, the bark of Butea superba, Roxb.

Pound all these together, squeeze out the juice and give about 8 ounces to drink for some three days. To be taken on an empty stomach.

(ee) *Lolo handi*, hot rice beer.

Get this from the liquor vendor and give to drink; if inefficacious, then

(ff) *Terel chal*, the bark of Diospyros tomentosa, Roxb.

Kaḍa beñjak,

Mañjurjhuṭi,

Caulia, Ruellia suffruticosa, Roxb.

Ṭompaṛ,

Kadam chal, the bark of Anthocephalus Cadamba, Benth. & Hook. f.

Atkir, Smilax ovalifolia, Roxb.

Boil and soak these, to be drunk daily with *mahũt guṛ*, refuse of molasses.

(gg) *Ḍuria hatkan*, Leea hirta, Herb. Banks.

Udal chal, the bark of Sterculia villosa, Roxb.

Sarjom chal, the bark of Shorea robusta, Gärtn.

Ul chal, „ „ „ Mangifera indica, L.

Kadam chal, „ „ „ Anthocephalus Cadamba, Benth. & Hook. f.

Corco chal, „ „ „ Casearea tomentosa, Roxb.

Hesak chal, „ „ „ Ficus religiosa, Willd.

Bir horeč, Atyllosia scarabædois, Benth.

Soak all these and give to drink with *cini*, sugar.

(hh) *Haḍpangla*,

Badgocak, Lygodium flexuosum, Sw.

Icak, Woodfordia floribunda, Salisb.

Sarjom chal, the bark of Shorea robusta, Gärtn.

Atnak chal, „ „ „ Terminalia tomentosa, W. and A.

Soso chal, „ „ „ Semecarpus Anacardium, L.

Hund baha rehel, the roots of Jasminum aborescens, Roxb.

Pound all these together and give to drink, and his urine will be as clear as a goat's, the pains will cease and complete recovery follow.

62. *Tamba band* (palsy or pain supposed to be caused by a witch's charm).

Medicines: (*a*) *Ąsąrią rẹhẹl*, the roots of Capparis horrida, L. f.

Jhiṅgur rẹhẹl thoṛa, a little of the roots of Arum campanulatum, Roxb.

Akaona rẹhẹl, the roots of Calotropis gigantea, R. Br.

Grind together, soak in a small earthen jar and smear on daily.

(*b*) *Ąsąrią rẹhẹl*, the roots of Capparis horrida, L. f.

Bando rẹhẹl, „ „ „ Spatholobus Roxburghii, Benth.

Tihon rẹhẹl, „ „ „ Canavalia ensiformis, DC.

Grind together and plaster over the whole body for 3 or 4 days.

63. *Lahor siṭkạ*. Lahore fever.

Symptoms. This is something that affects both men and women. They have slight fever, then the saliva dries up and there is intense thirst. This is *lahor siṭkạ*.

Medicines: (*a*) *Sọsọ chal*, the bark of Semecarpus Anacardium, L.

Mạṅjurjhuṭi rẹhẹl, the roots of

Nanha cạulią rẹhẹl, „ „ „ Ruellia suffruticosa, Roxb.

Grind these three and let the patient drink the juice three days and he will get well.

(*b*) *Gargạḍi rẹhẹl*, the roots of Coix lachryma, Willd.

Dak icạk rẹhẹl, the roots of Jussiæa suffruticosa, Linn.

Rạli rẹhẹl, the roots of Piper longum, Willd.

Jiṭhimond rẹhẹl, the roots of Clerodendron Siphonanthus, R. Br.

Darcini rẹhẹl, the roots of Laurus cinnamonum, Willd.

Grind these together and let the patient drink it.

(*c*) *Kadar rẹhẹl*, the roots of Asparagus racemosus, Willd.

Orop da, the bulb of Costus speciosa, Sm.

Misri cini, sugar-candy.

Mix the first two with the third, let the patient drink it and the temperature will become normal.

(*d*) *Dak icạk rẹhẹl*, the roots of Jussiæa suffruticosa, L.

Gargạḍi rẹhẹl, the roots of Coix lachryma, Willd.

Dare icạk rẹhẹl, the roots of Woodfordia floribunda, Salisb.

Grind these together and give to drink with sugar.

(*e*) *Thoṛa sọsọ chal*, a little of the bark of Semecarpus Anacardium, L.

Cạulią rẹhẹl, the roots of Ruellia suffruticosa, Roxb.

Grind, take the juice and give to drink with sugar for three days.

64. *Pilą*. Spleen.

Medicines: (*a*) *Kitạuri rẹhẹl sẹ sakam*, the roots or leaves of Plumbago Zeylanica, Willd.

Grind and mix with fowls' flesh, make into hand bread and give to eat.

(*b*) *Dạhu*, Artocarpus Lakoocha, Roxb.

Rub the sticky exudation over the spleen, and after grinding the bark give it to drink.

(*c*) *Sẹlẹp samanọm*, Gloriosa superba, L.

Batapi sindur, a preparation of red lead.

First apply the latter and over that smear the former as a plaster.

(*d*) If a patient has been suffering for from 3 to 5 years and no other remedy has proved efficacious, then the following may be tried, but with great care, as it is a poison, and an over-dose will prove fatal, *viz.*, *tutiạ*, sulphate of copper. For patients over 16 years of age give a piece the size of *rambṛa jañ*, a seed of Phaeseolus Mungo, var. Radiatus, L.

Cover this with *gại chale*, the cream of cow's milk and let him swallow it entire; it will melt gradually in the stomach and agitate it, and, as it were, knead the spleen thoroughly. The patient will burn and perspire profusely, and ease the bowels once or twice. When you see this let him take *gại toa jọjọ dahe mil pawa*, 8 ounces of sour curds of cows' milk, and he will feel relief. Give younger people in proportion.

65. *Kaṭ Pilạ*. (lit. Wood-spleen).

One "authority" says: This variety is similar to *poṭea pilạ* (66); the whole stomach is hard and distended as after a full meal; they can eat an enormous amount of rice and the stomach never subsides.

Medicines: (*a*) *Hiñ*, Ferrula asafœtida, Willd.

Hukạ dak, hookah water.

Sim bele, a hen's egg.

Mix together, roast and give to eat.

(*b*) *Corco chal*, the bark of Casearea tomentosa, Roxb.

Dhạniạ, Coriandrum sativum, L.

Boil and give to eat.

(*c*) *Teke caole mil pawa ataeme*, fry a pound of rice make from boiled paddy.

7 *gọṭẹn sọsọ jañ*, half roast 7 seeds of Semecarpus Anacardium, L.

Nim sakam ataeme, fry the leaves of Melia Azadirachta, L.

Pound these together fine, and give 3 spoonfuls every morning to eat.

(*d*) *Ghoṛa lạdạuṛi rẹhẹl*, the roots of Vitis tomentosa, Heyne.

Bana haṭak rẹhẹl, the roots of Oroxylon indicum, Benth.

Barañgọm rẹhẹl, the roots of Vernonia cineria, Less., or Glossogyne pinnatifida, DC.

Ạphim, opium.

Rạimạt lẹṇḍọñ, a kind of very large centipede.

Gẹgẹṭẹrẹñ, young centipedes.

Grind all these together, mix in *phuli pauṛa dak*, neat spirit, and make into pills, five of which to be taken every morning. If this does not cure, then burn him as described in *Laṛ pilạ*, No. 70.

66. *Poṭea pilạ*. Kala-Azar, or spleen permagnum.

One "authority" says: In this the stomach grows so as to look like a drum while the buttocks diminish in size; however much rice they may eat they are not satisfied, and whatever diet may be prohibited, that there is a great craving for.

Medicines: (*a*) *Phuṭiạ kạuḍi cun*, lime made from the small shells used in India as money.

Bẹrdọṛ rẹhẹt, the roots of Combretum nanum, Hamilt.

Mix and give to drink.

Akaona loṛe, the milky exudation of Calotropis gigantea, R. Br.

Sindur, red lead.

Mix and smear over the spleen.

(*b*) *Kalmeg rẹhẹt*, the roots of Andrographis paniculata, Nees.

Thoṛa ạphim, a little opium.

Mix and give to drink.

(*c*) *Kitạuri rẹhẹt*, the roots of Plumbago Zeylanica, Willd.

Kaḍa beṅjak rẹhẹt, the roots of

Haṭ rẹhẹt, the roots of Holarrhena antidysenterica, Wall.

Ạphim, opium.

Grind and make into 8 pills, one to be taken daily for eight days.

(*d*) *Jhiṅgur da*, the tuber of Arum campanulatum, Roxb.

Heat and apply as an ointment over the spleen.

(*e*) *Hiṅ*, the size of a fly's head of Ferrula asafœtida, Willd.

Rạsun bọhọk mit chimbṛi, one clove of a garlic.

Grind together and give to drink for eight days, and apply some as anointment over the spleen until it softens. Scratch over the spleen with *kũs ghãs*, Themuda gigantea, Haskel, so that the blood oozes into the scratches and then smear over them *akaona loṛe*, the milky exudation or Calotropis gigantea, R. Br.

(*f*) *Arak sindur*, genuine red lead.

Apply this and he will recover completely.

(*g*) *Bir buṭ rẹhẹt khudri*, a little bit of the roots of Flemingia congesta, Roxb.

Sohga, borax.

Rọl jaṅ, the seed of Terminalia Chebula, Retz.

Scrub the two former with the last so that some of the last is also intermingled, give a little to drink and smear some also over the spleen.

(*h*) *Rạimạt lẹnḍọṅ*, a kind of very large centipede.

Kitạuri rẹhẹt, the roots of Plumbago Zeylanica, Willd.

Mit'tan sosọ jan, a seed of Semecarpus Anacardium, L.
Kaḍa beṅjak rẹhẹl, the roots of
Kalmẹg, Andrographis paniculata, Nees.
Adagạthiạ ghās da, the bulb of Panicum repens, L.
Thoṛa ạphim a little opium.

Mix these together, make into pills and give to eat.

(i) *Ḍabha*, Citrus aurantium, Willd.
Phuṭiạ kạuḍi cun, lime made of the shells used in India as money.

Grind and mix both, then mix with *pạurạ*, spirits, and let him drink some every morning, or if inefficacious add a little *cuạ sosọ*, distilled Semecarpus Anacardium, L. and drink.

67. *Puni pilạ*. Spleen in atrophied infants.

Medicines: (a) *Akaona rẹhẹl*, the roots of Calotropis gigantea, R. Br.
Pẹa gol mạric, 3 black peppercorns.
Thoṛa goṭe rẹhẹl, a little of the roots of Croton oblongifolius, Roxb.
Thoṛa haṭ rẹhẹl, a little of the roots of Holarrhena antidysenterica, Wall.

Grind these together, make into pills and give daily to take.

68. *Khapra pilạ*. (See also No. 66) Spleen permagnum.

One 'authority' says: When this affection of the spleen begins there is pain, for the spleen is under the ribs, and when there is pain, it spreads to the whole stomach; when the spleen reaches up to the navel the pain is intense; if you then feel or press at the navel, you will find it slip away, and by this you will know it is *khapra pilạ*.

Medicines: (a) *Kaskọm jan*, cotton seed.
Kạtič talan sosọ, a little Semecarpus Anacardium, L.
Kạrhạni hoṛo, a variety of black paddy.
Kunạm da, the bulb of

Grind and make into hand bread.

(b) *Ghoṛa lạḍạuṛi da*, the bulb of Vitis tomentosa, Heyne.

Warm and give to drink, and apply some as an ointment over the spleen—an excellent remedy.

(c) *Bana haṭak chal*, the bark of Oroxylon indicum, Benth.
Baraṅgọm rẹhẹl, the roots of Vernonia cineria, Less., or Glossogyne pinnatifida, DC.
Thoṛa ạphim, a little opium.
Rạimạt lẹnḍọn, a kind of very large centipede.
Gẹgẹṭẹrẹn, young ones of above appearing in clusters.

Grind together, make into pills and give to eat; he will surely recover.

If it is a case of ordinary spleen disease,

(*d*) first trace the vein by feeling and then apply *sǫsǫ*, the seed of Semecarpus Anacardium, L.

to the vein, the back and all the nails on a Sunday; if you have correctly followed the vein this will effect a cure.

(*e*) *Hẹhẹl rẹhẹl*, the roots of Millettia auriculata, Baker.
Corco rẹhẹl, „ „ „ Casearea tomentosa, Roxb.

Grind these together, cook in *gại gǫtǫm*, melted butter of cows' milk, and give to drink, and after drinking it let him drink some cow's milk. For some time subsequently he must avoid eating the meat of buffaloes and rams, fish, plantains, jackfruit, milk and parched rice.

(*f*) *Corṛa chal*, the bark of
Kitạuri rẹhẹl, the roots of Plumbago Zeylanica, Willd.
Cun, lime burned from mussels.

First apply the lime externally, then after grinding the other two together smear over that; wait three days and then if there is no improvement,

(*g*) *Ghoṛa lada rẹhẹl*, the roots of Vitis tomentosa, Heyne.

Grind, warm slightly and give some to drink and plaster some over the spleen. Do so for three days; then if there is no amelioration,

(*h*) take the bark and two kinds of roots last mentioned, grind all together and after slightly warming smear over the spleen.

(*i*) *Buru ghoṛa lạdạuṛi*, Vitis tomentosa, Heyne, growing on hills.

Give the patient a little to drink, and after grinding some make it lukewarm and apply as a plaster over the spleen; he will get well.

(*j*) *Ạphim*, opium.
Kalmẹg, Andrographis paniculata, Nees.
Kitạuri rẹhẹl, Plumbago Zeylanica, Willd., the roots.
Kaḍa beṅjaḱ rẹhẹl, the roots of

Grind these and make them into balls the size of sheeps' or goats' excrement; then let the patient take these for 7 days, not more, as this medicine will work for a month.

(*k*) *Kitạuri rẹhẹl*, the roots of Plumbago Zeylanica, Willd.
Lẹnḍọṅ, a very large centipede, Spirocystus cilcylindricus.
2 *gan sǫsǫ jaṅ*, a couple of the seeds of Semecarpus Anacardium, L.

Take a little of the first of these and about three of the second, and grind all three together; make pills thereof and let him take these daily.

(*l*) *Kaḍa beṅjaḱ rẹhẹl*, the roots of
Kalmẹg 3 *tusạ*, 3 tips of Andrographis paniculata, Nees.
Jioti ghās ḍọg thoṛa, a little of the tips of a certain grass, Sesbania ægyptiaca, Pers.
About 8 oz. of the urine of a heifer.
Pạurạ, spirits.
Hiṅ, Ferrula asafætida, Willd.

Grind the first four with spirits and add asafætida as much as the size of a grain of *rambṛa*, Phaeseolus Mungo, var. Radiatus, Linn., and make him drink it; afterwards give him the rest of the remedy without the asafætida, the one dose of which will have its effects for about a month.

(m) *Haṭ rẹhẹt*, the roots of Holarrhena antidysenterica, Wall.
Goṭe rẹhẹt, „ „ „ Croton oblongifolius Roxb.
Pạclạ laṭha cip ciṛip rẹhẹt, the roots of
Lẹṇḍọṅ, Spirocystus cilcylindricus.
25 *gaṇḍa gol mạric*, 100 black peppercorns.

Mix and make into pills, to be taken daily until recovery.

(n) *Nawa sim bele*, new laid hen's egg.
Kitạuri rẹhẹt, the roots of Plumbago Zeylanica, Willd.

The former to be boiled with the latter and eaten daily.

(o) *Kitạuri*, Plumbago Zeylanica, Willd.
Lẹṇḍọṅ, Spirocystus cilcylindricus.
Họpọn macha sim, a smallish chicken.

The meat of the third to be cooked with the first two and eaten.

(p) *Kitạuri rẹhẹt*, the roots of Plumbago Zeylanica, Willd.
Mit sọsọ jaṅ, one seed of Semecarpus Anacardium, Linn.
Thoṛa hẹndẹ tilmiṅ, a little of the black variety of Sesamum orientale, Willd.
Caole ata, roasted rice.

Grind all these together and make into pills to be eaten daily.

For small children: (pp) *Akaona rẹhẹt*, the roots of Calotropis gigantea, R. Br. To be ground mixed with rice flour, made into hand bread and eaten. For adults: make about two oz. into a juice and add ten black peppercorns, and let them drink this daily until recovery.

As an unguent when the spleen is hard:—

(q) *Akaona*, Calotropis gigantea, R. Br.
Ạphim, opium.

Take about as much opium as the size of a grain of *rambṛa*, Phaeseolus Mungo, var. Radiatus, Linn., and about an ounce of the milk of the former, mix the two well together and apply externally to the spleen which will contract and get well.

(r) *Bir buṭ rẹhẹt*, the roots of Flemingia congesta, Roxb.
Rọl jọ, the fruit of Terminalia Chebula, Retz.
Sohga, borax.
Simbrit, shoots of Bombax malabaricum, DC.

First rub the first of above and take some of the juice; then rub the second with the third; then rub the last also, and mix the liquid of all together; give the patient some of this to drink and with some anoint over the spleen; recovery is sure.

(s) *Ḍhalka hạtkạn*, Leea macrophylla, Roxb.

After grinding mix it with rice flour, make into hand bread and give it to a child to eat; but an adult should drink it; the same remedy should be smeared daily over the spleen.

If an infant has *dud pilą*,

(*t*) *Tąṇḍi catǫm aṛak*, Desmodium triflorum, DC.
Sim kaṭa aṛak, Vitex peduncularis.
Piṭuą aṛak, Spermacoce hispida, Linn.

Grind all these, smear him with some and let him drink a little.

(*u*) *Sim kaṭa aṛak ręhęl*, the roots of Vitex peduncularis.
Tąṇḍi catǫm aṛak, Desmodium triflorum, DC.
Suruj mukhi aṛak ręhęl, the roots of Helianthus annuus, Willd.
Thoṛa muṅgą, a little Moringa pterygosperma, Gärtn.

Mix all these together and smear daily over the spleen, he will get well.

(*v*) *Jǫm jąnum ḍǫg pęa*, 3 shoots of Zizyphus Jujuba, Lamk.
Tąṇḍi catǫm aṛak ḍǫg, „ „ Desmodium triflorum, DC.

Take these and rub them fine (like tobacco) with dew and make into seven pills, and give them daily to a half grown child, one every day, to be swallowed with stale water.

(*w*) *Corco ręhęl*, the roots of Casearea tomentosa, Roxb.
Icąk ręhęl, „ „ „ Woodfordia floribunda, Salisb.

Grind together and give to drink.

(*x*) *Dudhiąni ręhęl*, the roots of Asclepias rosea, Roxb.

Cook and give to eat. If this is not successful, reduce to glowing coals *nim dare ḍąr gǫčak*, the dead branch of a Melia Azadirachta, L. tree, and placing a brass cup on the spleen apply these glowing coals.

(*y*) *Jǫm jąnum ḍǫg*, a shoot of Zizyphus Jujuba, Lamk.
Catǫm aṛak, Marsilia quadrifolia, L.

Grind these together and wet them with dew, add a little salt, make into pills and administer immediately.

69. *Jarǫ pilą.*

Symptoms. This is what we call the phase of spleen complaint, when a man has suffered for a long time from spleen and a number of our *ojhas* have given medicines till they are tired of it, without effecting a cure; the patient's arms and legs have become as thin as a rope, in fact only life is left.

Medicines: (*a*) First of all on Sunday morning smear his head well with *sasaṅ*, turmeric, Curcuma longa, Roxb., all over, for a couple of days; after that grind

Kiṭąuri ręhęl, the roots of Plumbago Zeylanica, Willd.

and make it into pills the size of goats' dung and mix therewith

Mit pawa moeda hǫlǫṅ, 8 oz. wheat flour.
Miṭaṅ sim bele, a hen's egg.

and make the whole into hand bread in leaves, put in the dew, and then give to eat in the morning. In 3 or 4 days he will be quite cured and put on flesh again.

70. *Laṛ pilạ.*

Symptoms. In this the spleen becomes enlarged under the ribs, where there is pain, and the patient shivers with cold as in *bhạlki ruạ* (54); it is not to be diagnosed by feeling; the fit of ague lasts a short time and then ceases.

Medicines: (*a*) *Akaona rẹhẹt*, the roots of Calotropis gigantea, R. Br. or C. procera, R. Br.

Kạhu botke, Bryonia lacinosa, L.

Karla da, the tuber of Momordica dioica, Roxb.

Ḍhela chal, the bark of Alangium Lamarckii, Thurs.

Phuṭiạ kạuḍi cun, lime made of the small shells used in India as money.

Grind all these together, squeeze out and after mixing with *pạurạ*, spirits, give to drink.

Should the skin becomes darkened in colour (*aṅgạura* supervene), then

(*b*) *Cọndọn kạti kaṭ*, a bit of the wood of Santalum album, L.

Rub on a stone and give what comes away to drink. If there should be dropsical symptoms

(*c*) *Dudhi loṭa rẹhẹt*, the roots of Ichnocarpus frutescens, R. Br.

Grind and give to drink.

This may also be given in cases of *kaṭ pilạ*.

(*d*) *Pea akaona sakam*, 3 leaves of Calotropis gigantea, R. Br. or C. procera, R. Br.

Miṭṭaṅ jivẹt cọḍgọć hako, a live fish, Ophiocephalus gachua.

Proceed as follows on a Sunday morning: First foment him once with each of the three leaves separately; then make the patient stand inside at the threshold of the door and you at the outside; let him feign to be bitten over the spleen by the fish three or five times; then after stringing the three leaves and the fish on a piece of string hang the whole up over the heat of the fireplace. In five days he will recover if this remedy acts; if not, then

(*e*) *Malhan sakam*, the leaves of Dolichos Lablab, L.

Lay these over the spleen, and spread over them a wet *dhuti* eight fold and over this again put a thin layer of *mat biti*, shredded bamboo, and set fire to these with *hẹsẹl aṅgra*, live coals of Anogeissus latifolia, Wall. Another man is to sit on the ground and stab with a stick a *họtọt*, Cucurbita lagenaria, purposelessly all the while until the patient feels pain, when all over the spleen is to be thrown away, and a blister will appear over the spleen, and he will recover.

71. *Banmara.*

Symptoms. Ascites with thin legs and pains in the joints of the legs.

Medicines: (*a*) *Gọċ dare reak̕ banda*, a parasitical plant found on a dead tree.
Kaṭkọm jaṅga rẹhẹl, the roots of Viscum attenuatum, DC.
Lag joṛa, Vanda Teres (?).
Gõṛẽ chal, the bark of Stephegyne parviflora, Korth.

Grind these together and smear on.

72. *Ạbhuạ.*

Symptoms. In this they swell up on one side and the other side remains normal.

Medicines: *Ạsạṛiạ*, Capparis horrida, L. f.
Lilkạthi, Polygala crotalarioides, Buch. and Ham.
Sealom, lichen.

Grind these together and plaster over the swollen part and invoke the spirit *Gosãe era.*

73. *Ruạ jaṛaokate mẽtãhãko bharao akan khan.* Facial œdema after long fever.

Medicines: (*a*) *Mithi*, Trigonella Fænumgraecum, Willd.

Grind and mix with *utiń sunum*, mustard oil, and let him anoint his face daily with this oil; then

(*b*) *Lag jọṛ*, Vanda Teres (?).
Gõṛẽ chal, the bark of Stephegyne parviflora, Korth.

Grind these two together and give a beer-leaf-cup full to drink, and plaster the remainder over the whole body.

(*c*) On Sunday morning make him cook some hot rice, make this into three balls and have a small earthenware pot full of water; then take the patient to the end of the village street and make him stand facing the sunrise; pour the pot of water over him and make him eat there two of the balls of rice while he puts down the third ball; then let him go straight home without looking back. If he acts thus this remedy will cure him.

74. *Mõk reak̕.* Swellings.

Medicines: *Cala bulạ*,
Bọd laṛ poha rẹhẹl, the roots of a shoot of Vitis adnata, Wall.

Grind and smear on.

75. *Udri.* Ascites, Dropsy and Anasarca.

Symptoms. This commences in the abdomen. It becomes thick at the navel and swells up puffily. Afterwards it spreads and the whole body distends like a drum.

Medicines: (*a*) *Bir malhan rẹhẹl*, the roots of Atyllosia mollis, Bth.
Sẹṅgẹl siń rẹhẹl, „ „ „ Tragia involucrata, Jacq.
Etka rẹhẹl, „ „ „ Mucuna pruriens, DC.
Dạtrạ rẹhẹl, „ „ „ Datura alba, Willd. or D. fastuosa, Willd.

Aṇḍia moron arak rehel, the roots of Gymnema hirsutus, W. and A., var. Decaisneanum, Wight.

Utri dudhi loṭa rehel, the roots of Cryptolepis Buchanani, R. and S.

Aṇḍia koṅgat rehel, the roots of Dregia volubils, Benth.

Take and mix equal quantities of all these, cook them in two pounds of mustard oil and anoint him therewith daily. Very early in the morning tie the first named on him.

An aperient: (*b*) *Datra rehel*, the roots of Datura alba, Willd. or D. fastuosa, Willd.

2 ounces of the juice to be extracted.

5 *gaṇḍa gol maric*, 20 black peppercorns.

Grind these and stir into two ounces of water; then add above two ounces of juice, strain and give to drink. A short time afterwards his bowels will begin to be moved; let him have some four motions, and if they do not then cease, mix some *jojo*, tamarinds, Tamarindus indica, L., and give about eight ounces to drink, when the evacuations will cease. He will become quite drunk and the eyes get bloodshot.

Then give *Kasmar chal*, the bark of Gmelina arborea, Roxb., and a little *Siṅ arak chal*, the bark of Bauhinia purpurea, L.

Grind small, mix with stale rice water and give about 8 ounces to drink. The other medicines to be smeared on the body. The aperient to be administered at intervals of ten to fifteen days until recovery.

(*c*) *Seṅgel siṅ rehel*, the roots of Tragia involucrata, Jacq.

Etka rehel, the roots of Mucuna pruriens, DC.

Aṇḍia moron arak rehel, the roots of Gymnema hirsutus, W. and A. var. Decaisneanum, Wight.

Datra rehel, the roots of Datura alba, Willd. or D. fastuosa, Willd.

Kukrucul baha rehel, the roots of Amaranthus frumentacens, Buch.

Eradom rehel, the roots Ricinus communis, L.

Utri dudhi loṭa rehel, the roots of Cryptolepis Buchanani, R. and S.

Kãrwãt rehel, the roots of Carissa Carandas, L.

Pound all these together with dew, to be obtained by drawing a clean cloth over the grass and squeezing it out. Plaster the entire body with the mixture until recovery.

Aperient to be given: (*d*) *Eradom dal*, the kernel of Ricinus communis, L.

Grind and make into balls half the size of those used in a cross-bow, and after stirring in eight ounces of hot water give to drink. If he has more than four motions mix tamarinds in stale rice water and give him four ounces to drink, which will bind him, and then let him bathe in cold water.

Various aperients: (*e*) *Bherṇḍa*, Jatropha Curcas, L.

Grind six of the fruits and stirring them in eight ounces of hot water give to drink. For children of 7 or 8 years old use only two of the fruits.

(*f*) *Kuṇḍo phọl*,

is an excellent aperient. For adults break one up into four ounces of water and give to drink. If he has more than four motions mix *jọjọ*, tamarinds, Tamarindus indica, L., in stale rice water and give to drink.

(*g*) *Eṭkẹć ḍạr*, a branch of Euphorbia antiquorum, L.

Pound and bruise this, toast it at the fire and squeeze out the water and after mixing 3 *gaṇḍa gol mạric*, 12 black peppercorns, make him drink four ounces hot. If the motions exceed four, give him sour curds of cow's milk.

(*h*) *Ḍhela chal*, the bark of Alangium Lamarckii, Thurs.

Extract the juice in eight ounces of water, add 12 black peppercorns and give to drink. To check the motions mix tamarinds in stale rice water, eight ounces, or give curds of cow's milk.

(*i*) *Jọjọ*, tamarinds, Tamarindus indica, L.

Draw off four ounces of very hot water, stir the tamarinds in this and give to drink; very shortly afterwards the bowels will begin to be moved. After some four motions give to drink *thoṛa sahṛa chal*, the bark of Streblus asper, Lour., and sour curds of cow's milk.

Steaming remedy: (*j*) *Akaona rẹhẹl*, the roots of Calotropis gigantea, R. Br.

Kāṛwāl rẹhẹl, the roots of Carissa Carandas, L.

Dạtrạ sakam, the leaves of Datura alba, Willd. or D. fastuosa, Willd.

Bir hoṛẹć, Atyllosia scarabædois, Benth.

Sinduạri sakam, the leaves of Vitex Negundo, L.

Tursi sakam, the leaves of Ocymum sanctum, Willd.

Bharbhạri sakam, the leaves of Ocimum basilicum, L. or O. canum, Sims.

Bana haṭak chal, the bark of Oroxylon indicum, Benth.

Kaera rẹhẹl, the roots of Musa paradisiaca. L.

Sẹṅgẹl siń rẹhẹl, the roots of Tragia involucrata, Jacq.

Etka rẹhẹl, the roots of Mucuna pruriens, DC.

Ul chal, the bark of Mangifera indica, L.

Buc chal, „ „ „ Cordia Myxa, L.

Pọjọ chal, „ „ „ Tetranthera monopetala, Roxb.

Saram lutur rẹhẹl, the roots of Clerodendron serratum, Spreng.

Cạili chal, the bark of Morinda exserta, Roxb.

Hemca aṛak, Enhydra fluctuans.

Pạni phol, Trapa bispinosa, Roxb.

Kaḍa bhosam, Oldenlandia paniculata (?).

Dak ghoṛa lada rẹhẹl, the roots of Vitis tomentosa, Heyne.

Kūs rẹhẹl, the roots of Themuda gigantea, Haskel.

Put all these into a new earthen pot and boil well. Make the patient lie down on a bed, cover him with a cloth which should hang down to the ground all round. Then putting the boiling water under the bed, steam him well until the perspiration drops from his body, when the swelling will subside.

(*k*) *Aṇḍiạ mọrọn aṛak rẹhẹt*, the roots of Gymnema hirsutus, W. and A., var Decaisneanum, Wight.
Sẹṅgẹl siṅ rẹhẹt, the roots of Tragia involucrata, Jacq.
Etka rẹhẹt, the roots of Mucuna pruriens, DC.
Sọsọ jaṅ bareage, two seeds of Semecarpus Anacardium, L.

Grind these together, make into pills and give to eat.

(*l*) *Koṅga*, Agave americana, L. } to be smeared
Utri dudhi, Cryptolepis Buchanani, R. and S. } on.
Bạṛ baha, the flower of Mimusops Elengi, L., to be drunk.
Bir malhan da, the bulb of Atyllosia mollis, Bth., to be hung on.

(*m*) *Bidhạnta chal*, the bark of Entada scandens, Benth.
Pio cẽṛẽ il, the feathers of the Oriolus melanocephalus.
Kunạm da, the bulb of
Haṛhat họtọt rẹhẹt, the roots of a bitter Cucurbita lagenaria.
Arak sutạm, red thread.

Grind to the consistency of porridge and plaster over the whole body. Some also to be drunk.

(*n*) *Orop da*, the tuber of Costus speciosa, Sm.
Matha aṛak rẹhẹt, the roots of Antidesma diandrum, Tulas.

Grind, heat and smear on.

Tọtnọpak chal, the bark of Eugenia operculata, Roxb.

Grind and give to drink.

(*o*) Plaster him with *gọd*, Aristolochia indica, Willd.

(*p*) *Tọtnọpak chal*, the bark of Eugenia operculata, Roxb.
Akaona sakam, the leaves of Calotropis gigantea, R. Br.

Put into an earthen pot, boil and steam the patient therewith.

(*q*) The same ingredients as in this No. 75 (*a*) with the addition of
Alagjạri rẹhẹt, the roots of Cuscuta chinensis, Lamk.
Sinduạri sakam, the leaves of Vitex Negundo, L.

but omitting *Aṇḍiạ koṅgat rẹhẹt*. Grind these together and boil in two pounds of mustard oil; anoint therewith the whole body from the face downwards and in three days the swelling will subside.

(*r*) The following or any one of them may be tied on the patient:
Bir malhan rẹhẹt, the roots of Atyllosia mollis, R. Br.
Etka rẹhẹt, the roots of Mucuna pruriens, DC.
Sẹṅgẹl siṅ rẹhẹt, the roots of Tragia involucrata, Jacq.
Kaera rẹhẹt, the roots of Musa paradisiaca, L.

(*s*) *Sęngęl siń ręhęl,* the roots of Tragia involucrata, Jacq.
Etka ręhęt, the roots of Mucuna pruriens, DC.
Kukṛucul baha ręhęl, the roots of Amaranthus frumentacens, Benth.
Eraḍǫm ręhęl, the roots of Ricinus communis, L.

Wring out a cloth wet with dew into a cup. With some of this water grind the above, then stir in the water and let all remain in the cup, and smear the patient with its contents.

(*t*) *Alagjaṛi nāṛī,* Cassytha filiformis, Roxb.
Sinduąri sakam, the leaves of Vitex Negundo, L.

Boil well in water, give a little to drink, and smear the rest of it over the whole body, when the swelling will at once subside.

(*u*) *Ul chal,* the bark of Mangifera indica, L.
Sęngęl siń ręhęl, the roots of Tragia involucrata, Jacq.
Etka ręhęt, the roots of Mucuna pruriens, DC.
Akaona ręhęl, the roots of Calotropis gigantea, R. Br. or C. procera, R. Br.
Dak reak kaḍa bhosam aṛak, Oldenlandia paniculata (?).
Pąni phǫl, Trapa bispinosa, Roxb.

Grind these and put them in a new earthen pot and after covering this with a leaf plate, boil them well and steam the patient while lying on a bed until he perspires.

(*v*) *Sǫsǫ jań 3 gan sę miltań,* 1 to 3 seeds of Semecarpus Anacardium, L.
Sęngęl siń ręhęl, the roots of Tragia involucrata, Jacq.
Etka ręhęl, the roots of Mucuna pruriens, DC.

Grind and make into pills, to be eaten daily; he will soon get well.

(*w*) *Bir malhan ręhęl,* the roots of Atyllosia mollis, Bth.

Grind and plaster over the whole body, and on Sunday tie the bass thereof on to his limbs.

When it begins in the face (Pąṇḍul udri),

(*x*) *Ghoṛa lądąuṛi ręhęl,* the roots of Vitis tomentosa, Heyne.

Grind, warm and smear over the whole body; rub a *tąrup alań,* leopard's tongue, on a stone and give him to drink.

When it begins at the navel,

(*y*) *Orop da,* the tuber of Costus speciosa, Sm.
Tǫlnǫpak chal, the bark of Eugenia operculata, Roxb.
Orsǫṛęń, Zingiber Cassumunar, Roxb. (?).
Ḍurą sań, Diascorea pentafylla, Willd.

Grind these together and smear on, and in three or four days he will get well.

One "authority" says: This follows after one is much reduced by fever; first the feet swell up, and afterwards the entire body swells up like a drum: it begins sometimes in the face or at the navel.

76. *Beraeti.* Ascites, or spleen (?).

Symptoms: In this the abdomen grows larger and the legs and arms become emaciated.

Medicines: (*a*) *Gaḍa kasmar ręhęt sę chal*, the roots of bark of Gmelina arborea, Roxb.

Grind, smear well with catgut or tie under the armpit.

Rąli ręhęt, the roots of Piper longum, L.

Grind and give to drink.

Bhuku chata, a termites' nest.

Dahe, curds

Mix and smear on daily.

77. *Hǫṛmǫ umbrąu ocoetako.*

This is to make lean people who eat well put on flesh.

Medicines: (*a*) *Moṭa sega*, the thick Mimosa rubicaulis, Lamk.

Moṭa ąṭkir, " " Smilax ovalifolia, Roxb.

Bhorkonḍ mañj, the heart of Hymenodictyon excelsum, Wall.

Ḍhiri kaṭkǫm, a crab found under stones.

Grind these together, cook in *utiñ sunum*, mustard oil, and give to eat; in five days he will be stout.

78. *Ṭan dhąt calak.* Slow pulse.

Medicines: *Dumur rasa*, the honey of the small honey bee.

Bhąbri chal, the bark of Embelia robusta, Roxb.

Cini, sugar.

Sahṛa chal, the bark of Streblus asper, Lour.

Saparǫm dare dak, the water from Nyctanthes Arbor-tristis, L.

Mare nañgle rapak rǫñgǫ, an old leathern yoke roasted to burning point.

Ato kundri datęl, the bulb of Cephalandra indica, Nand.

Mix these up together and give to drink for two or three days.

79. *Ṭaṭka rǫg.* Disease without premonitory symptoms.

Medicines: (*a*) *Mąhũt guṛ* ½ *powa*, 4 oz. refuse of molasses.

Siñjo sakam, 1 *powa*, 8 oz. leaves of Ægle Marmelos, Correa.

Gitil kaḍa 3 sę 4, 3 or 4 Gryllus monstrosus.

Grind together and give to drink for a couple of days or so.

80. *Koñka kuñkik.* Madness.

This may be due to many causes. Sometimes from fever, or from hard thinking the brain gets confused, or from demon possession, epilepsy or other causes.

One "authority" says: Those who are thus afflicted feel immensely strong, sometimes they run about, sometimes they walk about in a silly way and speak incoherently.

Medicines: *External administration*:—

(*a*) *Kāṛwāt ręhęl*, the roots of Carissa Carandas, L.
Gạbur ręhęl, „ „ „ Acacia Farnesiana, Willd.
Dạtrạ ręhęl, „ „ „ Datura alba, Willd. or D. fastuosa, Willd.
Boṅga bạri ręhęl, „ „ „ Typha angustifolia (?).
Sinduạri sakam, the leaves of Vitex Negundo, L.
Muṅgạ chal, the bark of Moringa pterygosperma, Gärtn.
Nạṅgrạuta ręhęl, the roots of Nardostachys jatamansi, DC.
Bana haṭak chal, the bark of Oroxylon indicum, Benth.

Get equal weights of all these, save more of the first named (for if the others are unobtainable this alone will prove serviceable), cook in mustard oil or preferably melted butter, and smear on daily.

Internal administration:—

(*b*) *Etka ręhęl*, the roots of Mucuna pruriens, DC.
Sęṅgęl siṅ ręhęl, the roots of Tragia involucrata, Jacq.
Goṭe ręhęl, the roots of Croton oblongifolius, Roxb.

Grind these three together, make into pills and give daily and apply the above (*a*) externally.

Superior remedy:—

(*c*) *Milṭaṅ carọriṅ*, one longicorn beetle.
3 *gurli jọ reak jaṅ*, the kernel of three fruits of

Grind these two small together, make into three pills and dry them. To be administered thus: For persons over 20 years of age one of these pills to be mixed in 1 *choṭak pạurạ*, two ounces of spirits, and drunk; for those of 12 to 16 years old half a pill in 1 oz. of spirits; of 10 years old one third of a pill in 1 oz. of spirits; of 7 to 9 years one fourth of a pill in 1 oz. of spirits; of 5 and 6 years one fifth of a pill in 1 oz. of spirits. This is a very poisonous remedy, and if too large a dose be given it may prove fatal. Patients will pass blood with their urine. Let them do so three or four times and then give some very sour curds of cows' milk. This will kill the poison in the medicine; mad people feel very hot in the body.

If after taking this medicine there are roaring or humming sounds in the ears, then

(*c*) *Rạṅgạini jạnum jọ jaṅtęl*, the kernel of the fruit of Solanum Jacquini, Willd.

Grind, cook in mustard oil and give to eat, when he will be all right.

(*d*) *Hund nāṛī chal*, the bark of Jasminum arborescens, Roxb.
Bando nāṛī chal, the bark of Spatholobus Roxburghii, Benth.
Kismis jọ, raisins.

Pound and crush the two barks and boil all with sugar, and give this daily.

(*e*) *Gại ghuṛạ aṛak*, Polygala chinensis, L.

Grind the entire plant, boil in mustard oil and anoint the face daily therewith.

(*f*) *Bayaṅ da*, the bulb of Dioscorea crispata, Roxb.
Etka jo, the fruit of Mucuna pruriens, DC.
Seṅgel siṅ rẹhẹl, the roots of Tragia involucrata, Jacg.
Hiṅ, Ferrula asafoetida, Willd.
Jhiṅgạ jo, the fruit of Luffa acutangula, Roxb.

To be smeared on.

(*g*) *Bọrlọm dare rẹhẹl*, the roots of
Jọrọ baṛe reak ḍog tẹl, a shoot of Ficus bengalensis, L.
Pan bhiṭuạk, the leaf stem of Piper Betle, L.
Cini, sugar.

First grind together *Gạbur baha*, the flower of Acacia Farnesiana, Willd., and *mẽṛhẽl ic*, some iron rust, and put it in a metal-locket; make a rope of the tail tuft of a black cow and tie this locket on to the rope. Then on Sunday morning before relieving nature in any way make him eat the medicine with the rust and whip him some five times as hard as you like with the rope.

(*h*) *Hoṛ ic*, human excrement.
Bir sukri ic, a wild pig's excrement.
Lumạm tọl tejo, a silkworm in its chrysalis stage.
Tạrup jọm sadọm khurạ, the hoof of a horse killed by a leopard.

Grind the first three and mix the fourth, and then give to drink. Let him neither speak nor run about, but stay perfectly still for some four hours.

(*i*) *Dạtrạ rẹhẹl*, the roots of Datura alba, Willd. or D. fastuosa, Willd.
Thoṛa ạphim, a little opium.
3 *se* 4 *gaṇḍa gan gol mạric*, 12 to 16 black peppercorns.

Grind all these together, and give to drink.

(*j*) *Kaskọm rẹhẹl*, the roots of Gossypium arboreum, L.
Caroṛiṅ, the longicorn beetle.
Gọc hoṛ khạpri reak, a bit of the skull of a dead man.
Toyo ic, jackals' excrement.
Mare naṅgle rapak rọṅgọ kate, an old leathern yoke thong, roasted to burning point.
Ḍaṅgra jaṅ, the bone of a bullock, } to be half roasted.
Sukri ḍhumbạk, pigs' excrement, }

Grind all these together; smear *guric*, cowdung, on the courtyard in front of the house, and on that offer this medicine to the spirits, naming them Duriạbarḍo and Nason Cạṇḍi, make some parallel lines with *sindur*, red lead, and after mixing in *dahe*, curds, give to drink, and he will get well.

81. *Rọhọṛ naṅjọm.* Atrophy, emaciation or cachexy. Believed by the Santals to be due to the action of witches.

Symptoms. In this a person without being ill gradually wastes away.

One "authority" says: In this the body will not get into good condition or fat, and even if they eat rice they continue to become emaciated.

Medicines: (*a*) *Sega ręhęl*, the roots of Mimosa rubicaulis, Lam.
Badgǫcak̓ ręhęl, the roots of Lygodium flexuosum, Sw.
Nanha dudhi lota ręhęl, the roots of Ichnocarpus frutescens, R. Br.

Grind and give to drink daily.

(*b*) *Katkǫm carẹč*, Rottboellia perforata, Corom. pl.
Kitą mańj, the heart of Phœnix acaulis, Buch.
Gaḍa surą, Cyperus tegetum, Roxb.
Icąk̓ ręhęl, the roots of Woodfordia floribunda, Salisb.

Grind and give to drink daily.

(*c*) *Cae cirota*, Gentiana cherayta, Roxb.
Jiṭhimond, Clerodendron Siphonanthus, R. Br.

Soak in water over night and in the morning after straining off the water give it to drink mixed with *misri cini*, sugar-candy. Scoop out a *sąru*, Celocasia antiquorum, Schott., and put in some *posta daṅa*, the seed of the opium poppy, and steam this. Then grind this and make into pills, some of the above water to be drunk with each pill.

(*d*) *Katkǫm carẹč ręhęl*, the roots of Rottboellia perforata, Corom. pl.
Sega jąnum ręhęl, the roots of Mimosa rubicaulis, Lam.
Sąuṛi ręhęl, the roots of Heteropogon contortus, R. and S.

Take a little of each of these, mix, grind and give to drink.

(*e*) *Seṛwaṅ ręhęl*, the roots of Vigna vexillata, Benth.
Raṅgąini jąnum ręhęl, the roots of Solanum Jacquini, Willd.

Grind together and give to drink.

(*f*) *Badgǫcak̓ ręhęl*, the roots of Lygodium flexuosum, Sw.
Hesak̓ jǫrǫ ḍog, tip of the aerial root of Ficus religiosa, Willd.
Baṛe jǫrǫ ḍog, tip of the aerial root of Ficus bengalensis, L.

Grind and mix these and give to drink.

(*g*) *Hąti ič*, elephant's excrement.
Sasaṅ, turmeric.
Buluṅ, salt.

Grind and mix these and plaster therewith.

(*h*) *Cąulią*, the roots of Ruellia suffruticosa, Roxb.
Badgǫcak̓, „ „ Lygodium flexuosum, Sw.
Kaḍa męt ręhęl, the roots of Premna herbacea, Roxb.
Kūs ręhęl, the roots of Themuda gigantea, Haskel.

Grind together and give to drink.

(*i*) the same as No. 208 (*d*).

(*j*) *Janhę naṅjom*, Polycarpæa corymbosa, Lamk.

Boṅga sarjom dak, the water of Ventilago calyculata, Tulasne.

Matkom rẹhẹl reak dak, the water of the roots of Bassia latifolia, Roxb.

Kaṭkom jaṅga, terel reak, the Viscum attenuatum, DC., found on the *terel*, Diospyros tomentosa, Roxb.

(*k*) *Icạk rẹhẹl*, the roots of Woodfordia floribunda, Salisb.

Gaḍa suṛạ rẹhẹl, the roots of Cyperus tegetum, Roxb.

Kaṭkom carẹc rẹhẹl, the roots of Rottboellia perforata, Corom. pl.

Kitạ mañj cetanre ọmọnok cip ciṛip rẹhẹl, the roots of Achyranthes aspera, L., growing from the heart of Phœnix acaulis, Buch.

Mix all these and give to drink with early success (a proved remedy).

(*l*) *Cae cirota*, Gentiana cherayta, Roxb.

Misri, sugar candy.

Kạliạ jirạ, Nigella indica, Roxb.

Jawan jirạ, Carum Ajowan, DC.

Lubui jirạ,

Put all these in a cup of water at night, and in the morning after pounding them a little, strain, add the sugar-candy and give to drink. Previously cook some *posta dana*, seeds of the opium poppy, grind them and make into pills, and whenever one of these is taken let him drink some of the above preparation. By following this course he will both be cured and regain strength.

This remedy is also good for *jarọ ruạ*, vide No. 56.

(*m*) The 3 ingredients specified in (*a*) above and

Icạk chal, the bark of Woodfordia floribunda, Salisb.

Ḍoḍhar, Adiantum lunulatum, Burm. or A. concinnum.

Saparọm rẹhẹl, the roots of Nyctanthes Arbor-tristis, L.

Edẹl mañj, the heart of Bombax malabaricum, DC.

Grind together and give to drink for a week.

82. *Bandọrgạli*. Cancer in the face.

Symptoms. This disease generally attacks the lower lip, cheeks or chin, and there is a profuse discharge of saliva. When the disease begins the lip or chin gradually continues to split, and if medicine is not quickly applied the sore will break out and in that case recovery is very doubtful.

One "authority" says: This begins like a pimple in the cheek, and later on developes into a sore that penetrates from outside to inside.

Medicines: (*a*) *Bir sọn*, wild hemp.

Alagjạṛi, Cuscuta chinensis, Lamk.

Grind the leaves of both of these and spread them over the spot and recovery will ensue.

(*b*) *Sirąuna* or *guklą*, Hygrophila spinosa, T. Anders.

Grind the bulb of this and apply it without heating. This may be used in both the early and the advanced stages of the sore.

(*c*) *Mǫsǫbǫr*, Barbadoes aloes.

Grind and apply this before the part swells or a sore breaks out.

(*d*) The earth with which the male bird imprisons the *camacakǫr* female (the black and white or grey hornbill) in its nest in a tree hollow, or a part of its body.
The root of *etka*, Mucuna pruriens, DC.
The root of *sęṅgęl siń*, Tragia involucrata, Jacq.
The root of *dare japak*, Scindapsus officinalis, Schott.
The kernel of the fruit of *bidhąnta*, Entada scandens, Benth.

Grind all these together and apply on the sore.

(*e*) *Ǫt banat*, lichen (on a stone).
The scraped husk of *saparǫm*, Nyctanthes Arbor-tristis, Linn.

Grind these together and sprinkle on the spot, and if it has burst inwardly stick a piece of paper on this.

(*f*) *Khayar mańj*, the pith or heart of Acacia Catechu, Willd.

Boil this down to the consistency of molasses and smear on the sore.

(*g*) *Dąre japak ręhęt*, the roots of Scindapsus officinalis, Schott.
Sǫ jǫtęt, the fruit of Eugenia Jambolana, Lamk.

Grind together and apply to the sore.

(*h*) *Dhūṛą̃*, resin of Shorea robusta, Gärtn.

Grind till it is like red lead, mix in a leaf cup of melted butter and add enough water rubbing all the time until it turns white like cream. Apply this to the sore.

(*i*) *Camacakǫr tuką*, the nest of the Hornbill bird.
Hęsęl tǫrǫć, the ashes of Anogeissus latifolia, Wall.
Sarjǫm jǫ, the fruit of Shorea robusta, Gärtn.

Grind these to a powder, sprinkle on the sore and cover with paper, and then

(*j*) *Gǫd*, Aristolochia indica, Willd.
Ńūṛūć jǫ reak dąl, the kernel of the fruit of Cassia Fistula, L.
Sealǫm, lichen.

Grind these with dew, no other water will do, and plaster on the sore. This remedy is applied after calling on the medicine man's goddess.

(*k*) The real specific for this disease is
Sahṛa banda, the parasitical air plant found on Streblus asper, Lour.

Two applications of this will result in a speedy cure.

83. *Ḍoho.* Tumours.

Medicines: (*a*) To soften: *nim sakam*, the leaves of Melia Azadirachta, L. Grind fine, heat, wrap in a piece of cloth and tie firmly on to the tumour.

(*b*) *Gại gọtọm*, melted butter of cows' milk.
Dhũṛạ̃, resin of Shorea robusta, Gärtn.
Nirbis, Kyllingia monocephala, L.
Selep samanọm, Gloriosa superba, Willd.
Terel dare reak̕ kaṭkọm jaṅga, Viscum attenuatum, DC., found on Diospyros tomentosa, Roxb.
Ạṭkuṛạ, Wrightia tomentosa, R. and S.
Buluṅ, salt.

Grind together, cook in melted butter of cows' milk, and apply externally. After softening pus will form, and to make it burst:

(*c*) *Mare ḍaṅgra jaṅ*, an old bullock bone.
Hoṛẹć, Dolichos biflorus, L.
Parwa ić, pigeons' dung.
Buluṅ, salt.

Grind together, plaster on the tumour, and it will soon burst.

84. *Ojo.* Boils.

One "authority" says: This usually begins like a pimple on the posterior, grows gradually to a large size and is painful.

Medicines: (*a*) Put fire to a piece of string used for the bottom of a bedstead and touch the head of the boil with this piece of burning string.

(*b*) Smear *loa loṛe*, the juice exuded from incision of the bark of Ficus glomerata, Roxb., on the swollen part.

(*c*) Grind *pọjọ chal*, the bark of Tetranthera monopetala, Roxb. and plaster it on.

(*d*) *Kolo da*, the bulb of Dioscorea dæmonum, Roxb.
Akaona loṛe, the exudation of Calotropis gigantea, R. Br.

To be smeared on.

(*e*) *Sirạm ṛẹhẹt*, the roots of Andropogon muricatus, Retz.
Ḍaṅgra jambe ḍaṭa, the jaw tooth of a bullock.

Grind the former, rub the latter on a stone, mix both and apply as a plaster. It will burst.

(*f*) *Gọtọm sunum*, melted butter.

If the boil will not burst then smear this on and it will cause it to do so. Then apply *jokha sakam*, the leaves of Sida humilis, Willd., when the pus may be squeezed out.

(*g*) When in the incipient stage apply (*b*) as above, which will check its growth; then

(h) Just touch the top once with a drop from *sǫsǫ*, the seed of Semecarpus Anacardium, L.

(i) When ripe prick a hole in the top and smear *jokha sakam*, the leaves of Sida humilis, Willd., all round and all the matter will be expelled.

85. *Bisphǫṛ.* Carbuncle.

Symptoms. This may appear on any part of the body, usually on the thigh or shin. At first small pimples appear, and afterwards it spreads all round, something hard arises from inside, it is very painful and there is a core within.

One "authority" says: This begins at first like a boil in the nape of the neck or middle of the back, and grows into a large sore which itches and causes a burning pain.

Medicines : (a) Smear *gǫtǫm*, melted butter, on, which will ripen it.

(b) *Gąṅgiṭ cun*, the lime obtained from nodular limestone.
Jhinuk cun, shell lime.
Thoṛa buluṅ, a little salt.

Mix and smear on.

(c) *Turąm rẹhẹl*, the roots of
Bhiḍi janatẹp rẹhẹl, the roots of Urena sinuata, L. or Triumfetta rhomboidea, Jac.
Maṭha aṛak̕ rẹhẹl, the roots of Antidesma diandrum, Tulas.

Grind these and plaster on, the sore will heal.

(d) *Kuclą jaṅ*, the seeds of Strychnos potatorum, Lin. f.

Grind and apply so that it may burst.

After bursting

(e) *Joka sakam*, the leaves of Sida humilis, Willd.
Pǫjǫ chal, the bark of Tetranthera monopetala, Roxb.

Grind and apply as a plaster.

(f) *Ąmbąitar jaṅ*, the bones of the snake Daboia Russellii, to burst it.
Bhorkoṇḍ baklak̕, the bark of Hymenodictyon excelsum, Wall.

Grind and dry, and making it into a powder dust it on.

(g) Get a piece of a waterpot that has been broken by an unmarried girl, rub it on a stone and apply what comes off with a feather to the sore, and see for three days whether it is drying up. If there is an increase of pus,

(h) *Mẹrlẹć chal*, the bark of Flacourtia Ramontchi, L'Herit.

Grind this fine to a powder and sprinkle on the sore, and it will check the discharge; and rub some of this also on the sore.

(i) *Akaṛ baha*, Limnophila Roxburghiana, G. Don.
Bherṇḍa loṛe, the exudation from Jatropha Curcas, L.

Grind the former, put some of the latter on it and grind a little more, and then smear the preparation on the sore; if there is pus wash it with *kạnji dak*, stale rice water, and adding a little water to the preparation squeeze it out into the cavity and in three days a cure will be effected.

(*j*) *Tejo mala rẹhẹt*, the roots of Cissampelos Pareira, L.

Baklak, the bark of trees that certain large caterpillars boring in trees cause to fall down.

Gạbur rẹhẹt chal, the bark of the roots of Acacia Farnesiana, Willd.

Gitil gãṛi, an insect that burrows in the sand in river beds.

Grind these together and boil in pure mustard oil. Clean the place, apply with a feather morning and evening.

86. *Hạmus.* Anæmia.

Symptoms. When one has suffered a long time from spleen, the blood in the body dries up causing the body to become pale.

Medicines: (*a*) Plaster him with *bir pan dare chal*, the bark of Monochoria plantaginea, Kunth.

(*b*) *Kadam*, Anthocephalus Cadamba, Bth. and Hook.

Kujri chal, the bark of Celastrus paniculatus, Willd.

Grind together and plaster therewith.

(*c*) *Kod sạkam*, the leaves of Eugenia Jambolana, Lamk.

Cook in mustard oil, and anoint with that oil.

(*d*) *Ọrsọṛiṅ da*, the bulb of Zingiber Cassumunar, Roxb. (?).

Kul jọm gại jaṅ, the bone of a cow killed by a tiger.

Bir họṛẹć, Atyllosia scarabædois, Benth.

The patient to be smeared with the first; the other two to be boiled and some of the water to be drunk.

(*e*) *Bana haṭak chal*, the bark of Oroxylon indicum, Benth.

Kạuhạ chal, the bark of Terminalia Arjuna, Bedd.

Ambṛa chal, „ „ „ Spondias mangifera, Pers.

Tạrup jọm gại jaṅ, the bone of cow killed by a leopard.

Boil the last in water and in that water mix the barks after grinding, and then the patient to drink some of it.

(*f*) *Arak meral sakam*, the leaves of Phyllanthus Emblica, L. which bears a red flower.

Bitkil cand rẹhẹt, the roots of Porana paniculata, Roxb.

Grind and smear over the whole body.

(*g*) *Tạrup jọmić reak jaṅ*, the bone of an animal killed by a leopard.

Haṭ jọ, the fruit of Holarrhena antidysenterica, Wall.

Haṛhat họṭọt, a bitter Curcurbita lagenaria, Willd.

Bãṛiạ̃ kạṇḍhum jọ, the fruit of Phyllanthus lanceolarius, Mull-Arg.

(h) *Tarup jom gai jan*, the bone of a cow killed by a leopard.

Boil this in water and with that water bathe him from head to foot, then

Kadam chal, the bark of Anthocephalus Cadamba, Benth. and Hook.

Ul chal, the bark of Mangifera indica, L.

Soso chal, „ „ „ Semecarpus Anacardium, L.

Grind together and smear over the whole body.

87. *Dorod*. Pain in any part of the body.

Medicines: (a) *Halim*, Lepidium sativum, L.

Dhalka hatkan, Leea macrophylla, Roxb.

Grind these and give a leaf cup full to drink and apply some to the seat of the pain.

(b) *Dhalka hatkan*, Leea macrophylla, Roxb.

Duria hatkan, Leea hirta, Herb. Banks.

Atnak chal, the bark of Terminalia tomentosa, W. and A.

Baru chal, „ „ „ Schleichera trijuga, Willd.

Jioli dog, a sprout of Sesbania ægyptiaca, Pers.

Grind these together very fine and after warming slightly plaster on to the seat of pain. Some two or three applications will cause the pain to cease.

88. *Hadi dorod*. Muscular pain from over-exertion.

Symptoms. If a man should work beyond his strength or lift anything very heavy, then he will get this, *i.e.* his limbs and whole body will ache.

One "authority" says: This commences in the neck. If one carries anything heavy on the head or shoulders a vein is strained or gets stiff. Then the body begins first to shiver and feel out of sorts, *i.e.* feverish. Then two or three days later one feels shooting pains in the limbs. Then there is pain in the neck, and if you are not soon rubbed it will become stiff. Then from this various complaints may result, *e.g. sagak* (q.v.), *betha* (q.v.), cough, spleen, convulsions, back-pain, intermittent fever, in fact all kinds of disorders may ensue. Therefore they call this the forerunner. And this is quite true. If the thick vein in the back gets *hadi* and it extends to the neck, there is headache, and if it extends downwards there is pain in the loins. Again, there is a small vein in the small of the back that runs to the stomach. If this gets *hadi* there is a feeling of repletion first and the food is not digested. Then follow diarrhœa and dysentery. Further, there is another small vein extending through the ribs to the spleen, and if this gets *hadi* spleen disease ensues. On this account they apply *soso*, the fruit of Semecarpus Anacardium, L. var. cuneifolia. There is also a vein between the scapulæ crossing to the chest, and if this gets *hadi*, *betha* (q.v.) will follow. There is also a small vein branching off from the big one in the lungs. If this gets *hadi* a cough will follow. Therefore many *ojhas* use *sǫsǫ* extensively. They employ it too in cases of cough. They look at the neck of the patient while he is coughing and apply *sǫsǫ* to the veins which they see swell up then. All these disorders are due to congestion of the blood. The blood courses continually through the veins, and if the flow of the blood in the veins is impeded disorder will ensue.

Medicines: (*a*) *Suruj mukhi aṛak*, Helianthus annuus, Willd.
Sim kaṭa aṛak, Vitex peduncularis.
Catǫm aṛak, Marsilia quadrifolia, L.

Grind these three and after warming a little plaster the whole body therewith. He will get well in some four days.

(*b*) *Mihndi sakam*, the leaves of Lawsonia alba, Lam.
Jǫjǫ sakam, " " " Tamarindus indica, L.
Kawẹl sakam, " " " Abrus precatorius, Willd.

Grind these, add a little salt, boil a little and plaster the whole body therewith.

(*c*) *Maṭha aṛak rẹhẹl*, the roots of Antidesma diandrum, Tulas.

Grind and plaster the whole body therewith.

(*d*) *Jǫjǫ jaṅ*, the seeds of Tamarindus indica, L.

Split, grind and apply after warming.

(*e*) Rub the whole body with *eraḍǫm sunum*, castor oil, and if the legs are contracted, mix a little salt with *loa loṛe*, the sticky juice exuded by Ficus glomerata, Roxb., and smear it on.

(*f*) *Akaona rẹhẹl*, the roots of Calotropis gigantea, R. Br.

Grind, warm a little and plaster therewith.

(*g*) *Ić ẹwẹr rẹhẹl*, the roots of Vitis latifolia, Roxb.

Grind to a very thin consistence, warm and apply to the painful parts: all pain will cease.

(*h*) *Dhonantori rẹhẹl ar sakam*, the roots and leaves of

Grind small, mix in water and let it drip over the whole body, when the pain will cease.

(*i*) *Jǫjǫ sakam sẹ dạl*, the leaves or the fruit kernel of Tamarindus indica, L.

Grind, warm and plaster this on.

(*j*) Add *bir jhuṅkạ*, Crotolaria calycina, Shrank., to the ingredients in (*a*) above and apply in same way.

(*k*) Mix some *isạbgul*, Plantago ispaghala, R. Fleming, with the milk of a black goat, grind and apply.

(*l*) Grind, warm and apply *hạlim*, Lepidium sativum, L.

(*m*) *Iskirem*, first of all massage the patient; if this does not suffice, then (*n*) *Tobak*, prick with a red hot iron; if this does not answer then apply

(*o*) *Sọsọ*, blister with the juice of the seeds of Semecarpus Anacardium, L. var. cuneifolia.

If this too is inefficacious, then

(*p*) *Jọjọ sakam sẹ dạl*, the leaves or kernel of the seed of Tamarindus indica, L.
Mihndi, Lawsonia alba, Lam.
Akaona chal, the bark of Calotropis gigantea, R. Br. or C. procera, R. Br.
Suruj mukhi, Helianthus annuus, L.
Arak sim kaṭa, the red Vitis peduncularis.
Bir jhuṅkụ, Crotalaria calycina, Shrank.
Ḍhalka catọm arak,
Hạlim, Lepidium sativum, L.

Grind these separately, mix together, equal quantities of each, heat or warm in a potsherd and plaster the whole body therewith, otherwise convulsions, paralysis of the tongue or hiccough may ensue, and there is an end of him.

89. *Sagak.*

Symptoms. This is like *hạḍi* (No. 88), results from that, and on feeling the pulse the indications are the same. They say, "There is poison in him or they have administered poison to him; how are we to get that out? then first the medicine will act.?"

Medicines: (*a*) First of all they bite them, or smear cowdung over the whole body, then after pronouncing spells and incantations they expel the poison, and then give

(*b*) *Sạuṛi rẹhẹt*, the roots of Heteropogon contortus, R. and S.
Kạṭkọm carẹć rẹhẹt, the roots of Rottboellia perforata, Roxb.
Icạk rẹhẹt, the roots of Woodfordia floribunda, Salisb.
Ḍoḍhar rẹhẹt, the roots of Adiantum lunulatum, Burm. or A. concinnum.
Kuṛit rama rẹhẹt, the roots of Zizyphus Oenoplia, Mill.

Grind these together and give to drink.

(*c*) *Mạric rẹhẹt*, the roots of Capsicum frutescens, Willd.
Lọpọn arak rẹhẹt, the roots of Terminalia bellerica, Roxb.

Put these in a leaf-cup with oil and pronounce incantations and then anoint the neck therewith; and holding a bit of the former of the above in the mouth, repeat incantations and blow on him, when the poison will come up. You must praise the *boṅgas* or spirits *Bisạ rạngi* and *Rọkọt kũạri* while blowing on him, and the poison will come up.

90. *Bãsli rog.*

Symptoms. This causes pain similar to rheumatism; they ache night and day. It begins in the limbs and gradually spreads through the whole body There are 18 varieties of this. In one, if it begins in an arm or leg, they tremble outright. In others it takes some 3,5,10,15, or 20 days to be fully developed. The limbs draw the whole body awry, or they are obliged to lie down with a thud.

Medicines: (*a*) *Bin lẹak gại gọtọm nạinu*, unmelted butter of cows' milk.
Tursi sakam mõṛẽ gaṇḍa, 20 leaves of Ocymum sanctum, Willd.

Grind the latter and mix with the former and rub daily with this. This will increase the pain, and after this take

Kaḍa beṅjak rẹhẹl, the roots of
Adhẹ, ginger, Zingiber officinale, Roscoe.

Grind these together and mix; plaster all the joints and cover with *kaera sakam*, the leaves of Musa paradisiaca, L., and wrap the whole in bandages.

(*b*) *Adagạṭhiạ ghãs da*, the bulbs of Panicum repens, L.
Bẹrẹl sasaṅ, raw turmeric, Curcuma longa, L.

Grind these together and plaster the whole of the arms and legs therewith.

(*c*) *Ạphim*, opium.
Dhũṛạ̃, resin of Shorea robusta, Gärtn.
Hiṅ, Ferrula asafætida, Willd.

Grind these together and smear all the limbs therewith.

(*d*) *Dạtrạ*, Datura alba, Willd. or D. fastuosa, Willd.
Kaḍa beṅjak,
Adagạṭhiạ ghãs da, the bulbs of Panicum repens, L.

Grind these together and extract about two ounces of juice, which mix with two ounces of *pạurạ*, spirits, and give to drink. If stupefaction should follow then mix

Kasmar chal, the bark of Gmelina arborea, Roxb.
Siṅ aṛak chal, „ „ „ Bauhinia purpurea, L.
Kạṅji dak, stale rice water

and give to drink.

(*e*) *Gại dahe urul oḍok nạinu*, the butter obtained by churning curds of cows' milk.
Mit gọṭẹc̓ tursi sakam, one leaf of Ocymum sanctum, Willd.

Put some of the former on the latter and let the patient eat this first. The butter must be unmelted. Then grind 12 of the same leaves, mix with the butter and smear it on, rubbing it in. You, the medicine applier, must be chaste and have no intercourse with women, and the patient must remain so also until he is cured. Do not let him eat any meat either. After rubbing him with above, then (*f*) *Kaḍa beṅjak*,

Adhẹ, Zingiber officinale, Roscoe.

Bẹrẹl sasaṅ, raw turmeric, Curcuma longa, Roxb.

Adagaṭhiạ ghās da, the bulbs of Panicum repens, L.

Grind these together fine and apply to all the joints that pain. Wrap in the leaves of *kaera*, Musa paradisiaca, L., and tie them firmly on until the medicine dries. Do this daily, and he will soon get well.

91. *Mackao.* Sprains, strains or wrenches.

Medicines: (*a*) *Ọr tiạr, sẹ iskir mardao baṛakeṭam, sẹm sọsọ tobak kela*,

You stretch the parts straight, or massage them, or blister by applying the juice of *sọsọ*, Semecarpus Anacardium, L. var. cuneifolia.

(*b*) apply as in No. 88 (p).

92. *Daṇḍa haso.* Pain in the loins.

Symptoms. This is characterised by a lacerating pain in the loins, in whatever attitude may be adapted.

Medicines: (*a*) *Poṇḍ kawẹl sakam*, the leaves of the white Abrus precatorius, L.

Grind and warm slightly and plaster warm on the loins.

(*b*) If this does not answer, let him be cupped.

(*c*) *Pọjọ*, Tetranthera monopetala, Roxb.

Bidhạnta, Entada scandens, Benth.

Kuclạ, Strychnos potatorum, Lin. f.

Grind together and plaster on.

93. *Hūk.* Pain in the loins. Lumbago.

Symptoms. This is a pain in the loins. It begins like *betha* (q.v.), but this is in the waist, whereas that is in the sides, and whoever has it is unable to walk from pain and stiffness.

Medicines: (*a*) *Laṭha cip ciṛip*,

Buluṅ, salt.

Grind these together and with it press the painful nerve.

(*b*) *Kaḍa beṅjak*,

Adagaṭhiạ ghās, Panicum repens, L.

Adhẹ, ginger, Zingiber officinale, Roscoe.

Grind these together and apply as a plaster, cover with *kaera sakam*, the leaves of Musa paradisiaca, L., and tie them on.

(*c*) *Chạtni chal*, the bark of Alstonia scholaris, R. Br.

Warm and apply this.

(*d*) *Bandphoṛa biṅ reak 3 jaṅ*, 3 bones of the Bungarus fasciatus snake.

String these on a string and tie them round the patient's waist.

(*e*) *Akaona rẹhẹt*, the roots of Calotropis gigantea, R. Br.

Grind small, heat and apply as a plaster.

(*f*) *Pipṛiañ rẹhẹl*, the roots of
Buluñ, salt.

Grind these together and press well down following carefully along the seat of pain.

(*g*) *Ẹḍhẹ cip ciṛip rẹhẹl*, the roots of an Achyranthes.

Add a little *buluñ*, salt, to these and grind them. Make the patient lie on the ground face downwards, and calling another man tell him to press this medicine down hard on the patient while you with a bit of stick make 7 lines on the ground beside one another calling out the numbers as you do so, one, two, three, etc. While you are doing so the other man presses him firmly down and then releases his hold and you rub out the marks or lines. Repeat this operation three, five or seven times and then make the patient stand up and cause him to crack his waist (like one's knuckles). If a cracking sound is emitted he will be cured there and then. Otherwise repeat the whole process for a couple of days. If this is not efficacious, then

(*h*) *Jioti*, Sesbania ægyptiaca, Pers.
Bạru chal, the bark of Schleichera trijuga, Willd.

Plaster him with these and he will get well.

94. *Bat*. Rheumatism.

Medicines: (*a*) *Bir pan rẹhẹl*, the roots of Monochoria plantaginea, Kunth.
Kaḍa mẹl rẹhẹl, „ „ „ Premna herbacea, Roxb.
Bạru banda rẹhẹl, „ „ „ the air plant found on Schleichera trijuga, Willd.
Telṅga ṭheṅga rẹhẹl, the roots of

Grind the first two and mix with melted butter of cows' milk and give to eat. Roast the second two to ashes and apply to the joints.

(*b*) *Akaona rẹhẹl*, the roots of Calotropis gigantea, R. Br.
Kāṛwāt rẹhẹl, „ „ „ Carissa Carandas, L.
Tọtnọpak chal, the bark of Eugenia operculata, Roxb.
Saram lutur rẹhẹl, the roots of Clerodendron serratum, Spreng.
Ul chal, the bark of Mangifera indica, L.
Chạtni chal, the bark of Alstonia scholaris, R. Br.

Grind these together, put in a new earthen pot and add water, cover with a leaf plate and boil well. Spread a cloth on the bed and after the patient has laid down on it cover him with a wrapper so that it hangs down all round and steam him with the medicine; do this for five or six days.

(*c*) *Gol mạric*, black pepper.
Kaḍa beṅjak rẹhẹl, the roots of

Pound these and give to drink daily.

(*d*) *Kāṛwāt rẹhẹl*, the roots of Carissa Carandas, L.
Akaona rẹhẹl, „ „ „ Calotropis gigantea, R. Br.
Ạsạṛiạ chal, the bark of Caparis horrida, L.f.

Ad sẹr gại gọtọm, 1 lb. clarified butter of cows' milk.

Ad sẹr tuṛi sunum, 1 lb. pure mustard oil.

Mix and boil all together, and rub him therewith some 30 days. If no better, then

(*e*) *Bẹrẹl sasań*, raw turmeric, Curcuma longa, Roxb.

Bẹrẹl adhẹ, raw ginger, Zingiber officinale, Roscoe.

Grind these together, and rub him daily therewith for a month.

(*f*) *Ad sẹr rạsun*, 1 lb. garlic.

Mil sẹr gại gọtọm, 2 lbs. clarified butter of cows' milk.

Boil these down together and make into pills the size of crossbow balls, and give three of them daily to eat for 40 or 80 days; you will cure cases of five years' standing. If the nerves of the arms and legs will not stretch out, then mix *pon chọṭak tạrpin sunum*, 8 oz. turpentine (spirits), warm it slightly and rub with it and foment him; he will assuredly get well.

(*g*) *Mandargọm sakam*, the leaves of Anona squamosa, L.

Tọlnọpak sakam, „ „ „ Eugenia operculata, Roxb.

Boil in water and steam and foment therewith.

If the patient is unable to stand

(*h*) *Pon chọṭak tạrpin sunum*, 8 oz. spirits of turpentine.

Bar chọṭak tuṛi sunum, 4 oz. pure mustard oil.

Mix and after warming slightly continue to smear it on until he can walk about.

Gạṭhiạ bat. Rheumatism in the joints.

(*i*) *Cip ciṛip rẹhẹl*, the roots of Achyranthes aspera, L.

Rạṅgạini rẹhẹl, the roots of Solanum Jacquini, Willd. half as much.

Tala poesa ọjọn arak sindur, the weight of half a pice genuine red lead.

Grind together and make into three pills the size of a hazel nut; dry and let him smoke them in a pipe three times, viz. 7 a.m., noon and 5 p.m.

(*j*) *Dạtrạ sakam reak rasa*, the juice of the leaves of Datura alba, Willd. or D. fastuosa, Willd.

Ạphim, opium.

Grind together, heat and apply, and foment.

(*k*) *Kaḍa mẹ̃l*, Premna herbacea, Roxb.

Bạru banda, the parasitical plant found on Schleichera trijuga, Willd

Telṅga ṭheṅga,

Sinduạri rẹhẹl, the roots of Vitex Negundo, L.

Reduce these to ashes which rub on the patient.

Ẹkẹn bat. Ordinary rheumatism.

(*l*) *Kaḍa beńjak rẹhẹl*, the roots of

Gol mạric, black pepper.

Grind these together and give to drink first; then

Akaona rẹhẹl, the roots of Calotropis gigantea, R. Br. or C. procera, R. Br.
Kāṛwāt rẹhẹl, the roots of Carissa Carandas, L.
Tọtnọpak chal, the bark of Eugenia operculata, Roxb.
Saram lutur rẹhẹl, the roots of Clerodendron serratum, Spreng.
Ul chal, the bark of Mangifera indica, L.
Chạtni chal, the bark of Alstonia scholaris, R. Br.

Put these in a pot, heat it and blow the smoke from them ou the patient.

95. *Bao bat.*

In this when the wind is from a certain direction, the pain begins and the veins are contracted. One must ascertain whence the wind is blowing, and if from the south-east, then apply the following:

Medicines: (*a*) *Sukri itil*, pigs' fat.
Jambro itil, the fat of the snake Zamenis mucosus.
Tọrhọl itil, „ „ „ „ guana.
Họrọ itil, „ „ „ a tortoise.

Melt these together and rub them on daily morning and evening.

96. *Họete sirjauk bat.* Rheumatism due to draught.

Symptoms. This rheumatism generally begins with pain in the fingers, knuckles, elbow joint, shoulder joint, loins, hip joint, the thigh or shin bones or other joints of the body, and there is a tingling pain in the soles of the feet, as if they had fallen asleep.

Medicines:

Steaming: (*a*) *Akaona rẹhẹl*, the roots of Calotropis gigantea, R. Br.
Kāṛwāt rẹhẹl, „ „ „ Carissa Carandas, L.
Tọtnọpak chal, the bark of Eugenia operculata, Roxb.
Asạṛiạ chal, the bark of Capparis horrida, L.f.
Saram lutur rẹhẹl, the roots of Clerodendron serratum, Spreng.
Chạtni chal, the bark of Alstonia scholaris, R. Br.
Sinduạri sakam, the leaves of Vitex Negundo, L.
Bir họṛẹč, Atyllosia scarabædois, Benth.
Ul chal, the bark of Mangifera indica, L.
Hesak chal, the bark of Ficus religiosa, Willd.

Grind these together, then put them in a new earthenware pot and after covering the top by tying on a leaf-plate boil it well. Spread a thin cloth over a rather high bed and let the patient lie on this and cover him with a sheet which should fall down to the ground on all sides. Then place the boiling medicines under the bed and pierce a small hole in the leaf plate so that the steam may escape, and steam the patient until the perspiration of the body is profuse. Steam him thus daily for 15 days.

To be smeared on:

(*b*) *Asaria chal*, the bark of Capparis horrida, L.f.
Kãrwãt rẹhẹt, the roots of Carissa Carandas, L.
Akaona rẹhẹt, the roots of Calotropis gigantea, R. Br.

Grind these together and boil in melted butter made of cows' milk and smear this on. The patient must abstain from buffalo milk and the butter made of it.

Internally: (*c*) Take about a pound of *rasun*, garlic, and grind it very carefully and cleanly. Then boil it in two pounds of cows' milk till the milk has boiled off. Make the residue into 25 pills, two of which are to be taken every day.

To be drunk with above:—

(*d*) *Kaḍa benjak rẹhẹt*, the roots of
Gol maric, black pepper.

Grind together and drink daily with the pills when swallowed.

To be plastered on:—

(*e*) *Bẹrẹl sasaṅ*, raw turmeric, Curcuma longa, Roxb.
Ḍuria hatkan, Leea hirta, Herb. Banks.
Adhẹ, ginger, Zingiber officinale, Roscoe.

Grind these together and plaster the whole limbs, somewhat more thickly over the joints, and wrap in *kaera sakam*, plantain leaves. If you wrap in the day time, remove them at night, and if at night then remove in the day time.

To be taken with (*e*):—

(*f*) *Kaḍa beṅjak rẹhẹt*, the roots of
Adagaṭhia ghãs rẹhẹt, „ „ „ Panicum repens, L.
Ḍamkaḍura rẹhẹt, the roots of

Grind these and give a little to drink daily with *paura*, spirits.

Other remedies:—

(*g*) *Datra rẹhẹt*, the roots of Datura alba, Willd. or D. fastuosa, Willd., take about an ounce of the juice of this.
Paura, spirits, about an ounce.
Pẹ ganḍa gan gol maric, about 12 black peppercorus.
Kaḍa beṅjak rẹhẹt, the roots of
Adagaṭhia ghãs rẹhẹt, „ „ „ Panicum repens, L.

Grind all these together and give to drink. Give in the morning and after doing so do not leave the patient alone or he will go out of his mind. This medicine will cause the eyes to become bloodshot and the saliva to dry up.

Then give: (*h*) *Kasmar chal*, the bark of Gmelina arborea, Roxb.
Siṅ arak chal, the bark of Bauhinia purpurea, L.
Thora cini, a little sugar.

Mix with *kạñji dak*, stale rice water, and give about 4 ounces to drink. Give three or four such doses till he comes to his senses.

If sores appear, then:—

(i) *Ạsạrịa chal*, the bark of Capparis horrida, L.f.
Kãṛwãl rẹhẹl, the roots of Carissa Carandas, L.
Simbrit, the fresh shoots of Bombax malabaricum, DC.

Grind these together, stir in melted butter of cows' milk made in June-July, and give with a burning "candle" as detailed in No. 197 (*c*). If sores appear in the mouth cook *ghi kuạri*, Yucca gloriosa, in melted butter of cows' milk, to be taken 15 days. Nothing but sago to be eaten; salt is strictly forbidden.

97. *Jaṅge bat.* (vide symptoms.)

Symptoms. This is when a man has walked very far and his thighs become rigid and he is unable to walk any more.

Medicines: (*a*) *Dạtrạ*, Datura alba, Willd. or D. fastuosa, Willd.
Adagạthiạ ghãs rẹhẹl, the roots of Panicum ṛepens, L.
Kaḍa beṅjak rẹhẹl, " " "

Extract 2 ounces of the juice of each of these, mix them with 2 ounces of *pạurạ*, spirits, and give to drink. If after becoming intoxicated he is restless and tries to rise, rub him well with *gại gọtọm*, melted butter of cows' milk, and the pain will cease and he will be able to walk. If intoxication continues, give him to drink a mixture of

Kasmar chal, the bark of Gmelina arborea, Roxb.
Siṅ aṛak chal, the bark of Bauhinia purpurea, L.
Kạñji dak, stale rice water

and it will disappear.

98. *Jhoṅji bat.*

Symptoms. In this the shins, thighs or the entire body feel numb, the skin turns red, and if you try to pinch them it does not pain them.

Medicines: (*a*) *Goṭe rẹhẹl*, the roots of Croton oblongifolius, Roxb.
Ẹḍhẹ rạṅgạini rẹhẹl, the roots of Solanum xanthocarpum, Schrad. et Wendl.

Grind these together and apply as an ointment where it has begun and cover with a thin cloth as a bandage. Give more of the same two ingredients mixed with *gẹl bar gol mạric*, 12 black peppercorns, to drink.

Sometimes the limbs become stiff, in which case:

(*b*) *Dạtrạ*, Datura alba, Willd. or D. fastuosa, Willd.
Kaḍa beṅjak,

Grind these and extract 2 ounces of the juice, which mix with

5 *gaṇḍa gol mạric*, 20 black peppercorns, and
1 *choṭak pạurạ*, 2 ounces spirits.

and give to drink. Rub well both the thigh nerves the whole way with melted butter of cows' milk. Should the medicine induce stupefaction then grind *kasmar chal*, the bark of Gmelina arborea, Roxb., and after mixing it with stale rice water give to drink and the stupefaction will cease.

(*c*) *Goṭe rẹhẹl*, the roots of Croton oblongifolius, Roxb.

Grind and apply to the numb parts and wrap in a plantain leaf till the medicine dries.

The following is an efficacious remedy in all kinds of rheumatism:

(*d*) *Jambṛo itil*, the fat of the Zamenis mucosus snake.
Boḍa itil, „ „ „ „ Python molurus snake.
Ḍaṅgra itil, „ „ „ „ a bullock.
Ayaṅ biṅ itil, „ „ „ „ cobra.
Mẹrọm kạsi itil, the fat of a castrated goat.
Haṛam tọrhọl itil, the fat of an old guana.
Sim itil, the fat of a fowl.

Mix all these fats together and apply and a cure is certain.

99. *Jhunkạ bat.*

Symptoms. In this kind of rheumatism the gait is unsteady and in walking the whole body trembles, and there is no energy in the limbs or any part of the body.

Medicines: (*a*) *Dạtrạ rẹhẹl*, the roots of Datura alba, Willd. or D. fastuosa, Willd.
Kaḍa beṅjak,
Gol mạric, black pepper.

Grind these together and extract in all about two ounces of juice, which mix with about two ounces of *pạurạ*, spirit, and give to drink. Should intoxication ensue, then mix *kasmar chal*, the bark of Gmelina arborea, Roxb., with stale rice water and give to drink, when the intoxication will disappear.

(*b*) *Dare katkọm jaṅga*, Viscum attenuatum, DC.
Bọkọm dạre chal, the bark of Melia Azadarach, L.
Ḍamka ḍurạ rẹhẹl, the roots of
Kaḍa beṅjak rẹhẹl, „ „ „
Adagạthiạ ghãs rẹhẹl, the roots of Panicum repens, L.
Ḍuriạ hạtkạn rẹhẹl, the roots of Leea hirta, Herb. Banks.
Cạuliạ rẹhẹl, the roots of Ruellia suffruticosa, Roxb.
Mạṅjur jhuṭi rẹhẹl, the roots of

Get all these properly and grind them, mixing them with *pạurạ*, spirit, and give to drink daily.

(*c*) *Bẹrẹl sasaṅ*, raw turmeric, Curcuma longa, Roxb., a whole lump,
Adhẹ, ginger, Zingiber officinale, Roscoe.

Grind these together and smear on daily.

100. *Mil kaṛ gǫc̆.* Hemiplegia.

Symptoms. This also is kind of *bat.* If it begins in the arm it will extend to the shoulder or the whole of that side will die, leg included. Or if it commences in the leg the whole of the leg and all the parts of the body on that side will die, *i.e.* be deprived of sensation.

This is of rare occurrence. People say if you beat an innocent person without cause it is a sin, as a punishment for which God sends this.

Medicines: (*a*) *Kaḍa beṅjak rẹhẹl*, the roots of
Adagạthiạ ghās da, the bulbs of Panicum repens, L.

Grind these together and smear on daily, leaving it thicker over the joints, and wrap and cover with *kaera sakam*, the leaves of Musa paradisiaca, L. Along with this mix *pẹ gaṇḍa gan gol mụric*, about a dozen black peppercorns, with the above ground ingredients and give to drink daily until recovery. Let him drink it for about a month.

(*b*) *Kāṛwāl rẹhẹl*, the roots of Carissa Carandas, L.
Akaona rẹhẹl, the roots of Calotropis gigantea, R. Br.
Chạtni chal, the bark of Alstonia scholaris, R. Br.
Ạsạriạ chal, the bark of Capparis horrida, L. f.
Saram lutur rẹhẹl, the roots of Clerodendron serratum, Spreng.
Sinduạri sakam, the leaves of Vitex Negundo, L.
Bir hǫrẹc̆, Atyllosia scarabædois, Benth.
Tursi sakam, the leaves of Ocymum sanctum, Willd.
Bharbhạri sakam, the leaves of Ocymum basilicum, L.
Dạtrạ sakam, the leaves of Datura alba, Willd. or D. fastuosa, Willd.
Bana haṭak chal, the bark of Oroxylon indicum, Benth.
Ul chal, the bark of Mangifera indica, L.

Put all these in a new earthenware pot, cover the top with a leaf plate and boil them well. Then after spreading a cloth over a somewhat high bed, let the patient lie down on it, and covering with a cloth descending on all sides to the ground steam him slowly. Do thus until he recovers.

(*c*) *Dhūṛā̤*, resin of Shorea robusta, Gärtn.
Hiṅ, Ferrula asafœtida, Willd.
Ạphim, opium.

Cook all these in melted butter of cows' milk and besmear him therewith.

(*d*) *Akaona rẹhẹl chal*, the bark of Calotropis gigantea, R. Br. or C. procera, R. Br.

Plaster him with this for a week to soften the veins; afterwards

(*e*) *Saram lutur rẹhẹl*, the roots of Clerodendron serratum, Spreng.
Tǫtnǫpak rẹhẹl, the roots of Eugenia operculata, Roxb.

Grind these together, boil in *utiṅ sunum*, mustard oil, and while doing so throw in a *rae kakaṛbak caṇḍbǫl*, chameleon's tail, and when all is cooked extract this tail, and let him anoint himself with the oil daily morning and evening. When the preparation is finished make more, as it will take a month to cure.

101. *Mirgi.* Epilepsy unspecified.

Medicines: (*a*) Make over to the patient a mixture of equal quantities of

Mĩhũ aḍo, calves' urine.

Hoṛ aḍo, human urine.

Muṅgạ tejo, the tassar silkworm.

Pạurạ, spirit.

As soon as the fit commences, immediately pour this mixture into his nose, and it will cause him to sneeze out the worm that is the cause of the malady.

(*b*) *Sẹṅgẹl siṅ rilkate*, ground Tragia involucrata, Jacq.

Dahe, curds.

Taben, rice soaked and flattened.

to be eaten.

Ạmbạitar biṅ reak itil, the fat of the snake Daboia Russellii,

to be smeared over the body.

Hiṅ, Ferrula asafœtida, Willd.

Huṭer baha reak rẹhẹl, the roots of Indigofera pulchella, Roxb.

Dạtrạ rẹhẹl, the roots of Datura alba, Willd. or D. fastuosa, Willd.

to be drunk.

(*c*) *Bilạti thamakur*, imported tobacco, one finger's length

Gol mạric, 5 black peppercorns.

Sirom rẹhẹl, one finger's length of the roots of Andropogon muricatus, Retz.

To be ground together into a fine powder and then with the help of a reed be blown into the nose of the patient. Thereafter the following to be eaten one day.

Kunạm rẹhẹl, the roots of

Hẹndẹ lilkạthi rẹhẹl, the roots of the black variety of Polygala crotalarioides, Buch. and Ham., 8-oz.

1 *pawa gan hẹndẹ horo hoḷoṅ*, about 8-oz. of flour made from black paddy.

to be made into hand bread.

(*d*) *Kunạm*,

Kạrhạni horo reak hoḷoṅ, the flour made from a certain variety of paddy.

To be made together into hand bread and eaten.

(*e*) *Tejo mala rẹhẹl*, the roots of Cissampelos Pareira, L.

Goṭe rẹhẹl, the roots of Croton oblongifolius, Roxb.

Hat̥ jo̥ jaṅ 2 gan, the stones of a couple of the fruit of Holarrhena antidysenterica, Wall.

Grind and pour into the patient's nose.

When there is unconsciousness with foaming and groaning,

(*f*) *Gol mạric*, black pepper.

Lọṅphul, cloves.

Kãṛwãl rẹhẹt, the roots of Carissa Carandas, L.

Thoṛa bọc, a little of the root stock of Acorus Calamus, Willd.

Mix and grind these and stir in *nirạ tuṛi sunum*, pure mustard oil, and anoint him daily from the forehead to the soles of the feet. As soon as the fit comes on drop two or three drops into his nose; he will certainly get well. *Forbidden diet*: any thing acid or sour, plantain and jack-fruit, the flesh of the *boaṛ hako*, a certain fish, of buffalo and sheep, in fact all meat should be eschewed until cured.

(*g*) *Muṅgạ dare rẹhẹtak̓ chal*, the bark of Moringa pterygosperma, Gärtn.

2 ana reak̓ ạphim, 2 annas worth of opium.

Grind together and make into thirty pills giving one daily for a month.

(*h*) *Duṇḍukil rẹhẹt*, the roots of Gardenia turgida, Roxb.

Bharbhạri jaṅ, the seeds of Ocimum basilicum, L.

20 *gaṇḍa gol mạric*, 80 black peppercorns.

Mix and grind these and stir in *pạurạ*, spirits, and as soon as the fit comes on drop two or three drops into his nose, and give a little daily to drink.

(*i*) *Bana hataṅ*, the brains of a bear.

Bilạti thamakur pon kạtup̓ gan, about 4 fingers' width or imported tobacco.

Gaṅja, Cannabis sativa, Willd.

2 ana reak̓ ạphim, 2 annas worth of opium.

Mix with mustard oil and pour into the nose when the attack begins.

(*j*) *Mirgi jel reak̓ harta*, the skin of a certain kind of deer.

Ṅ́ũṛũc̓ rẹhẹt, the roots of Cassia Fistula, L.

Niuri rẹhẹt, „ „ „ Elæodendron Roxburghii, W. and A.

Tale poha reak̓ da, the bulb of a seedling of Borassus flabelliformis, L.

Bhiḍi ạchim jo̥, the fruit of Centifida orbicularis, Lour.

42 *gaṇḍa gol mạric*, 168 black peppercorns.

Grind and mix with pure mustard oil and pour into his nose.

(*k*) *Salga chal*, the bark of Boswellia serrata, Wall.

Niuri chal se rẹhẹt, the bark or roots of Elæodendron Roxburghii, W. and A.

Gol mạric, black pepper.

Grind these together and mix with *pạurạ*, spirit, and when the fit commences pour into both nostrils.

(*l*) Kill a *cund*, musk rat, and put the body into a vessel so that it cannot be eaten; when decomposed larvae will emerge, which you must dry. Then take those and

Gitil gāṛī, Gryllus monstruosus.

Bheḍa bọhọkren tejo, the worms found in a ram's head.

Akaona tejo, the worm found on Calotropis gigantea, R. Br. or C. procera, R. Br.

Malhan ḍhomporen tejo, the creeping insects found in the lumps on the tendrils of Dolichos Lablab, L.

1 *ana reak gol mạric*, an anna's worth of black pepper.

Grind these together and mix in *utiń sunum*, mustard oil. Mix also the three ingredients of (*k*) above in this. Before the fit comes on pour this mixture once into the nose of the patient, and after the fit has begun do so again, and he will recover.

Prohibited diet: Plantains, jack fruit, buffalo meat, mutton, the flesh of *boaṛ hako*, a certain fish, *Callichrous pabo*.

When the fit occurs at full moon:—

(*m*) *Akaona darereko tahẹn jọṛko sọsrọć*, a grasshopper found in pairs on Calotropis gigantea, R. Br. or C. procera, R. Br.

Malhan sakamreko tahẹn tejo, the creeping insects found on Dolichos Lablab, L.

Grind both together and at the commencement of the fit pour into his nose, and if he sneezes well he will be cured; if he does not sneeze, repeat the operation at next full moon.

When the fit occurs the last day before new moon:

(*n*) *Bidhạnta rẹhẹl*, the roots of Entada scandens, Benth.

Qhọć aṛak rẹhẹl, „ „ „ Boerhaavia procumbens, Herb. Banks.

Akaona bandaren tejo, the caterpillar found on the parasitical plant on Calotropis gigantea, R. Br. or C. procera, R. Br.

Grind all these together, and as soon as the fit begins, pour into his nose.

(*o*) If this is inefficacious, mix (*m*) and (*n*) and proceed as in them.

(*p*) *Niuri chal*, the bark of Elæodendron Roxburghii, W. and A.

Goṭe rẹhẹl, the roots of Croton oblongifolius, Roxb.

Tejo mala rẹhẹl, the roots of Cissampelos Pareira, L.

5 *gaṇḍa gol mạric*, 20 black peppercorns.

Grind these fine to a powder which he must sniff up the nose daily. This medicine must be given to him after you have called on Kudrạ Cạṇḍi and Kal Cāora, the two self elected patron spirits; if the patient gets well, a fee of 5 rupees, and a sacrifice of a goat and a fowl, requisitioned from the patient, must be given.

102. *Hanak gujuk.* Epilepsy.

Medicines: *Akaona tejo*, the caterpillar found on Calotropis gigantea, R. Br.

Meral tejo, the caterpillar found on Phyllanthus Emblica, L.

Malhan tejo, the caterpillar found in the lumps on the tendrils of Dolichos Lablab. L.

Ạphim, opium.

Thamakur, tobacco.

Sạṅci mạric, black pepper.

Moṭa kaṭkọm carẹć, a thick Rottboellia perforata, Corom. pl.

103. *Judạ judạ mirgi rog.* Various forms of epilepsy.

Bana mirgi (lit. bear epilepsy, possibly some kind of non-epileptic convulsions).

Symptoms. When the fit commences they grunt like a bear and the eyes become quite red, and sometimes they becoming raving.

Medicines: (*a*) *Muṅgạ chal*, the bark of Moringa pterygosperma, Gärtn.

2 ana reak ạphim, two annas worth of opium.

Grind these together and make 15 pills, one to be taken daily.

(*b*) *Kãṛwãl rẹhẹl*, the roots of Carissa Carandas, L.

Gạbur chal, the bark of Acacia Farnesiana, Willd.

Boṅga bạri rẹhẹl, the roots of Typha angustifolia (?).

Dạtrạ rẹhẹl, the roots of Datura alba, Willd. or D. fastuosa, Willd.

Sinduạri rẹhẹl, *sẹ sakam*, the roots or leaves of Vitex Negundo, L.

Nạṅgrạuta rẹhẹl the roots of Nardostachys jatamansi, DC.

Ạṭi sahṛa chal, the bark of

Bana haṭak chal, the bark of Oroxylon indicum, Benth.

Thoṛa gan ạphim, a small quantity of opium.

Mix, cook in melted butter and smear over the whole body.

(*c*) *Gitil gãṛi*, Gryllus monstruosus.

Meralren tejo, the insect found on Phyllanthus Emblica, L.

Grind and make him sniff the mixture up into the nose.

(*d*) *Cẹrcẹṭẹć caṇḍbọl*, the tail of a gecko.

5 gaṇḍa gol mạric, 20 black peppercorns.

2 poesawak jãwãn, 2 pice worth of Carum Ajowan, DC.

Mit rọ bọhọk gaṅja, the size of a fly's head of Cannabis sativa, Willd.

Bhage thamakur, good tobacco.

Thoṛa bana hataṅ, a little of the brains of a bear.

Grind with or without pure mustard oil. Blow these at the commencement of an attack through a hollow cylinder into his nose, and he will assuredly get well. Mix also with above a little *sirom rẹhẹl*, the roots of

Andropogon muricatus, Retz. This is for a patient of 20 years old. *Forbidden diet*: Curry browned his life long, and the following for four or five years: plantains, jack fruit, buffalo meat, mutton, the flesh of the *boaṛ hako*, a certain fish, and cooked *bajṛa*, Sorghum vulgare, Pers.

104. *Bhalok Mirgi*. (lit. rabies-epilepsy).

Symptoms. It is uncertain when a fit of this comes on, but it may be recognized in the eyes which keep blinking rapidly; sometimes they scream out or exclaim ẽ! ẽ! and sometimes they tremble as if possessed by a spirit.

Medicines: (*a*) *Gaḍa gạ̃ri*, a certain water insect.

Bana hạtiạr, the penis of a bear.

Uchlạu tol hoṛ paṭwa, an intestinal worm vomited up by a human being.

Grind together and divide into two portions; one portion to be ground and mixed with the ingredients in No. 101 (p) and given to drink; the other to be filled into paper and when the fit commences poured into his nose. A couple of applications of this remedy will ensure a cure. The patron spirits are the same as in No. 101 (p).

105. *Hạrnạ mirgi*. (lit. deer-epilepsy).

Symptoms. In this they fling about one arm and one leg.

Medicines: *Mit choṭak gan dạtrạ rọs*, make about 2 oz. of the juice of Datura alba, Willd. or D. fastuosa, Willd.

Pẹ gaṇḍa gol mạric, 12 black peppercorns.

Mix and give to drink. If there is stupefaction then give

Kasmar chal, the bark of Gmelina arborea, Roxb.

Siṅ aṛak chal, the bark of Bauhinia purpurea, L.

to drink with stale rice water.

106. *Mit dọmte laṛaok ti jaṅga mirgi*. (lit. epilepsy with hands and legs moving simultaneously).

Symptoms. In this the limbs are contracted and foam issues from the mouth.

Medicines: Give both the pills and the external application detailed in 103 (*a*) and (*b*).

107. *Mit ti ar lutur laṛaok mirgi*. (lit. epilepsy in which one hand and one ear move).

Symptoms. At the commencement of each fit one arm, ear and eye twitch.

Medicines: (*a*) Give the remedies 103 (*a*) and (*b*).

(*b*) *Akaona banda*, the parasitical plant found on Calotropis gigantea, R. Br.

Muṅgạ banda, the parasitical plant found on Moringa pterygosperma, Gärtn.

Akaonareko tahẹn tejo, the caterpillars found on Calotropis gigantea, R. Br.
Bheḍa dereń dareren tejo, the insects found on Cassia Tora, L.
Malhan ḍhomporen tejo, the insects found on Dolichos Lablab, L.
Kaḍa ghurbạị ọtreko bhugạg, certain small insects making holes in the earth.
Gại ghurbại dare goṭatẹl, Polygala chinensis, L., the whole.
Dak uru, a water beetle.
Caya, Leptocorisa varicornis.
Cund canḍbọltẹl, the tail of a musk rat.
Gol mạric, black peppercorns.
Lọṅphul, cloves.
Bọc, the root of Acorus Calamus, Willd.
Kāṛwāl rẹhẹl, the roots of Carissa Carandas, L.

Grind all these, saturate then in mustard oil, let him sniff it up the nose and smear it on the whole head.

(*c*) *Duṇḍukil rẹhẹl*, the roots of Gardenia turgida, Roxb.
Bharbhạri jaṅ, the seed of Ocimum basilicum, L., or O. canum, Sims.
Lọṅphul, cloves.

Grind these, mix a little spirit and give to drink daily when well or the fit begins.

(*d*) Put nine pice into two ounces of water and grind
Kaḍa ghurbại, a certain insect
with that water and give to drink.

108. *Tọgọč urij reak*. (lit. rigidly closing jaws).

Medicines: (*a*) *Bẹrẹl sasaṅ*, raw turmeric, Curcuma longa, Roxb.

Burn him with this in the hollow behind the ear, force the teeth apart, rub the tongue with *etko hasa*, burnt clay from inside the fireplace, and rub the nerve on the nape of the neck with *utiṅ sunum*, mustard oil.

109. *Sir teṅgoyenre*. Cramp.

Medicines: *Terel jẹr*, the exudation from Diospyros tomentosa, Roxb.
Lọpọṅ jẹr, „ „ „ Terminalia bellerica, Roxb.
Dhūṛā̦ sarjọm reak, the resin from Shorea robusta, Gärtn.

Grind together and let him inhale it.

110. *Bại* (unspecified). Convulsions, cramps, an involuntary state or movement over which one has no control.

Medicines: (*a*) *Lọtọ jọ rọhọṛak*, the dried fruit of Randia dumetorum, Lam.

Grind and smear on him, and boiling some a little give him to drink, one day.

(b) *Jel deren*, a deer's horn.
Ak reak gabetel, the sediment on a bow (where it is caught).
Bele, a hen's egg.
Gol maric, black pepper.
Lumam, a silkworm.

To be mixed and eaten.

(c) *Ambaitar bin reak itil*, the fat of the snake Daboia Russellii.
Sengel sin, Tragia involucrata, Jacq.
Dahe, curds.
Taben, rice soaked and flattened.

The first to be smeared on, the second to be ground and eaten with the last two.

(d) *Gujha kaudhari*, 8 ounces of
Daho, curds.

To be both drunk and smeared on.

While the fit is on, put a ripe fruit of Luffa acutangula, Roxb. on a fire in a potsherd under the bedstead; it will emit smoke.

(e) *Hin*, Ferrula asafætida, Willd.
Bharbhari, Ocimum basilicum, L. or O. canum, Sims.
Ro, a fly.
Bindi, a spider.
Jel deren, a deer's horn, to be rubbed and mixed.
Gari bohok, a monkey's head.
Bet, a rattan, Calamus Rotang, L.
Ak mat, the scrapings of a bamboo bow.
Miru baha, Abutilon indicum, Don.

Grind all these together and give a little to drink. Then rub his mouth with the following:

Kalia jira, Nigella indica, Roxb.
Sinjo sakam, the leaves of Ægle Marmelos, Correa.
Gol maric, black pepper.

(f) *Guiha gandhari*,
Kaera rean dak, the water of a plantain.

Grind these together and stirring it into curds made from cows' milk, give a little to drink and rub over the whole body.

(g) *Buput dudhi rehet*, the roots of
Jhapni, Zornia diphylla, Pers. or Biophitum sensitivum, DC., the entire plant.

Grind together, give a little to eat and apply to the whole body.

For Dhinuk bai, when the muscles of the back are contracted:

(h) *Gundri gervel jo*, the fruit of
Dhiri kakra bohok, the head of a lizard.
Baghin rehet thora, a little of the roots of Mezoneurum cucullatum, W. and A.

Grind together and give to drink.

For *Sagum bai*:

(*i*) *Tarup jom sukri bohok*, the head of a pig eaten by a leopard.

Gari bohok, the head of a monkey.

Sadom jhin ghasao ńokkate, the scrapings from a horse's iron bit.

Dhubi ghās, Cynodon dactylon, Pers.

Grind together and give to drink.

If the limbs are cold,

Sar rehel, the roots of Saccharum Sara, Roxb.

Bhernda rehel, the roots of Jatropha Curcas, L.

Grind, stir into mustard oil and anoint therewith.

For *Tarka tarki bai*, spasms:

(*j*) *Bonga barchi rehel*, the roots of Leonates nepetœfolia, R. Br.

Gol maric, adults 4 peppercorns, children only 2.

Grind together and give to drink.

(*k*) *Bharbhari jan*, the seed of Ocimum basilicum, L. or O. canum, Sims.

2 *gan rasun*, a couple of garlic.

Grind together and rub or smear on the head and let him sniff a little up the nose.

(*l*) *Datra rehel*, the roots of Datura alba, Willd. or D. fastuosa, Willd.

Nanha dudhi lota rehel, the roots of Ichnocarpus frutescens, R. Br.

Grind together and give to drink and besmear him therewith; apply *ganja*, Cannabis sativa, Willd., to the fontanel.

(*m*) *Bir barni*, the roots of Clerodendron infortunatum, L.

Car sira rehel,

Gol maric, black pepper.

Grind together and give to drink, and if he is unable to speak, rub *etko hasa*, burnt clay from inside the fireplace, on his mouth and on the soles of his feet, and he will recover. Sit near the patient and see whether the *bai* takes any particular form.

III. *Alan obor bai*. (Paralysis of the tongue.)

Symptoms. This is a temporary paralysis of the tongue in which it adheres to the bottom of the mouth, and speech is impossible.

This is liable to occur when the patient is exhausted by illness, *i.e.* when he is moribund. If the tongue adheres to the bottom of the mouth, it is a sign one may give up hope, and people say, who knows? It is doubtful if he will survive.

Medicines: (*a*) *Maraṛ baha chal*, the bark of Erythrina indica, Lam.
Akaona rẹhẹl, the roots of Calotropis gigantea, R. Br.
Beṅgaṛ beṭahẹl, Solanum stramonifolium, Jacq.

Grind these together and cook in melted butter, then give to eat and smear therewith.

If obtainable:

(*b*) *Jhĩk poṭa*, the stomach of the Indian porcupine.
Cemeń bọhọk, the head of a mongoose.
Sọgọl bọhọk, „ „ „ the civet, Viverịcula malaccensis.

Roast the two latter to burning point and grind the first as it is therewith, and then cook and mix with (*a*).

(*c*) *Kạhu botke rẹhẹl*, the roots of Bryonia lacinosa, L.
Bir kundri rẹhẹl, „ „ „ Zehneria umbellata, Thw.
Ạphim, opium.
Gaṅja, Cannabis sativa, Willd.
Gurli jań,

Cook all these in mustard oil, give to eaṭ and smear therewith.

(*d*) *Eṭko hasa*, the burned clay from the inside of the fireplace.

This to be rubbed with the finger on the teeth and the tongue to be rubbed.

(*e*) *Jibhạ*,
Gol mạric, black pepper.

Grind together and give to drink, and the power of speech will return.

112. *Alań ọr bại.* (lit. convulsions with tongue drawn in).

Symptoms. After a complication of several of the already mentioned *bại* this kind may follow, i.e. the tendons of the whole body or of the tongue are contracted; they yawn continually, the eyes close, and they are unable to speak.

Medicines: (*a*) *Maraṛ baha chal*, the bark of Erythrina indica, Lam.
Akaona rẹhẹl, the roots of Calotropis gigantea, R. Br.
Goṭe rẹhẹl, the roots of Croton oblongifolius, Roxb.
Bhiḍi janaṭep rẹhẹl, the roots of Urena sinuata, L. or Triumfetta rhomboidea, Jacq.
Bar gẹl mõṛẽ gaṇḍa gol mạric, 100 black peppercorns.

Grind all these together and cook them in melted butter, then give to eat and smear him therewith.

113. *Bạghi sẹ bagha bại.* (lit. tiger or leopard convulsions).

Symptoms. In this people get angry like leopards or tigers for slight cause and sometimes they bite.

Medicines: (*a*) *Tayan jań*, the bone of a crocodile.
Tạrup jań sẹ bọhọk jań, the bone or skull of a leopard.

Rub these on a stone, give him to drink thereof and anoint him therewith.

(*b*) *Aphim*, opium, as much as a fly's head.
Gańja thoṛa, a little Cannabis sativa, Willd.

Take as much of these as equal in size to a grain of Cajanus indicus, Spreng., stir it about in a mussel shell full of water and give him to drink.

(*c*) *Dạtrạ rẹhẹl mit choṭak gan*, about 2 oz. of the roots of Datura alba, Willd. or D. fastuosa, Willd.
Pẹ gaṇḍa gol mạric, 12 black peppercorns.

Mix the juice obtained from the former with the latter, grind them together and give him to drink. If intoxication ensues, then grind

Kasmar chal, the bark of Gmelina arborea, Roxb. and
Siṅ aṛak chal, the bark of Bauhinia purpurea, L.

and give to drink with stale rice water, and he will recover.

114. *Bhalok bại*, (lit. rabies convulsions).

Symptoms. The neck is moved about, the mouth is constantly open, cannot in fact be shut, and there is continual dropping of saliva.

Medicines: (*a*) *Pạsi gọč seta bọhọk baeme*, keep the head of a dog that was strangled.

Rub this on a stone, give him to lick and smear the whole body therewith.

(*b*) *Gạbur chal*, the bark of Acacia Farnesiana, Willd.

Smear this over him and give him also a little of it to drink.

115. *Bhạṛwạ sẹ lumạm bại*, (lit. Attacus-caterpillar or silkworm convulsions).

Symptoms. In this they nod the head at intervals and throw the hands about.

Medicines: (*a*) *Oka darere kaḍako thapae, ona reak chal*, the bark of a tree that buffaloes strike.
Lumạm tejo, tọl bhitri khon gẹl tọl, the larva of a silkworm cut out from its chrysalis.

Grind these together and let him lick it, and smear a little over the whole body.

(*b*) If you can get the *bhạṛwạ tejo*, large caterpillars, principally those of *Attacus atlas* and *Attacus Selene*, roast them to burning point, give him to lick and also smear him therewith.

116. *Bindi bại*, (lit. spider convulsions, delirium febris).

Symptoms. They have a swinging gait like spiders and tremble.

Medicines: (*a*) *Gẹl gaṇḍa bindi gọčkom*, kill 40 spiders.
Nanha dudhi loṭa rẹhẹl, the roots of Ichnocarpus frutescens, R. Br.
Ṅũṛũč jọ reak gabe, the flesh of the fruit of Cassia Fistula, L.

Grind these three together, give to drink and smear over the whole body.

117. *Ceṅgha bại.* Colic (may be strangulation of the intestines).

Symptoms. Two thick nerves show up from the navel to the chest, and there is intense pain.

One "authority" says: This is very similar to *ḍhọnḍ bại* (No. 124), the difference being that in the latter a thick nerve is seen to rise on the surface, whereas this is absent in *ceṅgha bại*.

Medicines: (*a*) *Kạhu botke rẹhẹl*, the roots of Bryonia lacinosa, L.
Gol mạric, black pepper.
Thoṛa buluṅ, a little salt.

Grind together and give to drink at the commencement of the attack.

(*b*) *Haṭ rẹhẹl*, the roots of Holarrhena antidysenterica, Wall.
Tejo mala rẹhẹl, the roots of Cissampelos Pareira, L.
Kalmẹg 5 *ṭusạ*, 5 tips of Andrographis paniculata, Nees.
Jĩoti ḍọg, the tips of Sesbania ægyptiaca, Pers.
Hiṅ, Ferrula asafætida, the size of a grain of Phaseolus Mungo, Willd., var. radiatus, L.
Ạphim, opium, as much as a grain of Cajanus indicus, Spreng.
Mit' sẹr pạurạ, 2 lbs of spirit.

Soak all these and give a little to drink every day.

(*c*) *Kuclạ chal*, the bark of Strychnos potatorum, L. f.

Give one dr. of this to drink, and if it induces stupefaction then give
Kasmar chal, the bark of Gmelina arborea, Roxb., with sugar to drink.

(*d*) *Dhại da*, the bulb of Grislea tomentosa, Willd.
Gol mạric, black pepper.

Mix these and cook in cows' milk to do away with the itching and give to eat daily.

(*e*) *Kujri sunum*, the oil obtained from the seeds of Celastrus paniculatus, Willd.

Give about an iron spoonful of this, which is enough to cure.

(*f*) *Hukạ dak*, hookah water.
Poṇḍ rạsun, garlic.
Kalmẹg sakam, the leaves of Andrographis paniculata, Nees.

Grind all these together, make into pills and administer.

(*g*) *Pan khayar*, Acacia Catechu, Willd.
Jạmbir jọ, the fruit of Citrus medica, L.
Piṇḍe rẹhẹl, the roots of Randia uliginosa, DC.

Grind together and mix well with pure spirit and give to drink.

(*h*) *Bhạdoriạ rẹhẹl*, the roots of
Gol mạric 4, four black peppercorns.
Lilkạthi rẹhel, the roots of Polygala crotalarioides, Buch. and Ham.

Grind together and mix well with pure spirit and give to drink.

(*i*) *Pẹtcamṛa*, Helicteres Isora, L.
Tejo mala rẹhẹl, the roots of Cissampelos Pareira, L.

These are to be drunk.

Ạndia mọrọn aṛak, Gymnema hirsutus, W. and A., var. Decaisneanum, Wight.

Bạrsạ pakọṛ, Grewia sapida, Roxb.

These to be smeared on him.

(*j*) *Kạhu bòtke da*, the bulb of Bryonia lacinosa, L.

3 *gaṇḍa gol mạric*, 12 black peppercorns.

Thoṛa buluṅ, a little salt.

Grind these and give to drink.

(*k*) *Kalmẹg pẹ ṭusạ*, 3 tips of Andrographis paniculata, Nees.

Jīoti ḍọg, the tips of Sesbania ægyptiaca, Pers.

Haṭ rẹhẹt, the roots of Holarrhena antidysenterica, Wall.

Miṭ rọ bọhọk hiṅ, asafætida the size of a fly's head.

Grind these together, take the juice, add 8 ounces of *pạurạ*, spirits, strain and give 2 ounces to drink daily. *Forbidden diet*: the flesh of buffaloes, sheep and *boaṛ hako*, a certain fish, the fruit of the plantain and jack. *Icạk hako*, prawns or shrimps, are however permissible.

(*l*) *Miru baha rẹhẹt*, the roots of Abutilon indicum, Don.

Ḍhela chal, the bark of Alangium Lamarckii, Thws.

Grind these together mix with *pạurạ*, spirits, and give to drink.

(*m*) *Kạhu botke da*, the bulb of Bryonia lacinosa, L.

Pẹ gaṇḍa gol mạric, 12 black peppercorns.

Thoṛạ buluṅ, a little salt.

Kalmẹg, Andrographis paniculata, Nees.

3 *ṭusạ jīoti*, 3 tips of Sesbania ægyptiaca, Pers.

Thoṛa haṭ chal, a little of the bark of Holarrhena antidysenterica, Wall.

Miṭ rọ bọhọk gan hiṅ, Ferrula asafætida, Willd., about as much as the size of a fly's head.

Grind and mix these and strain so that you get about 8 ounces; mix this in 8 ounces *pạurạ*, spirits, and let him drink daily 2 ounces of this mixture until recovery.

N.B.—Some people give this last remedy for No. 124, *Dhọṇḍ bại*.

118. *Cihkạ bại*, (lit. starting convulsions).

(Delirium febris)

Symptoms. They continually start suddenly, get up and scream out.

Medicines: (*a*) *Cẹtẹr oka sẹčre ńūrok, ona sẹč reak chal chaḍaome.* Take off the bark in the direction that thunderbolts fall, cook it in oil and anoint him therewith.

(*b*) *Kul jaṅ*, the bone of a tiger.

Tayan bọhọk, the head of a crocodile.

Rub these and give him to drink.

(*c*) *Cẹtẹr dhiri*, a thunderbolt. Give as in(*b*).

119. *Corṭha bạị*, (lit. ill-behaviour convulsions).
(Delirium febris)

Symptoms. In this they get very angry; if you ask any question they commence abusing.

Medicines: (*a*) Keep the sheep's wool that cows vomit up, even if they die it will be found as a ball in their stomachs. Grind this and smear it over the whole body and give some to drink.

(*b*) *Bir karla da*, the bulb of the wild Momordica dioica, Roxb.
Pe ganḍa gol mạric, 12 black peppercorns.

Grind together and give to drink.

120. *Curi bai.*

Symptoms. They will speak to no one, remain silent and only look about.

Medicines: (*a*) *Sahel sakam rẹhẹl*, the roots of

Grind and give to drink.

(*b*) *Ọrsọreń da*, the bulb of Zingiber Çassumunar, Roxb. (?)
Gol mạric, black pepper.

Mix these and give him to drink, and plaster him therewith.

121. *Ḍabha bạị*, (lit. orange convulsions).

Symptoms. A swelling the size of a cup for holding oil or of an orange appears on the belly, and there is pain.

Medicines: (*a*) All the remedies under No. 117 are applicable in this.

(*b*) *Ṅũṛũč rẹhẹl*, the roots of Cassia Fistula, L.
Kamar cạpuạ reak mạilạ, the dirt from a blacksmith's bellows.

The former to be ground and given to drink, and the latter to be ground and smeared on the belly.

122. *Dãt kapaṭi bại.* Trismus (contraction of the muscles of the jaw).

Medicines: (*a*) *Hãṛũ jambe*, the jaw of a baboon.

Rub this and apply to his mouth. If not efficacious, take
Sạńci mạric, black pepper.

Grind and rub his teeth therewith.

123. *Dhinuk bại.* Tetanus, and possibly other convulsions.

Symptoms. This attacks people who are much weakened by illness, and when a fit of it is on they are bent like a bow and there is intense pain. Adults do not recover, children may.

Medicines: (*a*) *Ak reak mạilạ*, the dirt scraped off a bow where it is held.
Parkọm mạilạ, the dirt scraped off the wooden framework of a bedstead.
Tọl lumạm tejo, the silkworm in its chrysalis stage.

Grind these together and give to drink mixed with black pepper.

(b) *Gotom sunum*, clarified or melted butter.

Dhūṛā, resin of Shorea robusta, Gärtn.

Akaona rẹhẹt, the roots of Calotropis gigantea, R. Br.

Mix the first two to the consistency of butter and anoint the whole body therewith, and grind the last and plaster it on him.

(c) *Aphim*, opium.

Utiń sunum, mustard oil.

Gańja, Cannabis sativa, Willd.

Boil the first a little in the second and rub him with the preparation. Give him a little of the last to smoke.

(d) *Sukri ḍhumbak*, excrement of pigs.

Hati iċ, „ „ elephants.

Gadha iċ, „ „ asses.

Haṛhal hoṭol jań, the seeds of the bitter Cucurbita lagenaria.

Jhińga jań, the seeds of Luffa acutangula, Roxb.

Bir jhińga jań, the seeds of Luffa amara, R.

Mix these together, set fire to them in a large potsherd or something of the kind and let the smoke go on him.

(e) *Ropa ak*, a bow made of Bambusa Tulda, Roxb.

To be scraped, the scrapings set on fire and the patient smoked therewith.

(f) *Mal ak reak maila ar uṭi*, the dirt scraped off a bow of bamboo and a joint thereof.

Oka dare bayar kaḍa lengṛateye thapa akat, ona reak baklak, the bark of a tree that has been knocked by the left horn of a male entire buffalo.

Grind these together and smear the patient therewith.

124. *Dhoṇḍ bai.* (May be strangulation of the intestines.)

Symptoms. A nerve rises over the stomach across the body and there is pain.

One "authority" says: This begins in the stomach. A thick nerve rises from the breast to the navel, and there is intense pain causing the patient to writhe on his stomach and toss about.

Medicines: (a) All the remedies under No. 117 are applicable in this.

(b) *Mutha rẹhẹt*, the roots of Fimbrystylis monostachya, Hassk.

Upal baha ulḍha, the tuber of the lotus (*Nymphaea*).

Poraeni rẹhẹt, the root of Nelumbium speciosum, Willd.

Grind and give to drink.

(c) *Bokom baha rẹhẹt*, the roots of Melia Azadarach, L.

Akaona rẹhẹt, the roots of Calotropis gigantea, R. Br.

Bir ḍimbu rẹhẹt, the roots of

Give these to drink mixed with pure spirits.

N.B.—Use this remedy also in *kachma bai* and *paeṭhan bai*.

The only difference between *ḍabha bạai* and *paeṭhan bai* is that in the former the pain is stationary, whereas in the latter it moves about.

These remedies and those in No. 117 (*j* and *k*) may be applied in cases of *ḍabha bạai* and *paeṭhan bạai*.

(*d*) *Kalmẹg*, Andrographis paniculata, Nees.
Sẹkrẹć ḍọg, a leaf bud of Lagerstroemia parviflora, Roxb.
Gol mạric, black pepper.

Grind these together and give to drink.

This remedy may also be given for *ceṅgha bạai*, No. 117.

(*e*) First of all before bringing any medicine take
Kuiṇḍi sunum, oil from the kernel of Bassia latifolia, Roxb.

and rub him well with this from above downwards; if this does not cure, then

(*f*) *Piṇḍe rẹhẹl*, the roots of Randia uliginosa, DC.
Khayar, Acacia Catechu, L.
Pan sakam, the leaves of Piper Betle, L.
Cip' ciṛip rẹhẹl, the roots of Achyranthes aspera, L.

Grind all these together, mix with *pạura*, spirits, and give to drink.

125. *Dọrọd bạai*, (lit. internal pain convulsions).

Symptoms. This is when from the intense pain due to *hạḍi* or *betha* (q.v.) they run about and the neck is perfectly stiff.

Medicines: First extract the juice from a *tale ḍaṇḍil*, the stem of the leaf of Borassus flabelliformis, L.
Pẹa gol mạric, 3 black pepper-corns.
Lẹṇḍẹl, an earth-worm.
Miltạṅ bindi, a spider.
Culhạko potao gẹndrẹć reak dak, water from the rag with which the fireplace is wiped.

Grind these together and mix with above extracted juice, and give to drink; also smoke him from below with

Haṛhaṭ' hohọt', a bitter Cucurbita lagenaria, Willd. and
Jhiṅgạ jọ, the fruit of Luffa acutangula, Roxb.

126. *Gọmgọmi bạai*.

Symptoms. An unbroken silence is maintained.

Medicines: (*a*) *Sọgọt bọhọk*, the head of a civet, Vivericula malaccensis.
Cemeṅ bọhọk, „ „ „ a mongoose.

Rub on a stone and give him to lick. This will only change the form of *bạai*.

(*b*) Buy from a gipsy: *dhọnọsọṛ cẹṛẹ jaṅ sẹ họṛmọ hạtiṅ jähägem ṅam*, the bones or any part you may get of the body of a certain bird, Hydrocissa coronata.
Ruhi hako cũiạk, the scales of the fish Cyprinus denticulatus, Buch.
Sẹt mahakal jọ, Bryonia lacinosa, L., the white variety fruit.

Cook these in mustard oil and anoint therewith. Take a little of each of the ingredients and tying them on a string hang them round the neck as a necklace.

127. *Hạlmạn bạ̣i*, (lit. monkey convulsions).

Symptoms. In this they nod the head like monkeys and keep gnashing the teeth and embracing; there is a very great fear.

Medicines: (*a*) Rub the head of a monkey on a stone and mixing it with mustard oil plaster or anoint the entire body therewith.

(*b*) *Akaona rẹhẹl*, the roots of Calotropis gigantea, R. Br.
Maraṛ baha chal, the bark of Erythrina indica, Lam.
Gạ̣i gọlọm, melted butter made from cows' milk.

Cook the first two in the third and give some to eat as well as anoint him therewith.

128. *Hạṛdiạ bạ̣i.* Icterus.

Symptoms. In this the body, eyes and urine become yellow and continue thus for half or a whole month. It may attack both healthy and sick persons, and may prove fatal.

Medicines: (*a*) *Rọhọṛak sasaṅ bahatẹl*, the dried flower of Curcuma longa, Roxb.
Goṭe rẹhẹl thoṛa, a little of the roots of Croton oblongifolius, Roxb.
Ọmẹ chal, the bark of Miliusa velutina, Horask. fil. and Ths.

Grind together, make into pills and give daily as well as the next following.

(*b*) *Sega rẹhẹl*, the roots of Mimosa rubicaulis, Lam.
Nanha dudhi loṭa rẹhẹl, the roots of Ichnocarpus frutescens, R. Br.

Grind together and swallow the pills of above (*a*) with it.

(*c*) Wash the hands as follows:—
Ul chal, the bark of Mangifera indica.
Cun, shell lime.
Nirbis da, the bulb of Kyllingia monocephala, L.

Get some of the mango bark in the morning and mix the lime with them; stick the bulb in his ear. Make the patient gaze fixedly at the glow at sunrise and make him hold the prepared mango bark in the hand. Then pour water from a brass vessel several times on what he holds till it is quite clean. He will certainly get well.

(*d*) *Sega rẹhẹl*, the roots of Mimosa rubicaulis, Lam.
Badgọcak rẹhẹl, the roots of Lygodium flexuosum, Sw.
Nanha dudhi loṭa rẹhẹl, the roots of Ichnocarpus frutescens, R. Br.

Grind these three together and give to drink daily till recovery which is sure.

(*e*) Take a piece of *ul chal*, the bark of *Mangifera indica*, and smear on it some *cun*, shell lime. Make the patient stand facing the sun when he is rising resplendent and hold the lime smeared bark in his hand. Take a cup of water and pour it on his hand and continue doing so the while he is being rubbed by some one else. Then all the yellowness will be washed away by the bark. Grind some of it too and give him to drink. He will certainly get well, for I have cured many people thus.

129. *Harnạ bại*, (lit. deer convulsions).

Symptoms. They are in much trepidation, like deer, grind the teeth and move the upper lip as hares or horses in eating.

Medicines: (*a*) *Jel dereń*, a deer's horn.

Rub this on a stone and let him then lick it and rub it on his forehead.

(*b*) *Kāṛwāt rẹhẹl*, the roots of Carissa Carandas, L.
Utiń sunum, mustard oil.

Cook the former in the latter and anoint the whole body therewith.

130. *Hẹ̄kọ̄ṭ bại*. The rattling breathing and sound in extremis.

Symptoms. In this people hiccup emitting a sound like *hẹ̄kọ̄ṭ hẹ̄kọ̄ṭ*.

Medicines: (*a*) *Kul jań*, a tiger's bone.
Tayan bọhọk, a crocodile's skull.
Marak reak goṭa horṃọ sẹ ilko jọtọge, a peacock's whole body or the feathers, all.
Lọpọń chal, the bark of Terminalia bellerica, Roxb.
Jugi ḍuriạ rẹhẹl, the roots of
Ạphim, opium.

Roast the first two to burning point; grind the rest together and mix with the roasted bones, then give him to lick and also plaster him therewith.

(*b*) Grind *marak nạṇḍri*, the windpipe of a peacock and give to drink.

131. *Hikṭi bại*.

Symptoms. This affects women both in health and chiefly after childbirth. The head involuntarily trembles and nods, but in a short time it is over.

Medicines: (*a*) *Mirgi chal*, literally epilepsy bark; it is not a bark, but the skin of a species of deer.
Kāṛwāt rẹhẹl, the roots of Carissa Carandas, L.
Akaona rẹhẹl, the roots of Calotropis gigantea, R. Br.

Mix and grind and smear on, also cook in mustard oil and anoint the whole body therewith.

(*b*) *Gạrunḍi rẹhẹl*, the roots of Acternanthera sessilis, R. Br.
Haṭ jań, the stone of the fruit of Holarrhena antidysenterica, Wall.

Bharbhạri jaṅ, the stone of the fruit of Ocimum basilicum, L. or Ocimum canum, Sims.

Duṇḍukil rẹhẹl, the roots of Gardenia turgida, Roxb.

Grind fine with opium, make into pills and give daily.

132. *Jhạpni bạị.*

Symptoms. In this the eyes are fast closed.

Medicines: (*a*) *Jạnumanak sẹ bin jạnumanak jhạpni aṛak rẹhẹl sẹ sakamko*, the roots or leaves of either the thorny or thornless Zornia diphylla, Pers., or Biophytum sensitivum, DC.

5 *gaṇḍa gol mạric*, 20 black peppercorns.

Grind together, give to drink and smear the whole body therewith.

(*b*) *Jhạpni*, Zornia diphylla, Pers. or Biophytum sensitivum, DC.

Marak il reak mẹ̃ltẹl the eye of a peacock's feather.

Grind these together and smear over the whole body from the face downwards, and give some to lick.

133. *Kandọn bạị.* (lit. crying convulsions).

Symptoms. This affects chiefly babies, viz. they cry day and night.

Medicines: (*a*) *Bir sọn aṛak rẹhẹl*, the roots of

Bir jhuṅkạ aṛak rẹhẹl, the roots of Crotalaria calycina, Shrank.

Rereṅ, a cicada belonging to the species Platypleura.

Ghugri, the mole cricket, Gryllus gryllo-talpa.

Grind these all together, smear over the whole body, and let him lick a little.

(*b*) *Nanha dudhi loṭa*, Ichnocarpus frutescens, R. Br., to be given to smell.

(*c*) The dirt from a cart axle to be smeared on the forehead. If this fails, then mix with water the dirt from the arrow of the machine used for separating the seed from cotton and give to drink.

(*d*) *Kạuhạ chal*, the bark of Terminalia Arjuna, Bedd.

Doka chal „ „ „ Odina Wodier, Roxb.

Grind these and give to drink.

(*e*) *Gạ̃ṛi jambe*, the jaw bone of a monkey.

Sukri soṇḍa, a boar's tusk.

Cemeṅ ḍaṭa, the tooth of a mongoose.

Grind or rub these on a stone and give to drink what comes away.

134. *Kạuḍi ḍiạṅ bạị.*

Symptoms. In this people move about the arms and legs similar to the fluttering of the wings of the black winged kite.

Medicines: (*a*) Get the whole of a black winged kite or its feet and cook this in oil: or if only the feathers then roast these to burning point and stir about in oil. Anoint the whole body and give him to lick.

(*b*) *Rondoc arak dare*, Blumea Wightiana, DC.

Grind and plaster over the whole body.

135. *Kec mecao bai.* (lit. prancing convulsions).

Symptoms. In this the body twitches and they constantly try to get up, and sometimes the tongue is protruded with a lapping motion.

Medicines: *Sadom jhin merhel*, a horse's iron bit.
Gari bohok, a monkey's head.
Toya bohok, the head of a jay, Coracias indica.
Kaudi dian bohok, the head of a black winged kite.

Grind the last three together and add the water in which you have rubbed the first with a stone, and then give some to drink and smear some over the whole body.

136. *Khepa ar khipi bai.* (lit. raving mad convulsions; delirium febris).

Symptoms. In this the patient only laughs.

One "authority" says: If you happen to be near a person when a fit of this comes on, he will give you a sounding blow with a stick or his fist.

Medicines: (*a*) *Thora ganja*, a little Cannabis sativa, Willd.
Ro bohok in maran aphim, opium the size of a fly's head.

Make these into pills the size of a grain of Cajanus indicus, Spreng; stir these in about a mussel shell full of water and give him to drink. He will become intoxicated and lie still.

(*b*) *Nangrauta rehel*, the roots of Nardostachys jatamansi, DC.
Utin sunum, mustard oil.

Cook the former in the latter and smear the whole body therewith.
If he gets no better, then

(*c*) *Ad chotak gan datra rehel roskate*, take the juice of about an ounce of the roots of Datura alba, Willd. or D. fastuosa, Willd.
5 *ganda gol maric*, 20 black peppercorns.

Mix and give to drink. If he becomes intoxicated then mix
Kasmar chal, the bark of Gmelina arborea, Roxb.
Sin arak chal, the bark of Bauhinia purpurea, L.
and give to drink, when the intoxication will pass off.

(*d*) *Gol maric*, black pepper.
Adhe, Zingiber officinale, Roscoe.
Harhat hotol rehel, the roots of a bitter Curcurbita lagenaria.
Kadar rehel, the roots of Bonnaya veronicaefolia, Spreng.

Ḍimbu rẹhẹl, the roots of Ocimum basilicum, var. thyrsiflorum, L.

Grind these together and give to drink.

(*e*) *Kāṛwāl rẹhẹl*, the roots of Carissa Carandas, L.
Gạbur rẹhẹl, „ „ „ Acacia Farnesiana, Willd.
Nạṅgrạuta rẹhẹl, „ „ Nardostachys jatamansi, DC.

Grind these together, cook in oil and smear on the patient.

(*f*) *Lumạm tejo*, the larva of a silkworm, to be ṛoasted to burning point.
Bayar kaḍako thapa akat dare reak̓ chal, the bark of a tree knocked by a male entire buffalo.
Tejo mala rẹhẹl, the roots of Cissampelos Pareira, L.

Grind together and give to drink; with one breath bite off the bark of *eraḍọm*, Ricinus communis, L., and with one breath hang the bass of it on to his neck; and put a dot of *akaona loṛe*, the exudation from Calotropis gigantea, R. Br., on each one of all his nails.

The following may be given in all kinds of *bạì* :—

(*g*) *Kasmar rẹhẹl*, the roots of Gmelina arborea, Roxb.

Heat and plaster therewith.

(*h*) *Kāṛwāl rẹhẹl*, the roots of Carissa Carandas, L.

Plaster without heating.

(*i*) *Kāṛwāl sakam*, the leaves of Carissa Carandas, L.

Heat and plaster therewith.

Kikir bạì.

Symptoms. In this people scream *kikir kikir*, like the kingfisher.

Medicines: *Kikir cẹṛẹ̄ge gọjeme*, kill a kingfisher.
Karla da, the bulb of Momordica dioica, Roxb.

Cook these together and give to eat as well as plaster the whole body therewith and he will be cured.

Mẹtrẹć bạì. (Delirium febris; lit. teeth grinding convulsions).

Symptoms. In this the teeth are ground, the upper lip is protruded and moved about as by a horse in grazing, or both lips are moved as by a babe sucking at the breast.

Medicines: (*a*) *Jel dereṅ*, a deer's horn.
Sukri jambe, a pig's jaw bone.

Rub on a stone, give to drink and plaster the whole body therewith.

(*b*) *Adagạthiạ ghās da*, the bulbs of Panicum repens, L.
Kaḍa beṅjak̓ rẹhẹl, the roots of
Kạhu botke rẹhẹl, the roots of Bryonia lacinosa, L.
Beṅgaṛ betahet rẹhẹl sẹ jọ, the roots of Solanum stramonifolium, Jacq., or its fruit.

Rańgaini jo se rehel, the fruit or roots of Solanum Jacquini, Willd.

Cook these in melted butter and give to eat.

139. *Mocra mucri bai.* (lit. writhing convulsions).

Symptoms. In this they writhe and throw themselves about.

Medicines: (*a*) *Baghin rehel*, the roots of Mezoneurum cucullatum, W. and A.
Ato kundri, Cephalandra indica, Nand.
Tarpin sunum, Terebinthinæ oleum.
Daru, gunpowder.

Grind these together, mix in oil of turpentine, and rub it in on that side of the patient on which he tosses himself.

140. *Ńokor bai.* (? St. Vitus' dance).

Symptoms. In this they nod the head like *ńokor* bird (the red-start), the arms and legs tremble and they can grasp nothing with the hand.

Medicines: (*a*) *Nanha dudhi lota rehel*, the roots of Ichnocarpus frutescens, R. Br.
Sukri mutha da, the bulb of Scirpus monostachyos, Kön.
Dhubi ghãs rehel, the roots of Cynodon dactylon, Pers.
Mõrẽ ganda ro, 20 flies.
Ńokor cẽrẽ hormo reak jãhãtakge, any part of the body of the *ńokor* bird.

141. *Pajhar bai.* (lit. eagle convulsions).

Symptoms. In this people claw or scratch and clutch like eagles.

Medicines: (*a*) Get and keep the bones of an eagle from the knee downwards. Take a little of this, cook it in mustard oil and anoint the whole body and give him to lick.

(*b*) *Ghãrã ghãrĩ dare rehel*, the roots of

Grind with black pepper and give him to drink.

142. *Pãthã bai.*

Symptoms. There is an uncomfortable feeling in the stomach which moves about, and there is pain.

One "authority" says: Whereas in *dhond bai* (No. 124) the nerve rises in an upright direction, in this it does so transversely.

Medicines: (*a*) In this too all the remedies under No. 117 are applicable.

Forbidden diet:—

Bajra daka, the cooked preparation of Sorghum vulgare, Pers.
Handi, rice beer.
Kaera, plantains, Musa paradisiaca, L.
Kanthar, the fruit of Artocarpus integrifolia, L.
Kada ar bheda jel, the flesh of buffaloes and mutton.

Kesari dal, the split grain of Lathyrus sativus, L.
Kurmbi arak,
Bitkil toa, buffalo milk.
(*b*) *Mahadeb jata*.
Kedok arak, Argyreia speciosa, Sweet.
Capol, Desmodium cephalotes (?)
Bitkil cand, Porana paniculata, Roxb.

Pound the roots of all these together and give to drink.

If this does not avail, then

(*c*) take and mix with above the ingredients mentioned in No. 117 (*m*) and give to drink with *paura*, spirits.

143. *Rae kakarbak bai*. (lit. chameleon convulsions).

Symptoms. Chameleons (*rae kakarbak*) in walking extend the two front legs first and then the two hind ones with a jerky motion. Persons who have this *bai* have a similar gait.

Medicines: (*a*) Kill a chameleon and keep the tail or entire body. Take a little of this and cook it in oil, and anoint the patient therewith, but give him none to drink.

For internal administration:—

Bonga bari rehel, the roots of
Pea ponea gan gol maric, about 3 or 4 black peppercorns.

Grind together and give to drink.

144. *Ros bai*.

Symptoms. These are similar to those of *sugum bai*, No. 149; but the countenance is pale and speech indistinct.

Medicines: (*a*) *Rasun*, garlic.
Tejo mala rehel, the roots of Cissampelos Pareira, L.
Pea gol maric, 3 black peppercorns.

Grind and give to drink. If the teeth are clenched, then heat *berel sasan*, raw turmeric, Curcuma longa, Roxb., and burn him therewith in the hollow behind each ear.

145. *Sanipatik bai*.

Symptoms. This attacks women 5 or 10 days after giving birth to a child, when they start up suddenly as from a dream, give a loud scream and immediately lose consciousness.

Medicines: (*a*) *Suruj mukhi arak rehel*, roots of Helianthus annuus, Willd.
Surju muni rehel, the roots of
Bir lil rehel, the roots of wild indigo.
Sinduari chal, the bark of Vitex Negundo, L.
Kahu botke rehel, the roots of Bryonia lacinosa, L.
Pe ganda gol maric, 12 black peppercorns.

Mix and give to drink.

(*b*) *Bir lil sakam*, the leaves of wild indigo.
Kāṛwāl ręhęl, the roots of Carissa Carandas, L.
Nạṅgrạuta ręhęl, the roots of Nardostachys jatamansi, DC.
Sinduạri sakam, the leaves of Vitex Negundo, L.
Bana haṭak chal, the bark of Oroxylon indicum, Benth.
Ạṭi sahṛa chal, the bark of
Panjọṭ chal, the bark of Clerodendron phlomoides, Willd.
Pusi toa ręhęl, the roots of Euphorbia pilulifera, L.

Mix all these, give to drink and smear therewith.

(*c*) *Toyo karla jaṅ*, the kernel of
Gurli jaṅ, the kernel of
Karla da, the bulb of Momordica dioica, Roxb.
At da, „ „ „ Zehneria umbellata, Thw.

Mix all these with black pepper and give to drink, and after cooking a little of the same in mustard oil smear the whole body therewith.

146. *Selesa hẹ̄kọ̄ṭ bạ̄i.*

Symptoms. This is a very dangerous form of *bạ̄i*, in which the patient continually hiccoughs, and may easily prove fatal.

Medicines: (*a*) *Dare ṭipọć*,
Gạ̄i ghuṛạ, Polygala chinensis, L.
Kạṭić culuṅ rạṅgạini jạnum ḍọg, a bit of a sprout of Solanum Jacquini, Willd.

Grind together and stir in *luti rasa* or *dumur rasa*, honey of either of two kinds of small honey bees, and give to eat. If he can only swallow it once or twice he will recover.

147. *Siṭli bạ̄i.* (Collapse).

Symptoms. In this the entire body, limbs included, becomes as cold as ice.

One "authority" says: In this they become perfectly cold and the limbs are as soft as edible leaves. They lie perfectly quiet, and you can detect nothing amiss in their appearance, but if you feel them you find they are as cold as water.

Medicines: (*a*) *Adhẹ*, ginger.
Gol mạric, black pepper.
Tursi ręhęl, the roots of Ocymum sanctum, Willd.
Bharbhạri ręhęl, the roots of Ocymum basilicum, L. or O. canum, Sims.

Grind all these and give to drink.

(*b*) *Tursi*, Ocymum sanctum, Willd.
Bharbhạri sakam, the leaves of Ocymum basilicum, L. or O. canum, Sims.
Jhạpni ręhęl, the roots of Zornia diphylla, Pers. or Biophytum sensitivum, DC.

Adhe, ginger.

Gol maric, black pepper.

Grind all together and without warming plaster him therewith.

(*c*) *Maraṅ jhapni aṛak bin janumanak*, the thornless Zornia diphylla, Pers., or, Biophitum sensitivum, DC.

Janumanak jhapni rehel, the roots of the *jhapni* as above that has thorns.

Gol maric, black pepper.

Grind and mix, give to drink and plaster him therewith.

To warm the body :—

(*d*) *Kāṛwāt*, Carissa Carandas, L.

Plaster the whole body with this. After that plaster him with black pepper alone, and he will be all right.

(*e*) *Sar rehel* the roots of Saccharum Sara, Roxb.

Mota bhernda rehel, the roots of Jatropha Curcas, L.

Grind these together and smear over the whole body.

148. *Suar bai.* (lit. pig convulsions).

Symptoms. In this the patient foams at the mouth like pigs, the saliva forms into a mass and he makes a sound as of smacking in eating.

Medicines: (*a*) *Jambe se bohok jaṅ sukriak*, the jaw bone or skull of a pig that was killed by a tiger, or if unobtainable then that of any healthy pig.

Kahu botke rehel, the roots of Bryonia lacinosa, L.

Thora gan aphim, a small quantity of opium.

Grind these together, plaster the whole body therewith and let him eat a little.

149. *Sugum bai.* (lit. stealth convulsions).

Symptoms. In this the patient lies perfectly still, so that you think he is lying quietly, but repeated calls awaken no response.

Medicines: (*a*) *Dhiri kakṛa bohok*, the head of a certain lizard.

Saram babea bohok, " " Herpestes moticolus.

Grind these quickly and let him lick them.

(*b*) *Kaskom rehel*, the roots of Gossypium arboreum, L.

Kāṛwāt rehel, the roots of Carissa Carandas, L.

Kawel sakam, the leaves of Abrus precatorius, L.

Grind these together, warm slightly and plaster over the whole body.

150. *Tayan bai.* (lit. crocodile convulsions).

Symptoms. They make a noise like crocodiles, bite, creep on the stomach, blink the eyes and remain silent.

Medicines: (*a*) Roast the skull of a crocodile to burning point, stir it about in mustard oil, anoint him therewith and give him to drink.

(*b*) *Nạṅgrạuta rẹhẹl*, the roots of Nardostachys jatamansi, DC.
Kẹsọr da, the bulb of
Akaona rẹhẹl, the roots of Calotropis gigantea, R. Br.

Grind these together, cook in melted butter, give him to eat and anoint the whole body therewith.

151. *Taṛkha tạṛkhi bại.* (lit. writhing convulsions).

Symptoms. In this they toss about and writhe, the limbs are drawn up, and sometimes they scream.

Medicines: *Guṇḍri gẹrwẹl,*
Cupul jhạpni, Zornia diphylla, Pers.
Miltaṅ bindi, a spider.
Miltaṅ tala gol mạric, half a black peppercorn.

Grind all these together and smear over the whole body, and let him lick some.

152. *Ti hurlạ mirgi bại.*

Symptoms. They first swing about one arm and leg, afterwards the other; the eyes are fast closed for two or three days.

Medicines: (*a*) *Dạtrạ rẹhẹl mil choṭak rọsme*, take 2 oz. of the juice of the roots of Datura alba, Willd. or D. fastuosa, Willd.
Etka rẹhẹl, the roots of Mucuna pruriens, DC.
Thoṛa sẹṅgẹl siṅ rẹhẹl, the roots of Tragia involucrata, Jacq., a little of this.
Pẹ gaṇḍa gol mạric, 12 black peppercorns.

Grind together and give adults about 2 ounces and children a third of that. If there is stupefaction, then mix and give to drink with stale rice-water,
Kasmar chal, the bark of Gmelina arborea, Roxb.
Siṅ aṛak chal, „ „ „ Bauhinia purpurea, L.

153. *Ghao.* Any (open) sore.

Medicines: *Kuilạ*, charcoal.
Nim sakam, the leaves of Melia Azadirachta, L.

Grind, mix, heat, put in a piece of cloth and apply.

154. *Ạgyo ghao.*

Symptoms. This sore breaks out on the shin, thigh or elsewhere. It begins like a boil in many places and spreads deep; the pain is greater than that of a boil. Whereas a boil will get well of itself after bursting, this will not get well without medicine.

Medicines: (*a*) *Meral sakam*, the leaves of Phyllanthus Emblica, L.
Nim sakam, „ „ „ Melia Azadirachta, L.
Kaṇṭhaṛ sakam, „ „ „ Artocarpus integrifolia, L.

Fry to burning point, stir in mustard oil and apply as a plaster.

(*b*) When an unmarried girl lets fall and breaks an earthenware water-pot, bring that, rub a portion of it and smear on what is rubbed off; recovery will follow.

(*c*) Get hold of a potsherd that a certain snake (*tutri*, Eryx conicus) has turned out of its hole, rub this and smear the rubbings on.

155. *Bọhọk ghao* Sores in the head.

Medicines: (*a*) *Bạrni sakam*, the leaves of Clerodendron infortunatum, L.
Kana aṛak, " " " Commelyna bengalensis, L.

Or if these are unobtainable, then

Hạṇḍi mera, the refuse after brewing rice beer.
Kunạm da, the bulb of
Bọd laṛ, Vitis adnata, Wall.

Or failing this last, then in place of it

Sim bele, a hen's egg, and
Arak sindur, red lead.
Nanha pusi toa, Euphorbia thymifolia, Burm.

Grind together and apply as a plaster.

(*b*) *Agọire*, Dillenia scabrella, Roxb.
Cạr sirạ,

Roast both mixed in a potsherd to burning point, then grind and after mixing in mustard oil, apply with a feather.

Terelak mare baklak, the old dry bark of Diospyros tomentosa, Roxb.
Icạk baklak, the old dry bark of Woodfordia floribunda, Salisb.
Mare sarjọm reak baklak, the bark of an old Shorea robusta, Gärtn.
Ghugri, an entire mole cricket, Gryllus gryllo-talpa.
Puṭkạ, a puff-ball (Lycoperdon).

Wash the sore clean, apply mustard oil to it, and then after grinding all the above into a powder sprinkle it on to the sore.

156. *Boṅga khoda.*

(Possibly due to a sting; local acute swelling which breaks out into a slowly healing sore.)

Symptoms: There are several varieties of this: *hẹndẹge pusrik*, black pimples; *arakge pusrik*, red pimples; *lọ phoka leka phokak sẹ pusrik*, blisters as from burns, or pimples; *ghao gaḍaktako*, an ulcer either penetrating very deep or perforating, though it does not occasion much pain.

Medicines: In the black pimple variety,

(*a*) *Maraṛ baha chal*, the bark of Erythrina indica, Lam.

Grind and apply 3 or 4 times daily over the whole of the swelling, and make about an ounce of the juice of *bana haṭak chal*, the bark of Oroxylon indicum, Benth., and give to drink.

(*b*) *Mare nangle rapak rọngọeme*, roast an old leathern yoke-thong to burning point.

When a dog has stolen and eaten some raw rice and passes some of this out in his excreta, pick that out and keep it and roast or fry it to burning point.

Piṭuạ aṛak, Spemacoce hispida, L.

Piṇḍe chal, the bark of Randia uliginosa, DC.

Nanha dudhi loṭa rẹhẹl, the roots of Ichnocarpus frutescens, R. Br.

Dud baraṅgọm da, the bulb of

Ato piṇḍo da, „ „ „ Amorphophallus campanulatus, Blume.

Ghoṛa lada, Vitis tomentosa, Heyne.

Sạpin, Opuntia Dillenii, Haworth.

Dạtrạ rẹhẹl, the roots of Datura alba, Willd. or D. fastuosa, Willd.

Duṇḍukil rẹhẹl, the roots of Gardenia turgida, Roxb.

Nim chal sẹ sakam, the bark or leaves of Melia Azadirachta, L.

Fry all these to burning point and after stirring them in mustard oil apply as a plaster over the entire swollen part, which will subside in three hours and the pain will also cease quickly. This remedy is applicable in all the varieties of this complaint.

Before swelling occurs:—

(*c*) Plaster the warm excrement of a heifer who has not calved, over the pimples, and recovery will follow.

(*d*) *Nim chal sẹ sakam*, the bark or leaves of Melia Azadirachta, L.

Grind fine and apply without warming as a plaster; he will certainly get well.

If a sore breaks out:—

(*e*) *Hesak sakam ḍọg*, the budding leaves of Ficus religiosa, Willd.

Kadam sakam ḍọg, the budding leaves of Anthocephalus Cadamba, Bth. and Hook. f.

Meral chal, the bark of Phyllanthus Emblica, L.

Grind these to a coarse powder and sprinkle daily on the sores. Also boil the leaves of Melia Azadirachta, L. and wash the sores daily with that water.

(*f*) *Marań catọm aṛak*, Marsilea quadrifolia, L.

Grind and apply as a plaster without warming; efficacious.

(*g*) *Nim chal*, the bark of Melia Azadirachta, L.

Sọsọ chal, „ „ „ Semecarpus Anacardium, L.

Ńūṛūć jọ reak gabeṭẹt, the flesh of the fruit of Cassia Fistula, L.

Edẹl poha, a seedling of Bombax malabaricum, DC.

Grind these together and plaster over the swollen part near the sores; or fry to burning point into a powder and sprinkle it on; and if swollen, stir in oil and anoint.

(*h*) In all cases of this complaint:—

Niuri chal, the bark of Elæodendron Roxburghii, W. and A.

Ňũṛũč jọ reak gabetẹl, the flesh of the fruit of Cassia Fistula, L.

Grind together and apply without warming.

(*i*) *Candogaṛ gọd*,

Grind and apply without warming.

(*j*) The first two ingredients the same as the first two in No. (*b*).

Sạpin jạnum, Opuntia Dillenii, Haworth., also to be roasted to burning point.

Grind these three, or if the second is unobtainable, then the first and third and stir in pure mustard oil and smear him therewith. If you do this in the morning the swelling will go down by noon.

(*k*) If the patient vomits:

Nim rọs, the juice of Melia Azadirachta, L.

Maraṛ baha rọs, the juice of Erythrina indica, Lam.

Give this to drink.

(*l*) If there are any swellings, then grind the bark of *maraṛ baha*, Erythrinaindica, Lam., warm it and apply as an ointment, and he will get well at once.

(*m*) *Nim sakam*, the leaves of Melia Azadirachta, L.

Grind and apply without warming to the swellings.

(*n*) *Jokha sakam*, the leaves of Sida humilis, Willd., to be applied and

Ḍaṅgra jambe, the jawbone of a bullock to be rubbed on a stone and smeared on.

(*o*) *Hesak ḍọg*, the tip of Ficus religiosa, Willd.

Kadam ḍọg, ,, ,, Anthocephalus Cadamba, Benth. and Hook. f.

Meral chal, the bark of Phyllanthus Emblica, L.

Grind together and apply as an ointment without warming.

(*p*) If the sores become concave sprinkle on them a powder of

Mare naṅgle, an old leathern yoke thong.

Sạpin, Opuntia Dillenii, Haw.

(*q*) Or if these are stirred in mustard oil and applied, the sores themselves will get well. This is an excellent remedy.

(*r*) *Matkọm chal*, the bark of Bassia latifolia, Roxb.

Boṅga sarjọm chal, the bark of Ventilago calyculata, Tulasne.

Lọṭọ jọ, the fruit of Randia dumetorum, Lam.

Grind and apply as a plaster.

(*s*) Rice that has passed out in the excreta of a dog.

Wash and grind this, plaster some of this on the sore and give some to drink. Give this treatment for three days and a cure will follow.

(*t*) *Mare nańgle*, an old leathern yoke thong.

Sapin janum, Opuntia Dillenii, Haw.

Fry or roast these to burning point, burn *seta ić*, dogs' excrement, then grind all three together, stir in *utiń sunum*, mustard oil, and apply with a feather.

One "authority" says: This may begin in the toes or fingers, the parts affected becoming black as in tatoo marks. There is a burning pain, and if medicine be not quickly applied, it will continue to swell and become inflamed. If it extends to the throat death ensues.

157. *Dora ghao*. (*Dora* is the name of the cord worn by Santal males round the waist.)

Symptoms. This appears on the waist, round which little insects eat their way giving the sore the appearance of earth thrown up by the mole cricket.

Medicines: *Kahu botke rehel*, the roots of Bryonia lacinosa, L.

Aphim, opium.

Jurguda kaskom jań, the seeds of a certain variety of the cotton plant.

Kucla jań, the seeds of Strychnos potatorum, L.f.

Cook these in castor oil and apply daily.

158. *Dumur ghao*.

Symptoms. An excrescence appears on the body in appearance like the *dumur*, a species of wild honey bee, when in their hive.

Medicines: *Ot dhompo*, Lepidagathis cristata, Willd.

Bir kapu jo, the fruit of Dioscorea oppositifolia, L.

Tutri bińko odok kelhat, a piece of pottery unearthed by the *tutri* (Eryx conicus) snake.

Grind these together and apply to the sore.

159. *Gand ghao*. (Adenitis).

Symptoms. This appears in the groin and sometimes elsewhere, and occasionally it festers; it increases in size.

Medicines: (*a*) At the very commencement make the patient stand in the middle of the doorway and make as if to strike him with an axe, some three days; he will get well.

(*b*) *Loa lore*, the juice or gum exuded from Ficus glomerata, Roxb. on incision of the bark.

Buluń, salt.

Mix a little of the latter with the former and smear it on for two or three days, and he will get well.

(*c*) *Peaj*, onions.

Rẹthẹ ghoṛa lada rẹhẹl sẹ da, the roots or bulb of

Thoṛa mạric, a little chilli or capsicum, Capsicum frutescens, Willd.

Grind these and after warming a little apply.

To ripen it:—

(*d*) *Ḍaṅgra jambe ḍaṭa*, the jaw tooth of a bullock.

Rub this and smear it on.

To cause it to burst:—

(*e*) *Parwa ić*, pigeons' dung.

Hoṛẹć jaṅ, the seed of Dolichos biflorus, L.

Buluṅ, salt.

Grind these and smear over the sore.

To expel the pus:—

(*f*) *Pọjọ chal*, the bark of Tetranthera monopetala, Roxb.

Grind and plaster on, when the pus will come freely away.

(*g*) *Jokha sakam*, the leaves of Sida humilis, Willd.

These too if ground and applied as a plaster will cause the pus to come away on pressure.

(*h*) *Peaj*, onions.

Grind, warm and apply, and he will get well.

(*i*) *Cun*, shell lime.

Buluṅ, salt.

Loa loṛe, the gum exuded from Ficus glomerata, Roxb.

Mix and apply.

160. *Ghugri ghao.*

(? Adenitis scrofulosa colli).

Symptoms. This sore is similar to *hạsli* (No. 28, Le collier de Venus). This also appears all round the neck and descends to the breast and downwards, with the appearance of the earth cast up by the mole cricket (*ghugri*).

Medicines: (*a*) *Haṛhaṭ kundri da*, the bulb of the bitter Zehneria umbellata, Thew.

Ato kundri da, the bulb of Cephalandra indica, Nand.

Kạhu botke rẹhẹl, the roots of Bryonia lacinosa, L.

Gurli jaṅ, the seeds of

Jhiṅgạ jaṅ, „ „ Luffa acutangula, Roxb.

Bir jhiṅgạ jaṅ, the seeds of Luffa amara, R.

Haṛhaṭ họtọl jaṅ, the seeds of a bitter pumpkin, Cucurbita lagenaria, Willd.

Muṅgạ chal, the bark of Moringa pterygosperma, Gärtn.

Tutiạ thoṛa, a little sulphate of copper.

Cook in mustard oil and apply daily with a feather.

(b) *Mare nangle*, an old leathern yoke thong.

Ạṇḍiạ tale baha, the flower of the male Borassus flabelliformis, L.

Ọt ḍhompo, Lepidagathis cristata, Willd.

Biṇḍi muthạ ghās, Fimbristylis monostachya, Hassk.

Roast the first two and fry the last two, both to burning point, then grind all fine, stir in pure mustard oil and smear on.

161. *Kākbirạl ghao.* (Adenitis axillaris).

Symptoms. This appears first like a tumour in the armpit, and later it suppurates like a boil and is painful.

Medicines: (a) *Gại gọtọm sẹ gại toa chale*, melted butter made from cows' milk, or the cream of the same.

Apply on the sore and afterwards let a kitten or such like lick it off, recovery will follow.

(b) *Loa lore*, the gum exuded from Ficus glomerata, Roxb. on incision of the bark.

Buluṅ, salt.

Mix and smear on for some four days and the sore will subside.

(c) *Peaj*, onions.

Rạsun, garlic.

Ạphim, opium.

Gol mạric, black pepper.

Grind together and apply.

To ripen it:—

(d) *Gại gọtọm*, melted butter made from cow's milk.

Boi bindi jọ sẹ rẹhẹl chal, the fruit or the bark of the root of Randia dumetorum, Lamk.

Grind these together, boil and apply, and it will burst.

(e) *Parwa ić*, pigeon's dung.

Họrẹć jaṅ, the seed of Dolichos biflorus, L.

Buluṅ, salt.

Grind these together and apply to the top of the sore or drop a little on, and it will ripen.

To draw off the pus:—

(f) *Mạtha ạrak rẹhẹl*, the roots of Antidesma diandrum, Tulas.

Grind and apply and it will expel the pus.

(g) Smear some *toa*, milk, on the sore or swelling and let a cat lick it off.

162. *Ghurạ ghao.* (? Erisypelas).

Symptoms. Wherever this appears, be it in the leg, the shin, thigh, back or wherever it may be, it spreads all round.

Medicines: *Tutiạ*, sulphate of copper.

Muṅgạ dare tejo ganthar, the film of the insect found on Moringa pterygosperma, Gärtn.

Sẹlẹp samanọm rẹhẹl, the roots of Gloriosa superba, L.

Hāṛū awar nāṛī, Menispermum glabrum (?).

Grind all these, cook them in pure mustard oil and apply daily with a feather.

163. *Goda ghao.* (Sores in the legs in connection with oedema).

Symptoms. This begins in the legs, which swell up, and sometimes they break out into sores.

Medicines: (*a*) *Sẹṅgẹl siṅ rẹhẹl*, the roots of Tragia involucrata, Jacq.

Etka rẹhẹl, the roots of Mucuna pruriens, DC.

Bir malhan rẹhẹl, the roots of Atyllosia mollis, Bth.

Ạṇḍiạ mọrọn aṛak̓ rẹhẹl, the roots of Gymnema hirsutus, W. and A., var. Decaisneanum, Wight.

Kūs rẹhẹl, the roots of Themuda gigantea, Haskel.

Ạsạṛiạ chal, the bark of Capparis horrida, L.f.

Saram lutur rẹhẹl, the roots of Clerodendron serratum, Spreng.

Akaona rẹhẹl, the roots of Calotropis gigantea, R. Br.

Kāṛwāl rẹhẹl, „ „ Carissa Carandas, L.

Bana haṭak̓ rẹhẹl, the roots of Oroxylon indicum, Benth.

Bir hoṛẹc̓, Atyllosia scarabaedois, Benth.

Grind all these together and put into a new earthenware pot, covering all with a leaf plate. Add water and boil it well. Then spread a thin cloth over the bed, on which the patient must lie. Cover him with a thick sheet or such and let the cloth descend to the ground all round the bed like a curtain. Then steam the patient with the boiling medicines until the perspiration exudes profusely from his body. Repeat the operation until recovery.

(*b*) *Ạsạṛiạ chal*, the bark of Capparis horrida, L.

Kāṛwāl rẹhẹl, the roots of Carissa Carandas, L.

Simbrit, the fresh shoots of Bombax malabaricum, DC.

Grind all these and mix with melted butter of cow's milk. Take a length of a shoot of *jọm jạnum*, Zizyphus Jujuba, Lamk., as long as eight fingers placed side by side are broad, and wrap six fingers' breadth of this along with what you have ground. Then make the patient sit on a low stool, and making a ball of cowdung place it before him and stick the "candle" wrapped up with the medicine in the cowdung at the top. Then wrap the patient entirely up in a sheet and inside this set fire to the "candle." The patient must be careful not to look at the "candle" all the time you are lighting it and it is burning, but look in another direction; then the perspiration will exude profusely from his body. For people 40 to 60 years of age prepare 4 "candles" and apply for 4 days; the water will be expelled entirely from the body.

Before recovery there will be sores in the mouth. Then cook some *ghi kũạri*, Yucca gloriosa, in melted butter which he will eat. For 15 days the patient must eat no rice, curry, salt or sugar, but only sago.

164. *Jaṅ uri.*

Medicines: *Terel cẹtẹ*, the thin skin on the bark of Diospyros tomentosa, Roxb.

Doka chal, the bark of Odina Wodier, Roxb.

Grind with a stone and sprinkle on daily.

165. *Kadam baha ghao.*

Symptoms. This sore may appear on the back, breast, anywhere. A pimple comes up as in *boṅga khoda* (No. 156), but this differs from that. There is neither any swelling as in that, nor any pain. The sore bursts up from inside and expands on the surface like the flower of the *kadam*, Anthocephalus Cadamba, Bth. and Hook. f.

Medicines: (*a*) Make an ointment of *dhũṛã*, resin, and melted butter and apply daily with a feather.

(*b*) *Mare naṅgle*, an old leather yoke thong.

Aṇḍiạ tale baha, the flower of the male Borassus flabelliformis, L.

Sẹṅgẹl susurbaṅ chata, the nest of a certain wasp.

Saparọm chal, the bark of Nyctanthes Arbor-tristis, L.

Mạnikjọṛ,

Icạk rẹhẹl, the roots of Woodfordia floribunda, Salisb.

Fry these to burning point, stir in mustard oil and smear on with a feather.

166. *Kạr ghao.* (? Chronic scabies).

Symptoms. This is an eruption which appears in thick profusion on the legs, shins, feet, in fact in many places, in both children and adults. On ripening it is white and itches greatly so that they scratch the eruption itself.

Medicines: (*a*) *Muṅgạ rẹhẹl*, the roots of Moringa pterygosperma, Gärtn.

Tutiạ, sulphate of copper.

Boil in mustard oil and apply with a feather.

(*b*) *Mare naṅgle*, an old leathern yoke thong.

Aṇḍiạ tale baha, the flower of the male Borassus flabelliformis, L.

Corco chal, the bark of Casearea tomentosa, Roxb.

Nim chal, the bark of Melia Azadirachta, L.

Ọt ḍhompo, Lepidagathis cristata, Willd.

Bheḍa dereṅ rẹhẹl, the roots of Cassia Tora, L.

Sinduạri sakam, the leaves of Vitex Negundo, L.

Roast or fry all these to burning point, stir in mustard oil and anoint therewith.

(*c*) *Sẹlẹp samanọm rẹhẹl*, the roots of Gloriosa superba, L.
Hāṛū awar nāṛī, Menispermum glabrum (?).
Dare japak jọ, the fruit of Scindapsus officinalis, Schott.

Boil all these three well in oil and apply with a feather.

(*d*) Buy the real black pigment with which Hindus paint their goddess Kali black, and smear this on.

(*e*) *Bhage rambṛa*, sound Phaeseolus Mungo, var. radiatus, L.
Bẹrẹl adhẹ, raw ginger.
Bẹrẹl sasaṅ bọhọk, head of raw turmeric, Curcuma longa, L.

Grind these three very fine and plaster therewith, bandaging with rags. On the second day remove the bandage leaving the medicine there. Apply the plaster again for three or four days.

(*f*) The same as detailed in *Nạrgi ghao*, No. 169 (*b*).

(*g*) *Mare hukạ dak*, stale hookah water.
Citol hako, a certain fish.
Muṅgạ chal, the bark of Moringa pterygosperma, Gärtn.

Grind together and plaster on the sores.

(*h*) Smear *sukri itil*, pigs fat, on the sores.

(*i*) *Thamakur khaḍa*, the stems of the tobacco plant to be roasted to burning point, and then after adding
Puṭhi hako cūiāk, the scales of the fish Barbus stigma,

Grind both together, cook in *utiṅ sunum*, mustard oil, and apply daily.

(*j*) *Boṅga sarjọm chal*, the bark of Ventilago calyculata, Tulasne.

Grind and cook in *utiṅ sunum*, mustard oil, and sprinkle a little *cun*, lime, on, and

Sora, saltpetre.
Gọndhọk, sulphur.

Grind both these and stir them in *nạrkọṛ sunum*, cocoanut oil; then mix all the ingredients, and after washing the sores clean of an evening apply the mixture daily, and they will quickly dry up.

167. *Khaora ghao.*

Medicines: (*a*) *Akaona sakam ḍọgtẹl*, the tips of the leaves of Calotropis gigantea R. Br. or C. procera, R. Br.
Sinduạri sakam ḍọgtẹl, the tips of the leaves of Vitex Negundo, L.
Mạric ad pawa gan, 4 ounces Capsicum frutescens, Willd.
Gọndhọk mit anawak, an anna worth of sulphur.
Mit sẹr tuṛi sunum, 2 pounds pure mustard oil.

Pound the first four, put them in the last and boil well until it looks like water; while boiling add:—

Tutiạ, sulphate of copper.
Laṭha cip ciṛip rẹhẹl, the roots of
Pipṛiañ,
Sora, saltpetre.

Grind the saltpetre with the handle of a chisel, then rub the other three ingredients in the saltpetre, and then add this to the boiling mustard oil, and finally apply the mixture thinly to the sore.

168. *Khudạ jạurạ ghao.* (? Impetigo).

Symptoms. This sore is found in children from babyhood to some two years of age, or even in adults. It appears mostly in the face, cheeks, ears and head, first as pimples ripening white, and gradually spreads in clusters.

Medicines: (*a*) *Gạị gọtọm, nạinu urul tora*, melted butter from cows' milk prepared as soon as churned.
Marań catọm aṛak, the variety of Marsilea quadrifolia, L. that has reddish leaves.
Khode mamọn catọm aṛak.

Grind the two latter, mix with the first and apply daily.

169. *Nạrgi ghao.*

Medicines: (*a*) the same as No. 155 (*c*).
(*b*) *Terel opal cokak*, the surface bark of a sapling of Diospyros tomentosa, Roxb.
Mare sarjọm dareak chal, the bark of an old Shorea robusta, Gärtn.
Mare icạk dareak chal, the bark of an old Woodfordia floribunda, Salisb.
Ghugri, a mole cricket, Gryllus gryllo-talpa.
Puṭkạ, a puff-ball, Lycoperdon.

First of all clean the sore. Grind all the above together and then sprinkle some of this on the sore, cook more in oil and anoint the sore therewith.

(*c*) *Rạnu ran rẹhẹl*, the root of the ferment used to make rice beer.
Moṭa ạtkir rẹhẹl, the thick roots of Smilax ovalifolia, Roxb.
Sega rẹhẹl, the roots of Mimosa rubicaulis, Lam.

Grind together, cook in mustard oil and anoint the sore therewith.

170. *Koca nạrgi.*

Medicines: *Tejo ič*, the excreta of larvæ found on wattles.
Sẹkrẹč bhiṭuạk, the stem of the leaves Lagerstroemia parviflora, Roxb.
Kondro chal, the bark of Acacia Intsia, Willd.

Grind together, cook in mustard oil and anoint therewith. When the sore is very ripe, crush *murup rẹhẹl*, the roots of Butea frondosa, Roxb., and pour the fluid thus extracted into the sore.

171. *Phoka nạrgi ghao.*

Symptoms. This usually appears in the head as a blister like that from a burn, from which only watery matter issues and pimples arise profusely.

Medicines: (*a*) *Aṇḍiạ tale baha*, the flower of the male Borassus flabelliformis, L.

Mare naṅgle, an old leathern yoke thong.

Sẹṅgẹl susurbaṅ chata, the nest of the Pollestes hebraea wasp.

Piṭuạ aṛak, Spermacoce hispida, L.

Biṇḍi muthạ ghās rẹhẹt, the roots of Fimbristylis monostachya, Hassk.

Piṇḍạ chal, the bark of Randia uliginosa, DC.

Icạk rẹhẹt, the roots of Woodfordia floribunda, Salisb.

Mạnikjọṛ ghās dare,

Nim sakam, the leaves of Melia Azadirachta, L.

Hemca aṛak, Enhydra fluctuans.

Fry all these together to burning point, and after stirring in pure mustard oil smear therewith.

(*b*) *Nạrgi dare chal*, the bark of

Either fry this to burning point or pound it fine and apply.

(*c*) *Mare naṅgle*, an old leathern yoke thong.

Aṇḍiạ mọṛọn aṛak rẹhẹt, the roots of Gymnema hirsutus, W. and A., var. Decaisneanum, Wight.

Piṭuạ aṛak rẹhẹt, the roots of Spermacoce hispida, L.

Piṇḍạ dare chal, the bark of Randia uliginosa, DC.

Aṇḍiạ tale baha, the flower of the male Borassus flabelliformis, L.

Susurbaṅ chata, a wasps' nest.

Fry these together to burning point, and then after grinding stir in mustard oil, and apply with a feather.

(*d*) *Onẹ dare ḍarre bindi ganak leka ganthar gantharko oṛak idi*, the filmy substance like cobwebs spun by minute insects on the branches of trees.

Grind this small, cook in *utiṅ sunum*, mustard oil, and apply with a feather.

N.B.—Some people use this also for *uru ghao*, No. 179.

172. *Poca nạrgi ghao.*

Symptoms: This is a sore beginning in the head, which when it bursts emits a watery discharge that causes sores wherever it flows.

Medicines: (*a*) *Kuclạ jaṅ*, the seeds of Strychnos potatorum, Lin. f.

Khọdẹ mamọn calọm aṛak,

Roast to burning point, saturate in cocoanut or mustard oil, and apply.

(*b*) *Nanha dudhi loṭa*, Ichnocarpus frutescens, R. Br.
Tejo ganthar,
Mare naṅgle ata rọṅgọ, an old leathern yoke thong fried to burning point.

Stir in mustard oil and apply, half of it as a powder.

(*c*) *Toa chaletẹl*, the cream of milk.

Mix in water and smear on the greasy part of it.

N.B.—This is also good for pain in the loins.

(*d*) *Icạk rẹhẹt'*, the roots of Woodfordia floribunda, Salisb.
Nanha dudhi loṭa rẹhẹt, the roots of Ichnocarpus frutescens, R. Br.
Muthạ, Fimbrystylis monostachya, Hassk.

Grind these and cook them in mustard oil. Apply this oil to the sore with a feather, and make the solid ingredients into balls, which the patient must chew, swallowing the juice as in betel nut chewing.

(*e*) *Terel dare reak mare baklak*, the old bark of Diospyros tomentosa, Roxb.
Icạk dare reak rọhọṛ chal, the dried bark of Woodfordia floribunda, Salisb.
Mare sarjọm baklak, the bark of an old Shorea robusta, Gärtn.
Ghugri, a mole cricket, Gryllus gryllo-talpa.
Puṭkạ, a puff ball (Lycoperdon).

Grind together and make into a powder. Clean the sore and anoint first with oil, and then sprinkle the powder on.

173. *Nasọn ghao.*

Symptoms. This may occur or any part of the body. If you knock against anything and it swells up and afterwards a sore appears, while it pains as if one had been burnt, the sore spreads on the surface and deeper, or if a thorn has entered and it swells and becomes a sore this is *nasọn ghao.*

Medicines: (*a*) *Dud baraṅgọm*,
Marań catọm aṛak, Marsilea quadrifolia, L.

Grind these and apply daily, after first washing the place with water in which *nim sakam*, the leaves of Melia Azadirachta, L., have been boiled.

(*b*) *Akaona rẹhẹt*, the roots of Calotropis gigantea, R. Br.
Tutiạ, sulphate of copper.
Sẹlẹp samanọm rẹhẹt, the roots of Gloriosa superba, Willd.
Hạṛũ awar nạṛĩ, Menispermum glabrum.
Ạphim, opium.
Dhũṛạ̃, resin of Shorea robusta, Gärtn.
Dạtrạ rẹhẹt, the roots of Datura alba, Willd. or D. fastuosa, Willd.
Gańja, Cannabis sativa, Willd.

Grind all these, cook in pure mustard oil and anoint daily.

(c) *Sukri ghās rẹhẹl*, the roots of Scirpus monostachyos, Kön.
Pāuri uldhạ da, the bulb of a kind of lotus.

Grind together. Cover the sore with ***kadam sakam***, the leaves of Anthocephalus Cadamba, Bth. and Hook. f., and on the top of these place what you have ground. Then cover again with the same leaves and bandage the whole, removing it the next day. Do thus for two or three days, and all the matter will be expelled and the sore healed.

(d) *Monsa sir*, Euphorbia Ligularia, R.
Corṛa chal, the bark of
Jạnum dare chal, the bark of Zizyphus Jujuba, Lam.
Sạpin jạnum dare, Opuntia Dillenii, Haw.
Ẹtkẹč dare, Euphorbia antiquorum, L.
Biṇḍi muthạ ghās da, the bulbs of Fimbristylis monostachya, Hassk.
Piṭuạ aṛak, Spermacoce hispida, L.
Roṛa dare chal, the bark of Mallotus philippinensis, Müll. Arg.
Ạṇḍiạ tale baha, the flower of the male Borassus flabelliformis, L.
Mare naṅgle, an old leathern yoke thong.
Susurbaṅ chata, a wasps' nest.
Piṇḍạ dare chal, the bark of Randia uliginosa, DC.

Grind all these together and fry to burning point, then grind again to a powder and sprinkle it on.

(e) *Bọnkạpsi rẹhẹl*, the roots of Thespesia Lampas, Benth. & Hook. f.
Ič ẹwẹr da, the bulb of Vitis latifolia, Wall.
Tarse koṭạp rẹhẹl, the roots of Grewia villosa, Willd.
Bọd laṛ, Vitis adnata, Roxb.
Kamraj rẹhẹl, the roots of Buettneria herbacea, Roxb.
Seta kaṭa rẹhẹl, the root of Grewia polygama, Roxb.
Pẹṭ cambṛa rẹhẹl, the roots of Helicteres Isora, L.
Bherṇḍa dare, Jatropha Curcas, L.

Roast or fry all these to burning point, make to a powder which sprinkle on.

(f) *Sarjọm chal*, the bark of Shorea robusta, Gärtn.
Pọjọ chal, ,, ,, Tetranthera monopetala, Roxb.
Meral chal, ,, ,, Phyllanthus Emblica, L.
Dare bạṅki, ,, ,, Vanda Roxburghii, R. Br.
Mare naṅgle, an old leathern yoke thong.

Grind, fry to burning point and after saturating in mustard oil apply daily.

(g) *Sega jạnum rẹhẹl*, the roots of Mimosa rubicaulis, Lamk.
Tuliạ lọṅphul,

Grind these together with a little water and apply to the sore.

(*h*) *Ata ọhọč reak ṅọlhal*, the soot from a sherd that has been used for frying.

Hoṛẹč, Dolichos biflorus, L.

Gadha ič, donkey's excrement.

Mix these and grind fine like red lead and then plaster on the sore.

174. *Pạchiạri ghao.*

Symptoms. This may appear on any one. It appears as a blister from a burn, and when it bursts the sore spreads wherever the watery discharge flows.

Medicines: (*a*) *Ekasirạ dare chal*, the bark of Crataeva religiosa, Forst.

Grind and apply as an ointment, and the sore will dry up at once.

(*b*) *Meral chal*, the bark of Phyllanthus Emblica, L.

Grind and apply as an ointment, and he will get well.

(*c*) *Rọkọt cọndọn kaṭ*, blood coloured sandal wood.

Rub this and smear therewith, and it will dry up.

175. *Para ghao.*

(Sore due to mercurial poisoning).

Symptoms. The whole body is covered with red spots, each looking like a burn, and the skin over it very thin. If a person with this knocks against anything it hurts him, as if the whole body were one sore.

Medicines: (*a*) *Udạl sẹ ọdhra chal*, the bark of Sterculia villosa, Roxb.

Tẹlhẹč dare chal, „ „ Sterculia urens, Roxb.

Hopo baha dare chal, „ „ Cochlosperma gossypium, DC.

Sese baha dare chal, „ „ Sterculia colorata, Roxb.

Korkoṭ dare chal, „ „ Dillenia indica, L.

Bhorkoṇḍ dare chal, „ „ Hymenodictyon excelsum, Wall.

Sahar dare chal, the bark of Dillenia pentagyna, Roxb.

Mix these and grind together fine, add two ounces of melted butter of cows' milk and a little mustard oil, cook and besmear daily therewith.

(*b*) *Kạliạ jirạ*, Nigella indica, Roxb.

Dhạniạ, Coriandrum sativum, L.

Tilạị chal, the bark of Wendlandia tinctoria, DC.

Hoṇḍro chal, „ „ „

Icạk dare rẹhẹt chal, the bark of the roots of Woodfordia floribunda, Salisb.

Band lota nạṛī chal, the bark of Hippocratea arborea, Roxb.

Grind these together, make into pills after cooking and give to eat, or let him drink the same without cooking.

(*c*) *Hund baha chal*, the bark of Jasminum arborescens, Roxb.

Kujri nạṛī chal, „ „ „ Celastrus paniculatus, Willd.

Cook these in mustard oil and both give him some to drink and smear him with it.

176. *Ras bat ghao.* (may be clavus, corns).

Symptoms. This attacks the sole of the foot and the "sore" as it spreads goes deeper, so they cannot walk, only hobble or limp.

Medicines: (*a*) Apply the remedies detailed in No. 197.

(*b*) *Gẹgẹtẹrẹń*, a certain creeping insect that appears in clusters (Spirocystus cilcylindricus, while young.)

Grind these and give them to be eaten with *sạtu*, meal made from roasted grain, or something similar.

(*c*) *Mithi*, Trigonella Fœnum-græcum, Willd.
Simbrit, fresh shoots of Bombax malabaricum, DC.
Sora, saltpetre.
Gọndhọk, sulphur.
Tutiạ, sulphate of copper.

Grind these, cook in melted butter or pure mustard oil and apply to the cavity.

(*d*) *Mare nańgle*, an old leathern yoke thong.
Kedok aṛak rẹhẹl, the roots of Argyreia speciosa, Sweet.
Ọt ḍhompo, Lepidagathis cristata, Willd.
Piṇḍạ chal, the bark of Randia uliginosa, DC.
Saparọm chal, the bark of Nyctanthes Arbor-tristis, L.
Piṭuạ aṛak, Spermacoce hispida, L.
Biṇḍi muthạ, Fimbristylis monostachya, Hassk.

Fry these together to burning point, and then

Mithi, Trigonella Fœnum-græcum, Willd.
Tejpat, Laurus Cassia, Roxb.
Dhạniạ, Coriandrum sativum, L.
Kạliạ jirạ, Nigella indica, Roxb.
Susurbań chata, a wasps' nest.
Ạṇḍiạ tale baha, the flower of the male Borassus flabelliformis, L.

Fry these to burning point, grind and mix a little *gọndhọk*, sulphur, and then stir the whole in mustard oil and anoint therewith daily. Only the second of above, *kedok aṛak rẹhẹl* may be applied a an ointment.

(*e*) *Bir gońgha*, a forest snail.

Dry and grind this so that the patient does not know what it is, pour *utiń sunum*, mustard oil, on it and apply to the sore; afterwards

Bir rọkọć, a forest periwinkle.
Bir gońgha, a forest snail.
Sẹlẹp samanọm, Gloriosa superba, Willd.

Grind these together, plaster on to the sore and foment with fire till dry. Do this daily and in five days he will get well.

One "authority" says: This sore appears at the setting in of the rainy season and lasts throughout it, when it may heal spontaneously. During the hot weather the patient is quite free of it.

177. *Roga ghao.*

Symptoms. Sores break out over the whole body, which are very itchy, and a watery discharge issues from them.

Medicines: *Bọd laṛ banda*, a parasitical air plant found on Vitis adnata, Wall.

Grind this fine and cook it in *utiṅ sunum*, mustard oil, this oil to be rubbed on daily.

178. *Rọkọc̓ ghao.*

Symptoms. This sore appears on the shin, thigh, back of the hand or occasionally elsewhere. It looks like when four or five periwinkles cluster together, the sores run into one another and are conical on the top like periwinkles.

Medicines: (*a*) *Haṛhal họtọl jaṅ*, the seeds of a bitter pumpkin, Cucurbita lagenaria, Willd.

Ato jhiṅgạ jaṅ, the seeds of the cultivated Luffa acutangula, Roxb.

Bir jhiṅgạ jaṅ, the seeds of Luffa amara, Roxb.

Haṛhal kundri jaṅ sẹ da, the seeds or bulb of the bitter Zehneria umbellata, Thew.

Ato kundri da, the bulb of Cephalandra indica, Nand.

Kạhu botke rẹhẹt, the roots of Bryonia lacinosa, L.

Tutiạ, sulphate of copper.

Grind these, cook in mustard oil and apply daily with a feather.

(*b*) *Gạbur rẹhẹt*, the roots of Acacia Farnesiana, Willd.

Dak jẹr,

Sahṛa banda, the parasitical plant found on Streblus asper, Lour.

Kuṛil rama banda, the parasitical plant found on Zizyphus Oenoplia, Mill.

Grind and sprinkle some on the sore, and make some into pills to be eaten.

(*c*) *Meral sakam*, the leaves of Phyllanthus Emblica, L.

Fry to burning point, stir in mustard oil and apply with a feather.

(*d*) A sherd from a pot broken by a girl or a piece of pottery unearthed by the *tutri* (Eryx conicus) snake.

To be rubbed and the rubbings to be applied to the sore.

(*e*) *Muṅgạ banda*, the parasitical plant found on Moringa pterygosperma, Gärtn.

Bhorkonḍ banda, the parasitical plant found on Hymenodictyon excelsum, Wall.

Icąk banda, the parasitical plant found on Woodfordia floribunda, Salisb.

Janum banda, the parasitical plant found on Zizyphus Jujuba, Lam.

Grind all these together to a powder and sprinkle on.

(*f*) *Meral sakam*, the leaves of Phyllanthus Emblica, L.

Tutri biṅ kelhat, a piece of pottery unearthed by the *tutri* (Eryx conicus) snake.

Ḍangua kuṛi rapuṭ kelhat, a piece of pottery broken by an unmarried girl.

Fry the first to burning point, then grind all three together, stir in *utiṅ sunum*, mustard oil, and apply with a feather.

179. *Uru ghao.* Scaldhead. (? Tinea tonsurans).

Symptoms. This appears on and spreads over the whole head.

Medicines: (*a*) *Peaj*, onions.

Maric, Capsicum frutescens, Willd.

Nim sakam, the leaves of Melia Azadirachta, L.

Cook these in mustard oil and apply with a feather.

(*b*) The real way is to prick with a red hot iron the *uru eṅga* or lump that hangs about at the neck, and rec very will follow.

(*c*) Let the maternal uncle of the child bathe on a Sunday morning and then come and after wiping his feet wring out the water from his wet towel on the head of his nephew or niece as the case may be and a cure will result.

180. *Ugni jaura ghao.*

Symptoms. This sore may attack any one. It appears as a blister as from a burn and has a red appearance, causing a burning pain.

Medicines: (*a*) *Kucla jaṅ*, the kernel of Strychnos potatorum, Lin. f.

Nanha dudhi loṭa reheṭ, the roots of Ichnocarpus frutescens, R. Br.

Janum jhapni joto ge, the entire plant of the thorny variety of Zornia diphylla, Pers., or Biophitum sensitivum, DC.

Ṭanḍi catom aṛak, Desmodium triflorum, DC.

Eradom sunum, castor oil.

Roast the first and fry the second, both to burning point, mix all in the castor oil and apply daily.

(*b*) Saturate *korpur*, camphor, and *mithi*, Trigonella Fœnum-græcum, Willd., in *nạrkoṛ sunum*, cocoanut oil, and anoin him therewith.

(c) *Ekasirą dare chal*, the bark of Crataeva religiosa, Forst.

Grind and apply as an ointment without warming.

181. *Uri rǫg.* (Tubercular (?) fistula).

Symptoms. This sore occurs on the thighs, knees, buttocks and sometimes on the forearm. It swells up, but does not spread, and is extremely painful. The limbs or wherever the sore appears waste gradually away and still the discharge of pus does not cease. This differs from *palanią* which spreads deeper and is not painful.

Medicines: (a) *Udąl dare*, Sterculia villosa, Roxb.
Tęlhęč dare, Sterculia urens, Roxb.
Turąm,

Take the roots of these, warm them separately and apply.

(b) *Ghoṛa lada*, Vitis tomentosa, Heyne.
Duṇḍukil, Gardenia turgida, Roxb.
Kaḍa beňjak,

Grind these and apply them warm.

(c) *Sirąuna da*, the bulb of Hygrophila spinosa, T. Anders.

Grind and apply warm daily.

(d) *Ghoṛa lądąuṛi da*, the bulb of Vitis tomentosa, Heyne.

Warm and apply and he will certainly get well.

(e) *Edęl poha ręhęl*, the root of a sapling of Bombax malabaricum, DC.

Warm and apply; this is also efficacious.

(f) *Gańgiṭ cun*, the lime obtained from nodular or hydraulic limestone.

Apply on the swelling until it dissolves.

(g) *Udąl chal*, the bark of Sterculia villosa, Roxb.
Tęlhęč chal, „ „ „ Sterculia urens, Roxb.
Hopo baha chal, the bark of Cachlosperma gossypium, DC.

Warm and apply.

(h) If there is an open sore:—
Sahar chal, the bark of Dillenia pentagyna, Roxb.
Matkǫm chal, „ „ „ Bassia latifolia, Roxb.
Sarjǫm chal, „ „ „ Shorea robusta, Gärtn.
Meral chal, the bark of Phyllanthus Emblica, L.

Grind these together and sprinkle as a powder on the sore, and afterwards apply warm as an ointment.

(i) *Sikiom ręhęl*, the roots of Crinum zeylanicum, Roxb.
Bir sąru da, the tuber of Lasia heterophylla, Schott.
Kondro jąnum ręhęl, the roots of Acacia Intsia, Willd.
Terel cętę, the thin skin on the bark of Diospyros tomentosa, Roxb.

Grind these with *phuli pąurą*, neat spirits, and smear it on. If swollen, (*j*) *ukuṛil*, a wild bulbous plant.

Grind and plaster on.

If there is a burning pain:—

(*k*) *Khub lag bilạti thamakur*, very strong imported tobacco.

Grind with *hukạ dak*, hookah water, and palster on, when the pain will cease.

One "authority" says: This sore appears at any joint in the body. At first there is irritation, then a throbbing pain and swelling, and finally an intense burning pain.

182. *Lọ ghao.* Burns.

Medicines: (*a*) *Aṭen chal*, the bark of Combretum decandrum, Roxb. Anoint with this.

(*b*) *Boṅga bạrchi*, Leonates nepetæfolia, R.Br.

Roast to burning point and anoint therewith.

(*c*) *Sirom ṛẹhẹt*, the roots of Andropogon muricatus, Retz.
Atnak chal, the bark of Terminalia tomentos , W. and A.

Grind these and anoint therewith.

(*d*) *Murgạ rasa*, the juice of Pterocarpus Marsupium, Roxb.
Ńũṛũč ḍọg (*bale*), the young shoot of Cassia Fistula, Linn.

Mix these and apply.

(*e*) *Mẹṛọm itil reak sunum*, oil made from goats' fat.

Apply this.

(*f*) *Jạnum jhạpni ṛẹhẹt*, the roots of the thorny variety of Zornia diphylla, Pers., or Biophitum sensitivum, DC.
Eraḍọm sakam ḍọg, the tips of the leaves of Ricinus communis, L.

Grind these fine and cook in melted butter of cow's milk (or mustard oil) and apply daily with a feather.

(*g*) *Dhũṛạ̃*, resin of Shorea robusta, Gärtn.
Utiń sunum, mustard oil.

Mix these into an ointment and apply once a day, healing will follow.

(*h*) *Boḍa biń itil*, the fat of the snake Python molurus
Jambṛo biń itil, „ „ „ „ „ Zamenis mucosus.
Khạsi itil, „ „ „ a castrated goat.
Sim itil, „ „ „ a fowl.
Ḍaṅgra itil, „ „ „ a bullock.
Gạị gọṭọm thoṛa, a little melted butter made from cows' milk.

Mix all these together and smear on; the burning pain will be relieved and healing will follow.

(*i*) *Er hoṛẹč sakam*, the leaves of Dolichos biflorus, L.
Bir hoṛẹč sakam, „ „ „ Atyllosia scarabædois, Benth.

Tarọp dare sakam dọg, the tips of the leaves of Buchanania latifolia, Roxb.

Kạsi rẹhẹl, the roots of Saccharum spontaneum, L.

Fry all these to burning point and make them into a powder. Cover the burns first with cotton, then dust the powder on, and cover all with a bandage.

(*j*) *Akaṛ baha sakam*, the leaves of Limnophila Roxburghiana, G. Don.

Grind and plaster on.

(*k*) *Haṛhal hotọl rẹhẹl*, the roots of a bitter Cucurbita lagenaria, Willd.

Pound to shreds, cook in *utiṅ sunum*, mustard oil, plunge into a brass cup of cold water, and after squeezing it into a thin squash apply to the burn.

183. *Rọk ghao*. Wound from being gored.

Medicines: *Bir horẹć* (*bebak*), an entire Atyllosia scarabædois, Benth.

Get a new laid egg and breaking it into this mix the two thoroughly. If the entrails have protruded cut a pumpkin, Cucurbita lagenaria, and applying the medicine thereto push it carefully in. Otherwise simply apply the medicine to the wound.

184. *Sọbọk ghao*. Wound from being stabbed or crushed with the point or end of something with force (vulnus punctatum).

Medicines: (*a*) *Kaeru puṅgi*, the young conical as yet unopened leaf of a plantain.

Sẹkrẹć sakam, the leaves of Lagerstroemia parviflora, Roxb.

Matkọm dọg, the shoots of Bassia latifolia, Roxb.

Grind and apply as a plaster.

(*b*) *Khode baha rẹhẹl*, the roots of

Bọd laṛ poha rẹhẹl, „ „ „ a seedling of Vitis adnata, Wall.

Kamraj rẹhẹl, the roots of Buettneria herbacea, Roxb.

Hạḍ joṛa nạṛitẹl, the creeper Cissus quadrangularis, Willd.

Grind together and apply as a plaster.

If there is a fracture, for which this is also applicable, put splints over the plaster.

This may be used for both human beings and cattle.

185. *Jạnum rọk*. When stung by a thorn.

Medicines: (*a*) Apply *sọsọ*, the fruit of Semecarpus Anacardium, L.

and if you cannot extract the thorn, then

(*b*) *Akaona loṛe*, the exudation from Calotropis gigantea, R. Br. or C. procera, R. Br.

Drop this on and the same night it will come out.

186. *Tuṅ ghao.* Arrow wounds.

Medicines: (*a*) *Sạru da*, the tuber of Celocasia antiquorum, Schott.

Backọm lopol, Pollinia eriopoda, Hance, made into powder.

Sprinkle on the wound.

(*b*) If any one should wound another man with an arrow, the arrow sticking, he must get quickly *turạm*, grind it, smear it on the arrow and push the arrow away to one side, when the wound will at once heal up.

187. *Mak, tọhọl ar tuṅ ghao.*

Wounds caused by iron implements, by stumbling or by arrows.

Medicines: (*a*) *Suruj mukhi rẹhẹl*, the roots of Helianthus annuus, Willd.

Sim kaṭa aṛak, Vitex peduncularis.

Bir jhuṅkạ aṛak, Crotalaria calycina, Shrank.

Grind together and apply to the wound.

(*b*) *Turạm rẹhẹl*, the roots of

Seta kaṭa rẹhẹl, the roots of Gynandropsis pentaphylla, L.

Grind to a powder and sprinkle on.

(*c*) *Bạrsạ pakọṛ rẹhẹl*, the roots of Grewia sapida, Roxb.

Bọd laṛ rẹhẹl, „ „ „ Vitis adnata, Wall.

Grind together to a powder and sprinkle on.

(*d*) *Kamraj rẹhẹl*, the roots of Buettneria herbacea, Roxb.

Grind and apply.

Apply either of the following:—

(*e*) *Tarse koṭap rẹhẹl*, the roots of Grewia villosa, Willd.

(*f*) *Bọnkạpsi rẹhẹl*, the roots of Thespesia Lampas, Benth. and Hook. f.

(*g*) *Pọjọ chal*, the bark of Tetranthera monopetala, Roxb.

(*h*) *Sẹkrẹċ bhiṭuạk*, the stem of the leaves of Lagerstroemia parviflora, Roxb.

Grind very fine with water till it becomes like melted butter and apply to the sore where it must stay.

(*i*) First of all as soon as the wound is contracted urinate on it and dust some *cun*, lime, on.

(*j*) *Bọd laṛ rẹhẹl*, the roots of Vitis adnata, Wall.

Sẹkrẹċ ḍọg, a sprout of Lagerstroemia parviflora, Roxb.

Grind fine and plaster on.

(*k*) *Suruj mukhi rẹhẹl*, the roots of Helianthus annuus, Willd.

Ḍhalka catọm aṛak rẹhẹl, the roots of

Grind and mix these and plaster on.

If there is any watery discharge,

(*l*) *Mẹrlẹċ chal*, the bark of Flacourtia Ramontchi, L'Herit.

Grind to a powder and sprinkle it on.

N.B.—Even if there is a fracture this remedy is used and will join the parts again.

188. *Kasra.* Scabies.

One "authority" says: In this there are sores everywhere which itch excessively, even one's food is not digested. The real cause of it is dirt, in which insects make their appearance who continue spreading causing sores where they go.

Medicines: (*a*) *Konal pisrą*,
Joka, Sida humilis, Willd.
Gol mąric, black pepper.
Gǫndhǫk, sulphur.

Grind these together, cook in a brass vessel and apply with a feather to the parts affected.

(*b*) *Akaona dare rẹhẹl*, *sakam sẹ ḍǫg*, the roots, leaves or tips of Calotropis gigantea, R. Br., 4 oz.
Heñjel rẹhẹl, the roots of Solanum stramonifolium, Jacq., 4oz.
Sinduąri sakam ḍǫg, the tips of the leaves of Vitex Negundo, L., 2 oz.
Caole mąric, a kind of capsicum, resembling grains of rice.
Gǫndhǫk, sulphur, 2 pice worth.

Boil these in 8 ounces of mustard oil until the whole looks like water when it will be ready.

N.B.—This remedy is also applicable in *Khudą jąurą* (No. 168) and *Ugni jąurą* (No. 180).

(*c*) *Qt ḍhompo ghās*, Lepidagathis cristata, Willd.

Roast slightly to burning point at the fire and after stirring in mustard oil smear it on.

(*d*) Smear on *baṛe loṛe*, the sticky juice of Ficus bengalensis, L.
(*e*) Smear on *loa loṛe*, the sticky juice exuded by Ficus glomerata, Roxb.
(*f*) Smear on *akaona loṛe*, the sticky juice exuded by Calotropis gigantea, R. Br.
(*g*) Stick on the affected parts *goṭe sakam*, the leaves of Croton oblongifolius, Roxb.
(*h*) *Baglucą jǫ*, the fruit of Martynia diandra, Gloxin.
Jhiṅgą jañ, the seeds of Luffa acutangula, Roxb.

Distil and apply.

(*i*) Grind and apply *gǫndhǫk*, sulphur.
(*j*) *Tutią*, sulphate of copper.
Gǫndhǫk, sulphur.
Laṭha cip ciṛip rẹhẹl, the roots of
Pipṛiañ,
Cip ciṛip rẹhẹl, the roots of Achyranthes aspera, L.

Buy a new earthenware pot in which these must be rubbed, and grind them in it with the handle of a chisel, add some mustard oil and apply thinly with a feather.

(*k*) Wash the parts clean daily with warm water, and
Bagluca̦ sunum, oil of Martynia diandra, Gloxin.
Na̦rkō̦r sunum, cocoanut oil.

Take an equal quantity of each of these, shake in some *sindur*, red lead, and stir the whole into a thin mixture to be applied after washing the parts clean, and in three days they will dry up, a proved remedy.

(*l*) *Ede̦l je̦r*, the sticky exudation from Bombax malabaricum, DC.
Tuṛi, the seeds of Brassica campestris, L.
Sasaṅ, turmeric, Curcuma longa, Roxb.
Go̦ndho̦k thoṛa gan, a little sulphur.

Grind these together and apply to the sore parts.

189. *Da̦d*. Ringworm.

One "authority" says: In this minute pimples appear and spread, which itch excessively, especially when it is cold. Some persons can foretell by this itching when it is going to rain.

Medicines: (*a*) *Kedar sakam se̦ dare sudha̦*, the leaves of, or the entire Bonnaya veronicæfolia, Spreng.

Grind and smear on.

(*b*) *Coḍra chal*, the bark of

Grind and apply.

(*c*) *Ḍunḍukil re̦he̦l*, the roots of Gardenia turgida, Roxb.
Akaona re̦he̦l, the roots of Calotropis gigantea, R. Br. or C. procera, R. Br.
Etka re̦he̦l, the roots of Mucuna pruriens, DC.
Ka̦tič talaṅ corco re̦he̦l, a little of the roots of Casearea tomentosa, Roxb.

Grind these together, stir in *utiṅ sunum*, mustard oil, and let him anoint himself therewith.

N.B.—This remedy may also be used for the same complaint in cattle.

190. *Talsa*. Measles.

Medicines (*a*) *Ko̦de̦*, Eleusine corocana, Gärtn.

Make this into flour and smear it on, which will cause it to dry up, and make some into hand bread to be eaten.

(*b*) *Nim sakam*, the leaves of Melia Azadirachta, L.

Pound these and give to drink.

(*c*) *Ro̦l jo̦*, the fruit of Terminalia Chebula, Retz.
Lo̦po̦ṅ jo̦, „ „ „ Terminalia bellerica, Roxb.
Lil ka̦thi re̦he̦l, the roots of Polygala crotalarioides, Buch. and [Ham.

Soak these and give to drink daily morning and evening.

(*d*) *Sukri mulha rẹhẹl*, the roots of Scirpus monoṣtachyus, Kön.
Nanha dudhi loṭa rẹhẹl, the roots of Ichnocarpus frutescens, R. Br.

Grind together and give to drink daily, and it will obviate blood being mixed in the discharge.

Should the eruption go in:—

(*e*) *Sega rẹhẹl*, the roots of Mimosa rubicaulis, Lamk.
Kondro chal, the bark of Acacia Intsia, Willd.
Ạtkir rẹhẹl, the roots of Smilax ovalifolia, Roxb.

Grind together, mix with molasses and give to drink daily until the eruption reappears.

(*f*) First of all proceed as in No. 191 (*o*) to bring out the eruption all at once; then

(*g*) Spread *nim sakam*, the leaves of Melia Azadirachta, L. under him so that he lies thereon. Also use *kọdẹ*, Eleusine corocana, Gärtn., in both the ways detailed in (*a*) above.

N.B.—The eating of *họrẹć*, Dolichos biflorus, L., and of hot boiled rice is strictly forbidden.

If the eruption should go in, rub the skin of a *harba*, Manis pentadactyla, and let the patient lick it. Also in similar circumstances in *guṭi* (q.v.).

191. *Bọsọntọ sẹ Guṭi*. Small pox.

Medicines: (*a*) *Rańgạini jạnum*, Solanum Jacquini, Willd.
Nańgrạuta, Nardostachys Jatamansi, DC.

Boil and give to drink with sugar.

(*b*) *Gại toa*, cows' milk.
Gol mạric, black pepper.

Boil the former and give to drink with the latter.

(*c*) *Mare kọdẹ*, old Eleusine corocana, Gärtn.
Nim sakam, the leaves of Melia Azadirachta, L.

Grind together and plaster therewith. When the eruption is well developed
Kanṭhaṛ sakam, the leaves of Artocarpus integrifolia, L.

Fry to burning point and sprinkle on him.

(*d*) *Bạṛ baha*, the flower of Mimusops Elengi, L.

To be ground and drunk some three days.

Toyo sagak rẹhẹl, the roots of
Gọeṭha tọrọć, the ashes of dried cow dung.

Mix these and strew over the pustules.

(*e*) *Motam ol*, a certain edible mushroom.
Kocṛa jọ bẹrẹlak, unripe fruit of Bassia latifolia, Roxb.

To be mixed together and eaten two days.

To bring out the eruption:—

(*f*) *Mare kaskọm jań*, old cotton seed.

Grind with water and plaster over the whole body.

(g) *Ḍaṅ ghaṅgra*, a variety of Vigna Catiang.

Grind fine and plaster over the whole body.

When the pustules subside:—

(h) Let him eat *guạ*, Areca Catechu, L.

(i) *Motam ol*, a certain edible mushroom.

Kondro chal, the bark of Acacia Intsia, Willd.

Pound and give to drink, and when it has subsided, give the former alone to drink and plaster him therewith.

(j) *Kaḍa beṅjak rẹhẹl*, the roots of

Datrạ rẹhẹl, the roots of Datura alba, Willd., or D. fastuosa, Willd.

Turạm rẹhẹl, the roots of

Pound these and give an ounce of the juice extracted to drink. If stupefaction ensues then give *kasmar chal*, the bark of Gmelina arborea, Roxb., and *kạṅji dak*, stale rice water, to drink: Give this remedy at the commencement of the attack.

(k) The same as in (*d*) and (*e*) above, except that instead of the unripe fruit of Bassia latifolia, Roxb. substitute the unripe fruit of Musa paradisiaca, L.

(l) *Motam ol*, a certain edible mushroom.

Nim sakam, the leaves of Melia Azadirachta, L.

Caole mạric banda the parasitical plant found on the kind of capsicum resembling grains of rice.

Bir hoṛẹć dak (*teke kate*), the water after boiling Atyllosia scarabædois, Benth.

Dare cetan reak bhorkonḍ, Hymenodictyon excelsum, Wall., that has germinated in the stump of another tree.

Hesak banda, the parasitical plant found on Ficus religiosa, Willd.

Grind these together and give to drink. When the skin begins to peel off spread *nim sakam*, the leaves of Melia Azadirachta, L., on the bed and make the patient lie on them. If the pustules go inside, put the above *motam ol* and the eggs of the *ṭiṭiṛhić cẹṛẹ*, lapwing, Sarcicophorus bilobus or Lobivanellus Goensis, in rice and give to eat.

(m) *Kedok aṛak*, Argyreia speciosa, Sweet.

Kạliạ jirạ, Nigella indica, Roxb.

(n) *Kondro chal*, the bark of Acacia Intsia, Willd.

Sega chal, „ „ „ Mimosa rubicaulis, Lam.

Cạili chal, „ „ „ Morinda tinctoria, Roxb.

Turạm rẹhẹl, the roots of

Kaskọm bạṅgạura, cotton seeds.

Bạṛ chal, the bark of Mimusops Elengi, L.

Aṭkir rẹhẹl, the roots of Smilax ovalifolia, Roxb.

Nanha dudhi loṭa reheľ, the roots of Ichnocarpus frutescens, R. Br.

Kedar reheľ, the roots of Bonnaya veronicæfolia, Spreng.

Sarjom chal, the bark of Shorea robusta, Gärtn.

Boil all these together and give to drink daily. Add a little *guṛ*, molasses, as this causes a plentiful eruption. When such has taken place, spread a cloth on the bed and on this place the ashes of *nim sakam*, the leaves of Melia Azadirachta, L., after frying them to burning point, and scatter over these again rice flour or flour made from broken rice, and let the patient lie down on top of all. Strew daily over the pustules such ashes; or grind into a powder the roots of *turam*, and *baṛ chal*, the bark of Mimusops Elengi, L., and sprinkle this powder on the inflamed pustules. The erruption will be brought out by both cotton seeds and *motam ol*, a certain edible mushroom, and these will also heal the pustules.

(*o*) *Malhan*, Dolichos Lablab, L.

Ghaṅgra, Vigna Catiang.

To be made into curry and eaten; *guṛ*, molasses, also to be eaten; all these to be eaten to cause the eruption to come quickly.

When the eruption has fully come out, see if it is black on the top, for if so it is an indication it is about to go in again; then

(*p*) *Edel roṅga*, the knots on Bombax malabaricum, DC.

Loa sakam reak̕ jone, the warts on the leaves of Ficus glomerata, Roxb.

Seta ič caole, the grains of rice found in the excreta of a dog.

Motam ol, a certain edible mushroom.

Kulai ič, a hare's excrement.

Make him to drink these, and after grinding the first two of above, smear him therewith.

N.B.—He must on no account eat *horeč*, Dolichos biflorus, L., or the eruption will reappear.

(*q*) *Mahadeb jaṭa*,

Bir buṭ, Flemingia congesta, Roxb.

Grind these, give to drink with *phuli paura*, neat spirits. This remedy is to be given when the eruption is scanty. If the eruption goes in, then,

(*r*) *Motam ol*, a certain edible mushroom.

Edel roṅga, the knots on Bombax malabaricum, DC.

Kondro janum reheľ, the roots of Acacia Intsia, Willd.

Grind these and give to drink, and the eruption will come to the surface again.

To dry up the pustules: grind and mix,

(*s*) *Goeṭha toroč*, the ashes of dried cowdung and

Dhũrã, resin of Shorea robusta, Gärtn., and smear over the whole body.

To obviate pock marks:

(*t*) Smear the whole body with a mixture of *dhũṛạ̃*, resin of Shorea robusta, Gärtn. and

Dahe, curds.

As a prophylactic: (*u*) If there is a talk in the village that small pox has appeared or that many deaths from it are taking place, then all the leading men of the village meet in conclave and take counsel as to what measures to take to counteract it. And all will say, Let us make the effort, perhaps we shall succeed. The headman gets hold of a medicine man and all agree. Then the headman says, we must all become priests, i.e. sanctify ourselves ceremoniously.

Next morning all the village men assemble at the end of the village street; *miṭtaṅ guli pạthi mẹrọm*, a brown female kid, is brought; the medicine man brings with him a stick and the bark of both *bana haṭak*, Oroxylon indicum, Benth., and of *akaona*, Calotropis gigantea, R. Br. or C. procera, R. Br. He divides the barks into two portions, and calling on *Dhạrti mae*, and *Siṅ boṅga*, (*i.e.* mother earth and the sun) he makes them bury the bark here and there at the end of the village street, and they walk through the village holding the two sticks.

Then they take that brown female kid to the eastern boundary of the village and let her graze in the name of *Nag nạgin*. After she has grazed they walk round all the boundaries of the village with the kid and the two sticks. On returning to the place where she grazed they decapitate her and leave her body and the two sticks there; no one will eat her. If they continue well and the disease does not appear among them for a year, then a goat and pigeons are offered in sacrifice.

If before the above prophylactic measures are taken, a case of small pox should appear, then all the senior men in the village assemble quickly and say, Come let us send away the disease, so that it may not go beyond this man or spread further. The following is the method used to attain this. They make all the dwellers in the village without distinction take medicine. This is

(*v*) *Gol mạric*, black pepper.

Adwa caole, rice made from sun-dried, not boiled paddy.

Ẹdẹl roṅga, the knots on Bombax malabaricum, DC.

These are ground together and then eaten, when no small pox will occur.

The following is given to the patient already attacked:

(*w*) *Gargạḍi rẹhẹl*, the roots of Coix lachryma, Willd.

Laṭha cip ciṛip rẹhẹl, the roots of

Grind these two together; let an unmarried girl spin a thread of cotton, on to which the medicine is tied, and it is then tied on to the patient, and calling on the spirits *Nag nạgin* and *Kạli mae* the disease is dismissed. In this way the disease is confined to the one person and will not spread. If he is the victim of witches he will die, but if it is due to an epidemic he will recover.

192. *Chucundari.* Chancre (a venereal sore), also syphilis in its first stage.

Symptoms. Men get this. Small pimples appear on the surface or point of the penis which develop into a sore.

Medicines (*a*) *Andia moron arak rehel*, the roots of Gymnema hirsutus, W. and A., var. Decaisneanum, Wight.

Berel gua jo, a fresh areca nut, Areca Catechu, L.

Pan sakam, the leaves of the Piper Betle L.

Kalia jira, Nigella indica, Roxb.

Grind all these together, cook them in mustard oil or melted butter and apply with a feather.

(*b*) *Ulič alan arak*, parsley.

Mandargom sakam, the leaves of Anona squamosa, L.

Bir jhunka arak, Crotalaria calycina, Shrank.

Jira, carraway seed, Carum Carui, L.

Jawan, Carum Ajowan, DC.

Mithi, Trigonella Fænum-græcum, Willd.

Dhania, coriander seed, Coriandrum sativum, L.

Thora tutia, a little sulphate of copper.

Grind all these together to a powder and sprinkle it on.

(*c*) *Icak rehel*, the roots of Woodfordia floribunda, Salisb.

Grind to a powder and apply.

(*d*) *Datra jo*, the fruit of Datura alba, Willd. or D. fastuosa, Willd.

Cip cirip rehel, the roots of Achyranthes aspera, L.

Cook in oil and smear on.

(*e*) *Amaegom rehel*, the roots of

to be ground and smeared on.

(*f*) *Dak horo rean bohok*, the dried head of a water tortoise, Trionix gangeticus.

Etkeč chal, the bark of Euphorbia antiquorum, L.

Sekra janum chal, the bark of Zizyphus rugosa, Lamk.

Kidiň katkom gota hormo, the entire body of a scorpion.

Soso chal, the bark of Semecarpus Anacardium, L.

Grind together and plaster on, or cook in oil and anoint with the oil.

(*g*) *Dare japak nariak mañjtel*, the pith of Scindapsus officinalis, Schott.

Nanha dudhi lota rehel, the roots of Ichnocarpus frutescens, R. Br.

Andia moron arak rehel, the roots of Gymnema hirsutus, W. and A., var. Decaisneanum, Wight.

Grind together, boil in pure mustard oil, add a little melted butter and then apply with a feather.

(*h*) *Bẹrẹl guạ*, a fresh areca nut, Areca Catechu, L.

Ạṇḍiạ mọrọn aṛak rẹhẹl, the roots of Gymnema hirsutus, W. and A., var. Dicaisneanum, Wight.

Sarjọm chal, the bark of Shorea robusta, Gärtn.

Mandargọm sakam, the leaves of Anona squamosa, L.

Grind these together to a powder. Boil in water *nim sakam*, the leaves of Melia Azadirachta, L., and wash the sore clean with that water. Then fill up the sore with the powder; he will assuredly get well.

(*i*) *Bir hoṛẹč rẹhẹl*, the roots of Atyllosia scarabædois, Benth.

Moṭa koṅga rẹhẹl, the roots of Agave americana, L.

Goṭe rẹhẹl, the roots of Croton oblongifolius, Roxb.

Dry these, grind them to powder and sprinkle or dust them on the sore.

(*j*) *Horọ bọhọk*, the head of a tortoise.

11 *Gol mạric*, 11 black peppercorns.

Half roast or roast the former to burning point, then grind both together, and then after cooking in *utiṅ sunum*, mustard oil, let him apply it to the sore, and he will be well in five days.

One "authority" says: This appears as a corrosive sore at the base of the penis, and if medicine is not applied quickly, the penis will drop off and they will be eunuchs for life. Sometimes if the sore penetrates internally it is fatal.

193. *Gurmi*. Syphilis.

Symptoms. This generally attacks immoral persons, and is sometimes inherited by children. It is usually contracted by intercourse with prostitutes. It begins with sores on the surface of the penis, and gradually spreads over the whole body. In appearance the reddish pustules are like those of small pox.

Medicines: (*a*) *Eṭkẹč dare reak maṅj*, the pith of Euphorbia antiquorum, Linn.

Akaona rẹhẹl, the roots of Calotropis gigantea, R. Br.

Ạṇḍiạ mọrọn aṛak rẹhẹl, the root of Gymnema hirsutus, W. and A., var. Decaisneanum, Wight.

Etka rẹhẹl, the roots of Mucuna pruriens, DC.

Sạpin jạnum sokam, the leaves of Opuntia Dillenii, Haw.

Bandphoṛa biṅ jaṅ, the bones of the Bungarus fasciatus snake.

Roast or fry all these to burning point, mix all together and boil in mustard oil, and then apply with a feather.

(*b*) *Caole ata rọṅgọeme*, roast or fry rice to burning point.

Sarjọm dare ḍhompo ṭhenak chal, sẹ mare dare reak chal chaḍaome, remove the bark on the excrescence of a Shorea robusta, Gärtn, or the bark of an old tree.

Dhūṛã, resin of Shorea robusta, Gärtn.

Thoṛa tutiạ, a little sulphate of copper.

First boil some leaves of the *nim*, Melia Azadirachta, Linn., in water and with that bitter water wash the parts clean, and then after you have ground all the above to powder sprinkle it over the parts.

(*c*) *Mare amṭha*, a little old dried flesh of the mango fruit.

Tutiạ, sulphate of copper.

Bilạti thamakur, imported tobacco.

First wash with the *nim* water as in above (*b*), then grind these three ingredients with hookah water and apply the mixture as an ointment.

(*d*) *Powa bhor taṛpin sunum*, 8 oz. Terebinthinæ oleum.

Ad powa ulin̈ sunum, 4 oz. mustard oil.

First wash with *nim* water as in (*b*) and (*c*), and then anoint with this mixture, and the sores will dry up.

(*e*) *Nạrkọṛ sunum ad powa*, 4 oz. cocoanut oil.

Karbolik mõṛẽ ṭhọp, 5 drops carbolic acid.

After first cleaning anoint with this mixture.

(*f*) *Ạṇḍiạ moṛọn aṛak ṛẹhẹl*, the roots of Gymnema hirsutus, W. and A., var. Decaisneanum, Wight.

Dare japak man̈jge, the pith of Scindapsus officinalis, Schott.

Nanha dudhi loṭa ṛẹhẹl, the roots of Ichnocarpus frutescens, R. Br.

Wash with *nim* water as above. Boil the above three in a mixture of mustard oil and melted butter and apply with a feather.

(*g*) *Icạk ṛẹhẹl*, the root of Woodfordia floribunda, Salisb.

Ọskọrbul,

Grind the first fine to a powder and sprinkle it on. Grind the second with hot water on a stone or sherd and apply to the sores with a feather.

(*h*) *Rọsọ kạpur*, a farthing's worth of white sublimate or muriate of mercury.

Simbrit, the fresh shoots of Bombax malabaricum, DC.

Kạgji nimbu ṛẹhẹl, the roots of Citrus acida, Roxb., a good quantity.

Grind these together and make into pills, three of which to be taken daily until the lips break out in sores. Then take the bark of *baṛ dare*, Mimusops Elengi, L., bruise and boil it in water, and let the patient rinse the mouth with that water daily until recovery.

(*i*) *Ran̈gạini ṛẹhẹl*, the roots of Solanum Jacquini, Willd.

Joka sakam, the leaves of Sida humilis, Willd.

Kasmar chal, the bark of Gmelina arborea, Roxb.

Cip ciṛip ṛẹhẹl, the roots of Achyranthes aspera, Linn.

Sẹkrẹć ḍọg, the shoots of Lagerstroemia parviflora, Roxb.

Grind together, warm in mustard oil and immerse therein and mixing well apply with a feather.

(j) *Ạtkir rẹhẹl*, the roots of Smilax ovalifolia, Roxb.

Nanha dudhi loṭa rẹhẹl, the roots of Ichnocarpus frutescens, R. Br.

Sarjọm chal, the bark of Shorea robusta, Gärtn.

Kundri chal, „ „ „ Zehneria umbellata, Thew.

Sega chal, „ „ „ Mimosa rubicaulis, Lamk.

Kadar rẹhẹl, the roots of Bonnaya veronicæfolia, Spreng.

Nim chal, the bark of Melia Azadirachta, L.

Boil all these thoroughly together and give to drink daily.

(k) The same, with the omission of *dhũṛạ̃*, resin, as No. (b) above, and to be applied in same way.

(l) *Mare jọjọ*, the old fruit of Tamarindus indicus, L.

Tutiạ, sulphate of copper.

Thoṛa bilạti thamakur sakam, a little of the leaves of imported tobacco.

Grind with *hukạ dak̔*, hookah water, and after washing the sore clean, plaster the medicine you have ground on it.

The pain caused must be borne.

(m) Immediately dry *sarjọm chal*, the bark of Shorea robusta, Gärtn., and sprinkle or dust on the sore which will gradually dry up. This causes no pain.

(n) *Bandphoṛa biń rapak̔ rọńgọeme*, roast to burning point the bones of the Bungarus fasciatus snake.

Etka rẹhẹl, the roots of Mucuna pruriens, DC.

Aṇḍiạ mọrọn aṛak̔ rẹhẹl, the roots of Gymnema hirsutus, W. and A., var. Decaisneanum, Wight.

Dare japak̔ mańjiẹl, the pith of Scindapsus officinalis, Schott.

Nim sakam, the leaves of Melia Azadirachta, L.

Sinduạri sakam, the leaves of Vitex Negundo, L.

Nanha dudhi loṭa rẹhẹl, the roots of Ichnocarpus frutescens, R. Br.

Grind these together, cook in melted butter of cows' milk and smear on.

(o) *Para dak̔*, quicksilver water.

Sanam jạt mọsọla, one of each kind of all sorts of spices.

Sọsọ jań, the seed of Semecarpus Anacardium, L.

Roast the last to burning point, fry the spices slightly, and after grinding and mixing both add the first, and make into seven pills to be taken for seven days, when the mouth will develop sores. The medicine must then be discontinued, he must brush the teeth with a twig of *bherṇḍa*, Jatropha Curcas, L., and wash the mouth with water in which *bạṛ chal*, the bark of Mimusops Elengi, L., has been boiled. Recovery will follow in 15 days' time.

(*p*) *Sindrit*, fresh shoots of Bombax malabaricum, DC.
Rǫsǫmuni,
Rǫs sindur, factitious cinnabar.
Sora, saltpetre.

Grind these together, stir in *utiń sunum*, mustard oil, and apply to the sores.

(*q*) *Nanha dudhi loṭa rẹhẹl*, the roots of Ichnocarpus frutescens, R. Br.
Ǫt ḍhompo, Lepidagathis cristata, Willd.
Kasmar chal, the bark of Gmelina arborea, Roxb.
Rąńgąini rẹhẹl, the roots of Solanum Jacquini, Willd.
Jokha sakam, the leaves of Sida humilis, Willd.

Grind all these together, cook in *utiń sunum*, mustard oil, and apply with a feather to the penis. Also give the following *internally*:

(*r*) *Sarjǫm baha*, the flowers of Shorea robusta, Gärtn.
Sasań baha, " " " Curcuma longa, Roxb.
Bońga sarjǫm chal, the bark of Ventilago calyculata, Tulasne.

Grind these together, mix in *guṛ*, molasses, and give to drink.

Gurmi is a name sometimes used also for other diseases than syphilis, *viz.*, gonorrhœa, and any kind of eczema penis et scroti.

One "authority" says: There is no certainty as to the origin of this. Some people say if you have connection with a woman given to promiscuous intercourse you will contract this or swollen testicles. Occasionally I have seen people who are not fornicators suffering from this. It is said to be contracted thus: If you walk over a place where a syphilitic person has made water, the exhalation from this, from the action of the sun, will infect you.

194. *Maejiu hoṛ kuṭhi gąrmi*. (? Women's gonorrhœa, or cystitis.)

Symptoms. A burning sensation in the abdomen at micturition.

Medicines: (procurable at medicine vendors.)
Kąṭlą jẹr,
Cae cirǫta, Gentiana Cherayta, R.
Meral jǫ, the fruit of Phyllanthus Emblica, Linn.
Dhiri ghās,
Thoṛa mithi, a little Trigonella Fænum-græcum, Willd.

Soak all these in a cup of water, taking of the first a ball about the size of a pea. Then in the morning after grinding squeeze out and give this water to the patient to drink.

195. *Hąsli ghao*. A tertiary manifestation of syphilis on the neck and chest. "Le collier de Venus."

Medicines: (*a*) *Rẹṭhẹ bǫd laṛ rẹhẹl chal*, the bark of the root of a small Vitis adnata, Wall.
Caole ata, roasted rice.

Roast the rice to burning point and roast the bark also or dry it in the sun. Then grind both together and making it into a powder apply to the sore.

(*b*) *Dhũṛã*, resin of Shorea robusta, Gärtn.

Nim sakam, the leaves of Melia Azadirachta, Linn.

Kahu botke rẹhẹt, the roots of Bryonia lacinosa, Linn.

Bir kundri da, the tuber of Zehneria umbellata, Thew.

Pọrọl jhiṅgạ jaṅ, the seeds of Luffa acutangula, Roxb.

Ato jhiṅgạ jaṅ, the seeds of the garden variety of same.

Sẹlẹp samanọm rẹhẹt, the roots of Gloriosa superba, Willd.

Aṇḍiạ mọrọn aṛak rẹhẹt, the roots of Gymnema hirsutus, W. and A., var. Decaisneanum, Wight.

Nanha dudhi loṭa rẹhẹt, the roots of Ichnocarpus frutescens, R. Br.

Kedok aṛak rẹhẹt, the roots of Argyreia speciosa, Sweet.

Daṛe japak manjhẹt, the pith of Scindapsus officinalis, Schott.

First cook the resin in mustard oil and make it into a kind of butter. Then boil and cook all the other ingredients in this preparation and anoint the place therewith.

(*c*) *Mare naṅgle*, an old leather thong used for binding the yoke to the plough beam.

Aṇḍiạ tale baha, the flower of the male Borassus flabelliformis, L.

Ọt ḍhompo ghãs, Lepidagathis cristata, Willd.

Binḍi muthạ rẹhẹt, the roots of Fimbristylis monostachya, Hassk.

Roast the first two to burning and fry the second two to burning ; then mixing all grind them fine. If there is much liquid discharge make into a powder and dust it on, otherwise mix it with pure mustard oil and apply with a feather to the sore.

(*d*) *Gurli sẹ toyo karla da jaṅ*,

Bir kundri, Zehneria umbellata, Thew. } both
Ato kundri, Cephalandra indica, Nand. } bitter.

Kahu botke rẹhẹt, the roots of Bryonia lacinosa, Linn.

Nim chal, the bark of Melia Azadirachta, Linn.

Sẹlẹp samanọm rẹhẹt, the roots of Gloriosa superba, Willd.

Muṅgạ chal, the bark of Moringa pterygosperma, Gärtn.

Pusi pan rẹhẹt, the roots of Ehretia lævis, Roxb.

Grind all the first seven together, boil them in the oil of the *ṭhaḍiạ* variety of Brassica campestris, Linn., mixing also the last named and apply daily.

(*e*) *Rọsọ kạpur*, one tola, the weight of a rupee of a white sublimate or muriate of mercury.

Lọbọṅ, cloves, 84 pieces.

Goṭe rẹhẹt, 1½ dr. of the root of Croton oblongifolius, Roxb.

Grind these with goats' milk, no water, and make into pills the size of hares' dung. Four of these pills to be eaten the first day and two daily the four following days till the patient begins to slaver, and then no more. The pills to be taken before meals, and only water that has been boiled and cooked to be drunk. The sore is not to be touched the whole time.

When there is a slight sore in the mouth and the saliva flows freely, then

Bạṛ chal, the bark of Mimusops Elengi, L.
Bubla chal, the bark of Acacia arabica, Willd.

to be boiled together and the water to be used for washing the mouth out.

This medicine may also be used for syphilitic sores, gonorrhœa and rheumatism.

(*f*) *Murgạ banda*, parasitical plant found on Pterocarpus Marsupium, Roxb.
Terel cẹtẹ, the thin skin on the bark of Diospyros tomentosa, Roxb.
Kaṭkọm jaṅga, Viscum attenuatum, DC.

Grind, boil in mustard oil and anoint the sore therewith.

(*g*) *Gaḍa gạṛi*, a certain water insect.

To be roasted, made into a powder and sprinkled on the sore.

(*h*) *Rọkọc̓ jel*, the flesh of small molluscs or periwinkles.

To be cooked in mustard oil and smeared on the sore.

(*i*) *Kamraj rẹhẹt*, the roots of Buettneria herbacea, Roxb.
Saoraj jọ reak̓ jaṅ, the stone of the fruit of Vernonia anthelmintica, Roxb.
Rọhọṛ sarjọm chal, the dried bark of Shorea robusta, Gärtn.

Grind a little of all these together with water and apply to the spot.

(*j*) *Dhũṛạ*, resin of Shorea robusta, Gärtn.
Turạm,

Grind these together and after boiling in *utiṅ sunum*, mustard oil, pour into a cup of water and apply the butter-like scum that rises to the surface.

(*k*) *Kujri chal rẹhẹt reak̓*, the bark of the roots of Celastus paniculatus, Willd.
Mạṅjur jhuṭi rẹhẹt, the roots of
Laṭha cip̓ ciṛip̓ jọ, the fruit of

Grind these together, cook in *utiṅ sunum*, mustard oil, and apply with a feather.

(*l*) *Bir baraṅgọm*, Glossogyne pinnatifida, DC.
Mare naṅgle, an old leather yoke thong.

Roast the latter to burning point, then grind along with the former, cook in *utiṅ sunum*, mustard oil, and

Sar rẹhẹt, the roots of Saccharum Sara, Roxb.
Ṅũṛũc̓ jaṅ reak̓ dạl, the kernel of the seed of Cassia Fistula, L.

Grind these with *sisir dak*, dew, and mix with the previous cooked remedy and apply with a feather.

One "authority" says: This commences on the neck, chest, collar bone or nape of the neck, and wherever the watery discharge spreads the sores will follow.

196. *Taru landup*. (Perforating ulcer of the palate.)

Symptoms. This commences in the nose and the sores eat away in the palate upwards and the nose downwards, and the speech becomes nasal.

Medicines: (*a*) *Naksuri dare reak jo se chal tanak*, the fruit, bark or such of
Bonkapsi jan, the seed of Thespesia Lampas, Benth. & Hook. f.
Saparom chal, the bark of Nyctanthes Arbor-tristis, L.
Icak rehet, the roots of Woodfordia floribunda, Salisb.
Manikjor ghās,
Dhiri banda,
Jotamansi rehet, the roots of Nardostachys Jatamansi, DC.
Rangaini janum rehet, the roots of Solanum Jacquini, Willd.
Serwan rehet, the roots of Vigna vexillata, Benth.
Gote rehet, the roots of Croton oblongifolius, Roxb.
Nanha dudhi lota rehet, the roots of Ichnocarpus frutescens, R. Br.

Grind all these and cook them in pure mustard oil and let the patient sniff it up the nose. (Mix *kia baha*, Pandanus odoratissimus, Willd., and *maran catom arak*,)

(*b*) If you can, get hold of an unborn hare, extract it entire from the mother, and dry it.
Kulai ic, hare's excrement.
Kulai uptel, hare's hair.
Jhik pota se iltel, the stomach or quills of a porcupine.

Grind all these fine into a powder, which dust on to the sore.

Forbidden diet: Boiled rice, milk or curds (*dahe*), salt, vegetables, pulse, etc.; only flour made from roasted grain, otherwise the sore will develop further.

(*c*) *Oskorbul*,
Simbrit, fresh shoots of Bombax malabaricum, DC.
Barni baha, Clerodendron infortunatum, L.

Grind these together and make into 5 pills the size of sheeps' or goats' excrement, one pill covered in cream from cows' milk to be taken daily. If the mouth develops sores, cook *ghi kuari*, Yucca gloriosa, in melted butter and rub it on the tongue. Diet same as in (*b*) above.

(*d*) *Ot oponom*, Angelica glauca, Edgew.

Cut a disc of this the size of the cavity or hole (similar to the disc of potsherd used in the game called *kati*). Grind fine together

Kuḷai tarọp rẹhẹl, the roots of
Bọd laṛ rẹhẹl, the roots of Vitis adnata, Wall.

Push into the cavity and fix above disc and then rub on these ground medicines.

Bhạbri, Embelia robusta, Wall.
Mare panahi kuṭrạ, a piece of an old shoe.
Bọd laṛ rẹhẹl, the roots of Vitis adnata, Wall.

Grind these three together and apply as a plaster.

Hạṛũ jọmak jinis, something of which a hamunan has eaten.
Tale gele, the male flower of Borassus flabelliformis, L.

Roast these to burning point and after grinding them small stir in *kạñji dak*, stale rice water, and let him apply this daily.

The man who provides the medicine must not see the patient for two weeks, but send the medicine by some one else, and in that period the patient will be cured.

One "authority" says: This begins with a small pimple on the palate which gradually becomes bigger like a boil; when ripe it emits a rotten odour and as it increases it makes a hole, so that it is difficult to eat food or drink water, and it may spread so that the nose falls in.

197. *Paeṭhaniạ ghao.*

Symptoms. This results from rheumatism, and sometimes if one person in the house gets it, then as in small pox the whole household is infected. Our ancestors say this is the penalty of sexual immorality; if any one sins in that way he will get it.

Medicines: (*a*) *Akaona*, Calotropis gigantea, R. Br.
Ạsạṛiạ chal, the bark of Capparis horrida, L. f.
Ạṇḍiạ mọrọn aṛak, Gymnema hirsutus, W. and A., var. Decaisneanum, Wight.
Ạṇḍiạ koṅgat rẹhẹl, the roots of Dregia volubilis, Benth.

Boil these in mustard oil and smear on.

By steaming:

(*b*) *Akaona rẹhẹl*, the roots of Calotropis gigantea R. Br.
Kạṛwạ̃l rẹhẹl, ,, ,, ,, Carissa Carandas, L.
Ạsạṛiạ chal, the bark of Capparis horrida, L.
Sinduạri sakam, the leaves of Vitex Negundo, L.
Bir họṛẹc̃, Atyllosia scarabædois, Benth.
Bana haṭak chal, the bark of Oroxylon indicum, Benth.
Saram lutur rẹhẹl, the roots of Clerodendron serratum, Spreng.
Sasaṅ bọhọktẹl, a knot of turmeric, Curcuma longa, L.
Tọtnọpak chal, the bark of Eugenia operculata, Roxb.
Gote chal, ,, ,, ,, Croton oblongifolius, Roxb.
Karam chal, ,, ,, ,, Adina cordifolia, H. f. and B.
Kasmar chal, ,, ,, ,, Gmelina arborea, Roxb.

Grind all these, put them in a new earthen pot, cover them with a leaf-plate and boil well. Then after spreading a thickish cloth over a bed make the patient lie thereon and cover him with a sheet or blanket so that it falls on all sides of the bed down to the floor. Then put the boiling medicines underneath the bed and steam him until the perspiration pours from his body. By so doing his sore will dry up.

(c) *Asaṛiạ chal*, the bark of Capparis horrida, L.
Kãṛwãt rẹhẹt, the roots of Carissa Carandas, L.
Simbrit, fresh shoots of Bombax malabaricum, DC.

First grind the first two fine together, then add the third and grind all three mixing them well. Then mix some of the first in melted butter. Then tear a strip of cloth about the width of two fingers and dip it in melted butter. Take a new shoot of *jọm jạnum*, Zizyphus Jujuba, Lamk., as long as the width of eight fingers placed bẹside one another, and plaster on the length of six fingers' breadth the medicines already ground and mixed. Then wrap round this the soaked strip of cloth, leaving two fingers' breadth free. Then get a handful of cowdung and stick the free two fingers' breadth of the swathed medicine into this, and make the patient sit on a low stool close to this and cover him with a sheet. Then set fire to the "medicine stick" or "candle." The patient must not look at it burning, but remain covered till it has burnt out. Burn such a "candle," one on each of three or four days, by which time he will get sores in the mouth, and sometimes the tongue protrudes. Then cook some *ghi kũạri*, Yucca gloriosa, in melted butter and smear this on his tongue and lips; then the sores in the mouth and stomach will get well.

198. *Palaniạ ghao*. A chronic progredient sore, a carbuncle on the back.

Symptoms. This sore appears mostly in the back, shoulder blade or ribs. At first an excrescence comes up, which later festers internally, and afterwards breaks out in three or four places into a sore. If medicine is not applied it will penetrate deeper.

Medicines: (a) *Sarjọm chal* (*haṛam dare*) the bark of an old Shores robusta, Gärtn.
Meral chal, the bark of Phyllanthus Emblica, L.
Bhạbri rẹhẹt, the roots of Embelia robusta, Roxb.
Biṇḍi muthạ ghãs rẹhẹt, the roots of Fimbristylis monostachya, Hassk.
Sukri muthạ ghãs da, the bulb of Scirpus monostachyus, Kön.
Hesak̃ ḍọg, the budding leaves of Ficus religiosa, Willd.
Kadam sakam ḍọg, the budding leaves of Anthocephalus Cadamba, Bth. and Hook. f.

Grind all together into a powder and sprinkle it daily on the sore after having daily washed it with water in which the leaves of *nim*, Melia Azadirachta, L., have been boiled.

(*b*) *Suruj lẹwẹr baha*, Helianthus annuus, L.
Mare naṅgle, an old leathern yoke thong.
Dare bạṅki, Vanda Roxburghii, R. Br.
Dhiri banda ghãs,
Akaona rẹhẹl, the roots of Calotropis gigantea, R. Br.

Grind these together to a powder and dust it on the sore.

(*c*) *Tarse koṭap rẹhẹl*, the roots of Grewia villosa, Willd.
Mọsọbọr, Barbadoes aloes.
Bẹrẹl sasaṅ bọhọk, head of raw turmeric, Curcuma longa, Roxb.

After washing the wound with water as in (*a*) above, grind these together and apply daily.

(*d*) *Bir jhuṅkạ*, Crotalaria calycina, Shrank.
Bir sọn sakam, the leaves of
Mandargọm sakam, the leaves of Anona squamosa, L.
Kạhu botke rẹhẹl, the roots of Bryonia lacinosa, L.
Sukri muthạ ghãs da, the bulb of Scirpus monostachyus, Kön.
Dhubi ghãs da, the bulbs of Cynodon dactylon, Pers.
Kaṇṭhaṛ sakam, the leaves of Artocarpus integrifolia, L.
Amsopori dare rẹhẹl chal, the bark of the roots of Psidium Guava, Raddi.
Hesak̔ chal, the bark of Ficus religiosa, Willd.

Fry these to burning point and make a powder to be dusted on daily.

(*e*) *Bheḍa dereṅ rẹhẹl*, the roots of Cassia Tora, L.
Baglucạ jọ, the fruit of Martynia diandra, Gloxin.
Karam chal, the bark of Adina cordifolia, H. f. and B.
Korkoṭ chal, „ „ „ Dillenia indica, L.
Sahar chal, „ „ „ Dillenia pentagyna, Roxb.
Gõṛẽ dare chal, the bark of Stephegyne parvifolia, Korth.
Sekra dare chal, „ „ „ Zizyphus rugosa, Lamk.
Sẹkrẹc̔ dare chal, „ „ „ Lagerstroemia parviflora, Roxb.
Hesak̔ chal, „ „ „ Ficus religiosa, Willd.
Terel chal, the bark of Diospyros tomentosa, Roxb.
Icạk̔ chal, „ „ „ Woodfordia floribunda, Salisb.

Grind a little of all these and sprinkle it on.

(*f*) *Buru ghoṛa lada*, Vitis tomentosa, Heyne.
Ẹdẹl poha, a seedling of Bombax malabaricum, DC.
Ic̔ çvẹr da, the bulb of Vitis latifolia, Roxb.
Bọd laṛ nạ̃ṛi, Vitis adnata, Wall.

Fry these to burning point and make a powder to be dusted on daily after washing the sore.

(*g*) *Ḍoka rẹhẹl chal*, the bark of the root of Odina Wodier, Roxb.
Janhe lobok̔, the bran of Paspalum scrobiculatum, L.
Kạṅji, stale rice water.

Wash with the last, pound the first two very fine and sprinkle on daily.

(*h*) *Gaḍa gāṛī*, a certain water insect.
Mohlom, ointment.

Grind and mix and apply to the sore.

(*i*) *Ḍaṅgra harta reak naṅgle*, a yoke rope of ox leather.

Roast to burning point, grind fine and sprinkle dry on the sore.

(*j*) *Sarjom chal, haṛam dare reak*, the bark of an old Shorea robusta, Gärtn.
Meral chal, the bark of Phyllanthus Emblica, L.
Corco chal, ,, ,, ,, Casearea tomentosa, L.
Bhabri rehel, the roots of Embelia robusta, Roxb.
Campa rehel, ,, ,, ,, Michelia champaca, L.
Piṇḍa chal, the bark of Randia uliginosa, DC.
Nim chal, ,, ,, ,, Melia Azadirachta, L.
Mare naṅgle rapak roṅgo, an old leathern yoke thong roasted to burning point.
Suruj lewer baha, the flower of Helianthus annuus, L.

Collect all these and fry or roast them all, as may be feasible, to burning point. Then grind them to a powder and sprinkle this powder on.

(*k*) *Kujri chal*, the bark of Celastus paniculatus, Willd.
Baṛ chal, ,, ,, ,, Mimusops Elengi, L.
Terel chal, ,, ,, ,, Diospyros tomentosa, Roxb.
Hesel chal, ,, ,, ,, Anogeissus latifolia, Wall.
Corco chal, ,, ,, ,, Casearea tomentosa, L.
Soso chal, ,, ,, ,, Semecarpus Anacardium, L.
Totnopak chal, the bark of Eugenia operculata, Roxb.
Sekreč chal, ,, ,, ,, Lagerstroemia parviflora, Roxb.
Hesak chal, ,, ,, ,, Ficus religiosa, Willd.
Kadam chal, ,, ,, ,, Anthocephalus Cadamba, Benth. and Hook. f.

Grind to a powder and sprinkle on.

(*l*) *Bonkapši rehel*, the roots of Thespesia Lampas, Benth. and Hook. f.
Petcambṛa rehel, ,, ,, ,, Helicteres Isora, L.
Tarse koṭap rehel, the roots of Grewia villosa, Willd.
Barsa pakoṛ rehel, the roots of Grewia sapida, Roxb.
Seta kaṭa rehel, ,, ,, ,, Grewia polygama, Roxb.

Grind all these to a powder and apply.

(*m*) As this appears first like a boil, *ojo*, treat it first as such; if this fails, then you may know it is this complaint and proceed with
Merleč chal, the bark of Flacourtia Ramontchi, L'Herit.
Janhe lobok, the bran of Paspalum scrobiculatum, L.

Gundli lobok, the bran of Panicum miliare, Lamk.
Iṛi lobok, „ „ „ Panicum Crus-galli, L.

Dry the first named and grind it to a powder, then grind and mix the others therewith and sprinkle the mixture daily on the sore.

199. *Nākrisạ.* (? Syphilitic ulcer in the nose).

Symptoms. A pustule forms inside the nose, bursts and becomes a sore.

Medicines: (*a*) *Kidiń baha ṛeheṭ*, the roots of Ipomæa Quamoclit, L.
Tirṛạ da, the bulbs of Pueraria tuberosa, DC.

Grind and let him drink some and sniff some up the nose.

(*b*) *Arak̃ purại*, the red variety of Basella alba, Willd.

Cook in mustard oil and let him sniff it up the nose.

(*c*) *Moṭa purại aṛak, sakamṭeṭ, nạṛī ṭeṭ*, the leaves and tendrils of Basella alba, Willd.

Pound and squeeze into the nose, repeating until cured.

(*d*) *Kọnḍẹń da*, the bulb of Eriosema chinensis, Voq.
Tirṛạ ḍọg, the tips of Pueraria tuberosa, DC.

Grind together and give to drink and make him sniff some up the nose.

(*e*) *Moṭa purại sakam ar nạṛiṭeṭ*, the stem and leaves of a thick Basella alba, Willd.

Pound slightly and squeeze into the nose, repeating till he is well, which will be very quickly.

(*f*) *Họrọ bọhọk̃*, the head of a tortoise.

Grind and cook in *utiń sunum*, mustard oil, or even without cooking, and let him sniff it up the nose. Further, grind together

Kọnḍẹń da, the bulb of Eriosema chinensis, Voq.
Tirṛạ da, „ „ „ Pueraria tuberosa, DC.

and let him take a little thereof every day; take also an iron ladle full of each of *utiń sunum*, mustard oil, and water, put them in a cup and churn them together with a piece of twig used as a toothbrush and rub it well into the forehead.

200. *Hẹrẹl pọrdhọl.* (? Spermatorrhoea).

Symptoms. In this men pass blood in the excreta, something white, discharged from the urethra. It occurs twice or thrice monthly.

Medicines: (*a*) *Ẹdẹl poha*, a seedling of Bombax malabaricum, DC.
Misri, sugar-candy.

Cut the former into round slices and eat with the latter, and for two or three days drink cold water. No intercourse with women is permissible.

(*b*) *Miru baha ṛẹheṭ*, the roots of Abutilon indicum, Don.
Haṭ ṛẹheṭ thoṛa, a little of roots of Holarrhena antidysenterica, Wall.
Ạphim thoṛa, a little opium.

Grind these three and make into 5 pills. Brush the teeth daily with a twig of the second of above three and take one of these pills. Make a hole at the foot of a *loa dare*, Ficus glomerata, Roxb., in which bury a small vessel and after severing one of the roots of the tree let the juice therefrom drop into this vessel. This juice to be drunk by the patient.

(*c*) *Edel poha rehel*, the roots of a seedling of Bombax malabaricum, DC.
Hat rehel, the roots of Holarrhena antidysenterica, Wall.
Miru baha rehel, the roots of Abutilon indicum, Don.
Aphim, opium.

Grind these all together and make into pills to be taken daily.

N.B.—Women suffering from menorrhagia have also been cured by this remedy.

Herel hor pond pordhol. (? Gonorrhoea, ? Spermatorrhoea).

Symptoms. In this something white escapes along with the urine and by degrees the body becomes emaciated.

Medicines: (*d*) *Hesak chal*, the bark of Ficus religiosa, Willd.
Kũs ghãs rehel, the roots of Themuda gigantea, Haskel.
Bir horeć rehel, „ „ „ Atyllosia scarabædois, Benth.
Mahũt gur, the refuse of molasses.

Pound the first three together and after boiling well with the last give to drink daily.

(*e*) *Badam jo reak gabe*, the kernel of almonds.
Pe ganda gol maric, 12 black peppercorns.

Grind together, mix with 8 ounces *paura*, spirits, and give 2 ounces daily to drink.

(*f*) *Campa rehel*, the roots of Michelia champaca, L.

Boil and give to drink like tea daily for some 15 days and he will assuredly recover.

201 *Pondgeko racatere.* (White-coloured urine.)

Medicines: (*a*) *Kaera dak*, the juice of Musa paradisiaca, L.
Cini se misri, sugar or sugar-candy.
Mahabari boc, Zingiber Zerumbet, Roscoe.
Posto dana, seed of the opium poppy.

Take a little of each of these, grind, warm and give to drink.

(*b*) *Hesak chal*, the bark of Ficus religiosa, Willd.
Kasi ghãs rehel, the roots of Saccharum spontaneum, L.

Grind these together and boil well with *mahũt gur*, the refuse of molasses, and give to drink daily; recovery is certain.

(*c*) *Lopon arak*, Aerua lanata, L.
Adwa caole, rice made from sun-dried, not boiled paddy.

Grind these together, make into hand bread and put out in the dew; let her eat it the following morning and do so for three consecutive days; then proceed with

(*d*) *Campa rẹhẹl*, the roots of Michelia champaca, L.
Rọkọt condọn kaṭ, blood coloured sandalwood.
Joba baha rẹhẹl, the roots of Hibiscus rosa-sinensis, L.
Arak upạl baha rẹhẹl, the roots of Nymphæa rubra, Roxb.

Grind, mix, boil in water and let her drink for about a fortnight; then

(*e*) *Huṭer baha rẹhẹl*, the roots of Indigofera pulchella, Roxb.
Pọṇḍ kawẹt rẹhẹl, „ „ „ the white Abrus precatorius, L.
Cihũṭ laṛ rẹhẹl, the roots of Spatholobus Roxburghii, Benth.
Adagạthiạ rẹhẹl, the roots of Panicum repens, L.

Grind and give to drink. If this is ineffective then

(*f*) Take all the ingredients in (*d*) and (*f*) grind together and give to drink.

If there is internal pain:

(*g*) *Cạili rẹhẹl*, the roots of Morinda exserta, Roxb.
Hạlim, Lepidium sativum, L.
Jioti, Sesbania ægyptiaca, Pers.
Ḍuriạ hạtkạn, Leea hirta, Herb. Banks.

Grind these together, warm and apply as a plaster below the navel; if applied for three days he will get well.

202. *Racateak bọndlenre.* Retention of urine.

Medicines: (*a*) *Bandphoṛa biṅ jaṅ*, a bone of the Bungarus fasciatus snake.
Milṭẹn ghugri, a mole cricket, Gryllus gryllo-talpa.
Rọhọe malhan rẹhẹl, the roots of a cultivated Dolichos Lablab, L.

Rub the first on a stone and mix the rubbings with the ground product of the other two and give to drink, when the patient will urinate at once.

(*b*) *Muṅgạ dare chal sẹ rẹhẹl chal*, the bark of Moringa pterygosperma, Gärtn., or of its roots.
Are gaṇḍa gol mạric, 36 black peppercorns.

Grind, mix and apply over the abdomen, and the patient will urinate at once.

After or during childbirth the urine is retained, and both then and in fevers this remedy is efficacious.

(*c*) *Gilil gạ̃ṛi*, Gryllus monstruosus.
Mạhũt guṛ, the refuse of molasses.

Mix and give to drink.

(*d*) *Pọṇḍ sega rẹhẹl*, the roots of the white Mimosa rubicaulis, Lamk.

Pound and crush to pieces, boil and give to drink.

203. *Ṭhọp ṭhọpko racatere.* Dysuria.

Medicines: *Aṇḍiạ mọrọn aṛak da*, the bulb of Gymnema hirsutus, W. and A., var. Decaisneanum, Wight.

Bana haṭak chal, the bark of Oroxylon indicum, Benth.
Adagaṭhia̹ rẹhẹl, the roots of Panicum repens, L.

Mix and grind these and give to drink.

204. *Jhala sẹ Setoṅ lagao.* Dysuria, nearly always caused by excessive perspiration.

Medicines: (*a*) *Aṭkir rẹhẹl*, the roots of Smilax ovalifolia, Roxb.
Kadar rẹhẹl, the roots of Bonnaya veronicæfolia, Spreng.
Boṅga sarjọm rọs, the juice of Ventilago calyculata, Tulasne.
Sarjọm rọs, the juice of Shorea robusta, Gärtn.
Tarọp chal, the bark of Buchanania latifolia, Roxb.
Terel rẹhẹl, the roots of Diospyros tomentosa, Roxb.
Mẹrọm mẽl chal, the bark of Ixora parviflora, Vahl, or Olax nana, Wall.
Rọl chal, the bark of Terminalia Chebula, Retz.
Lọpọṅ chal, the bark of Terminalia bellerica, Roxb.
Kaṭić kadar rẹhẹlṭẹl, the bark of a small Bonnaya veronicæfolia, Spreng.

Collect all these and give to drink.

(*b*) *Hẹsẹl dare chal*, the bark of Anogeissus latifolia, Wall.
Kauha̹ dare chal, „ „ „ Terminalia Arjuna, Bedd.
Gaḍa terel chal, „ „ „ Diospyros montana, Roxb.

Grind together and give to drink.

(*c*) *Ńũṛũć bale ḍọg reak mańj*, the pith of a fresh shoot of Cassia Fistula, L.

Grind fine, mix with sugar and give to drink.

(*d*) *Họṛẹć*, Dolichos biflorus, L.

Make this into a curry to be eaten some five days.

(*e*) The best medicine of all for this is *lọlọ ca*, hot tea, the drinking of which is followed by an immediate cure; but this we have only learnt lately.

(*f*) *Nãṛi murup chal*, the bark of Butea superba, Roxb.
Suruj mukhi baha rẹhẹl, the roots of Helianthus annuus, L.
Ńũṛũć bale ḍa̹r reak mańj, the pith of a young branch of Cassia Fistula, L.

Grind these, mix with *cini*, sugar, and give to drink.

If blood is passed with the urine, then

(*g*) *Matkọm chal*, the bark of Bassia latifolia, Roxb.
Lọpọṅ chal, „ „ „ Terminalia bellerica, Roxb.
Ṭa̹ṇḍi ma̹ric, found in the rice fields, the leaves resembling those of Capsicum frutescens, Willd.
Thoṛa ka̹uḍi cun, a little lime made of the shells used as money in India.

Grind and mix these, add a little *mare guṛ*, old molasses, or *cini*, sugar, and give to drink.

One "authority" says: This follows being long or walking long in the sun. Generally it will result from drinking water before the body has cooled down after exposure to the sun.

205. *Māyāmgeko pesabre.* Hæmaturia.

Medicines: (*a*) *Mare jhaṇṭireko tahẹn tejo*, creeping insects found in old wattles.

Mare sea sąuṛi tọrọc̓, the ashes of rotten Heteropogon contortus, R. & S.

Kāṛā kąuḍi cun, lime made of the shells used as money in India.

First grind the insects with water; then mix and stir up with the other two ingredients, strain and give to drink.

(*b*) Cut all round the inside of *Arakak̓ lạṭu peaj*, a large red onion; then insert a little *ạphim*, opium, in the hollow, envelope all in earth and bake in the fire. When the earth is scorched, pull it out of the fire and give the onion to eat. Should stupefaction ensue, toast *kaera ḍhạṇḍkil*, the stalk of Musa paradisaica, L., at the fire, squeeze out and collect the water from it and give him that water to drink.

(*c*) *Rọl chal*, the bark of Terminalia Chebula, Retz.

Cīhūṭ chal, „ „ „ Spatholobus Roxburghii, Benth.

Ḍoka chal, „ „ „ Odina Wodier, Roxb.

Muṅgạ chal, „ „ Moringa pterygosperma, Gärtn.

Duṇḍukil chal, the bark of Gardenia turgida, Roxb.

Paḍer chal, „ „ „ Stereospermum suaveolens, DC.

Grind these together and give to drink.

(*d*) *Nanha dudhi loṭa rẹhẹl*, the roots of Ichnocarpus frutescens, R. Br.

Malhan nāṛī ḍhomporeko tahẹn 2 *sẹ* 3 *tejo*, 2 or 3 of the creeping insects found on the lumps on the tendrils of Dolichos Lablab, L.

Tejo mala rẹhẹl, the roots of Cissampelos Pareira, L.

Mix, grind and give to drink.

(*e*) Grind *ńūṛūc̓ dọg*, a shoot of Cassia Fistula, L. and give to drink with sugar.

(*f*) *Bir haṭ rẹhẹl*, the roots of Holarrhena antidysenterica, Wall. (?)

Bir jhuṅkạ rẹhẹl, the roots of Crotalaria calycina, Shrank.

Grind these with water and give to drink.

(*g*) *Edẹl poha*, a seedling of Bombax malabaricum, DC.

Atnak̓ poha sẹ chal, a seedling or the bark of Terminalia tomentosa, W. and A.

Mạhūt guṛ, the refuse of molasses.

Mix and give to drink.

206. *Khaṛak muth.* Gravel.

Symptoms. In this the urine is red or blood is passed, and occasionally white also, and there is intense pain.

Medicines: (*a*) *Bhạbri rẹhẹl*, the roots of Embelia robusta, Roxb.

Bạrni rẹhẹl, the roots of Clerodendron infortunatum, L.

Paṛọ da, the bulb of Curcuma angustifolia, Roxb.

Arak̕ sẹ poṇḍ meral sakam, the leaves of either the red or white Phyllanthus Emblica, L.

Tursi sakam, the leaves of Ocimum sanctum, Willd.

Ạṭkir rẹhẹl, the roots of Smilax ovalifolia, Roxb.

Grind these and take the juice, and give to drink with *mạhũt guṛ*, the refuse of molasses; mix also a little *sora*, saltpetre.

(*b*) *Mạhũt guṛ*, the refuse of molasses.

Sora, saltpetre.

First smear the former on the abdomen, then after pounding the latter fine sprinkle it over and cover with a piece of white paper; in a little while he will urinate.

(*c*) *Orop̕ da*, the tuber of Costus speciosa, Sm.

Give this to drink and apply to the abdomen.

(*d*) *Hesak̕ chal*, the bark of Ficus religiosa, Willd.

Bir hoṛẹć, Atyllosia scarabædois, Benth.

Kũs rẹhẹl, the roots of Themuda gigantea, Haskel.

Lọṅphul, cloves.

Cini, sugar.

Grind the first three and boil well, then mix the last two and give to drink.

(*e*) *Tejo mala rẹhẹl*, the roots of Cissampelos Pareira, L.

Haṭ jọ jaṅ, the stone of the fruit of Holarrhena antidysenterica, Wall.

Grind and give to drink.

(*f*) *Hạlim*, Lepidium sativum, L. to be thrown into the mouth.

Cae cirota, Gentiana cherayta, Roxb.

Jiṭhimond rẹhẹl, the roots of Clerodendron Siphonanthus, R. Br.

The two latter to be steeped in a little water, this water to be drunk with an admixture of sugar-candy, and the two steeped ingredients to be thrown into the mouth.

(*g*) *Binḍi muthạ ghãs rẹhẹl*, the roots of Fimbristylis monostachya, Hassk.

Bharbhạri jaṅ the seed of Ocimum basilicum, L., or O. canum, Sims.

Extract the juice of the former and steep the latter in it, and then give to drink; the pain will cease.

(*h*) *Ato kundri datẹl*, the bulb of Cephalandra indica, Nand.
Bhạbri chal, the bark of Embelia robusta, Roxb.
Sahṛa chal, „ „ „ Streblus asper, Lour.

Grind together and stir in water. Take some of the juice of the *sarjọm dare*, Shorea robusta, Gärtn., mix it with the other water. Then strain this water and add *cini*, sugar, and *dumur rasa*, the honey of the small honey bee, and stir in it *mare naṅgle rapak rọṅgọkate*, an old leathern yoke thong roasted to burning point, the whole forming about a tumblerful of water, to be drunk once a day for three days.

(*i*) *Kạpu da*, the tuber of } to be drunk
Jĩoti, Sesbania ægyptiaca, Pers. } with spirits.
Ñụṛũc jọ, the fruit of Cassia Fistula, L.

(*j*) *Kawẹl rẹhẹl*, the roots of Abrus precatorius, L.
Mạhũt guṛ, the refuse of molasses.
Sora, saltpetre (the size of a pill).
Gọndhọk, sulphur („ „ „ „)
Opal terel dare reak jẹr, the exudation from a sapling of Diospyros tomentosa, Roxb.
Khayar jẹr, the exudation from Acacia Catechu, Willd.

Grind, stir in the refuse of molasses and give to drink.

(*k*) *Kadar nạ̃ṛĩ*, Asparagus racemosus, Willd.
Ạtkir, Smilax ovalifolia, Roxb.
Cini, sugar.
Mạhũt guṛ, the refuse of molasses.
Matha aṛak, Antidesma diandrum, Tulas.
Bheḍwa, Hibiscus cancellatus, Roscoe, var. fusiformis, Willd.

(*l*) *Bhạbri rẹhẹl*, the roots of Embelia robusta, Roxb.
Paṛọ da, the bulb of Curcuma angustifolia, Roxb.
Arak meral sakam, the leaves of the red Phyllanthus Emblica, L.
Atnak chal, the bark of Terminalia tomentosa, W. and A.
Bạrni rẹhẹl, the roots of Clerodendron infortunatum, L.
Tursi sakam, the leaves of Ocymum sanctum, Willd.
Ạtkir rẹhẹl, the roots of Smilax ovalifolia, Roxb.
Thoṛa rambṛa jaṅ, a few seeds of Phæseolus Mungo, var. Radiatus, L.
Nạ̃ṛĩ murup rẹhẹl, the roots of Butea superba, Roxb., or
Murup dare chal, the bark of Butea frondosa, Roxb.

Extract about 2 pounds of the juice of all these collectively, mix a little *sora*, saltpetre, and after stirring in *mạhũt guṛ*, the refuse of molasses, give him 2 ounces to drink at intervals, and soon afterwards he will urinate.

(*m*) Apply *mạhũt guṛ*, the refuse of molasses, on the abdomen up to the navel, and after sprinkling *sora*, saltpetre, thereon rub him, and then cover with a piece of white paper. He will urinate soon afterwards, and even if he has not done so for about a couple of days he will soon get relief.

(*n*) *Orop da*, the tuber of Costus speciosa, Sm.

Extract the juice of this and after mixing with the refuse of molasses give him to drink. Grind the tuber small and apply as an ointment.

(*o*) *Muṅgạ dare chal sẹ rẹhẹl*, the bark or roots of Moringa pterygosperma, Gärtn.
Pẹ gaṇḍa gol mạric, 12 black peppercorns.

Grind together and apply as an ointment on the abdomen; must not be taken internally.

(*p*) *Bhạbri jaṅ*, the seed of Embelia robusta, Roxb.
Haṭ jaṅ, ,, ,, ,, Holarrhena antidysenterica, Wall.

Grind, mix and give to drink, when he will urinate at once.

(*q*) *Patal kohṇḍa reak da*, the tuber of Pueraria tuberosa, DC.
Kamraj rẹhẹl, the roots of Buettneria herbacea, Roxb.
Upạl baha arakak, Nymphæa rubra, Roxb.
Mạhūt guṛ, the refuse of molasses.

Take the water from the first (like melted hail inside), and grind the next two, mix all together and give to drink once a day for three days.

(*r*) *Bhạbri chal*, the bark of Embelia robusta, Roxb.
Paṛọ da, the tuber of Curcuma angustifolia, Roxb.
Arak' meral sakam, the leaves of the red Phyllanthus Emblica, L.
Atnak chal, the bark of Terminalia tomentosa, W. and A.
Bạrni rẹhẹl, the roots of Clerodendron infortunatum, L.
Tursi sakam, the leaves of Ocymum sanctum, Willd.
Ạṭkir rẹhẹl, the roots of Smilax ovalifolia, Roxb.
Ramṛa jaṅ, the seeds of Phæseolus Mungo, var. Radiatus, L.
Nạṛī murup rẹhẹl, the roots of Butea superba, Roxb.

Pound all these together and take about two pounds of the juice, and mix a little *sora*, saltpetre, and *mạhūt guṛ*, refuse of molasses, therewith and give about a ladle full at intervals to drink. Apply also externally (*m*) as above.

(*s*) *Jugiạ rẹhẹl*, the roots of Cordia Macleodii, H. f. and T.
Kiṭạ maṅj, the heart of Phœnix acaulis, Buch.
Makaṛkenda rẹhẹl, the roots of Diospyros embryopteris, Pers.
Gaḍa terel, Diospyros montana, Roxb.
Dhiri banda,
Suntas,
Mạhūt gur, refuse of molasses.

Grind these together, then grind *adwa caole*, rice made from sun-dried, not boiled, paddy into meal, and after mixing it with above make into hand bread and put out into the dew, after which it is to be eaten. Do this daily and in three or four days it will be evident whether it is efficacious or not.

207. *Ekasiṛa.* Orchitis, Epidydimitis, or (so mostly) Hydrocele.

Symptoms. This is a very bad and troublesome male complaint, from which many men have to suffer all their life if medicine be not quickly applied.

Medicines: (*a*) *Aṇḍia moṛon aṛak ṛeheḷ*, the roots of Gymnema hirsutus, W. and A., var. Decaisneanum, Wight.

To be cooked in melted cows' butter and the place to be anointed therewith. If no such melted butter is to be had, apply the roots nevertheless only.

(*b*) *Akaona ṛeheḷ*, the roots of Calotropis gigantea, R.Br.

Daṭra ṛeheḷ, „ „ „ Datura alba, Willd. or D. fastuosa, Willd.

Aṇḍia moṛon aṛak ṛeheḷ, the roots of Gymnema hirsutus, W. and A., var. Decaisneanum, Wight.

Cook all these in melted cows' butter and apply externally, he is sure to get well.

(*c*) *Poṇḍ akaona ṛeheḷ*, the roots of the white-flowered Calotropis gigantea, R.Br.

To be ground and mixed with old rice water, and then applied externally to the spot.

(*d*) *Bir goṅgha*, the shell of a forest snail.

Leṇḍoṅ, the skeleton of a dead centipede.

Phuli paura, neat spirits.

Karhani hoṛo reak adwa caole, the rice made from the sun-dried product of a variety of black paddy.

Goṭe ṛeheḷ, the roots of Croton oblongifolius, Roxb.

Grind together and mixing it with neat spirit, make the patient drink it.

(*e*) *Aṇḍia moṛon aṛak ṛeheḷ*, the roots of Gymnema hirsutus, W. and A., var. Decaisneanum, Wight.

Apply as an ointment to the spot and he will surely get well.

(*f*) The same as in the preceding (*e*) and

Akaona ṛeheḷ, the roots of Calotropis gigantea, R.Br.

Daṭra ṛeheḷ, „ „ „ Datura alba, Willd. or D. fastuosa, Willd.

Dhũṛã, resin of Shorea robusta, Gärtn.

Gol maric thoṛa, a little black pepper.

Grind all these together, cook in melted butter of cows' milk and smear on; recovery is sure to follow.

(*g*) On Saturday evening put out *mit laṭi sutam*, a skein of thread, in the dew; on Sunday morning twist it into a cord of five strands and tie this in one breath to the big toe of the foot on the side that pains him, and make three striped marks across his forearm with *soso*, the fruit of Semecarpus Anacardium, L., and he will recover if the complaint is due to the wind; otherwise proceed with the following:

(*h*) First of all let him pretend to scratch himself with *bardũṛũč rama*, a bat's claws or nails, and then
Bhiḍi ạchim, Centifida orbicularis, Lour.
Mulạ, Raphanus sativus, L.
Bilạti thamakur, imported tobacco.

Grind these, pour on some *loa loṛe*, the sticky exudation from Ficus glomerata, Roxb., and cook the whole in *utiṅ sunum*, mustard oil, and let him smear this oil on, when he will recover provided it is not chronic, or it will take some time. This remedy is intended for application before it reaches a chronic stage.

(*i*) *Hãṛũ ič*, a baboon's excrement.
Kulại ič, a hare's „
Piskạ da, the tuber of Dioscorea oppositifolia, L.
Ekasirạ rẹhẹl, the roots of Crataeva religiosa, Forst.

Grind these with *sisir dak*, dew, and then
Bilạti thamakur, imported tobacco.
Gọč lẹnḍọṅ, the skeleton of a dead centipede.
Gạṅgiṭ cun, lime from nodular or hydraulic limestone.
Ạṇḍiạ mọrọn aṛak rẹhẹl, the roots of Gymnema hirsutus, W. and A., var. Decaisneanum, Wight.
Akaona rẹhẹl, the roots of Calotropis gigantea, R. Br., or C. procera, R. Br.
Dạtrạ rẹhẹl, the roots of Datura alba, Willd. or D. fastuosa, Willd.
Dhũṛã, resin of Shorea robusta, Gärtn.
Gol mạric, black pepper.

Cook all these in *gại gọtọm*, melted butter from cows' milk, and apply.

One "authority" says: In this the private parts swell up so that walking is difficult. It may arise from two causes, either from leading a licentious life, or from the wind being in a certain direction which causes pain and sets up the complaint.

208. *Gidrạko punik*. Infantile atrophy.

Symptoms. This occurs in infants both when the mother's milk is secreted and when it dries up. Whatever remedy is applied to the mother should also be applied to the child.

Medicines: (*a*) *Bẹrẹl sasaṅ bọhọk*, a knot of raw turmeric, Curcuma longa, R.
Ạṇḍiạ mọrọn aṛak rẹhẹl. the roots of Gymnema hirsutus, W. and A., var. Decaisneanum, Wight.

Grind these two together and saturate them with mustard oil. In the evening anoint or smear the child all over with this and let it stay till 9 o'clock the following morning. Then wash it off and give a fresh application of the same to stay on till the evening. Repeat this process daily till the child is well.

For the mother grind only the roots of the latter of above and make into pills to be administered thus. Let her take a mouthful of unboiled rice made from boiled paddy and chew and eat this after taking into the mouth one of the pills. This to be repeated daily for 7 or 8 days, then her milk will flow and the child put on flesh. Take the upper bark or roots of *bhorkonḍ dare*, Hymenodictyon excelsum, Wall., smash them into a pulp and smear the entire body of the child for about half a month.

(*b*) *Nanha pusi toa*, Euphorbia thymifolia, Burm.

Grind the whole plant and smear the child with this daily, giving the mother some of the same to drink, and you will see her milk will flow and the child get well.

(*c*) *Ḍel cẽṛẽ bele*, the egg of the humming bird.

To be broken, stirred together and a spoonful to be taken by the child.

(*d*) *Bhorkonḍ dare cetan reaṅ ręhęl*, the roots of Hymenodictyon excelsum, Wall.

Kuṛil rama cetan reaṅ cip ciṛip, Achyranthes aspera, L., found growing over Zizyphus oxyphylla, Edgew.

To be ground together and smeared on the child.

(*e*) *Ạnḍiạ mọrọn aṛak ręhęl*, the roots of Gymnema hirsutus, W. and A., var. Decaisneanum, Wight.

Bęręl sasaṅ bọhọk, a knot of raw turmeric, Curcuma longa, Roxb.

Give to drink along with *męrọm toa*, goats' milk, an immediate cure will follow.

(*f*) Grind the two ingredients of (*e*) above and saturate with *nirạ tuṛi sunum*, pure mustard oil. Anoint the child therewith every morning, wash it off at noon, smear it on again. At 3 P.M. again wash it off and re-apply letting it stay all night. Then in the morning wash it off and repeat the process daily till recovery.

(*g*) *Dare cetan bhorkonḍ chal, ręhęl sę sakam*, the bark, roots or leaves of Hymenodictyon excelsum, Wall., growing on trees.

Grind and saturate with turmeric in mustard oil and apply as in (*f*) above.

(*h*) Same as (*g*) preceding and

Sasaṅ bọhọk, a knot of turmeric, Curcuma longa, Roxb.

Adagạthiạ ręhęl, the roots of Panicum repens, L.

Stir after grinding in mustard oil and anoint therewith daily after bathing.

(*i*) *Bhuku chata*, a termites' nest.

Grind with the milk of a black cow who has also a black calf, stir in the same milk and smear on daily after bathing.

(*j*) *Bęręl sasaṅ bọhọk*, a knot of raw turmeric, Curcuma longa, L.

Saturate in mustard oil, and after washing off the first that you smeared on smear this on every evening.

(*k*) *Dare cetan bhorkonḍ chal*, the bark of Hymenodictyon excelsum, Wall., growing on trees.

Guriċ gaṇḍar, the larvæ of beetles found in middens of cowdung.

Ọp̣ọnọm, Angelica glauca, Edgew.

Bọhọk̄ sasań, a knot of turmeric, Curcuma longa, Roxb.

Grind these together, smear the child therewith, and girdle him with *alagjaṛi*, Cassytha filiformis, Roxb. If this alone is not efficacious apply along with it

(*l*) *Adagaṭhiạ*, Panicum repens, L.

Hẹndẹ gại toa, the milk of a black cow.

209. *Gidrạko ahak̄.* (Believed due to the evil eye.)

Symptoms. This is a spell cast generally on children; but sometimes also on adults. After it children cry, sometimes vomit, and after that have watery evacuations.

Medicines: (*a*) *Eraḍọm laṛtẹl*, the peeled bark of Ricinus communis, L.

With one breath bit off a strip of this and tie it on the child.

(*b*) *Ambṛa jań*, the seed of Spondias mangifera, Pers.

Take one of these that people have sucked and thrown away, grind it and give to drink; recovery is sure.

(*c*) *Laṭha cip̣ ciṛip̣ rẹhẹl*, the roots of

3 *gol mạric*, 3 black peppercorns.

Mix these and give to drink, and with the plant itself make a pass three times downwards and stick behind the ear, all in one breath.

(*d*) *Ḍhaḍra haṭak*, an old worn out winnowing fan.

Mil kuṭrạ ṭhuṭki jọnọk̄ jeleń uṭạrak̄ 3 *carẹċ*, the 3 longest bits of an old worn out broom.

Milṭań sọsọ jań, a seed of Semecarpus Anacardium, L.

Let the child touch these and then the mother with one breath make three passes over the child, and then let the medicine giver take all and throwing them on the top of their roof go straight home.

210. *Bale gidrạko uchlạu.* Infants' vomiting.

Medicines: (*a*) *Jạnum jạmbir chal*, the bark of a thorny Citrus medica, L.

Kaera sakam, a leaf of Musa paradisiaca, L.

Dhiri kaṭkọm jańga sẹ họṛmọtẹl, the leg or body of a crab found under stones.

Ulḍhạ da, the tuber of a Nymphæa.

Wrap the first in the second and warm it, and squeeze the water out into a cup. Take the juice of the last two, and give all to drink.

(*b*) *Toyo sagak̄ rẹhẹl*, the roots of

Jạnum aṛak̄ rẹhẹl, „ „ „ Amaranthus spinosus, Willd.

Grind these together and give to eat with *ńẹlẹ rasa*, honey.

211. *Bale gidrạ toageko cidir khan.* (When babies pass milky stools.)

Medicines: *Sikuạr rẹhẹl*, the roots of

Grind and make to drink.

212. *Bale gidrạ goh.* (Infants' summer diarrhoea.)

Symptoms. Infants pass black motions.

Medicines: (*a*) *Ńũṛũć chal*, the bark of Cassia Fistula, L.

Hẹmsagọr da, the bulb of Cotyledon laciniata, Willd.

Thoṛa cun, a little lime.

Nim chal, the bark of Melia Azadirachta, L.

Grind and mix these, and after warming a little plaster the stomach and whole body, or the mother too may drink it.

(*b*) *Lọpọṅ aṛak*, Aerua lanata, L.

Wrap in leaves, roast in embers and give the mother to eat.

213. *Sea sahẹl.* Foul breath. (Ozaena ?)

Symptoms. In this the breath is offensive and there is a mucous discharge from the nose resembling lichen or mould in colour.

Medicines: (*a*) Cook *goṭe chal*, the bark of Croton oblongifolius, Roxb., in mustard oil, and make into pills to be eaten.

(*b*) *Goṭe chal*, the bark of Croton oblongifolius, Roxb.

Cuṭiạ bardũṛũć, a kind of small bat.

Cook in mustard oil, let him sniff some up the nose, and smear some over the face. Let him also eat a little.

One "authority" says to grind above first, using the roots instead of the bark of the former, otherwise the same, and to apply three or four times.

214. *Dọyọk.* Nausea and vomiting.

Medicines: (*a*) *Bardũṛũć ulạwak*, what a bat has spat out.

Ạimại satekore upko sọgẹkak, the hairs that women stick into the eaves of a house.

Singe the hairs and then grind both together and give to drink.

If this is not efficacious then mix with above

(*b*) *Puṭki rẹhẹl*, the roots of Scirpus rotundus.

(*c*) *Marak pĩńc reak mẹ̃l*, the eye of a peacock's tail.

Tale ḍạnḍil, the stem of the leaves of Borassus flabelliformis, L.

Foment the latter and extract the juice, and in this mix the former and after mixing *dumur rasa*, the honey of the small honey bee, give to drink.

215. *Uchlạu.* Vomiting.

Medicines: *Uṭki rẹhẹl*, the roots of

Tursi sakam (*thoṛa*), a few leaves of Ocymum sanctum, Willd.

Grind together and give to drink.

216. *Sereṛ sereṛ aikauk.* Nausea.

Symptoms. This may arise when one sees something one longs for being eaten, or without known cause, or from the presence of worms in the stomach.

Medicines: *Nim sakam*, the leaves of Melia Azadirachta, L.
Sinjo sakam, the leaves of Ægle Marmelos, Correa.
Soso jaṅ, the seeds of Semecarpus Anacardium, L.

Fry and dry the first two, and half roast the third, 3 seeds for a child or 5 to 7 seeds for an adult. Take also some *khoi ata*, rice parched in a particular way; then make all into a meal and give every morning 3 to 5 leaf-spoons full to eat, which will cure.

217. *Dub ḍubia.*

Symptoms. There is a feeling of repletion in the stomach the result of over-eating, which may induce diarrhoea.

Medicines: (*a*) *Kuinḍi sunum*, oil obtained from the seed of Bassia latifolia, Roxb.

Rub this over the stomach and apply *lolo toroć*, hot ashes, to the navel, when the stomach will relax.

(*b*) *Pudin aṛak*, mint, Mentha sativa, Willd.
Buluṅ, salt.

A mixture of these to be eaten.

218. *Laćre kusur tahẹnre julap ran.*

An aperient in cases of stomach derangement, specially indigestion.

Medicines: *Ẹtkẹć loṛe tala choṭak gan*, about an ounce of the sticky exudation of Euphorbia antiquorum, L.
2 *sẹ* 3 *gan mutha da*, some 2 or 3 bulbs of Fimbristylis monostachya, Hassk.

Grind the latter and mix with former. Grind also *thoṛa buluṅ*, a little salt, and *thoṛa sasaṅ*, a little Curcuma longa, Roxb., and mix with above and *tala pawa gan hoṛo caole reak holon*, about two ounces of rice flour, and after baking in leaves give to eat. After eating a little hot water must be drunk three or four times, when watery motions will commence. Continue the hot water drinking until the desired number of motions have been passed, and when it is wanted to stop them drink some cold water which will stop them. The *ẹtkẹć loṛe* must be fresh, as if stale it will be poisonous.

219. *Kosa sẹ jhaṛa bako phirau.* Constipation or obstruction.

Medicines: (*a*) *Misri cini*, sugar-candy.
Adhẹ, ginger, Zingiber officinalis, Roscoe.
Gol maric, black pepper.

Grind all these together and let the patient eat it.

(*b*) *Jāwān jira*, Carum Ajowan, DC. & Carum Carui, L.
Bẹrẹl adhẹ, raw ginger.

Choṭa hạrlạ, Terminalia Chebula, Retz.
Biṭ buluṅ, a factitious salt containing sulphur.

Grind these together and let him eat it, drinking about four ounces of hot water, and the bowels will be opened.

(*c*) *Bẹrẹl adhẹ*, raw ginger.
Ca, tea.

Mix and boil together and let the patient drink it after mixing salt in it, and he will be all right.

220. *Pithi rọg*. ? Urticaria and Dyspepsia.

Medicines: *Sasaṅ baha*, the flower of Curcuma longa, Roxb.
Hẹmsagọr, Cotyledon laciniata, Willd.
Sọsọ jaṅ, the seed of Semecarpus Anacardium, L., var. cuneifolia.
Cẹrcẹṭẹc̓, a lizard.
Paṅjọt sakam, the leaves of Clerodendron phlomoides, L. fil.
Kasmar chal, the bark of Gmelina arborea, Roxb.
Moṭa dare japak̓, Scindapsus officinalis, Schott.
Dare bạṅki, Vanda Roxburghii, R. Br.
Bana haṭak̓, Oroxylon indicum, Benth.
Buc chal, the bark of Cordia Myxa, L.

Pound all these, mix and give to drink.

221. *Kạchmạ*. (lit. tortoise.)

Symptoms. A hard swelling arises in the stomach like a small brass cup or a tortoise, hence the name.

Medicines: *Adagạthiạ rẹhẹl*, the roots of Panicum repens, L.
Jhankaṛa rẹhẹl, „ „ „ Thysanolæna acarifera, Nees.
Poṇḍ rạsun, white garlic.
Kạhu botke da, the bulb of Bryonia lacinosa, L.
Gol mạric, black pepper corns.
Thoṛa buluṅ atakate, a little salt fried.

Grind all together and give to drink, or else mix with some *pạurạ*, spirits, and give a little every morning to drink until recovery.

222. *Paṭha sẹ Koema*. (Constipation, obstruction.)

Symptoms. In this there is a swelling in the stomach like a young frog.

Medicines: (*a*) *Kạhu botke da*, the bulb of Bryonia lacinosa, L.
Adhẹ, ginger.
Mọrọn aṛak̓ da, the bulb of Gymnema hirsutus, W. and A., var. Decaisneanum, Wight.
Gol mạric, black pepper.

Grind these with water and make into pills to be swallowed.

(*b*) *Hesak chal*, the bark of Ficus religiosa, Willd.

Grind and give to drink.

(*c*) *Bidhạnta chal*, the bark of Entada scandens, Benth. Pound with water and give to drink; then shortly afterwards stir *buluṅ*, salt, in a brass-cup full of water that is sold for 8 annas, and let him drink it.

(*d*) *Ato piṇḍạ da*, the bulb of Amorphophallus campanulatus, Blume.
Kalmẹg, Andrographis paniculata, Nees.
Kạhu botke da, the bulb of Bryonia lacinosa, L.
Saoraj, Vernonia anthelmintica, Roxb.

Grind these and when the swelling rises give some to drink mixed with half a leaf-cupful of either *pạurạ*, spirits, or hot water.

223. *Puṭi*. Constipation with meteorismus.

Medicines: (*a*) *Laṭha cip cirip*,
Gol mạric, black pepper.

Grind and give to drink.

(*b*) *Lọṭọ jọ*, the fruit of Randia dumetorum, Lam.

Grind, warm and smear all round the navel, and give a little to drink.

(*c*) *Nanha lẹṇḍẹl aṛak*,

Grind and give to drink with *bạli guṛ*, crystallized raw sugar.

(*d*) Roasted *siṅjọ sakam*, leaves of Ægle Marmelos, Correa.
Thoṛa kalmẹg rẹhẹl, a little of the roots of Andrographis paniculata, Nees.
Buluṅ, salt.
Khạḍi tọrọć, the ashes of Indian corn cobs.
Saoraj, Vernonia anthelmintica, Roxb.

Mix these and give to drink.

(*e*) *Lọṭọ jọ*, the fruit of Randia dumetorum, Lam.
Kuiṇḍi kaṛe, oilcake left after extracting the oil from the kernel of Bassia latifolia, Roxb.
Nun juạn, salt and Carum Ajowan, DC.
Kạliạ jirạ, Nigella indica, Roxb.
Siṅjọ sakam, the leaves of Ægle Marmelos, Correa.

Fry, grind and give to drink.

(*f*) *Goṭe rẹhẹl*, the roots of Croton oblongifolius, Roxb.
Buluṅ, salt.

Grind these together and give to drink daily, and he will get well.

(*g*) *Sega rẹhẹl*, the roots of Mimosa rubicaulis, Lamk.
Badgọcak rẹhẹl, the roots of Lygodium flexuosum, Sw.
Nanha dudhi loṭa rẹhẹl, the roots of Ichnocarpus frutescens, R. Br.

Grind these together and give to drink daily, a quick recovery will follow.

(*h*) *Kuṇḍi kaṛe*, oilcake left after extracting the oil from the kernel of Bassia latifolia, Roxb.

Pudin aṛak, mint, Mentha sativa, Willd.

Warm the former and apply as a plaster over the stomach and give the latter to eat. Wait and see if gas is voided; if not, then proceed to

(*i*) *Tursi sakam*, the leaves of Ocymum sanctum, Willd.

Haṭ dạl, the kernel of the fruit of Holarrhena antidysenterica, Wall.

Goṭe rẹhẹl, the roots of Croton oblongifolius, Roxb.

Pea gol mạric, 3 black peppercorns.

Saoraj, Vernonia anthelmintica, Roxb.

Grind all these together and give to drink; it will be followed by the voidance of the gas and a loose motion.

224. *Rọs piti ruạ*. (Indigestion.)

Symptoms. This may occur in either children or adults. If one has eaten a surfeit of anything savoury, from that day the humours of the body increase, and later they get sick. They vomit bile freely and have a severe headache.

Medicines: (*a*) *Sega rẹhẹl*, the roots of Mimósa rubicaulis, Lam.

Pound and give to drink, when the humours will be absorbed or dissipated.

(*b*) 25 *gaṇḍa gol mạric*, 100 black peppercorns.

Laṭha cip ciṛip,

Adhẹ, ginger, Zingiber officinalis, Roscoe.

Bọc, the root of Acorus Calamus, Willd.

Grind these and make into pills, one to be taken each morning, noon and evening.

For children: *Darcini*, cinnamon.

Adhẹ, ginger.

Ṅẹlẹ rasa, honey.

Grind the first two together, mix with the third and give to eat.

225. *Sukạn pit*. (Indigestion.)

Symptoms. If a person eats a meal after the usual time his bowels will be confined, *i.e.* they will not be moved as usual. He will get headache at sunrise, have catarrh and cough.

Medicines: (*a*) Boil *gại toa*, cows' milk, with *guṛ*, molasses, or *cini*, sugar, and let him drink it warm, and on his bowels being moved he will get well.

(*b*) *Laṭha cip ciṛip rẹhẹl*, the roots of

Pẹ gaṇḍa gol mạric, 12 black peppercorns.

Thoṛa gulạñj baha dare chal, a little of the bark of Plumeria acutifolia, Poiret.

Pound all these, extract 2 ounces of the juice and give to drink, which will open the bowels.

226. *Ič ado bondok.* Retentio urinæ et fæcum.

Medicines: (*a*) Add to the ingredients detailed in No. 223 (*h*) and (*i*)
Dare cetan hesak rehet chal, the bark of the surface roots of Ficus religiosa, Willd.

Grind all together, and give to drink.

If the patient is a baby take only
(*b*) *Saoraj*, Vernonia anthelmintica, Roxb.

Grind and let the child lick it.

(*c*) *Bonga sarjom rehet chal*, the bark of the roots of Ventilago calyculata, Tulasne.
Sukri dhumbak, pig's excrement.

Grind these together, stir in *utin sunum*, mustard oil, and apply over the whole abdomen.

227. *Sokhao.* Parching thirst.

Symptoms. In this the saliva dries up and there is intense thirst, sometimes without fever.

Medicines: (*a*) *Dak icak rehet*, the roots of Jussiæa suffruticosa, Linn.
Gargadi rehet, „ „ „ Coix lachryma, Willd.
Gol maric, black pepper.
Bar chimbri gan rasun, about a couple of clusters of garlic.

Grind these four together and let the patient drink the juice, he will get well.

(*b*) *Jithimond*, Clerodendron Siphonanthus, R. Br.
Halim, Lapidium sativum, Linn.

Soak both in water, and let the patient drink that water, he will get well.

228. *Tetan maraok.* (to quench thirst).

If you are suffering from parching thirst chew
Jithimond, Clerodendron Siphonanthus, R. Br.

and swallow the juice, which will quench the thirst.

229. *Lač haso.* Stomach-ache.

Medicines: (*a*) *Hat rehet, jan, jo se chal*, the roots, seed, fruit or bark of Holarrhena antidysenterica, Wall.
Sahra chal, the bark of Streblus asper, Lour.
Tejo mala rehet, the roots of Cissampelos Pareira, L.

Grind and give to drink.

(*b*) *Dhela chal*, the bark of Alangium Lamarckii, Thws.
Sahra chal, „ „ „ Streblus asper, Lour.
Bir catom arak rehet, the roots of

Grind and give to drink.

(*c*) *Pẹtcambṛa rẹhẹl*, the roots of Helicteres Isora, L.
Kuclạ, Strychnos potatorum, Lin. f.

Rub these with water, add 2 or 3 *hạlim jań*, seeds of Lepidium sativum, L., and give to drink.

(*d*) *Kạńji dak*, stale rice water.
Küs rẹhẹl, the roots of Themuda gigantea, Haskel.
Teke caole sok lopol, the powdery remains of rice boiled prior to husking after it has been cleaned.

Grind the second with the first and after mixing the third give to drink.

(*e*) *Ạtkuṛạ chal*, the bark of Wrightia tomentosa, R. and S.
should be added to each of the above.

(*f*) *Kalmẹg*, Andrographis paniculata, Nees.
Pańjọt, Clerodendron phlomoides, Willd.

Grind and give to drink. May also be used for colic.

(*g*) *Tejo mala rẹhẹl*, the roots of Cissampelos Pareira, L.

To be chewed and then swallowed.

230. *Tẹmẹć lać haso.* Colic.

Medicines: (*a*) *Jọm jạnum dare chal*, the bark of Zizyphus Jujuba, Lam.

Extract the juice from this, add a little *buluń*, salt, and give to drink; an immediate cure will follow.

(*b*) *Jọm jạnum rẹhẹl*, the roots of Zizyphus Jujuba, Lam.

Grind, mix well with *buluń*, salt, and give to drink.

N.B.—This may also be given for ordinary stomach-ache.

231. *Khokraok leka lać haso.* Griping pains in the stomach.

Medicines: (*a*) *Jọm jạnum rẹhẹl*, the roots of Zizyphus Jujuba, Lam.
Sarjọm chal, the bark of Shorea robusta, Gärtn.

Grind these and after squeezing out the juice give to drink.

(*b*) *Tạṇḍi catọm aṛak*, Desmodiun triflorum, DC.
Dare japak, Scindapsus officinalis, Schott.

These two to be chewed and the juice swallowed.

232. *Lać hạḍ hạḍ sạḍere.* When there is a rumbling noise in the stomach.

Medicines: (*a*) Grind *pọjọ chal*, the bark of Tetranthera monopetala, Roxb.

And if there is great pain grind *bẹrdọṛ rẹhẹl*, the roots of Combretum nanum, Hamilt., and give to drink.

(*b*) *Terel cẹtẹ*, the thin skin on the bark of Diospyros tomentosa, Roxb.

Grind with water and give to drink.

(*c*) *Tejo mala rẹhẹl*, the roots of Cissampelos Pareira, L.

To be chewed and the juice swallowed.

(*d*) *Kalmẹg*, *Pańjọt*, } same as No. 229 (*f*).

233. *Khakharni lac haso.*

Medicines: *Terel rehel*, the roots of Diospyros tomentosa, Roxb.

Bonkapsi rehel, the roots of Thespesia Lampas, Benth. & Hook. f.

Petcambra jo, the fruit of Helicteres Isora, L.

Grind these three together and take the juice, and give to drink with the milk of *hende merom*, a black goat: he will speedily get well.

234. *Ringor rongor lac haso.* (Chronic stomach-ache).

Medicines: *Murga chal*, the bark of Pterocarpus Marsupium, Roxb.

Satsayar, Dalbergia latifolia, Roxb.

Jom lar chal, the bark of Bauhinia Vahlii, W. and A.

Cihut lar chal, „ „ „ Spatholobus Roxburghii, Benth.

Atnak chal, „ „ „ Terminalia tomentosa, W. and A.

Caole ata rongo, rice fried to burning point.

Sinjo sakam, the leaves of Ægle Marmelos, Correa.

Boil all these together, and give the water to drink daily; speedy cure.

235. *Khala dobha.*

Symptoms. This arises in the stomach, is very painful, and the stomach heaves and falls greatly in breathing and the ribs seem to recede. (Only children).

Medicines: *Dabha jo reak rasa*, the juice of the fruit of Citrus Aurantium, Willd.

Dare tipoc,

Gai ghura, Polygala chinensis, L.

Kaudi cun, lime made from the shells used as money in India.

Grind together and give to drink.

236. *Pande then haso buka latarre.*

Symptoms. This pain in the abdomen below the navel may result from *hadi* (No. 88), owing to a *sir* being strained with some congestion of blood.

Medicines: *Gote rehel*, the roots of Croton oblongifolius, Roxb.

Ohoc arak rehel, the roots of Boerhaavia procumbens, Herb. Banks.

Miltan gol maric, 1 black peppercorn.

Grind these together and give a little to drink, and plaster some over the abdomen.

237. *Nar betha.* (? biliary colic).

Symptoms. In this there is intense piercing pain at the navel causing the patient to be doubled up, and if medicine be not given quickly it may prove fatal.

Medicines: Till the following can be got, rub the patient with oil vigorously and afterwards burn him with the point of a red hot sickle; then procure

Ạsạrią, Capparis horrida, L.f.
Bana hatạk, Oroxylon indicum, Benth.
Riḍe, Casearia tomentosa, Roxb.
Lilkạthi, Polygala crotalarioides, Buch. and Ham.
Ḍhela, Alangium Lamarckii, Thws.
Karam ṭusạ, a shoot of Adina cordifolia, H. F. and B.
Kod ṭusạ, „ „ „ Eugenia Jambolana, Lamk.
Guą, Areca Catechu, L.
Pan, Piper Betle, L.
Tojo mala, Cissampclos Parcira, L.
Kạhu botke, Bryonia lacinosa, L.
Suruj mukhi, Helianthus annuus, Willd.
Lilibichi,
Arak upḍal baha, Nymphæa rubra, Roxb.
Mahũt guṛ, refuse of molasses.

Grind all these together and mix them, and give to drink thrice daily, viz. morning, noon and evening, and he will get well in three days.

238. *Ponḍ risạ sẹ gurjukaṭa.* Prolapsus ani, also Fistula ani.

Symptoms. This disease has its origin in the tenesmus of dysentery, and results in *prolapsus ani*.

Medicines: (*a*) *Kabab cini*, Cubebs piper.
Ramṛa, Phæseolus Mungo, var. Radiatus, L.
Dhũṛã, resin of Shorea robusta, Gärtn.
Darcini, cinnamon.

Stir these in *gọtọm sunum*, melted butter, and smear on, and then after warming your foot push in the protuberance with it.

(*b*) *Kumbiṛ baha*, the flower of Careya arborea, Roxb.
Họrọ bọhọk, the head of a tortoise.

The latter to be roasted and eaten and some of it to be ground with the former into a powder and eaten.

(*c*) *Ọhọć aṛak rẹhẹl*, the roots of Boerhaavia procumbens, Herb. Banks.
Hẹndẹ mẹrọmak māyām, the blood of a black goat.

Cook or boil these together and give to eat.

(*d*) *Ḍhela poha rẹhẹl*, the roots of a seedling of Alangium Lamarckii, Thws.

Mix this with the milk of an entirely white cow who has also a white calf, 16 oz. for an adult and half that for a child, boil and give to drink for three days.

(*e*) *Gạrunḍi aṛak, sakam sẹ rẹhẹl*, the leaves or roots of Acternanthera sessilis, R. Br.

Laṭha cip ciṛip ręhęt, the roots of
Ḍhąkni aṛak,

Grind these together and give to eat after mixing up with *taben*, rice soaked and flattened, *dahe*, curds, and a little salt.

(*f*) *Kaḍęčte tejoko oṛag, ona kaḍęč*, the sticks with which certain insects make their "house."
Kaskǫm bąṅgąura, cotton seeds.

Fry the latter to burning point, reduce both by grinding to a powder, and after anointing the spot with melted butter, sprinkle the powder on and foment.

(*g*) *Hǫręč dąl*, the split pulse of Dolichos biflorus, L.
Sasaṅ, turmeric, Curcuma longa, Roxb.

Cook together and give to eat.

(*h*) *Dub biląsi ręhęt*, the roots of
Bęręl adhę, raw ginger, Zingiber officinalis, Roscoe.
Kąlią jiṛą, Nigella indica, Roxb.
Jawan jiṛą, Carum Ajowan, DC. & Carum Carui, L.

Grind, boil in milk to the consistency of porridge and give to eat.

(*i*) *Bir buṭ*, Flemingia congesta, Roxb.
Saram lutur, Clerodendron serratum, Spreng.
Bǫnkąpsi, Thespesia Lampas, Benth. & Hook. f.

Grind and give to drink for three days.

(*j*) *Terel cętę*, the thin skin on the bark of Diospyros tomentosa, Roxb.

Grind small, cook in *gǫtǫm*, melted butter of cows' milk and give to eat.

239. *Bhąlki lač haso.* (Colic ? biliary).

Medicines: (*a*) *Haṭ chal, jǫ sę jaṅ*, the bark, fruit or kernel of Holarrhena antidysenterica, Wall.
Sahṛa chal, the bark of Streblus asper, Lour.
Tejo mala ręhęt, the roots of Cissampelos Pareira, L.

Grind these and give to drink.

(*b*) *Ḍhela chal*, the bark of Alangium Lamarckii, Thws.
Sahṛa chal, " " " Streblus asper, Lour.
Bir catǫm aṛak ręhęt, the roots of

Grind these and give to drink.

(*c*) *Pętcambṛa ręhęt*, the roots of Helicteres Isora, L.
Kucla, Strychnos potatorum, Lin. f.

Rub these two in water, add two or three seeds of *hąlim*, Lepidium sativum, L., and give to drink.

(*d*) *Kąṅji dak*, stale rice water.
Kũs ręhęt, the roots of Themuda gigantea, Haskel.
Teke caole reak sok lopot, the powdery remains of cleaned rice that was boiled when it was paddy.

Grind the second with the first and then mixing with the third give to drink.

(*e*) *Aṭkuṛạ chal*, the bark of Wrightia tomentosa, R. and S.

A little of this is to be added to each of the above four remedies.

Khokraoko leka hak̃so khan. If there are griping pains:

(*f*) *Jǫm jạnum rẹhẹl*, the roots of Zizyphus Jujuba, Lamk.
Sarjǫm chal, the bark of Shorea robusta, Gärtn.

Grind these together, squeeze out and give to drink.

(*g*) *Tạṇḍi catǫm aṛak*, Desmodium triflorum, DC.
Dare japak̃, Scindapsus officinalis, Schott.

Let him chew these and swallow the juice.

(*h*) *Pǫjǫ chal*, the bark of Tetranthera monopetala, Roxb.

Grind and give to drink, and if he has severe pain:

Bẹrdǫṛ rẹhẹl, the roots of Combretum nanum, Hamilt.

Grind and give to drink.

(*i*) *Terel cẹṭẹ*, the thin skin on the bark of Diospyros tomentosa, Roxb.

Grind with water, mix with the milk of a black goat and give to drink.

(*j*) *Tejo mala rẹhẹl*, the roots of Cissampelos Pareira, L.

To be chewed and swallowed.

(*k*) *Kalmẹg*, Andrographis paniculata, Nees.
Pańjǫt, Clerodendron phlomoides, Willd.

Grind and give to drink.

240. *Lac̓ oḍokok̓.* Ordinary diarrhoea.

Medicines: (*a*) *Kod ṭusạ*, a shoot of Eugenia Jambolana, Lamk.

Grind and make into a thin soup, add *mẹrǫm toa*, goats' milk, and give to drink.

(*b*) *Gote rẹhẹl*, the roots of Croton oblongifolius, Roxb.
Haṭ rẹhẹl, „ „ „ Holarrhena antidysenterica, Wall.
Ambṛa chal, the bark of Spondias mangifera, Pers.
Tejo mala rẹhẹl, the roots of Cissampelos Pareira, L.
Sadǫm ic̓, horse dung.

Grind all together and give to drink.

241. *Birsạha lac̓ oḍok.* Watery diarrhoea.

Medicines: (*a*) *Bir sẹ tạṇḍi catǫm aṛak rẹhẹl*, the roots of or the roots of Desmodium triflorum, DC.

Grind and give to drink.

(*b*) *Piṇḍe chal*, the bark of Randia uliginosa, DC.
Hẹsẹl ḍǫg, a tip or bud of Anogeissus latifolia, Wall.
Terel dǫg, „ „ „ „ „ Diospyros tomentosa, Roxb.
Aphim mit rǫ bǫhǫk, opium the size of a fly's head.

Arak meral sakam, the leaves of the red Phyllanthus Emblica, L.

Grind these and give to drink.

(c) *Terel jo̜ reak gabe*, the flesh of the fruit of Diospyros tomentosa, Roxb.

Cihũṭ laṛ re̜he̜l, the roots of Spatholobus Roxburghii, Benth.

Rot chal, the bark of Ougeenia dalbergioides, Benth.

Ga̜ruṇḍi re̜he̜l, the roots of Acternanthera sessilis, R. Br.

Grind these with water very thin, squeeze out and after sprinkling a little lime on give him to drink.

(d) Grind the kernel of the fruit of Shorea robusta, Gärtn. and give him to drink.

Ja̜num lobok, the ground stones of Zizyphus Jujuba, Lamk.

and let him eat the latter also.

(e) *Ḍoka chal*, the bark of Odina Wodier, Roxb., to be ground and drunk.

(f) *Adagaṭhia̜ da*, the bulb of Panicum repens, L.

Kalme̜g thoṛa, a little Andrographis paniculata, Nees.

Cato̜m aṛak re̜he̜l, the roots of Marsilia quadrifolia, L.

Grind and give to drink.

(g) *Baṛe chal*, the bark of Ficus bengalensis, L.

Sahṛa chal, „ „ „ Streblus asper, Lour.

Sarjo̜m chal, „ „ „ Shorea robusta, Gärtn.

Bo̜d laṛ re̜he̜l, the roots of Vitis adnata, Wall.

Kedok aṛak re̜he̜l, the roots of Argyreia speciosa, Sweet.

Grind and give to drink.

(h) *Ambṛa chal*, the bark of Spondias mangifera, Pers.

Khode baha re̜he̜l, the roots of

Capot re̜he̜l, „ „ „ Desmodium cephalotes.

Haṭ jo̜ reak da̜l, the kernel of the fruit of Holarrhena antidysenterica, Wall.

Grind and give to drink.

(i) *Ḍoka chal*, the bark of Odina Wodier, Roxb.

Nun jua̜n, salt and Carum Ajowan, DC.

Siṅjo̜ sakam, the leaves of Ægle Marmelos, Correa.

(j) Make three or four holes in a *peaj*, onion, and insert some *a̜phim*, opium, therein, cook in the fire and give to eat. Also give the juice of *kod*, Eugenia Jambolana, Lamk. to drink.

(k) *Bana haṭak re̜he̜l*, the roots of Oroxylon indicum, Benth.

Ul chal, the bark of Mangifera indica, L.

Sahṛa chal, the bark of Streblus asper, Lour.

Ḍhalka cato̜m aṛak re̜he̜l, the roots of

Suruj mukhi nāṛī rehet, the roots of Helianthus annuus, Willd.

Grind these together, mix in a 4 anna brass-cupful of water, add a little *cun*, shell lime, and after stirring well give to drink. After drinking three times he should recover, but if not, then add the following and give to drink:

(*l*) *Terel jer*, the sticky exudation of Diospyros tomentosa, Roxb.
Rol chal, the bark of Terminalia Chebula, Retz.
Ḍodhar, Adiantum lunulatum, Burm. or A. concinnum.

242. *Sea bele lekako oḍokokre.* When the excreta are like rotten eggs.

Medicines: (*a*) *Aṇḍia moron arak rehet*, the roots of Gymnema hirsutus, W. and A., var. Decaisneanum, Wight.

Grind and give it to him to lick.

(*b*) *Goṭe rehet*, the roots of Croton oblongifolius, Roxb.

Grind and give him to drink daily.

243. *Kitạ kaṭao.*

If there is an epidemic of cholera, small pox or cattle disease which has reached your neighbourhood, you call on the people of your village to take measures to ward it off. If no one will listen to you then you yourself, or with as many more as will act with you, take action to ward it off from your own house or houses; this is called *kitạ kaṭao*.

Procedure: *Akaona ṭhenga ar chal*, a stick and the bark of Calotropis gigantea, R. Br., or C. procera, R. Br.

Take these with as many as you intend, and after naming *Dharti mae* offer in sacrifice a *hende kaloṭ*, a black pullet; dig a hole and bury the pullet in it with

Akaona chal, the bark of Calotropis gigantea, R. Br. or C. procera, R. Br.
Ḍunḍukil chal, the bark of Gardenia turgida, Roxb.
Bana haṭak chal, „ „ „ Oroxylon indicum, Benth.

and in the name of the spirits *Bon duạr* and *Kạlinath* make strokes of red lead and repeat the *mantar* formula. If you remain immune for a year you offer sacrifice. Cp. p. 143–4.

244. *Hawa duk se marań laċ oḍok.* Cholera.

Medicines: (a) *Ul chal*, the bark of the mango tree, Mangifera indica, L.
Sarjom chal, the bark of Shorea robusta, Gärtn.
Kadam chal, „ „ „ Anthocephalus Cadamba, Benth. and Hook. f.

Grind these three together, squeeze out the juice and give this with a little shell lime very quickly to drink. If there is no amelioration then give the juice of the first two mixed with opium the size of a pea to drink.

(*b*) *Sahṛa chal*, the bark of Streblus asper, Lour.
Ḍoka chal, „ „ „ Odina Wodier, Roxb.

Take the juice of both, mix with opium the size of a pea and give to drink.

(c) *Haṭ chal*, the bark of Holarrhena antidysenterica, Wall.

Tejo mala ręhęt, the roots of Cissampelos Pareira, Linn.

Grind these together, squeeze out the juice and mixing with opium the size of a pea, give to drink.

(d) *Atnak̄ chal*, the bark of Terminalia tomentosa, W. and A.

Hęsęl chal, „ „ „ Anogeissus latifolia, Wall.

Lọpọṅ chal, „ „ „ Terminalia bellerica, Roxb.

Mix these and give to drink.

(e) *Terel jẹr*, the resin of Diospyros tomentosa, Roxb.

Ul koyo reak̄ dạl, the pulverised kernel of a mango stone.

Mix and grind the size of a pea of the former with the latter, when the purging, vomiting and suppression of urine, if the last has occurred, will cease at once.

Gulạṅj baha ręhęt chal, the bark of the roots of Plumeria acutifolia, Poiret.

Akaona ręhęt, the roots of Calotropis gigantea, R. Br.

Chạtni chal, the bark of Alstonia scholaris, R. Br.

Gol mạric, black pepper.

Grind these together and plaster the abdomen therewith and give a little to drink.

(f) *Jhiṅjiṭ chal*, the bark of Bauhinia retusa, Roxb.

Grind and squeeze out the juice and give some 2 ounces of the juice to drink, he will be stopped.

(g) *Niuri chal*, the bark of Elæodendron Roxburghii, W. and A.

Grind about 3 ounces of this, squeeze out the juice and give to drink. If this be ineffective, then mix the same quantity of

Bir hoṛẹć, Atyllosia scarabædois, Benth.

and give to drink.

(h) *Goṭe ręhęt*, the roots of Croton oblongifolius, Roxb.

Sega ręhęt, „ „ „ Mimosa rubicaulis, Lam.

Grind these two and give about 2 ounces to drink.

(i) *Terel chal*, the bark of Diospyros tomentosa, Roxb.

Hęsęl chal, „ „ „ Anogeissus latifolia, Wall.

Grind and give to drink.

To quench the thirst in cholera:

(j) *Ul chal*, the bark of Mangifera indica, L.

Sarjọm chal, „ „ „ Shorea robusta, Gärtn.

Kadam chal, „ „ „ Anthocephalus Cadamba, Benth. and Hook. f.

Hesak̄ chal, „ „ „ Ficus religiosa, Willd.

Ḍoka chal, „ „ „ Odina Wodier, Roxb.

Ambṛa chal, the bark of Spondias mangifera, Pers.

Orop chal, „ „ „ Costus speciosa, Sm.

Kadar ṛẹhẹt, the roots of Bonnaya veronicæfolia, Spreng.

Nanha dudhi loṭa ṛẹhẹt, the roots of Ichnocarpus frutescens, R. Br.

Bir hoṛẹć, Atyllosia scarabædois, Benth.

Bana haṭak chal, the bark of Oroxylon indicum, Benth.

Mix a little of all these and give to drink, when the thirst will be quenched.

(*k*) *Nim chal,* the bark of Melia Azadirachta, L.

Haṛam siṅjo chal, „ „ „ an old Ægle Marmelos, Correa.

sẹ sakam, or its leaves.

Sarjọm dhũṛạ̃, the resin of Shorea robusta, Gärtn.

Ul koyo reak dạl, the pulverized kernel of a mango stone.

Grind all these, *i.e.* first the two barks and take their juice, then mix and add the last two, and give the mixture to drink. If the above mentioned ingredients are not soon obtainable in order to quench the thirst, then anyhow get

(*l*) *Hesak chal,* the bark of Ficus religiosa, Willd.

Ḍoka chal, „ „ „ Odina Wodier, Roxb.

Grind them together and give a little at a time to drink.

If blood is present in cholera:—

(*m*) *Bir buṭ ṛẹhẹt,* the roots of Flemingia congesta, Roxb.

Binḍi muthạ ṛẹhẹt, the roots of Fimbristylis monostachya, Hassk.

Nanha dudhi loṭa ṛẹhẹt, the roots of Ichnocarpus frutescens, R. Br.

Seta kaṭa ṛẹhẹt, the roots of Grewia polygama, Roxb.

Bạrsạ pakoṛ ṛẹhẹt, „ „ „ Grewia sapida, Roxb.

Sukri muthạ ṛẹhẹt da, the bulb of the roots of Scirpus monostachyus, Kön.

Tarse koṭap, Grewia villosa, Willd.

Kamraj ṛẹhẹt, the roots of Buettneria herbacea, Roxb.

Sikuạṛ ṛẹhẹt, „ „ „

Grind all these, or as many of them as are obtainable, together and give to drink, or make into pills to be swallowed.

(*n*) *Haṭ jo reak jaṅ sẹ dạlṭẹt,* the stone or kernel of the fruit of Holarrhena antidysenterica, Wall.

Tejo mala ṛẹhẹt, the roots of Cissampalos Pareira, Linn.

Mix these and give to drink. This is an excellent remedy.

For those whose eyes get yellow in cholera:—

(*o*) *Isor muli gọd,* Aristolochia indica, Willd.

Lọpọṅ chal, the bark of Terminalia bellerica, Roxb.

Adagạthiạ ṛẹhẹt, the roots of Panicum repens, Linn.

Ul chal, the bark of Mangifera indica, L.
Sarjom chal, „ „ „ Shorea robusta, Gärtn.

Grind these and extract the juice which give to drink mixed with opium.

For those whose eyes become red or bloodshot:—

(*p*) *Isor muli god*, Aristolochia indica, Willd.
Sahra chal, the bark of Streblus asper, Lour.
Sarjom chal, „ „ „ Shorea robusta, Gärtn.
Ul chal, „ „ „ Mangifera indica, L.

Pound these and extract about an ounce of the juice, which is to be mixed with opium the size of a pea and drunk.

To be used as a prophylactic at the cholera season :

(*q*) *Atnak chal*, the bark of Terminalia tomentosa, W. and A.
Jom lar chal, „ „ „ Bauhinia Vahlii, W. and A.
Cihut lar chal, „ „ „ Spatholobus Roxburghii, Benth.
Jhinjit chal, „ „ „ Bauhinia retusa, Roxb.
Hesak chal, „ „ „ Ficus religiosa, Willd.
Sarjom chal, „ „ „ Shorea robusta, Gärtn.
Ul chal, „ „ „ Mangifera indica, L.
Doka chal, „ „ „ Odina Wodier, Roxb.
Tarop chal, „ „ „ Buchanania latifolia, Roxb.
Niuri chal, „ „ „ Elæodendron Roxburghii, W. and A.
Bana hatak chal, the bark of Oroxylon indicum, Benth.
Makarkenda chal, „ „ „ Diospyros embryopteris, Pers.
Bir horeć, Atyllosia scarabædois, Benth.
Sega rehel, the roots of Mimosa rubicaulis, Lam.
Gote rehel, „ „ „ Croton oblongifolius, Roxb.
Atkir rehel „ „ „ Smilax ovalifolia, Roxb.
Nim chal, the bark of Melia Azadirachta, R.
Sinjo chal, „ „ „ Ægle Marmelos, Correa.
Kadar rehel, the roots of Bonnaya veronicæfolia, Spreng.
Asaria chal, the bark of Capparis horrida, Linn. f.
Saram lutur rehel, the roots of Clerodendron serratum, Spreng.
Gabur chal, the bark of Acacia Farnesiana, Willd.
Nangrauta rehel, the roots of Nardostachys Jatamansi, DC.
Korkot rehel se chal, the roots or bark of Dillenia indica, Linn.
Armu chal, the bark of Bursera serrata, Wall.
Ato pinda chal, the bark of Amorphophallus campanulatus, Bl.
Gõrẽ chal, „ „ „ Stephegyne parvifolia, Korth.
Edel chal, „ „ „ Bombax malabaricum, DC.
Baru chal, „ „ „ Schleichera trijuga, Willd.
Hesel chal, „ „ „ Anogeissus latifolia, Wall.
Terel chal, „ „ „ Diospyros tomentosa, Roxb.

Matkom chal, the bark of Bassia latifolia, Roxb.

Karam chal, „ „ „ Adina cordifolia, H. F. and B.

Pound and lacerate all these and soak them in water, and give the children daily a small quantity to drink.

Pills to be taken by healthy people when cholera is epidemic:—

(*r*) *Biṇḍi muthạ ghās*, Fimbristylis monostachya, Hassk.

Sukri muthạ ghās, Scirpus monostachyus, Kön.

Adagạthiạ ghās, Panicum repens, L.

Nanha dudhi loṭa rẹhẹl, the roots of Ichnocarpus frutescens, R. Br.

Bir buṭ rẹhẹl, the roots of Flemingia congesta, Roxb.

Kaḍa beṅjak rẹhẹl, the roots of

Kalmẹg, Andrographis paniculata, Nees.

Haṭ rẹhẹl, the roots of Holarrhena antidysenterica, Wall.

Saram lutur rẹhẹl, the roots of Clerodendron serratum, Spreng.

Kamraj rẹhẹl, the roots of Buettneria herbacea, Roxb.

Seta kaṭa rẹhẹl, the roots of Grewia polygama, Roxb.

Nim chal sẹ sakam, bark or leaves of Melia Azadirachta, L.

Siṅjọ chal sẹ sakam, „ „ „ „ Ægle Marmelos, Correa.

Bạrsạ pakọṛ rẹhẹl, the roots of Grewia sapida, Roxb.

Paṅjọl rẹhẹl „ „ „ Clerodendron phlomoides, Willd.

Ạṭkir rẹhẹl, „ „ „ Smilax ovalifolia, Roxb.

Sẹroaṅ rẹhẹl, „ „ „ Vigna vexillata, Benth.

Campa rẹhẹl, „ „ „ Ochna squarrosa, L.

Bhạbri rẹhẹl, „ „ „ Embelia robusta, Roxb.

Sarjọm chal sẹ dhũṛạ̃, the bark or resin of Shorea robusta, Gärtn.

Jọm laṛ chal, the bark of Bauhinia Vahlii, W. and A.

Cĩhũṭ chal „ „ „ Spatholobus Roxburghii, Benth.

Ạphim 4 ana reak, 4 annas worth of opium.

Pạurạ 1 sẹr, 2 pounds spirit.

Grind all these and then mix in the opium and spirit. If the epidemic is very severe give only one pound of the spirit.

What persons taking medicine to cholera patients should do:—

(*s*) *Isor muli gọd sakam*, the leaves of Aristolochia indica, Willd.

Adhẹ, ginger.

Mix and keep in the mouth like a quid of tobacco.

(*t*) *Rạsun*, garlic.

Tursi, Ocimum sanctum, Willd.

Bharbhạri sakam, the leaves of Ocimum basilicum, Linn., or O. canum, Sims.

Grind together, cook with mustard oil and anoint the entire body therewith. You should not apply the medicine yourself, let them do it themselves, neither should you eat their food or drink their water.

(u) *Sondhaeni rẹhẹl sẹ sakam*, the roots or leaves of Tylophora longifolia, Wight.

Chew and keep in the mouth swallowing the juice.

(v) *Bir buṭ rẹhẹl*, the roots of Flemingia congesta, L.
Pẹtcambṛa rẹhẹl, „ „ „ Helicteres Isora, L.

Grind together and give to drink with a spoonful of spirit.

Cihũṭ laṛ, Spatholobus Roxburghii, Benth.
Kaḍa mẽl, Premna herbacea, Roxb.
Jao, barley, Hordeum vulgare, L.
Ramṛa, Phæseolus Mungo, var. radiatus, L.
Sahṛa rẹhẹl, the roots of Streblus asper, Lour.

All these to be ground together and then drunk.

If he recovers then he should eat

Dahe, curds.
Taben, rice soaked and flattened.

Or if not quickly obtainable let him drink

Baṛe rẹhẹl, the roots of Ficus bengalensis, L.
Gõṛẽ rẹhẹl, „ „ „ Stephegyne parvifolia, Roxb.

(w) *Baṛe jọrọ ḍọg tẹl*, a shoot of the aerial root of Ficus bengalensis, L.

Crush this with water, and squeezing out the water give some to drink, after which the patient must lie still for some time.

(x) *Mare taben*, old soaked and flattened rice.
Seta aṇḍir rẹhẹl, the roots of Grewia polygama, Roxb.
Sikuaṛ rẹhẹl, the roots 1½ inch thick of
Kamraj rẹhẹl, „ „ of Buettneria herbacea, Roxb., 4 ounces.

Grind together, make into pills, the size of hares' excrement and give for two or three days.

(y) *Aphim*, opium.
Phuli paura, neat spirits.
Bẹrdọṛ rẹhẹl, the roots of Combretum nanum, Hamilt.
Tarse kotap, Grewia villosa, Willd.
Utri dudhi, Cryptolepis Buchanani, R. and S.
Buc chal, the bark of Cordia Myxa, Linn.
Bir eraḍọm, the wild Ricinus.
Jọm laṛ rẹhẹl, the roots of Bauhinia Vahlii, W. and A.
Murgạ chal, the bark of Pterocarpus Marsupium, Roxb.
Rot chal, „ „ „ Ougeenia dalbergioides, Benth.
Cĩhũṭ laṛ rẹhẹl, the roots of Spatholobus Roxburghii, Benth.
Goṭe rẹhẹl, the roots of Croton oblongifolius, Roxb.

Haṭ chal, the bark of Holarrhena antidysenterica, Wall.
Bir ḍimbu ṛeheṭ, the roots of
Tejo mala ṛeheṭ, „ „ „ Cissampelos Pareira, L.
Bir jhunkạ da, the tuber of Crotalaria calycina, Shrank.
Ul chal, the bark of Mangifera indica, L.
Kadam chal, „ „ Anthocephalus Cadamba, Bth. and Hook. f.
Sasaṅ baha, the flower of Curcuma longa, Roxb.
Paṅjọṭ, Clerodendron phlomoides, Willd.

Grind all these together and soak them in about a quart of spirit, make into pills and give three of them a day.

If there is a burning sensation in the chest, then grind

Mẹrlẹć sakam, the leaves of Flacourtia Ramontchi, L'Herit.

and apply them as a plaster to the chest.

(z) *Arak ạṭkir*, the red Smilax ovalifolia, Roxb.
Bạrsạ pakọṛ, Grewia sapida, Roxb.
Nanha dudhi loṭa ṛeheṭ, the roots of Ichnocarpus frutescens, R. Br.
Goboriạ dudhi loṭa ṛeheṭ, the roots of
Cĩhũṭ laṛ ṛeheṭ, the roots of Spatholobus Roxburghii, Benth.
Rot chal, the bark of Ougeenia dalbergioides, Benth.
Jọm laṛ ṛeheṭ, the roots of Bauhinia Vahlii, W. and A.
Tejo mala ṛeheṭ, „ „ „ Cissampelos Pareira, L.
Meral chal, the bark of Phyllanthus Emblica, Linn.
Bir jhuṅkạ ṛeheṭ, the roots of Crotalaria calycina, Shrank.

Grind all these together, soak them in spirit and eat.

(aa) *Kamraj ṛeheṭ*, the roots of Buettneria herbacea, Roxb.
Sikuạr ṛeheṭ, „ „ „
Tarse koṭap ṛeheṭ, the roots of Grewia villosa, Willd.
Rọsọmuni,
Gol mạric, 84 black peppercorns.

Grind together and compel the patient to drink it.

(bb) *Ạphim*, opium.
Hẹsẹl chal, the bark of Anogeissus latifolia, Wall.
Piṇḍe jọ, the fruit of Randia uliginosa, DC.
Nun juạn, salt and Carum Ajowan, DC.
Terel jọ, the fruit of Diospyros tomentosa, Roxb.
Ḍuṇḍukiṭ, Gardenia, turgida, Roxb.

(cc) *Cĩhũṭ laṛ*, Spatholobus Roxburghii, Benth.
Sahṛa chal, the bark of Streblus asper, Lour.
Bir buṭ, Flemingia congesta, L.

(dd) *Jiṭhimond*, Clerodendron Siphonanthus, R. Br.
Darcini, cinnamon.
Sũṭ, dry ginger.

Pipol, Piper longum, Willd.
Dhũṛã, resin of Shorea robusta, Gärtn.
Gọd, Aristolochia indica, Willd.
Nim banda, the parasitical plant found on Melia Azadirachta, L.
Tuṛi sunum, mustard oil.

(*ee*) *Ul chal*, the bark of Mangifera indica, L.
Sarjọm chal, „ „ Shorea robusta, Gärtn.

Mix the juice of these and add a little shell lime, and give to drink every hour.

(*ff*) *Sahṛa chal*, the bark of Streblus asper, Lour.

Take the juice of this, add opium the size of a pea, and after mixing them give to drink and the evacuations will cease.

(*gg*) *Tejo mala rẹhẹt*, the roots of Cissampelos Pareira, L.
Sẹroaṅ rẹhẹt, „ „ „ Vigna vexillata, Benth.
Haṭ chal, the bark of Holarrhena antidysenterica, Wall.

Take the juice of these, add some opium and give to drink.

If the bowels and urine are both stopped plaster these on the abdomen :

(*hh*) *Akaona chal*, the bark of Calotropis gigantea, R. Br.
Muṅgạ chal, „ „ „ Moringa pterygosperma, Gärtn.
Gol mạric, black pepper.

(*ii*) *Isor muli gọd*, Aristolochia indica, Willd.

Give this to drink, it will cure.

(*jj*) *Sahṛa chal*, the bark of Streblus asper, Lour.
Thoṛa haṭ chal, a little bark of Holarrhena antidysenterica, Wall.

Mix and give to drink, or, take the roots of these, mix about 6 ounces and add opium the size of a mustard seed, and give 6 ounces to drink at intervals, and the thirst and purging will cease.

If the burning sensation in the body does not stop,

(*kk*) *Ul chal*, the bark of Mangifera indica, L.
Sarjọm chal, „ „ „ Shorea robusta, Gärtn.
Hesak chal, „ „ „ Ficus religiosa, Willd.
Ambṛa chal, „ „ „ Spondias mangifera, Pers.
Doka chal, „ „ „ Odina Wodier, Roxb.
Ṡahṛa chal, „ „ „ Streblus asper, Lour.
Nim chal, „ „ „ Melia Azadirachta, L.
Siṅjọ chal, „ „ „ Ægle Marmelos, Correa.

Soak all these in water, pound them and after adding a little opium give to drink.

Sometimes there is a complication in cholera of *khaṛak muth*, kidney gravel, also, evidenced by inability to void urine and to ease the bowels. In such case (*ll*) *Akaona rẹhẹt*, the roots of Calotropis gigantea, R. Br.

Grind, heat and give a little to drink, warm, at a time, and then both stools and urine will come away like blood.

(*mm*) If blood is present in the evacuations give no hard or brittle medicines, or they will be fatal, but:

Sẹroañ, Vigna vexillata, Benth.
Seta kaṭa rẹhẹt, the roots of Grewia polygama, Roxb.
Biṇḍi muthạ ghãs rẹhẹt, the roots of Fimbristylis monostachya, Hassk.
Bạrsạ pakọṛ rẹhẹt, the roots of Grewia sapida, Roxb.

Pound all these together and give to drink raw, recovery is sure.

(*nn*) *Ul chal*, the bark of Mangifera indica, L.
Sarjọm chal, „ „ „ Shorea robusta, Gärtn.
Kadam chal, „ „ „ Anthocephalus Cadamba, Benth. and Hook. f.
Ḍoka chal, „ „ „ Odina Wodier, Roxb.
Ambṛa chal, „ „ „ Spondias mangifera, Pers.
Bir họṛẹč sakam, the leaves of Atyllosia scarabædois, Benth.
Ạṭkir rẹhẹt, the roots of Smilax ovalifolia, Roxb.
Nanha dudhi loṭa rẹhẹt, the roots of Ichnocarpus frutescens, R. Br.
Turạm rẹhẹt, the roots of

Pound all these non-bitter ingredients together, boil in an earthenware pot and give that water to drink.

(*oo*) *Kamraj rẹhẹt*, the roots of Buettneria herbacea, Roxb.
Tarse kọṭap rẹhẹt, the roots of Grewia villosa, Willd.

Whichever of these you can get give to drink raw.

N.B.—There is always intense thirst in these attacks, but however importunate the appeals for water, none whatever must be given or it may prove fatal.

(*pp*) *Haṭ chal*, the bark of Holarrhena antidysenterica, Wall.
Ḍhela chal, „ „ „ Alangium Lamarckii, Thws.
Tarọp chal, „ „ „ Buchanania latifolia, Roxb.
Saram lutur rẹhẹt, the roots of Clerodendron serratum, Spreng.
Tejo mala rẹhẹt, the roots of Cissampelos Pareira, L.

Grind together and give to drink. If it does not cease, then

(*qq*) *Gabla chal*, the bark of Acacia arabica, Willd.
Kasmar chal, „ „ „ Gmelina arborea, Roxb.
Nim chal, „ „ „ Melia Azadirachta, L.
Ul chal, „ „ „ Mangifera indica, L.
Ḍhela chal, „ „ „ Alangium Lamarckii, Thws.
Tarọp chal, „ „ „ Buchanania latifolia, Roxb.

Edẹl poha rẹhẹt, the roots of a seedling of a Bombax malabaricum, DC.

Boil these together and after grinding the following to a powder mix with that water and give to drink :—

Gol maṛic, black pepper.
Lọṅphul, cloves.
Kabab cini, Cubeba officinalis, Miqu.

When the cholera has stopped he will feel hot in the body ; give then *gạidahe*, curds of cows' milk, to drink.

(*rr*) *Karhạni hoṛo*, a certain variety of black paddy.

Fry this and pound it into bran and give to eat ; make him drunk with *pạurạ*, spirits, and make him drink a little more after eating above. This to be given in the initial stage, so that he may not be afraid. If he survives for 10 hours he will be all right. The great thing is there should be no fear and this is to attain that ; then

(*ss*) *Bạrsạ pakọṛ*, Grewia sapida, Roxb.
Bẹrdọṛ, Combretum nanum, Hamilt.
Tarse koṭap, Grewia villosa, Willd.

Grind these together ; heat *bẹrẹl sọsọ*, raw Semecarpus Anacardium, L., and drop two drops into above ground mixture ; also drop two drops of *utiṅ sunum*, mustard oil ; add about 16 ounces *dahe*, curds, stir all well together and give to drink.

In former times our forefathers used to bind the evil powers so that cholera and small-pox might not enter the village. On the first of the month of *Mag*, they would have a village council and all consult together. They would fix a day saying, On such and such a day we shall do thus ; let no one be absent.

On the appointed day when all are assembled it is said, We all have to be priests, and purify ourselves before setting to work, let no one hang back or be false ; and those of you who won't be priests, make it known on that morning or you will get into trouble. And you, so and so, first of all bathe yourselves in the morning, you will have to grind the medicines. And for the work on that day get the sacrifices ready, and we will all raise a subscription for the price of them. The sacrifices are a black female kid and a back pullet. On that day we shall all gather at the end of the village street and sacrifice them.

The heads of that kid and pullet are buried there, and going to the foot of some tree, they promise the *boṅgas* or spirits of the village boundaries ; "Let no trouble or misfortune enter or intrude into this village befalling man or beast. If we continue all right for a year we shall satisfy you to repletion."

After repeating this formula the medicines are given to be ground, viz :—

(*tt*) *Phuli pạurạ*, neat spirit,
Ramṛa, Phaeseolus Mungo, var. radiatus, L.

Adwa caole, rice made from sun-dried, not boiled, paddy.
Aphim, opium.
Sikuar,
Tarse koṭap, Grewia villosa, Willd.
Barsa pakor, Grewia sapida, Roxb.
Bir eradom, the wild castor oil plant.
Campa, Michelia champaca, L.
Ḍunḍukil, Gardenia turgida, Roxb.
Bana haṭak, Oroxylon indicum, Benth.
Asaria, Capparis horrida, L.
Hiñjor, Barringtonia acutangula, Gärtn.
Ruhen, Soymida febrifuga, Juss.
Binḍi mutha, Fimbristylis monostachya, Hassk.
Cĩhũṭ lar, Spatholobus Roxburghii, Roxb.
Kaḍa mẽl, Premna herbacea, Roxb.
Ponḍ murut,
Ambṛa, Spondias mangifera, Pers.
Sahṛa banda, parasitical plant found on Streblus asper, Lour.
Meral banda, „ „ „ on Phyllanthus Emblica, L.
Bhorkonḍ banda, „ „ „ Hymenodictyon excelsum, Wall.
Ḍunḍukil banda, parasitical plant found on Gardenia turgida, Roxb.
Icak banda, parasitical plant found on Woodfordia floribunda, Salib. (Loranthus Buddeoides, Wedd.)
Pinḍe banda, parasitical plant found on Randia uliginosa, DC.
Soso banda, „ „ found on Semecarpus Anacardium, L.
Baru banda, „ plant found on Schleichera trijuga, Willd.
Kamraj, Buettneria herbacea, Roxb.
Sondhaeni, Tylophora longifolia, Wight.
Sese baha, Sterculia colorata, Roxb.
Ato eradom, Ricinus communis, L.
Laṭha cip ciṛip,
Bariar phul,
Kũs, Themuda gigantea, Haskel.
Lopoñ arak, Aerua lanata, L.
Sahṛa chal, the bark of Streblus asper, Lour.
Buluñ, salt.
Dare japak, Scindapsus officinalis, Schott.
Sãoraj, Vernonia anthelmintica, Roxb.
Tejo mala, Cissampelos Pareira, L.

Pan muhri, the seed of Pimpinella anisum, L.
Mọsọla, spices.
Jirạ, Carum Carui, L.
Ul chal, the bark of Mangifera indica, L.
Kạuḍi cun, shell lime.
Nanha gọd,

All these are ground together, mixed with *phuli pạurạ*, neat spirits, and made into balls. Then taking them to the foot of that tree, they are there divided into as many portions as there are households in the village. Then after making a soup of the flesh of that kid and rice, and eating this they leave that place. The medicine man makes some flour water in a leaf cup and puts those portions of medicine into a winnowing fan. Then the entire village male population move off together and begin at the house at the end of the village; first he sprinkles their water pots with that flour water; then calling the wife of the head of that household he gives her their portion of the medicine and says, This medicine we have prepared to protect the village; give it to as many people as are in the house and they are to eat it; omit no one. And in this way they all go along together and repeat the operation at each house.

In this way formerly in our forefathers' time the village was in one way under control, and therefore no kind of trouble could easily effect an entrance. In those days too they did not die while strong or as children, only when they became old men or women. In those days also trouble and sickness did not show themselves as now. Then too there was no spite or tale-bearing. But now there is a great deal of both; trouble and sickness too are increased. What are we to do?

If all went well with us the year through, then what had been vowed was given, and thus they would fulfil their vows. In this way they would act year by year to ward off cholera and small-pox.

(*uu*) *Tarse koṭap*, Grewia villosa, Willd.
Sikuạr,
Barañgọm, Vernonia cineria, Less., or Glossogyne pinnatifida, DC.
Ato piṇḍe, Amorphophallus campanulatus, Blume.
Gol mạric, black pepper.
Hẹndẹ mẹrọm toa, the milk of a black goat.
Sahṛa rẹhẹt, the roots of Streblus asper, Lour.

Grind these and give to drink.

If his stomach makes a noise:

Kạhu botke rẹhẹt, the roots of Bryonia lacinosa, L.
Jạnum ḍọg, a sprout of Zizyphus Jujuba, Lam.
Nim sakam, the leaves of Melia Azadirachta, L.

Plaster him over with these.

If his stomach swells up:

Ghugri, Gryllus gryllo-talpa.

Thoṛa haṭ chal, a little of the bark of Holarrhena antidysenterica, Wall.

Thoṛa karhạni hoṛo ata, a little fried paddy of a certain black variety.

Grind together, make into a ball and give to eat.

If when there are no more evacuations he seems about to collapse:

Nim kaḍẹč, twigs of Melia Azadirachta, L.

Heat these and wrap round both his arms and both his legs.

If the saliva dries up:

Kạsi sakam, the leaves of Saccharum spontaneum, L.

Turạm da, the bulb of

Guạ, Areca Catechu, L.

Grind these and give to drink; or if these are not readily obtainable, then

Akaṛ baha, Limnophila Roxburghiana, G. Don.

Tursi sakam, the leaves of Ocymum sanctum, Willd.

Oroṗ da, the bulb of Costus speciosa, Sm.

Grind these, mix with *cini*, sugar, and give to drink; or give him to eat *jiṭhimond*, Clerodendron Siphonanthus, R. Br.

If he has gripes: grind *pẹṭcambṛa*, Helicteres Isora, L., and plaster it on the stomach and give a little to drink. You must invoke the spirits *Kạli mae*, *Nag nạgin*. The sacrifices to be offered in the event of recovery are a black goat and two pairs of pigeons.

If there is pain in the stomach:

(*vv*) *Nanha gọd*,

Ul chal, the bark of Mangifera indica, L.

Sarjọm chal, the bark of Shorea robusta, Gärtn.

Thoṛa cun, a little shell lime.

Stir together a little and give to drink.

(*ww*) *Sahṛa chal*, the bark of Streblus asper, Lour.

Thoṛa ạphim, a little opium.

Tejo mala, Cissampelos Pareira, L.

Sẹṛoañ, Vigna vexillata, Benth.

Haṭ chal, the bark of Holarrhena antidysenterica, Wall.

Mix the juice of these in opium and give to drink.

(*xx*) *Niuri chal*, the bark of Elæodendron Roxburghii, W. and A.

Jhinjiṭ chal, „ „ „ Bauhinia retusa, Roxb.

To be drunk.

If both urine and evacuations are stopped

(*yy*) *Akaona chal*, the bark of Calotropis gigantea, R. Br. or C. procera, R. Br.

Muṅgą chal, the bark of Moringa pterygosperma, Gärtn.
Gol mąric, black pepper.

Grind these and plaster over the abdomen; or

(*zz*) grind all the ingredients prescribed to be drunk together, and give to drink.

245. *Marań kuthą lać haso sę amsam.* Dysentery.

Symptoms. In this blood is passed with the excrement and there is great pain in the abdomen and navel. In this complaint no bitter medicine whatever should be given, otherwise death will certainly ensue. Astringent, viscid or slimy medicines should be administered.

Medicines: (*a*) *Biṇḍi muthą ghās rẹhẹl*, the roots of Fimbristylis monostachya, Hassk.

Sukri muthą ghās rẹhẹl, the roots of Scirpus monostachyus, Kön.

Nanha dudhi loṭa rẹhẹl, the roots of Ichnocarpus frutescens, R. Br.

Piṭuą aṛak, Spermacoce hispida, Linn.

Sim kaṭa rẹhẹl, the roots of Vitex peduncularis.

Suruj mukhi aṛak rẹhẹl, the roots of Helianthus annuus, Willd.

Duṇḍukil rẹhẹl, the roots of Gardenia turgida, Roxb.

Paḍer rẹhẹl, the roots of Stereospermum suaveolens, DC.

Turąm rẹhẹl, „ „ „

Tipọć rẹhẹl, „ „ „

Piṇḍą dare chal, the bark of Randia uliginosa, DC.

Babla chal, „ „ „ Acacia arabica, Willd.

Pańjọt chal, „ „ „ Clerodendron phlomoides, Willd.

Atnak chal, „ „ „ Terminalia tomentosa, W. and A.

Aṇḍią mọrọn aṛak rẹhẹl, the roots of Gymnema hirsutus, W. and A., var. Decaisneanum, Wight.

Cihūṭ laṛ, Spatholobus Roxburghii, Benth.

Jọm laṛ dare chal, the bark of Bauhinia Vahlii, W. and A.

Barańgom rẹhẹl, the roots of Vernonia cineria, Less. or Glossogyne pinnatifida, DC.

Kalią kuąr sẹ gąi mulą rẹhẹl, the roots of

Muć aṛak rẹhẹl, the roots of Polygonum plebejum, Br.

Pusi toa rẹhẹl, the roots of Euphorbia pilulifera, Linn.

Dud barańgọm rẹhẹl, the roots of

Bąrsą pakọṛ rẹhẹl, „ „ „ Grewia sapida, Roxb.

Seta kaṭa rẹhẹl, „ „ „ Grewia polygama, Roxb.

Tarse koṭap rẹhẹl, „ „ „ Grewia villosa, Willd.

Maṭha aṛak rẹhẹl, „ „ „ Antidesma diandrum, Tulas.

Hạlim, Lepidium sativum, L.
Murgạ dare chal, the bark of Pterocarpus Marsupium, Roxb.
Rot chal, „ „ „ Ougeenia dalbergioides, Benth.
Kedok̇ aṛak̇ rẹhẹl, the roots of Argyreia speciosa, Sweet.

Pound all these small and boil them in about four pounds of water in a new vessel, and soak them; to be drunk daily.

(*b*) *Turạm*,
Ṭipọć,
Aṇḍiạ mọrọn aṛak̇, Gymnema hirsutus, W. and A., var. Decaisneanum, Wight.

Grind these and mix them with flour making it into unleavened or hand bread and give to eat. If the two latter ingredients are unobtainable, then give the first only.

(*c*) *Campa rẹhẹl*, the roots of Ochna squarrosa, L.
Aṭkir rẹhẹl, „ „ „ Smilax ovalifolia, Roxb.
Ḍhalka hạtkạn rẹhẹl, the roots of Leea macrophylla, Roxb.
Tarse koṭap rẹhẹl, „ „ „ Grewia villosa, Willd.
Babla chal, the bark of Acacia arabica, Willd.
Pañjọt chal, „ „ „ Clerodendron phlomoides, Willd.

Pound all these, boil in a new vessel and give daily to drink.

(*d*) *Hạlim*, Lepidium sativum, L.
Maṭha aṛak̇ rẹhẹl, the roots of Antidesma diandrum, Tulas.

Grind these together, make into unleavened or hand bread with flour and give to eat.

(*e*) *Murgạ chal*, the bark of Pterocarpus Marsupium, Roxb.
Rot chal, „ „ „ Ougeenia dalbergioides, Benth.
Jugiạ chal, „ „ „ Cordia Macleodii, H. f. and T.
Nạṅgrạuta rẹhẹl, the roots of Nardostachys Jatamansi, DC.
Atnak̇ chal, the bark of Terminalia tomentosa, W. and A.
Dare murup̣ chal, „ „ „ Butea frondosa, Roxb.
Ḍurạ da, the bulb of
Bayañ da, „ „ „ Dioscorea crispata, Roxb.
Piskạ da, „ „ „ Dioscorea oppositifolia, L.

Mix water with these and pound them, boil them and give daily to drink.

(*f*) *Bọnkạpsi rẹhẹl*, the roots of Thespesia Lampas, Benth. and Hook. f.
Pẹtcambṛa rẹhẹl, „ „ „ Helicteres Isora, L.
Saparọm chal, the bark of Nyctanthes Arbor-tristis, L.
Icạk̇ rẹhẹl, the roots of Woodfordia floribunda, Salisb.
Ḍuriạ hạtkạn rẹhẹl, the roots of Leea hirta, Herb. Banks.

Pound and boil these and give daily to drink.

(*g*) *Khode baha aṛak̇*,
Muć aṛak̇ rẹhẹl, the roots of Polygonum plebejum, Br.

Grind, mix with flour and make into unleavened or hand bread and give to eat.

(*h*) *Bele sinjo*, the ripe fruit of Ægle Marmelos, Correa.

Misri, sugar candy.

Mix up the former in hot water with the latter, *i.e.* make a sherbet, and give to drink.

(*i*) *Lopon arak*, Ærua lanata, Linn.

Roast these in an envelope of leaves and give to eat.

(*j*) *Amsam dhiri*, stone beads of reddish, greyish and other colours.

To be rubbed on a stone in water, which is then given to children to drink, *i.e.* child patients.

(*k*) *Campa rehel*, the roots of Michelia champaca, L.

Badam jo gabetel, the kernel of almonds.

Makarkenda jo, the fruit of Diospyros embryopteris, Pers.

Rokot condon, blood coloured sandal wood, Santalum album, L.

Arak upal baha, Nymphaea rubra, Roxb.

Arak raj baha, the red variety of Nerium odorum, Soland.

Halim, Lepidium sativum, L.

Parch or fry dry the last. Grind small and mix all the ingredients and make into pills, which should be dissolved in hot water just before being drunk.

(*l*) *Ul chal*, the bark of Mangifera indica, L.

Ambra chal, ,, ,, ,, Spondias mangifera, Pers.

Sahra chal, ,, ,, ,, Streblus asper, Lour.

Mix and grind these and give to drink.

(*m*) *Seta kata rehel*, the roots of Grewia polygama, Roxb.

Bãriã kandhum rehel, the roots of Phyllanthus lanceolarius, Mull-Arg.

11 *gol maric*, eleven black peppercorns.

Grind these together and give to drink.

(*n*) Grind *arak upal baha*, Nymphaea rubra, Roxb., and give to drink.

(*o*) Make him drink about a pound of buffalo milk as soon as it has been taken from the animal.

To cause the pain at the abdomen and navel to cease :—

(*p*) *Darcini*, cinnamon.

Rokot condon kat, blood coloured sandal wood, Santalum album, L.

Sũt, dry ginger.

Roast these three slightly and after grinding give a little to drink and apply externally over the abdomen and navel.

(*q*) *Pond dhiri*, feldspar or quartz.

Karkat dog, a shoot of Zizyphus xylopyra, Willd.

First heat the former red hot and throw it into water when it will fall to pieces. Then grind it with the latter and apply to the abdomen and navel.

(*r*) *Akaona lor̥e*, the milky exudation of Calotropis gigantea, R.Br. Smear this over the abdomen and navel.

Prohibited articles of diet:—

(*s*) *J̣el*, meat.
Hako, fish.
Munga ar̥ak, the leaves of Moringa pterygosperma, Gärtn.
Kur̥mbi ar̥ak, a certain potherb.
Gạndhạri ar̥ak, Amaranthus gangeticus, var. angustifolia, L.
Gạrunḍi ar̥ak, Acternanthera sessilis, R. Br.
Ạlu, potatoes.
Bengar̥, Solanum Melangena, L.
Kesari dạl, Lathyrus sativus, L.
Buṭ dạl, Cicer arietinum, L.
Rambr̥a dạl, Phaeseolus Mungo, var. radiatus, L.
Maṭọr dạl, Pisum arvense and P. sativum, L.
Har̥hat karla, the bitter var. of Momordica dioica, Roxb.
Hẹrẹm tij, anything sweet.
Toa, milk.
Khạjạri, parched rice.
Mạsri dạl, Ervum Lens, L.

The only *dạl* (or split grain) allowed is *họrẹć*, Dolichos biflorus, L.

(*t*) *Ambr̥a chal*, the bark of Spondias mangifera, Pers..
Ạtkur̥ạ rẹhẹt chal, the bark of the roots of Wrightia tomentosa, R. and S.
Tejo mala rẹhẹt, the roots of Cissampelos Pareira, L.

Pound these together and of the resultant water give ½ oz. daily for three days.

If there is no amelioration, then

Karkaṭ sakam, the leaves of Zizyphus xylopyra, Willd.
Kạliạ jirạ, Nigella indica, Roxb.

Grind these together and give to drink.

(*u*) *Bir buṭ*, Flemingia congesta, L.
Ạtkir rẹhẹt, the roots of Smilax ovalifolia, Roxb.
Bir cạmuk da, the tuber of

Cook in mustard oil and give to eat.

(*v*) *Arak meral sakam*, the leaves of the red Phyllanthus Emblica, L.
Campa rẹhẹt, the roots of Michelia champaca, L.
Ạnḍiạ mọrọn ar̥ak rẹhẹt, the roots of Gymnema hirsutus, W. and A., var. Decaisneanum, Wight.
Sarjọm chal, the bark of Shorea robusta, Gärtn.

Seta aṇḍir rẹhẹl, the roots of Grewia polygama, Roxb.

Sahṛa chal, the bark of Streblus asper, Lour.

Biṇḍi muthạ rẹhẹl, the roots of Fimbristylis monostachya, Hassk.

Bheḍwa datẹl, the tuber of Hibiscus cancellatus, Roscoe, var. fusiformis, Willd.

Collect all these and let him drink them with hot water.

(*w*) *Ḍoka*, Odina Wodier, Roxb.

Murgạ, Pterocarpus Marsupium, Roxb.

Atnak̄ chal, the bark of Terminalia tomentosa, W. and A.

Sarjọm chal, „ „ „ Shorea robusta, Gärtn.

Guạ, Areca Catechu, L.

Utri dudhi loṭa, Cryptolepis Buchanani, R. and S.

Koṅga, Agave americana, L.

Rạli, Piper longum, Willd.

Bir eraḍọm, the wild Castor oil plant.

Jhik poṭa, a porcupine's stomach.

Siṭkạ,

Kedok̄ aṛak̄, Argyreia speciosa, Sweet.

Gargạḍi, Coix lachryma, Willd.

Ạṭkir, Smilax ovalifolia, Roxb.

(*x*) *Nanha pusi toa rẹhẹl*, the roots of Euphorbia thymifolia, Burm.

Pạtni bele rẹhẹl, the roots of Helianthus annuus, Willd.

Ạṭkir rẹhẹlak̄ gabeṭẹl, the flesh of the roots of Smilax ovalifolia, Roxb.

Baṛe jọrọ reak̄ bale ḍọg, the fresh shoot of an aerial root of Ficus bengalensis, L.

Ạphim, opium, about the size of fly's head.

Grind these together and make into pills the size of hares' excrement; give one such pill three times a day.

(*y*) *Biṇḍi muthạ rẹhẹl*, the roots of Fimbristylis monostachya, Hassk.

Bir baraṅgọm rẹhẹl, the roots of Glossogyne pinnatifida, DC.

Ọpọnọm rẹhẹl, the roots of Angelica glauca, Edgew.

Ḍuṇḍukil rẹhẹl, „ „ „ Gardenia turgida, Roxb.

Toyo caṇḍbọl rẹhẹl, the roots of Desmodium gangeticum, DC.

Bir jhuṅkạ rẹhẹl, „ „ „ Crotalaria calycina, Shrank.

Pound these and squeeze out the juice, which the patient is to drink.

(*z*) *Biṇḍi muthạ*, Fimbristylis monostachya, Hassk.

Tikin siṅ,

Icạk̄ sakam, the leaves of Woodfordia floribunda, Salisb.

(*aa*) *Ẹtkẹć*, Euphorbia antiquorum. L.
Buluṅ, salt.
Ghikūạ̃ri, Yucca gloriosa.
Arak upạl, Nymphaea rubra, Roxb.

(*bb*) *Campa rẹhẹt*, the roots of Michelia champaca, L.
Terel jọ, the fruit of Diospyros tomentosa, Roxb.
Haṭ rẹhẹt, the roots of Holarrhena antidysenterica, Wall.
Goṭe rẹhẹt, „ „ „ Croton oblongifolius, Roxb.
Paḍer rẹhẹt, „ „ „ Stereospermum suaveolens, DC.
Sạuṛi rẹhẹt, „ „ „ Heteropogon contortus, R. and S.
Bọd laṛ baklak, the bark of Vitis adnata, Wall.
Pạtni bele, Helianthus annuus, Willd.
Sọ dare reak chal, the bark of Eugenia Jambolana, Lamk.

Grind and mix all these and give to drink. Afterwards let him eat *pan*, the leaf of Piper Betle, L., and *khayar*, Acacia Catechu, Willd.

(*cc*) *Ḍunḍukit rẹhẹt*, the roots of Gardenia turgida, Roxb.
Seta pan, Monochoria plantaginea, Kunth.
Binḍi muthạ da, the bulb of Fimbristylis monostachya, Hassk.
Ul chal, the bark of Mangifera indica, L.
Ḍoka chal, „ „ „ Odina Wodier, Roxb.
Ambṛa chal, „ „ „ Spondias mangifera, Pers.

Grind and give to drink.

(*dd*) *Surju muni rẹhẹt*, the roots of
Turạm rẹhẹt, „ „ „

Grind these, make into pills to be eaten.

(*ee*) *Binḍi muthạ*, Fimbristylis monostachya, Hassk.
Ambṛa chal, the bark of Spondias mangifera, Pers.

Mix these with some *cun*, lime, and give to drink.

(*ff*) *Terel jọ*, the fruit of Diospyros tomentosa, Roxb.
Daka, boiled rice.
Taben, rice soaked and flattened.

Mix these thoroughly and give to eat.

Oḍokok jọkhẹć hasokore. When there is pain at stool.

(*gg*) *Lẹbẹt cẹnḍẹń jạnum rẹhẹt*, the roots of trodden down Zizyphus Jujuba, Lamk.
Tejo mala rẹhẹt, the roots of Cissampelos Pareira, L.
Miru baha rẹhẹt, „ „ „ Abutilon indicum, Don.
Sarjọm chal, the bark of Shorea robusta, Gärtn.
Buc chal, „ „ „ Cordia Myxa, L.
Buḍhi gạsić rẹhẹt, the roots of Pavetta indica, L., var. tomentosa, Roxb , or Callicarpa macrophylla, Vahl.
Tẹrẹl ḍọg, a shoot of Diospyros tomentosa, Roxb.

Mix, grind and give to drink.

(*hh*) *Campa rẹhẹl*, the roots of Michelia champaca, L.
Haṭ rẹhẹl, „ „ „ Holarrhena antidysenterica, Wall.
Paḍer rẹhẹl, „ „ „ Stereospermum suaveolens, DC.

Grind and give to drink.

(*ii*) *Turạm rẹhẹl*, the roots of
Aṇḍiạ mọrọn aṛak rẹhẹl, the roots of Gymnema hirsutus, W. and A., var. Decaisneanum, Wight.
Ṭipọć rẹhẹl, the roots of
Kedok aṛak rẹhẹl, the roots of Arygyreia speciosa, Sweet.
Bạrsạ pakọṛ rẹhẹl, „ „ „ Grewia sapida, Roxb.
Seta kaṭa rẹhẹl, „ „ „ Grewia polygama, Roxb.
Thoṛa ḍuṇḍukil rẹhẹl, the roots of Gardenia turgida, Roxb. (a little).
Thoṛa paḍer rẹhẹl, the roots of Stereospermum suaveolens, DC. (a little).
Baraṅgọm rẹhẹl, the roots of Vernonia cineria, Less., or Glossogyne pinnatifida, DC.
Biṇḍi muthạ rẹhẹl, the roots of Fimbristylis monostachya, Hassk.
Sukri muthạ rẹhẹl, the roots of Scirpus monostachyus, Kön.
Nanha dudhi loṭa rẹhẹl, the roots of Ichnocarpus frutescens, R. Br.
Ḍhalka hạtkạn rẹhẹl, the roots of Leea macrophylla, Roxb.
Maṭha aṛak rẹhẹl, the roots of Antidesma diandrum, Tulas.
Hạlim, Lepidium sativum, L.
Gại mulạ sẹ hạliạ kuạri mulạ rẹhẹl, the roots of

Boil all these and after cooling give to drink; persevere with this for 15 to 26 days, giving it some 5 times in the day and some 6 times at night. The evacuations will have the appearance of the medicine, but still keep on with it. If there is pain at the navel smear *akaona loṛe*, the sticky exudation of Calotropis gigantea, R. Br., on daily and the pain will cease. Until recovery a gruel of *sạgu dana*, sago, should be taken flavoured with salt or sugar, but no rice. The water drunk should be warm, not cold.

N.B.—The last named of above has thin tendrils and leaves and yields a sticky exudation like that of *kedok aṛak*, Argyreia speciosa, Sweet, while the bulb is like that of *bheḍwa*, Hibiscus cancellatus, Roscoe, var. fusiformis, Willd.

For children.

(*jj*) *Turạm rẹhẹl*, the roots of
Baraṅgọm rẹhẹl, the roots of Vernonia cineria, Less., or Glossogyne pinnatifida, DC.

Make into hand bread with wheat flour and give to eat daily until recovery.

(*kk*) *Ḍhalka hạtkạn*, Leea macrophylla, Roxb.

Make into hand bread with wheat flour and give to eat.

(*ll*) *Ṭipọč da*, the bulb of

Make into hand bread with wheat flour and give to eat.

(*mm*) *Tilmiń sakam*, the leaves of Sesamum orientale, Willd.

Soak in water and give that water to drink. Knead the leaves and squeeze out the water which will be viscid, and give that water to drink.

For pain at the navel :—

(*nn*) Roast *poṇḍ dhiri*, quartz, to burning point, throw it into water when it will splutter and crack and become loose. Taking it out grind with *jạnum ḍọg*, a shoot of Zizyphus Jujuba, Lam., and it will swell up. Apply that as an ointment to the navel. Give also to drink

Tarse koṭọp rẹhẹl, the roots of Grewia villosa, Willd.
Kamraj rẹhẹl, the roots of Buettneria herbacea, Roxb.

(*oo*) *Jọm laṛ chal*, the bark of Bauhinia Vahlii, W. and A.
Cihũṭ laṛ rẹhẹl, the roots of Spatholobus Roxburghii, Benth.
Kadam chal, the bark of Anthocephalus Cadamba, Benth. and Hook. f.
Sarjọm chal, the bark of Shorea robusta, Gärtn.
Hesak chal, „ „ „ Ficus religiosa, Willd.
Ḍoka chal, „ „ „ Odina Wodier, Roxb.
Ambṛa chal, „ „ „ Spondias mangifera, Pers.
Bir hoṛẹč, Atyllosia scarabaedois, Benth.
Campa rẹhẹl, the roots of Michelia champaca, L.
Pańjọt dare chal, the bark of Clerodendron phlomoides, Benth.
Bẹrdọṛ rẹhẹl, the roots of Combretum nanum, Hamilt.
Ạtkir rẹhẹl, „ „ „ Smilax ovalifolia, Roxb.

Grind all these and boil well, then throw away the barks and give to drink daily. Give no boiled rice to eat till the child asks for it, for if eaten the medicines will not act promptly. Give only a gruel of sago with the addition of salt. This disease is a sequel of measles. There is nothing bitter in the medicines, they are only insipid.

(*pp*) *Murgạ chal*, the bark of Pterocarpus Marsupium, Roxb.
Satsayar chal, „ „ „ Dalbergia latifolia, Roxb.
Jọm laṛ chal, „ „ „ Bauhinia Vahlii, W. and A.
Cihũṭ laṛ chal, „ „ „ Spatholobus Roxburghii, Benth.
Atnak chal, „ „ „ Terminalia tomentosa, W. and A.
Caole ata rọńgọ, rice fried to burning point.
Sińjọ sakam, the leaves of Ægle Marmelos, Correa.

Boil all these together, and give the water to drink daily: he will surely recover.

(*qq*) *Campa rẹhẹl*, the roots of Michelia champaca, L.
Haṭ rẹhẹl, „ „ „ Holarrhena antidysenterica, Wall.
Paḍer rẹhẹl, „ „ „ Stereospermum suaveolens, DC.

Grind these together and give to drink.

(*rr*) *Biṇḍi muthạ da*, the bulb of Fimbristylis monostachya, Hassk.

Ambṛa chal, the bark of Spondias mangifera, Pers.

Grind these together, squeeze through a cloth and after mixing with *kāṛā kạuḍi cun*, the lime from the small shells used as money in India, give to drink.

(*ss*) *Ọhọc aṛak ṛẹhẹt*, the roots of Boerhaavia procumbens, Herb. Banks.

Aṭkir ṛẹhẹt, „ „ „ Smilax ovalifolia, Roxb.

Icạk ṛẹhẹt, „ „ „ Woodfordia floribunda, Salisb.

Tejo mala ṛẹhẹt, „ „ „ Cissampelos Pareira, L.

Grind together and give to drink.

(*tt*) *Mare taben*, old rice soaked and flattened to be washed seven times.

Ghoṛa lạdạuṛi, Vitis tomentosa, Heyne.

Biṇḍi muthạ, Fimbristylis monostachya, Hassk.

Grind the last two together and mix with the first into a clammy mixture, and give for three days, when a cure will follow. If on gōing to stool there should be prolapsus ani, then give

(*uu*) *Muthạ da*, the bulb of

Biṇḍi muthạ da, the bulb of Fimbristylis monostachya, Hassk.

Arak upạl baha da, the bulb of Nymphæa rubra, Roxb.

Baṛe baha ṛẹhẹt, the roots of Pentapetes phoenicia, L.

Grind and mix these and give to drink, or mix with above and give to eat.

If no gas is expelled,

(*vv*) *Jọm jạnum ṛẹhẹt*, the roots of Zizyphus Jujuba, Lam.

Pound and give to drink.

If the urine cannot be voided,

(*ww*) *Dare cetan reak hesak ṛẹhẹt chal*, the bark of the roots of Ficus religiosa, Willd., growing on another tree.

Pound and give, and normal conditions will return.

If there is an internal scraping pain, *i.e.* as if there was no more excrement to come away, then

(*yy*) *Muthạ da*, the bulb of Fimbristylis monostachya, Hassk.

Suruj mukhi ṛẹhẹt, the roots of Helianthus annuus, L.

Grind together and give to drink.

246. *Māyām ar suluc leka oḍokok.*

Blood and slime in the excretions.

Medicines: *Campa ṛẹhẹt*, the roots of Michelia champaca, L.

Terel jọ, the fruit of Diospyros tomentosa, Roxb.

Haṭ ṛẹhẹt, the root of Holarrhena antidysenterica, Wall.

247. *Khok.* Cough.

Medicines: (*a*) *Pipol*, Piper longum, Willd.

Dumur rasa, the honey of the small honey bee.

Grind these together and let him eat some every morning.

(*b*) *Rọhọṛ adhẹ*, dried ginger, Zingiber officinalis, Roscoe.

Grind fine, mix with melted butter and sugar and after warming a little give to drink.

(*c*) Touch the uvula with the fruit of *sọsọ*, Semecarpus Anacardium, L.

When the phlegm is tenacious:—

(*d*) *Ṭhạḍiạ tuṛi*, a variety of Brassica campestris, L.

Rạṅgạini rẹhẹt, the roots of Solanum Jacquini, Willd.

Sasaṅ bọhọk, a knot of turmeric, Curcuma longa, Roxb.

To be drunk.

(*e*) *Beṅgaṛ beṭahet rẹhẹt*, the roots of Solanum stramonifolium, Jacq.

Adagạṭhiạ rẹhẹt, the roots of Panicum repens, L.

Kũs and *kạsi*, Themuda gigantea, Haskel, and Saccharum spontaneum, L.

Badgọcak, Lygodium flexuosum, Sw.

Biṇḍi muthạ, Fimbristylis monostachya, Hassk.

Bạṛ chal, the bark of Mimusops Elengi, L.

Banat arakak, a bit of a red woollen blanket.

Bir baraṅgọm, Glossogyne pinnatifida, DC.

Sẹga jạnum rẹhẹt, the roots of Mimosa rubicaulis, Lamk.

Cạuliạ, Ruellia suffruticosa, Roxb.

Kadar, Bonnaya veronicæfolia, Spreng.

Dhiri banda,

Etka rẹhẹt, the roots of Mucuna pruriens, DC.

Ạṇḍiạ goṅgha, the shell of a male snail.

Upel baha arakak, Nymphæa rubra, Roxb.

Kamraj, Buettneria herbacea, Roxb.

Grind these together, cook in oil, and after making into pills give to eat.

(*f*) *Adagạṭhiạ rẹhẹt*, the roots of Panicum repens, L.

Kạsi rẹhẹt, " " " Saccharum spontaneum, L.

Beṅgaṛ beṭahet rẹhẹt, the roots of Solanum stramonifolium, Jacq.

Kũs rẹhẹt, the roots of Themuda gigantea, Haskel.

Arak upạl baha, Nymphæa rubra, Roxb.

Banat arakak, bit of a red woollen blanket.

Etka rẹhẹt, the roots of Mucuna pruriens, DC.

Bạṛ chal, the bark of Mimusops Elengi, L.

Rọl jọ, the fruit of Terminalia Chebula, Retz.

Grind all these together, cook in melted butter and give to eat. Give most of the third of above named roots.

(g) *Nanha dudhi loṭa rẹhẹt*, the roots of Ichnocarpus frutescens, R. Br.

Musnạ jaṅ, the seeds of Linum usitatissimum, L.

Boil each separately in a brass cup of the size sold for 8 annas and strain; boil again, mix and then give to drink.

(h) *Lilkạthi*, Polygala crotalarioides, Buch. and Ham.

Gol mạric, black pepper.

Tursi sakam, the leaves of Ocymum sanctum, Willd.

Adwa caole, rice made from sundried, not boiled, paddy.

Grind all these together and give to drink.

(i) *Hẹsẹl chal*, the bark of Anogeissus latifolia, Wall.

Sẹkrẹċ chal, ,, ,, ,, Lagerstroemia parviflora, Roxb.

Let him chew these daily; if the patient is an infant plaster *joka sakam*, the leaves of Sida humilis, Willd., on the fontanel.

If the cough seems to be bronchial or asthmatic:

(j) bring a little of the bark of each of all the trees in the forest, grind this along with some *gol mạric*, black pepper, make into pills and give one pill daily each forenoon and one each afternoon.

248. *Ṭhae khok*. Dry cough.

Medicines: *Gol mạric* (4), 4 black peppercorns.

Lilkạthi rẹhẹt, the roots of Polygala crotolarioides, Buch. and Ham.

Grind together, cook in oil and give to drink.

249. *Selesa*. (Bronchitis or a cold or a chill.)

Symptoms. If a person bathes for a long time in water, and then his head gets hot and thereby cold strikes his chest or lungs, he will wheeze, and the middle of the head, where an infant's fontanel is, will become as hot as fire. Both children and adults may get this. Some people get from this *Pạchiạri betha* (pneumonia). These have a pain in the chest and all the ribs, they breathe with difficulty and experience a piercing pain. The Santals when suffering from *Pạchiạri betha* call it a stabbing by the evil spirits, but it is a consequence of *selesa*.

Medicines: (a) *Laṭha cip ciṛip rẹhẹt*, the roots of

Sũṭ and *pipol*, ginger and Piper longum, Willd.

Darcini, cinnamon.

Adagạthiạ ghãs da, the bulbs of Panicum repens, L.

Grind all these small and after mixing with *ńẹlẹ rasa*, honey, give to eat.

(b) *Chạtni chal*, the bark of Alstonia scholaris, R. Br.

Haṭ chal, ,, ,, ,, Holarrhena antidysenterica, Wall.

10 *goṭẹċ gol mạric*, 10 black peppercorns.

Mix the juice extracted from these and give to drink.

Bẹrẹl sasaṅ, raw turmeric, Curcuma longa, Roxb.

Mạric, chilli, Capsicum frutescens, Willd.

Grind these and after shaving over the fontanel, apply there.

If there is pain in the chest or ribs:

(*c*) *Rại tuṛi*, Brassica campestris.

Grind and apply without heating (a sinapism).

(*d*) *Isạbgul*, Plantago ispaghala, R. Fleming.

Grind and apply warm

(*e*) *Chạtni chal*, the bark of Alstonia scholaris, R. Br.

Mix with the milk of a black goat and apply warm.

(*f*) *Tejo mala rẹhẹl*, the roots of Cissampelos Pareira, L.

5 *gol mạric*, 5 black peppercorns.

Grind together and give to drink.

250. *Khok manda*. Cough and cold.

Medicines: (*a*) *Rạsun*, garlic.

Adagạthiạ ghās da, the bulbs of Panicum repens, Linn.

Buluṅ, salt.

Grind these together, make into pills to be taken daily, and the cold will certainly get well.

(*b*) *Nawa sim bele*, new laid fowl's egg.

Buluṅ, salt.

Mạric, chilli, Capsicum frutescens, Willd.

Sasaṅ, turmeric, Curcuma longa, Roxb.

To be cooked together and taken 3 or 4 times, when he will get well.

(*c*) *Beṅgaṛ beṭahel jọ*, the fruit of Solanum stramonifolium, Jacq.

Gại gọtọm, melted butter made from cows' milk.

The former to be cooked in the latter and then eaten.

(*d*) *Adagạthiạ ghās da*, the bulbs of Panicum repens, Linn.

Ẹdhẹ raṅgạini jạnum, dareko jọko, the entire plant and fruits of Solanum xanthocarpum, Schrad. et Wandl.

Boil these together and after adding salt make the patient drink it.

(*e*) *Sọsọ*, Semecarpus Anacardium, Linn., var. cuneifolia.

Grind with roasted rice and let the patient eat it.

(*f*) *Hẹṅjẹl jọ*, the fruit of Solanum stramonifolium, Jacq.

Caole ata, roasted rice.

Both to be roasted, then ground together and eaten with the addition of a little salt.

(*g*) *Adagạthiạ da*, the bulbs of Panicum repens, Linn.

To be cooked in oil and eaten.

(*h*) *Rạṅgạini jạnum rẹhẹl, dare, sakam*, the entire plant, roots and leaves of Solanum Jacquini, Willd.

Adagạthiạ ghās da, the bulbs of Panicum repens, L.

Boil these together and give to drink with salt every morning till recovery.

(*i*) *Mare jọjọ ar amṭha*, the old fruit and inspissated juice of Tamarindus indica, L.

First brown this like curry, then add 8 ounces water and 2 ounces *misri*, sugar-candy, and after boiling well till amalgamated, give to drink.

(*j*) *Hẹsẹl chal*, the bark of Anogeissus latifolia, Wall.

Sẹkrẹč chal, „ „ „ Lagerstroemia parviflora, Roxb.

Let him chew these daily.

(*k*) *Adagaṭhiạ da*, the bulb of Panicum repens, L.

Pọstọ dana, the seeds of the opium poppy.

Lọṅphul, cloves.

Jawan, Carum Ajowan, DC.

Biṭ buluṅ, factitious salt containing sulphur.

Grind all these together fine, make into pills the size of a small pea, one pill to be eaten every morning, and a little *gañja*, Cannabis sativa, Willd. to be licked.

(*l*) *Rạṅgạini jạnum rẹhẹl ar sakam*, the roots and leaves of Solanum Jacquini Willd.

Adagaṭhiạ, Panicum repens, L.

Boil these together, and after adding salt to be drunk.

(*m*) *Jọjọ amṭha*, the dried flesh of the fruit of Tamarindus indica, L.

Boil in 8 ounces of water, add a little *misri*, sugar-candy, and give to drink.

251. *Kạṭič gidrạko mandak*. Cold in infants.

Medicines: (*a*) *Adagaṭhiạ ghãs*, Panicum repens, Linn.

Darcini, cinnamon.

Sũṭ, dry ginger.

Pipol, Piper longum, Willd.

Grind these together, then mix with *ṅẹlẹ rasa*, honey, and let them lick it. Babies to lick honey only.

(*b*) *Thoṛa darcini*, a little cinnamon.

Sũṭ, dry ginger.

Grind together, stir in honey of either the ordinary or humble bee and give to lick.

(*c*) *Hẹñjẹl rẹhẹl*, the roots of Solanum stramonifolium, Jacq.

Sọsọ jaṅ milṭẹn gan, about one seed of Semecarpus Anacardium, L.

Caole ata rọṅgọak, rice fried to burning point.

Grind all together and give to eat like a porridgy mess.

(*d*) *Darcini*, cinnamon.

Sũṭ, dry ginger.

Grind and mix with honey of the ordinary or small bee and give it a little *gañja*, Cannabis sativa, Willd., to lick, and smear a little on the fontanel.

(*e*) *Joka sakam*, the leaves of Sida humilis, Willd.
Grind and plaster on the fontanel and some to be licked.

252. *Dhọ̃k.* Phthisis previous to hæmoptysia, also bronchitis and asthma.
Medicines: (*a*) *Kạhu botke rẹhẹl*, the roots of Bryonia lacinosa, L.
Campa rẹhẹl, „ „ „ Michelia champaca, L.
Grind these together, cook in melted butter and give to eat.

(*b*) *Cae cirota*, Gentiana cherayta, Roxb.
Kọrpur, camphor.
Elaci, cardamums, Alpinia cardamomum, Roxb.
Mahabạri bọc, Zingiber zerumbet, Roscoe.
Darcini, cinnamon.
Sũṭ pipol, dry ginger and Piper longum, Willd.
Kabab cini, Cubeba officinalis, Miqu.
Gol mạric, black pepper.
Mix a little of each of these, grind dry and give to eat.

(*c*) *Lọṅphul*, cloves.
Phọṭ kạpur,
Cirota, Gentiana cherayta, Roxb.
Pipol, Piper longum, Willd.
Darcini, cinnamon.
Kabab cini, Cubeba officinalis, Miqu.
Adagạthiạ rẹhẹl, the roots of Panicum repens, L.
Mahabạri bọc, Zingiber zerumbet, Roscoe.
Gol mạric, black pepper.

Grind these together, cook in mustard oil and give to eat. Afterwards let him eat *pan sakam*, the leaves of Piper Betle, L., with *khayar*, Acacia Catechu, L.

(*d*) Bring the heart of all kinds of trees from the forest and boil in a new vessel; strain off the blood coloured water and boil that water down. Then let him eat the residue very early in the morning. This will cause him to vomit. When he is exhausted with vomiting let him eat hot boiled rice with *gại dahe*, curds made from cow's milk.

(*e*) *Sũ hako im*, the liver of a porpoise, Delphinus Gangeticus.
Poṇḍ rạṅgaini rẹhẹl, the roots of the white Solanum xanthocarpum, Schrad. et Wendl.
Tạrup nạṇḍri, a leopard's windpipe.
Khikṛi nạṇḍri, a fox's windpipe.
Grind and mix these and after cooking in mustard oil give to eat.

(*f*) *Kạsi rẹhẹl*, the roots of Saccharum spontaneụm, L.
Matkọm mañj, the heart of Bassia latifolia, Roxb.
Kaṇṭa siris mañj, the heart of Albizzia myriophylla, Bl.

Boil all these down in a new vessel to the consistency of the raw molasses made from Bassia latifolia, Roxb. and after grinding *ul banda*, the parasitic plant found on the mango tree, mix this, make into pills and give to eat.

(g) *Ọrsọṛẹñ da*, the bulb of Zingiber Cassumunar, Roxb.
Kaṇṭa kucạ aṛak,
Kaṇṭa sạru da, the bulb of Lasia heterophylla, Schott.
Orop da, „ „ „ Costus speciosa, Sm.
Bẹṛẹl sasaṅ, raw turmeric.
Gol mạric, black pepper.
Sanam lekan gọṛọm mọsọla thoṛa thoṛa, mix a little of all kinds of pungent spices.

Grind to a powder and give to eat.

When blood is mixed:

(h) *Arak upạl baha sẹ uldhạtẹl*, the flower of Nymphœa rubra, Roxb., or the tubers of the same.
Poṇḍ rạṅgaini dare sẹ rẹhẹl sakam jọtọge, the roots, leaves or entire white Solanum xanthocarpum, Schrad. et Wendl.

Cook in melted butter of cows' milk, mixing also *paḍeṛ chal*, the bark of Stereospermum suaveolens, DC., make into pills to be taken daily.

(i) the same as (a) above till the cough ceases when
(j) the same as (b) above with the addition of *ghọr*, buttermilk, until recovery.
(k) *Adagạthiạ da*, the bulb of Panicum repens, L.
Kạhu botke da, „ „ „ Bryonia lacinosa, L.
Binḍi muthạ rẹhẹl, the roots of Fimbristylis monostachya, Hassk.
Sukri muthạ rẹhẹl, the roots of Scirpus monostachyus, Kön.
Campa baha, Michelia champaca L.

Grind all these together, mix with *matkọm mañj reañ guṛ*, molasses extracted from the heart of Bassia latifolia, Roxb., cook the whole and give about a spoonful only to drink as it is a very powerful medicine.

(l) *Sũṭ*, dry ginger.
Pipol, Piper longum, Willd.
Sinid baha,
Dhela chal, the bark of Alangium Lamarckii, Thws.
Gol mạric, black pepper.
Campa baha, Michelia champaca, L.

Grind all these together and give to eat without cooking. *Forbidden diet*: Browned curries, pork, curry of the fruit or leaves of Cucurbita moscheta, Duchesne, buffalo meat, mutton, and the leaves of *Kantha aṛak*, Euphorbia granulata, Forsk.

(m) *Kạsi rẹhẹl*, the roots of Saccharum spontaneum, L.
Karsaṛe rẹhẹl, the roots of Thysanolaena acarifera, Nees.

Tarop rehel reak chal, the bark of the roots of Buchanania latifolia, Roxb.

Matkom dare reak manj, the heart of Bassia latifolia Roxb.

Grind together, cook in mustard oil, make into pills and give to eat.

(*n*) *Hũnd baha rehel*, the roots of Jasminum arborescens, Roxb.

Nanha dudhi lota rehel, the roots of Ichnocarpus frutescens, R.Br.

Mahabari boc, Zingiber zerumbet, Roscoe.

Sũt, dry ginger.

Pipol, Piper longum, Willd,

Gol maric, black pepper.

Kalia jira, Nigella indica, Roxb.

Lonphul, cloves.

Grind all together and give to eat.

(*o*) *Adhe*, ginger, Zingiber officinalis, Roscoe.

Etkeć lore, the sticky exudation of Euphorbia antiquorum, L.

Hemsagor, Cotyledon laciniata, Willd.

Karsare da, the bulb of Thysanolæna acarifera, Nees.

(*p*) *Kasi da*, the bulb of Saccharum spontaneum, L.

Moron arak rehel, the roots of Gymnema hirsutus, W. and A., var. Decaisneanum, Wight.

Kalmeg, Andrographis paniculata, Nees.

Bengar betahel, Solanum stramonifolium, Jacq.

(*q*) *Kasi ghãs rehel*, the roots of Saccharum spontaneum, L.

Kasmar chal, the bark of Gmelina arborea, Roxb.

Dhela chal, the bark of Alangium Lamarckii, Thws.

Sekreć sakam, the leaves of Lagerstroemia parviflora, Roxb.

Chatni chal, the bark of Alstonia scholaris, R.Br.

Arak raj baha, the red var. of Nerium odorum, Soland.

Matkom chal, the bark of Bassia latifolia, Roxb.

Pound all these and put them in a new earthen pot with about a pint of water. Cover with a leaf plate and boil thoroughly. Drain off the water and add to it the following after grinding them small and throwing away the barks :—

Darcini, cinnamon.

Kabab cini, Cubebs piper.

Pipol, Piper longum, Willd.

Sũt, dry ginger.

Thora boc, a little of the root stock of Acorus Calamus, Willd.

Elaci, Alpinia cardamomum, Roxb.

Then boil thoroughly again after covering with a leaf plate, as the remedy will lose its efficacy if the steam escapes. Some 4 to 8 ounces will remain, which give for about a week. When the cough is easier, discontinue it and give the following for about a couple of days:

Hęndę buluṅ, black salt.
Khạiri buluṅ, brown or dirty coloured salt.
Biṭ buluṅ, a factitious salt containing sulphur.
Poṇḍ buluṅ, white salt.
Raṅgạini jạnum rẹhẹt, the roots of Solanum Jacquini, Willd.
Adagạthiạ ghās da, the bulb of Panicum repens, L.

To be ground together and made into pills. If the cough returns stop the medicine. If the three following medicines are bought in Calcutta and given in succession, he will certainly get well:—

Sasarǫ,
Darka ristu,
Sǫmęsǫṅ rǫsayǫn.

Kạsi dama, asthma:—

(r) *Kạsi rẹhẹt*, the roots of Saccharum spontaneum, L.
Kūs rẹhẹt, " " " Themuda gigantea, Haskel.
Kǭc bel chal, the bark of Feronia Elephantum, Correa.
Kaḍa beṅjak rẹhẹt, the roots of
Ạṇḍiạ mǫrǫn ạṛak rẹhẹt, the roots of Gymnema hirsutus, W. and A., var. Decaisneanum, Wight.
Sūṭ, dry ginger.
Pipol, Piper longum, Willd.
Lǫṅphul, cloves.
Pǫstu, poppy seed.
Hạlim, Lepidium sativum, L.
Raj baha, Nerium odorum, Soland.
Bir karla rẹhẹt, the roots of the wild Momordica dioica, Roxb.

Make into pills without cooking and give daily in the morning and he will recover.

Dama dhǭk, asthma.

(s) *Hūnd baha rẹhẹt*, the roots of Jasminum arborescens, Roxb.
Ghi kūạ̄ri rẹhẹt, " " " Yucca gloriosa, or
Nanha dudhi loṭa rẹhẹt, the roots of Ichnocarpus frutescens, R. Br.
Rǫhǫṛ adhẹ, dried Zingiber officinalis, Roscoe.
Pipol, Piper longum, Willd.
Mahabạri bǫc, Zingiber zerumbet, Roscoe.
21 *gaṇḍa gol mạric*, 84 black peppercorns.

Grind all these together and make into pills, one of which to be taken thrice daily.

If the wheezing does not cease,

(*t*) *Caulia rehel*, the roots of Ruellia suffruticosa, Roxb.

Pound and give the liquid to drink daily.

Khadar khodor dhok, bronchitis.

Symptoms. There is a rattling or wheezing sound in breathing.

(*u*) *Hasa arak*,
Tol lumam tejo, a silkworm chrysalis.

Grind together and give to drink.

253. *Raj rog, thae khok ar kasi dhok.*

Consumption (*i.e.* hæmoptysis), dry cough and bronchitis.

Symptoms. This begins with a cough which is very severe; what is eaten is not digested, there is much vomiting. Such is the case in dry cough and bronchitis, and when it has lasted some time it developes into consumption and blood is brought up when coughing.

Medicines: (*a*) There are eight kinds of salt, viz.
Bit buluṅ, a factitious salt containing sulphur.
Khairi buluṅ, brown or dirty coloured salt.
Hende buluṅ, black salt.
Pond buluṅ, white salt.

The names of the other kinds I do not know, but if you ask the shopkeeper for them he will give you.

Darcini, cinnamon.
Kabab cini, Cubeba officinalis, Miqu.
Cae cirota, Gentiana cherayta, Roxb.
Sũt, dry ginger.
Adhe, Zingiber officinalis, Roscoe.
Pipol se roli jo, Piper longum, Willd.
Juṅgi phol jo,
Jutri phol jo,
Boro elaci jo, large cardamums.
Chota elaci jo, small cardamums.

Grind all these together very fine, dry, i.e. without any water. Then kill a young pigeon and fry its meat in mustard oil. Add the 8 kinds of salt and spices you have mixed, about two mussel shells full, and when the cooking is done let this suffice to be taken once a day for four days with a meal. Repeat this treatment daily for one or two months and recovery will follow.

(*b*) The 8 kinds of salt mentioned in (*a*)
Orop dare reak jaṅ, the stone of Costus speciosa, Sm.
Edhe raṅgaini janum rehel, the roots of Solanum xanthocarpum, Schrad. et Wendl.
Heñjel rehel, the roots of Solanum stramonifolium, Jacq.
Adagathia ghãs da, the bulb of Panicum repens, Linn.

Grind these four ingredients together, mix with the different kinds of salt and make into pills to be eaten daily till the cough stops, when the medicine is to cease.

(c) *Darcini*, cinnamon.
Kabab cini, Cubeba officinalis, Miqu.
Pipol, Piper longum, Willd.
Sohga, borax.

Grind these four together into a powder, then mix with sugar-candy and grind, to be swallowed as a powder with the help of a little warm water.

(d) *Kitą dąl*, the kernel of Phoenix acaulis, Buch. } to be mixed
Dahe, curds. } together and
Taben, rice soaked and flattened. } eaten daily.
Bąṛ baha chal, the skin of the flower of Mimusops Elengi, L.
Raj baha arakak, the red variety oleander, Nerium odorum, Soland.
Upąl bahateḽ, the flower of the lotus, Nymphæa Lotus, Willd.
Sąphur rẹhẹl,
Parwa mayām, pigeon's blood.
Pąuną,
Kaṇṭa sąru, Lasia heterophylla, Schott.
Adagąṭhią, Panicum repens, Linn.
Rǫl jǫ, the fruit of Terminalia Chebula, Retz.
Khayar ǫjǫn, Acacia Catechu, Willd.
Niuri dare, Elæodendron Roxburghii, W. and A.
Kąṭić talań sẹṅgẹl siń, a little of Tragia involucrata, Jacq.
Bhuku chata, a termites' nest.

To be eaten nine days.

(e) *Arak raj baha*, the red oleander flower, Nerium odorum, Soland.
Hẹndẹ mẹrǫm reak māyām, the blood of a black goat.
Dherkaete gẹḍẹ māyām, especially ducks' blood.

To be made into a soup and taken.

(f) *Arak upąl baha*, the red lotus flower, Nymphaea rubra, Roxb.
Bir campa rẹhẹl, the roots of Ochna squarrosa, Willd.
Khayar mańj, the heart of Acacia Catechu, L.
Matkǫm mańj, ,, ,, ,, Bassia latifolia, Roxb
Hẹndẹ sim māyām, the blood of a black fowl.

All to be boiled together and drunk.

When there is a copious expectoration of blood:

(g) *Hẹndẹ sim māyām*, the blood of a black fowl,
Hẹndẹ mẹrǫm māyām, the blood of a black goat.

To be drunk.

(*h*) *Kạhu botke*, Bryonia lacinosa, Linn.
Campa, Michelia champaca, L.
Haṛhal hoṭoṭ, a bitter pumpkin, Cucurbita lagenaria, Willd.
Sega jạnum, Mimosa rubicaulis, Lamk.
Adagạthiạ, Panicum repens, Linn.

To be cooked with melted butter.

(*i*) *Jạphir phọl*,
Banat araḱak, thick European made woollen red cloth.
Upạl baha araḱakge, the red lotus flower, Nymphaea rubra, Roxb.
Jaephọl, nutmeg.

Grind all these together, cook in melted butter and then to be eaten.

If a woman with a cough has no milk then give her to eat

(*j*) *Banda*, a parasitical plant.

If a woman will not stay with her coughing husband then make her eat

(*k*) *Ḍaharreko ńamok pọṭọm tejo*, a chrysalis found on the roads, or those found on trees will also do.

(*l*) *Kạhu botke*, Bryonia lacinosa, Linn.
Campa, Michelia champaca, L.

Let the patient eat these first, and then proceed with

Bọc, Acorus Calamus, Willd.
Cirota, Gentiana cherayta, Roxb.
Kuṛ,
Kaphọr, camphor.
Elaci, Alpinia cardamomum, Roxb.
Mahabạri bọc, Zingiber zerumbet, Roscoe.
Sũṭ, dry ginger.
Pipol, Piper longum, Willd.
Gol mạric, black pepper.
Darcini, cinnamon.
Kabab cini, Cubeba officinalis, Miqu.
Basọk, Justicia Adhatoda, L.

Grind all these together and make into pills to be taken. Give only a little, not much.

(*m*) *Baṛ chal*, the bark of Mimusops Elengi, L.
Arak upạl baha da, the tuber of the red Nymphaea rubra, Roxb.
Adagạthiạ rẹhẹt, the roots of Panicum repens, Limn.
Banat arakak, thick European made woollen red cloth.
Kạsi rẹhẹt, the roots of Saccharum spontaneum, Linn.
Kũs rẹhẹt, „ „ „ Themuda gigantea, Haskel.
Kaṇṭa kucạ rẹhẹt, the roots of Mimosa rubicaulis, Willd.

Aṇḍiạ mọrọn aṛak rẹhẹt, the roots of Gymnema hirsutus, W. and A., var. Decaisneanum, Wight.

Lọṅphul, 4 or more cloves.

Jiṭhimond chal, the bark of Clerodendron Siphonanthus, R. Br.

All these to be ground together, boiled in mustard oil and eaten.

(*n*) *Kondro chal*, the bark of Acacia Intsia, Willd.

Jugi ṭupri rẹhẹt, the roots of

Lodam chal, the bark of Symplocos racemosa, Roxb.

Grind together and give to drink with boiling water.

(*o*) *Miru baha rẹhẹt*, the roots of Abutilon indicum, Don.

Thoṛa haṭ chal, a little bark of Holarrhena antidysenterica, Wall.

Arak joba baha, the red flower of Hibiscus rosa-sinensis, L.

Arak raj baha, „ „ „ „ Nerium odorum, Soland.

Arak upạl baha, „ „ „ „ Nymphaea rubra, Roxb.

Grind these all fine together, then add 2 annas worth of *ạphim*, opium, and grind again; make into pills of which 3 to be taken daily. If this does not cure, then

(*p*) *Biṭ buluṅ thoṛa*, a little of the factitious sulphur containing salt.

Poṇḍ buluṅ thoṛa, a little white salt.

Darcini, cinnamon.

Kabab cini, Cubeba officinalis, Miqu.

Sũṭ, dry ginger.

Pipol jọ, Piper longum, Willd.

Kạliạ jirạ, Nigella indica, Roxb.

Lubui jirạ,

Jawan jirạ, Carum Ajowan, DC.

Sẹ jọtọ mọsọla ran mesalme, or mix all spices.

Grind all these very fine. First fry the meat of a *parwa*, pigeon, in mustard oil till it frizzles, then add a mussel shell full (about a dessert spoonful) of what you have ground. If the oil seems drying up, add a little more until cooked. Give this to eat for some five days and recovery is sure to follow.

(*q*) *Salọk misri*, a kind of sugar-candy.

Mix this with cow's milk and boil; make into pills of which three to be taken daily for three days.

(*r*) *Kọbọl jọ*,

Rọkọt cọndọn, blood coloured sandal wood.

Rọs mạnik,

Rọs sindur, a sort of factitious cinnabar.

Jaephọl, nutmeg.

Chobṛa,

Elaci, Alpinia cardamomum, Roxb.
Jiṭhimond, Clerodendron Siphonanthus, R. Br.
Mahabạri bọc, Zingiber zerumbet, Roscoe.
Họrtoki, the fruit of Terminalia Chebula, Retz.
Juṅgi họrtoki (*rọl*), Terminalia Chebula, Retz. (?).

Grind together, mix with the blood of a *risạ sim*, fowl with bristling or up standing feathers, and make into 9 pills to be taken. For 21 days let him eat exclusively pulses as curry. If this is ineffective give the preceding one (*p*).

(*s*) *Raj baha*, Nerium odorum, Soland.
Pạni phọl, Trapa bispinosa, Roxb.
Arak upạl, Nymphaea rubra, Roxb.
Sũṭ, dry ginger.
Pipol, Piper longum, Willd.
Boṅga bạri,

(*t*) *Bọnkạpsi jaṅ*, the kernel of Thespesia Lampas, Benth. and Hook. f.
Haṭ jaṅ, the kernel of Holarrhena antidysenterica, Wall.
Nạṅgrạuta rẹhẹl, the roots of Nardostachys jatamansi, DC.
Adagạṭhiạ da, the tuber of Panicum repens, L.
Kũs rẹhẹl, the roots of Themuda gigantea, Haskel.
Kạhu botke da, the tuber of Bryonia lacinosa, L.
Gạiphọl,
Kanda sạru da, the tuber of a var. of Celocasia antiquorum, Schott.
Mahabạri bọc, Zingiber zerumbet, Roscoe.
Kabab cini, Cubeba officinalis, Miqu.
Jawan, Carum Ajowan, DC.
Gol mạric, black pepper.
Pipol, Piper longum, Willd.
Kalmẹg, Andrographis paniculata, Nees.

Grind all these together, boil in *utiṅ sunum*, mustard oil, and give to eat. If he has bronchial asthma, then cook above ingredients in melted butter and give to eat.

(*u*) *Kạsi rẹhẹl*, the roots of Saccharum spontaneum, L.
Tarọp rẹhẹl, „ „ „ Buchanania latifolia, Roxb.
Matkọm maṅj, the heart of Bassia latifolia, Roxb.
Karsaṛe, Thysanolaena acarifera, Nees.
Cạuliạ, Ruellia suffruticosa, Roxb.

Grind these together, cook in *utiṅ sunum*, mustard oil and give to eat three times a day.

(*v*) *Miru baha rẹhẹl*, the roots of Abutilon indicum, Don.
Thoṛa haṭ chal, a little of the bark of Holarrhena antidysenterica, Wall.

Arak joba baha, the red Hibiscus rosa-sinensis, L.
Arak raj baha, „ „ Nerium odorum, Soland.
Arak upal baha, „ „ Nymphaea rubra, Roxb.

Grind all these to a fine powder, then add a little *aphim*, opium, and grind again, make into pills, of which three to be taken daily.

(*w*) *Bit bulun*, a factitious salt containing sulphur.
Pond se panga bulun, white salt.
Joto lekan mosola, all kinds of spices.

Mix these with the ingredients mentioned in the previous one (*u*) make into pills of which three to be taken daily.

(*x*) *Pe sakam pan*, 3 leaves of Piper Betle, L.
Thora khayar, a little Acacia Catechu, L.
Kūs rehel, the roots of Themuda gigantea, Haskel.
Arak upal baha, the red Nymphaea rubra, Roxb.
Bare baha, Pentapetes phoenicia, L.
Arak gandhari, the red Amarantus gangeticus, var. angustifolia, L.
Saram māyām, the blood of the sambar stag, Rusa aristotelis.
Caole maric rehel, the roots of a kind of capsicum, the fruit-like grains of rice.
Lonphul, cloves.
Kalia jira, Nigella indica, Roxb.
Terel cete, the thin skin on the bark of Diospyros tomentosa, Roxb.

Grind all these along with the ingredients in (*u*) above, mixing them, cook in *gai gotom*, melted butter from cow's milk, to be eaten every morning.

254. *Pathri rua se betha.*

(? Pleurisy; supposed to be caused by a witch's charm.)

Symptoms. In this there is intense pain in the chest, as if it were splitting; the pain shifts about in the chest and is not stationary, and sometimes the breathing is stopped.

Medicines: *Badgocak rehel*, the roots of Lygodium flexuosum, Sw.
Sega rehel, „ „ „ Mimosa rubicaulis, Lam.
Kondro janum rehel, the roots of Acacia Intsia, Willd.
Kadar rehel, the roots of Asparagus racemosus, Willd.
Salga jer se chal, the sticky exudation or bark of Boswellia thurifera, Colebroke.

Grind together, mix with water and give to drink.

255. *Betha.*

(Intercostal neuralgia, Pleurisy, Pneumonia.)

Symptoms. This is an aggravated form of *hadi*. If one lifts anything very heavy or something of the kind, it is followed by a sharp pain under the ribs or in the chest.

Medicines: (*a*) *Ḍhalka hạtkạn*, Leea macrophylla, Roxb.
5 *gọṭẹć gol mạric*, 5 black peppercorns.

Extract the juice of the former, mix with the latter and plaster therewith, giving also a little to drink.

(*b*) *Ḍuriạ hạtkạn*, Leea hirta, Herb. Banks.
Sạṇḍi saba hạtkạn,

Grind these separately, plaster and give some to drink.

(*c*) *Chạtni chal*, the bark of Alstonia scholaris, R.Br.
10 *gọṭẹć gol mạric*, 10 black peppercorns.

Extract the juice of the former, mix and give to drink, and warming some a little plaster therewith.

(*d*) *Gaḍa terel*, Diospyros montana, Roxb.
Kạuhạ chal, the bark of Terminalia Arjuna, Redd.
Bạru chal, „ „ „ Schleichera trijuga, Willd.
Ạsạṛiạ chal, „ „ „ Capparis horrida, L. f.
Ruhen chal, „ „ „ Soymida febrifuga, Juss.
Jhiṅgur da, the bulb of Arum campanulatum, Roxb.
Dare japak jọ, the fruit of Scindapsus officinalis, Schott.
Maṭha aṛak chal, the bark of Antidesma diandrum, Tulas.
Akaona rẹhẹt, the roots of Calotropis gigantea, R. Br.

Grind whichever of these you can get and apply as a plaster and give to drink any of the first five, but the remainder may only be applied as a plaster.

(*e*) *Ghoṛa lada rẹhẹt*, the roots of Vitis tomentosa, Heyne.

Warm a little of this and apply to the painful part. Then cutting into thin slices mix with 12 black peppercorns and after cooking in mustard oil give to eat daily. Even if of years' standing it will cure.

(*f*) *Ẹdẹl chal*, the bark of Bombax malabaricum, DC.
Jur juri da, the bulb of

Grind together and smear on. If there is no alleviation, then

Tọlnọpak chal sẹ rẹhẹt, the bark or roots of Eugenia operculata, Roxb.

Boil and smear on.

Bhạbri chal, the bark of Embelia robusta, Roxb.
Ḍunḍukil rẹhẹt, the roots of Gardenia turgida, Roxb.
Ạṇḍiạ mọrọn rẹhẹt, the roots of Gymnema hirsutus, W. and A., var. Decaisneanum, Wight.
Terel poha rẹhẹt, the roots of a seedling of Diospyros tomentosa, Roxb.
Poṇḍ họṛẹć, white Dolichos biflorus, L.

Cook these in melted butter and give to eat.

(*g*) *Hạtkạn chal*, the bark of Leea macrophylla, Roxb.
Ruhen chal, „ „ „ Soymida febrifuga, Juss.
Ḍuriạ hạtkạn rẹhẹl, the roots of Leea hirta, Herb. Banks.
Jĩoti, the entire Sesbania aegyptiaca, Pers.

Grind together, some to be drunk, some to be smeared on.

If the pain does not cease, then afterwards

Coḍra chal, the bark of

Grind and smear on.

(*h*) *Dhạlka hạtkạn*, Leea macrophylla, Roxb.
Ḍuriạ hạtkạn, Leea hirta, Herb. Banks.
Ruhen, Soymida febrifuga, Juss.

Grind together and plaster therewith. The patient to eat hand bread made of the millet Eleusine corocana, Gärtn.

(*i*) *Ghoṛa lada rẹhẹl*, the roots of Vitis tomentosa, Heyne.
Moṭa hạtkạn, Leea macrophylla, Roxb.

(*j*) *Ḍuriạ hạtkạn*, Leea hirta, Herb. Banks.
Bạru chal, the bark of Schleichera trijuga, Willd.
Corco chal, „ „ „ Casearea tomentosa, Roxb.
Jĩoti, Sesbania aegyptiaca, Pers.
Goṭe chal, the bark of Croton oblongifolius, Roxb.

(*k*) *Ruhen chal*, the bark of Soymida febrifuga, Juss.
Ghoṛa lạdạuṛi da, the bulb of Vitis tomentosa, Heyne.
Kạuhạ chal, the bark of Terminalia Arjuna, Bedd.
Bherṇḍa loṛe, the exudation from Jatropha Curcas, L.
Bạru chal, the bark of Schleichera trijuga, Willd.
Sahar chal, „ „ „ Dillenia pentagyna, Roxb.

Grind these together, warm somewhat and apply to the seat of pain.

(*l*) *Jel dereń*, a deer's horn.

Grind fine, warm slightly and apply to the painful part.

If there is pain in the chest

(*m*) *Ḍhalka hạtkạn da*, the tuberous root of Leea macrophylla, Roxb.

Grind fine with water, and after warming slightly plaster on to the painful part, and if it stays thus all day it will do no harm.

256. *Pạchiạra betha.* Pneumonia.

Medicines: (*a*) *Muṅgạ dare sẹ rẹhẹl chal*, the bark of the tree or roots of Moringa pterygosperma, Gärtn.
3 *gaṇḍa gol mạric*, 12 black peppercorns.

Grind together and apply without warming.

(*b*) *Rạsun*, garlic.

Grind and apply without warming, and when this begins to cause pain remove it, otherwise it may cause the skin to break.

(*c*) ***Rại tuṛi***, **Brassica campestris, L.**

Grind and apply without warming.

(*d*) ***Ṭhạḍiạ tuṛi***, a variety of Brassica campestris, L.

Luṭni tuṛi, „ „ „ „ „ „

Grind together and apply; a complete cure will soon follow.

(*e*) *Dare japak iọ*, the fruit of Scindapsus officinalis, Schott.

Warm and apply.

(*f*) *Ič ẹwẹr da*, the bulb of Vitis latifolia, Roxb.

Grind, warm and apply.

Pạchiạ betha (on the right side).

(*g*) *Jọnọk carẹč*, a broom splinter.

First break this in two and make passes over the patient repeating charms; and then

(*h*) *Hạlim*, Lepidium sativum, L.

A little to be drunk and a little to be smeared on; if this is not enough, then mix

(*i*) *Ḍhalka hạtkạn*, Leea macrophylla, Roxb.

and apply

(*j*) *Ḍuriạ hạtkạn*, Leea hirta, Herb. Banks.

Jĩoti mil khudri gan, a little bit of Sesbania aegyptiaca, Pers.

Smear the former only on, and the latter to be drunk.

(*k*) *Kọdẹ piṭhạ*, hand bread made of Eleusine corocana, Gärtn.

Joṇḍra dak mạṇḍi, gruel of Zea Mays, L.

Both to be eaten; rice gruel will not do.

(*l*) *Muṅgạ chal*, the bark of Moringa pterygosperma, Gärtn.

Pẹ gaṇḍa gol mạric, 12 black peppercorns.

Grind both together and plaster on the painful part.

257. *Suk betha*. (? Pleuritis exsudativa.)

Symptoms. There is a pain in the ribs or sides, which gradually increases and the breath comes heavily.

Medicines: (*a*) *Ḍhalka hạtkạn rẹhẹt*, the roots of Leea macrophylla, Roxb. Grind, warm and apply to the seat of pain. If the pain is deep seated then cut the above into slices and after mixing 3 *gaṇḍa gol mạric*, 12 black peppercorns, cook in mustard oil and give to eat, when the pain will rise to the surface.

(*b*) *Bạru chal*, the bark of Schleichera trijuga, Willd.

Heat and apply as an ointment, and after mixing black pepper with its juice give to drink.

(*c*) *Ruhen chal*, the bark of Soymida febrifuga, Juss.

Warm and apply as an ointment and give some also to drink.

(*d*) *Sim kaṭa hạtkạn*,

Warm and apply.

(e) *Asaria chal*, the bark of Capparis horrida, L. f.

Warm and apply and after mixing black pepper give some to drink.

(f) *Ghora ladauri da*, the bulb of Vitis tomentosa, Heyne.

Warm and give to drink, and cut some into slices, add 12 black peppercorns and cook in mustard oil and then give to eat; the pain will come to the surface.

(g) *Gada terel chal*, the bark of Diospyros montana, Roxb.

Warm and apply.

(h) *Sandi saba rehel*, the roots of Briedelia stipularis, Bl.

Warm and apply.

(i) *Sandi saba hatkan rehel*, the roots of

Warm and apply.

(j) *Duria hatkan se dhalka hatkan rehel*, the roots of Leea hirta, Herb. Banks., or Leea macrophylla, Roxb.

Dare japak jo, the fruit of Scindapsus officinalis, Schott.

Etka rehel, the roots of Mucuna pruriens, DC.

Jioti dog, the tips of Sesbania aegyptiaca, Pers.

Baru chal, the bark of Schleichera trijuga, Willd.

Grind all these and plaster on the painful part.

If all these are unobtainable quickly, then

(k) *Dhalka hatkan*, Leea macrophylla, Roxb.

Halim, Lepidium sativum, L.

Grind and mix both these and give a little to drink and plaster a little where it pains.

258. *Murhuć jom.* Leprosy.

Medicines: (a) *Koronj sunum*, the oil obtained from the seeds of Pongamia glabra, Vent.

Raekakarbak candbol, the tail of a chameleon.

Jhurjhuria, the tinsel looking chrysalis of a certain butterfly (one).

Hende tilmiń (1 *pai gan*), about 1 lb. of the black Sesamum orientale, Willd.

Soso (5 *gan*), about 5 fruits of Semecarpus Anacardium, L.

Gidi im, the liver of a vulture.

Pulverise the last three together and give to eat. Cook in the first named the two following ingredients and anoint therewith daily.

(b) *Simbrit*, fresh shoots of Bombax malabaricum, DC.

Rosomuni,

Ros sindur, a sort of factitious cinnabar.

Sora, saltpetre.

Batapi sindur, a preparation of red lead.

Sinduran rote, a kind of frog with red coloured head.

Grind all these together fine, mix into three or four pounds of pure oil made from *ṭhạḍiạ tuṛi*, a var. of Brassica campestris, L., and stir all together. The patient to anoint himself therewith daily. If the oil comes to an end add more.

Proscribed: meat and fish of any kind; beer and spirits; complete abstention from sexual intercourse is essential.

Permitted diet: the split fruit of *hoṛeč*, Delichos biflorus, L., *mạsri*, Ervum lens, L., *raheṛ*, Cajanus indicus, Spreng.

If there are open sores on the limbs, then grind all the above together and cook in above oil, and anoint therewith, when he will recover.

After recovery he will feel numb, and then give:—

(*c*) *Pọstu dana*, poppy seed.
Lọṅphul, cloves.
Gol mạric, black pepper.
Kạliạ jirạ, Nigella indica, Roxb.
Ghikũạri, Yucca gloriosa.

Grind together, mix with pure *gọlọm*, melted butter from cows' milk, and anoint therewith daily. Further let him boil the following together and bathe and wash the hands in the water:—

Gabla chal, the bark of Acacia arabica, Willd.
Kạuhạ chal, „ „ „ Terminalia Arjuna, Bedd.

259. *Dhaot.* Sexual inopia.

Symptoms. This is where there is an absence of all desire for sexual intercourse in either sex with the other.

Medicines: (*a*) *Monkha*, 2 ounces.
Kismis, 2 „ raisins.
Choṛa, 8 „
Kạbligọlọr, 2 „
Pistạ, 2 „ poppy seeds.
Bidạm, 2 „
Gukhur kaṭa, 1 „
Rạsun, 1 „ garlic.
Misri, 8 „ sugar candy.

Boil all these together in about two pounds of milk and make 30 pills. Then let the patient swallow one of these pills with half a pound of milk daily for 30 days. Then the former desire will return.

260. *Mãyõ koṛa.* Male impotency.

Medicines: (*a*) *Aṇḍiạ mọrọn aṛak̓ rẹhẹl*, the roots of Gymnema hirsutus, W. and A., var. Decaisneanum, Wight.
Sẹṅgẹl siń rẹhẹl, the roots of Tragia involucrata, Jacq.
Baraṅgọm rẹhẹl, „ „ „ Vernonia cineria, Less., or Glossogyne pinnatifida, DC.
Aṇḍiạ ghaṛwa, a male sparrow.

Grind the first three and cook into a curry with the sparrow, and give to eat. He should eat only *rambṛa dal*, the pulse of Phaeseolus Mungo, var. radiatus, L.

(*b*) On Sunday kill a *gaḍa cạńcir*, Motacilla luzoniensis, make a cup of its feathers in which he should eat his curry; dry the bird itself and cutting off a piece of it cook this in mustard oil and besmear the whole body therewith.

(*c*) *Sẹṅgẹl siń rẹhẹt*, the roots of Tragia involucrata, Jacq.
Kũs rẹhẹt, the roots of Themuda gigantea, Haskel.
Kọrpur, camphor.

Grind together and make into pills and let him take these for about a month.

261. *Bạńjhi*. Barrenness in women.

Remedies: (*a*) Certain insects make lumps or knots on the branches of the *meral* tree, Phyllanthus Emblica, Linn., in appearance like the fruit of the *meral*. Saying the names of boy and girl break off the lumps on the branches of two trees leaving a lump on each. Then get two of the insects.
Nirạ sindur, genuine red lead.
Binḍi muthạ ghãs da, the bulb of Fimbristylis monostachya, Hassk.
Sukri muthạ ghãs da, the bulb of Scirpus monostachyus, Kön.
2 *lọṅphul*, 2 cloves.
Bale gidrạ reak bukạ, the navel of a newly born infant, if the midwife can keep it; if not then get
Hẹndẹ mẹrọm họpọn bukạ, the navel of a black kid.
2 *bhelaonḍi*, 2 balls of sheep's or goat's dung.

Grind all these together, make into pills and give the woman to eat.

(*b*) This may be due to disease, or to the influence of malign spirits, or to the man being infructuous. First of all, they exorcise the spirits, then they make a low footstool of the wood of the *sọsọ*, Semecarpus Anacardium, L. and buy a new *kanḍa*, full sized earthenware waterpot, and a new *khạnḍi*, a woman's full sized cloth. At grey dawn on Sunday they take the husband and wife to the end of the village street, the woman carrying above pot full of water on her head along with her. The medicine man removes the obstruction by passing a mottled fowl three times round them. The woman seats herself on above stool, and at sunrise they pour the pot of water over her. Then she changes her cloth, putting on the above new one and leaving the old wet one there, and then goes straight home without looking back. The man too after beating the pot to pieces goes straight home. Then the rest of the party follow there leaving the wet cloth where it was abandoned. After reaching the house the medicine man naming the Sun god, gives an ear of paddy to the woman who puts it into the front fold of her cloth. After a little while he tells her to look at the ear of paddy. They look at it to see how many of the ears have fallen off and tell her so many of her children will die by and by. Afterwards he gives her medicine, viz.,

Nahelre janamak ol, a mushroom that has sprung up on a plough.

Oka kanthar khub joka ona darere arakge baisaukok, onam husil chadaoa, the scraped off red excrescence that appears on a richly fruit-bearing Artocarpus integrifolia, L.

Meral dareren tejo, the insects described at the beginning of this above.

Having got these he tells her, "I won't give you the medicine to-day; first of all both of you become priests (i.e. they must sleep apart on mats on the floor, a ceremonial purification), and I will give it you to-morrow morning." Both husband and wife do as they are told. Next morning he grinds together the above ingredients, and after smearing cowdung on the courtyard in front of the house he names the spirits *Garbhu* and *Kũãr* and puts strokes of red lead on the prepared spot, and the medicine also he offers there, and after pronouncing an invocation he gives her the medicine to drink. He gives her it to drink for five Sundays, and they wait for a month to see if she has conceived. If not, the spirits are exorcised again. When she bears a child it is named after the medicine man.

262. *Bahu jemon aloe dar*. To prevent the wife running away.

Medicines: (*a*) *Okatakre daka tukuc ko ãrgoe bindi*, the soot of a straw-ring on which cooking pots are placed when taken off the fire.

Datauni reak hatar gidi ictel, the fibres of a wooden tooth-brush spat out after using it.

Kadec' tejo, a certain caterpillar.

Grind these together and give them to her without her being aware of it on a Sunday, and she won't run away any more.

(*b*) If a woman will not stay with her husband then make her eat

Daharreko ñamok' potom tejo, a chrysalis found on the road, or those found on trees will also do.

263. *Kukhi marao reañ*. To shut up the womb.

Medicines: (*a*) *Pan rehel*, the roots of Piper Betle, L.

Mañgri hako baha, the gills of Macropteronotus magur (fish).

Aphim, opium.

Grind these together and give to eat, after which she will bear no more children.

264. *Gidrąjoñ reañ.* To get children.

Medicines: (*a*) *Meralren tejo*, the caterpillar found on the Phyllanthus Emblica, L.

Kuñkąlren tejo ar oṛaktęt' hǫ̃, the clay house and caterpillars stored in it by a species of wasp.

Grind these together and give to drink.

Gąbur chal, the bark of Acacia Farnesiana, Willd.

To be put in a hollow metal receptacle and worn on the string or girdle round the waist by both husband and wife.

(*b*) *Kuṇḍel tejo*, a certain caterpillar.

Kaḍęć tejo, " "

Kuñkąl tejo ar oṛaktęt, } as above in (*a*)
Meralren tejo, }

Grind together and make into pills, three to be taken on the morning of the Sunday after the cessation of the menses and three more on the following Sunday morning.

(*c*) *Gątur baha ręhęt*, the roots of

Ato reañ muñgą chal, the bark of a village Moringa pterygosperma, Gärtn.

Grind these together and put into a hollow metal receptacle, which should be worn attached to the string or girdle round the waist, or to a thread amulet suspended on the arm.

N.B.—Midwives are in the habit of taking a piece of the umbilical cord of a newly born male child, drying it and giving it to a woman who only gives birth to girls.

265. *Ritu hoyok.* To cure Amenorrhoea.

(Medicine to produce regular menses.)

Medicines: (*a*) *Ponḍ peaj*, white onions.

Rąsun, garlic.

Adhę, ginger, Zingiber officinalis, Roscoe.

Rǫkǫt cǫndǫn kaṭ, blood coloured sandal wood.

Boil all these together and let her drink it daily for about a week.

(*b*) One "authority" prescribes the same ingredients as above, but says they are to be pounded to pieces, then boiled in a one rupee brass cup of water, to be drunk daily every morning for a week, the preparation being renewed if necessary.

266. *Pǫrdhǫl.* Menorrhagia or Flooding.

Symptoms. An abnormally profuse discharge of the menses.

Medicines: (*a*) *Arak upąl baha*, Nymphaea rubra, Roxb.

Joba baha, Hibiscus rosa-sinensis, Linn.

Suruj mukhi ręhęt, the roots of Helianthus annuus, Willd.

Makaṛkenda jo̤ reak gabe, the flesh of the fruit of Diospyros embryopteris, Pers.

Marāṛ baha, Erythrina indica, Lam.

Mackundạ baha, Pterospermum acerifolium, Willd.

Saparo̤m baha se̤ sakam, chal, the flower, leaf or bark of Nyctanthes Arbor-tristis, Linn.

Boil all these together, give the patient to drink daily and the discharge will gradually cease.

(*b*) *Arak upạl baha*, Nymphaea rubra, Roxb.

Joba, Hibiscus rosa-sinensis, Linn.

Mackundạ baha, Pterospermum acerifolium, Willd.

Ro̤ko̤t co̤ndo̤n, blood coloured sandal wood.

Suruj mukhi re̤he̤l, the roots of Helianthus annuus, Willd.

Grind all these together, make into pills and let her take them daily.

(*c*) *Miru baha*, Abutilon indicum, Don.

Haṭ chal, the bark of Holarrhena antidysenterica, Wall.

Sahṛa chal, ,, ,, ,, Streblus asper, Lour.

Ạphim, opium.

Grind a little of the first three with some opium and make pills. After cleaning the teeth with twigs of the second of above, let her take the pills, swallowing them with the juice of figs. The fig juice to be obtained thus: sever the root of the tree (Ficus glomerata, Roxb.) and receive the juice that will exude in a small earthen vessel. Take about a quarter of a gallon and let her swallow the pills as above daily with some of this.

(*d*) *Ḍabha jo̤ reak gabe*, the flesh of the fruit of Citrus Aurantium, Willd.

Joba baha, Hibiscus rosa-sinensis, Linn.

Arak upạl baha, Nymphaea rubra, Roxb.

Pe̤ gạṇḍa gol mạric, 12 black peppercorns.

Grind all together and make 21 pills. Then let her take one 3 times a day with about an ounce of spirit, and she will certainly get well.

(*e*) *Arak upạl baha*, Nymphaea rubra, Roxb.

Suruj mukhi re̤he̤l, the roots of Helianthus annuus, Willd.

Joba baha, Hibiscus rosa-sinensis, Linn.

Raj baha, Nerium odorum, Soland.

Mackundạ baha, Pterospermum acerifolium, Willd.

Miru baha re̤he̤l, the root of Abutilon indicum, Don.

Ạphim, opium.

Grind all these together, make into pills and give daily, when she will certainly recover.

(*f*) *Campa re̤he̤l*, the roots of Michelia champaca, L.

Ro̤ko̤t co̤ndo̤n, blood coloured sandal wood.

Makaṛkenda jo̜ reak gabe, the flesh of the fruit of Diospyros embryopteris, Pers.

Ica̜k re̜he̜t, the roots of Woodfordia floribunda, Salisb.

Grind all these fine together, omitting the last named if unobtainable, and after boiling them in water, give the patient to drink. Every time it is drunk add to the mixture saltpetre and *ako̜rkora*, Anthemis pyrethrum. Among all the remedies for this complaint enumerated above these last two are the most important. They have been tried and proved efficacious. Both the thirst and burning will cease.

(*g*) *Upa̜l baha*, Nymphaea lotus, Willd.

Po̜rdho̜l baha,

Sa̜luk baha, the flower of Nymphæa rubra, Roxb.

Collect together and give to drink for three days.

(*h*) *Podho bahate̜t*, the flower of

21 *gaṇḍa gol ma̜ric*, 84 black peppercorns.

Grind and give to drink twice.

(*i*) *Patal kohṇḍa*, Pueraria tuberosa, DC.

Ato kundri, Cephalandra indica, Nand.

Sora, saltpetre.

Guṛ, molasses.

O̜po̜no̜m, Angelica glauca, Edgew.

Rambṛa ja̜num,

Cato̜m aṛak, Marsilia quadrifolia, L.

Grind together and give to drink.

(*j*) *Upa̜l baha da*, the bulb of Nymphaea rubra, Roxb.

Banat arakak, thick European made woollen red cloth.

Ba̜ṛ chal, the bark of Mimusops Elengi, L.

Kho̜de̜ baha da, the bulb of

Bo̜d laṛ poha re̜he̜t, the roots of a seedling of Vitis adnata, Wall.

Kamraj re̜he̜t, the roots of Buettneria herbacea, Roxb.

Grind and give to drink.

(*k*) *Huṭer baha re̜he̜t*, the roots of Indigofera pulchella, Roxb.

Ṭa̜ṇḍi cato̜m aṛak re̜he̜t, the roots of Desmodium triflorum, DC.

Oṛsa aṛak re̜he̜t, the roots of Commelyna suffruticosa, Bl.

Karhani hoṛo reak adwa caole, the rice made from the sun-dried grain of a variety of black paddy.

Ma̜hũt guṛ, the refuse of molasses.

Grind all but the last together, mix in the last and give to drink.

(*l*) *Kaḍe̜č tejo*, a certain caterpillar.

Ho̜ro̜ bo̜ho̜k, the head of a tortoise.

(m) *Campa rẹhẹl*, the roots of Michelia champaca, L.
Rọkọt cọndọn kaṭ, blood coloured sandal wood.
Joba baha, Hibiscus rosa-sinensis, L.
Arak upạl baha, Nymphaea rubra, Roxb.

Grind all these, boil them together in water and give to drink for 15 days.

(n) *Arak upạl baha ar datẹl*, the flower and bulb of Nymphaea rubra, Roxb.
Suruj mukhi rẹhẹl, the roots of Helianthus annuus, Willd.
Joba baha, Hibiscus rosa-sinensis, L.
Thoṛa ạphim, a little opium.

Collect these, make into pills and give to eat daily.

(o) *Miru baha rẹhẹl*, the roots of Abutilon indicum, Don.
Haṭ rẹhẹl, the roots of Holarrhena antidysenterica, Wall.
Edẹl poha rẹhẹl, the roots of a seedling of Bombax malabaricum, DC.
Thoṛa sahṛa chal, a little of the bark of Streblus asper, Lour.
Ạphim, opium.

Grind together, make into pills to be eaten.

(p) *Mackundạ baha*, Pterospermum acerifolium, Willd.
Gaḍa terel jọ, the fruit of Diospyros montana, Roxb.
Turạm rẹhẹl, the roots of
Rọkọt cọndọn kaṭ, blood coloured sandal wood.

Grind together, and make into pills of which one to be taken daily.

(q) *Campa rẹhẹl*, the roots of Michelia champaca, L.
Arak upạl baha da ar baha, the tuber and flower of Nymphaea rubra, Roxb.
Murup chal, the bark of Butea frondosa, Roxb.
Murgạ chal, „ „ „ Pterocarpus Marsupium, Roxb.

(r) *Karhani hoṛo caole*, rice made from a certain variety of black paddy.
Bhaya bhagwa rẹhẹl, the roots of Polygonum plebejum, Br.
Ḍhalka catọm aṛak rẹhẹl, the roots of
Tale mañj, the heart of Borassus flabelliformis, L.

Grind these together, mix with *guṛ*, molasses, and give to drink.

267. *Gọrọb Pọrdhọl.*

Symptoms. In this women during pregnancy get a discharge resembling blood or ash water.

Medicines: *Icạk rẹhẹl*, the roots of Woodfordia floribunda, Salisb.
Bhạbri rẹhẹl, „ „ „ Embelia robusta, Roxb.
Saparọm chal, the bark of Nyctanthes Arbor-tristis, L.
Rọkọt cọndọn kaṭ, blood coloured sandalwood.
Eḍhẹ campa rẹhẹl, the roots of

Mix and grind these to a powder, boil and give the patient slightly warm to drink.

268. *Gọrọb sitkạ.*

Symptoms. This occurs during pregnancy. Sometimes the lower extremities ache and the pain spreads up to the whole body. They swell up as in dropsy, and the appearance is the same as in dropsy and the saliva dries up.

This is *gọrọb* or *dud siṭkạ.*

Medicines: (*a*) Slice into round pieces the roots of *ẹdẹl poha*, a seedling of Bombax malabaricum, DC., and mixing it with something sticky as sugar, let the patient eat this for about 15 days.

Boil the same medicine with the refuse of molasses, smear the body therewith for about 15 days, and she will get well.

(*b*) An unguent.

Sẹṅgẹl siṅ rẹhẹt, the roots of Tragia involucrata, Willd.
Etka rẹhẹt, " " " Mucuna pruriens, DC.
Bir malhan rẹhẹt, " " " Atyllosia mollis, Bth.
Utri dudhi loṭa, " " " Cryptolepis Buchanani, R. and S.
Alagjạṛi rẹhẹt, " " " Cuscuta chinensis, Lamk.

After grinding these five kinds of roots together boil them in mustard oil and anoint the whole body daily.

(*c*) *Ṭampa ṭurạ mit rẹhẹt*, one root of
Cạuliạ bar rẹhẹt, two roots of Ruellia suffruticosa, Roxb.

Let her chew these, not more, and swallow the juice twice, and then expel the roots from her mouth.

Kuṛi ṭukuć bele, the egg of the Lobivanellus goensis.
Atnak chal, the bark of Terminalia tomentosa, W. and A.
Gaḍa icạk rẹhẹt, the roots of Woodfordia floribunda, Salisb. growing near rivers.

Grind and mix these together, mix with lukewarm water and rub it into her head.

269. *Gọrọb họrko ṭan ruạlenre.* Continuous fever during pregnancy.

Medicines: (*a*) *Nim sakam*, the leaves of Melia Azadirachta, Linn., to be boiled, the water to be drained off and then with the addition of *mạhũt guṛ*, molasses refuse, to be drunk like tea. All the symptoms will disappear and no harm ensue.

(*b*) *Kaḍa beṅjak rẹhẹt*, the roots of

An infusion of these may be drunk daily without injury. Molasses refuse may be added to this.

270. *Gidrạ hako pako bako hoe họtlen khan.* Protracted labour.

Medicines: (*a*) *Cip ciṛip rẹhẹt sẹ daretẹt*, the roots or entire plant of Achyranthes aspera, L.

Stick this into the top of the doorway while holding your breath, and as soon as ever the child is born remove it; otherwise all kinds of things will be discharged.

(*b*) The midwife may demand the production of a "thunderbolt," i.e. an implement of the stone age, believed by the Santals to be a "thunderbolt". It may be made use of in three ways, which, however, may be combined. One is to rub the "thunderbolt" against a stone, generally that on which they grind their spices, having first poured water on this. The water, which will contain something of the "bolt," is then given to the woman to drink. Another way is to keep the "bolt" above the head of the woman and pour water over it in such a manner that it flows down on her forehead and face, The third way is to put the stone into the eaves just outside the door; and care must be taken that the person performing this operation holds his breath. This last precaution is absolutely necessary for the desired effect of the application of this kind of "medicine." Probably this holding of the breath is meant to secure the efficacy of the remedy by keeping it free from any defilement from extraneous influences. When a "thunderbolt" is not procurable, twigs of certain trees (e.g. as stated in (*a*) above) may be used for the same purpose and in the same manner, or even a bullet that has been shot from a gun.

(*c*) *Tursi ręhęt*, the roots of Ocymum sanctum, Willd.

Dig this up partially and then with one breath pull it out and tell the midwife also with one breath to insert it in the mother's hair of the head.

(*d*) *Akaona ręhęt*, the roots of Calotropis gigantea, R. Br., or C. procera, R. Br.

5 *gotęć gol maric*, 5 black peppercorns.

Extract about 2 ounces of the juice of the former, add the latter and give some to drink, and after warming the rest apply it over the abdomen.

(*e*) *Laṭha cip ciṛip ręhęt*, the roots of

Gol maric, black pepper.

Grind and give some to drink, and after grinding the rest very small apply as an ointment to the abdomen.

(*f*) Stick *baṛe baha ręhęt*, the roots of Pentapetes phoenicia, L. in the head of the mother.

After the child is born and if the afterbirth does not come away, then let her drink the above roots together with *gol maric*, black pepper.

If fever ensues then

Saram lutur rẹhẹl, the roots of Clerodendron serratum, Spreng.
Sẹlẹp samanọm, Gloriosa superba, Willd.

Grind these and after warming a little smear over the navel.

(*g*) Pour water over a "thunderbolt" (as described in (*b*) above) on the woman, or if such be unobtainable then over a chip of a tree that has been struck by lightning.

(*h*) Fetch the husband's elder brother, let him stand quite nude in the doorway and shake out his loin apron and the hair of his head; if this does not answer, then

(*i*) Invoke the spirits *Ulum pạikạ* and *Julum pạikạ* and scatter some uncooked grains of rice, and do with *tursi sakam rẹhẹl*, the roots of Ocymum sanctum, Willd., as detailed in (*c*) above.

Protracted labour is sometimes considered due to misbehaviour on the part of the woman. Women friends will gather round the woman in labour. If they think that it is unduly protracted they will urge the poor woman to name the men with whom she may have had illicit intercourse.

271. *Maejiu họṛ gidrạko hoyoktakore racate bọndlenre.* Retention of urine during parturition.

Medicines: *Muṅgạ chal rẹhẹl*, the roots of Moringa pterygosperma, Gärtn.
Pẹ gaṇḍa golmạric, 12 black peppercorns.

Grind together and place on the abdomen without heating.

272. *Baha baṅ oḍoklen khan.* When the afterbirth does not come away.

It might be noted that the afterbirth is buried inside the house in a corner, care being taken that it is buried below the space between two rafters, and not below a rafter.

Medicines: (*a*) *Kaṇṭhaṛ baha sẹ ḍọgṭẹl*, the flower or shoot of Artocarpus integrifolia, L.
Hãṛũ reak ãwãr, the afterbirth of a monkey, obtainable from Bir họṛ, a small Muṇḍa tribe who eat monkeys.

Grind together and give to drink.

If the afterbirth of a monkey is unobtainable, then

(*b*) *Cip ciṛip rẹhẹl*, the roots of Achyranthes aspera, L.
Kaṇṭhaṛ baha, the flower of Artocarpus integrifolia, L.

Grind together and give to drink.

273. *Họṛmọ algaolen khan gidrạ hoekate.* *Prolapsus uteri* after childbirth.

Medicines: (*a*) *Dak họrọ bọhọk*, the head of a tortoise, Trionix gangeticus.
Bạṛiạ̃ kaṇḍhum rẹhẹl, the roots of Phyllanthus lanceolarius, Mull-Arg.

Mare kaskǫm dare rẹhẹt, the roots of an old cotton plant, Gossypium arboreum, L.

Backǫm reak tulạm, the cotton of Pollinia eriopoda, Hance. (found at the base of the plant).

Grind together, give her a little to drink and let her also apply a little herself to her private parts. Let her place a fire of *mẹrǫm bhelaoṇḍi*, goats' dung, under her bed.

(*b*) First let the midwife foment her and try to replace the womb; if unsuccessful,

(*c*) *Hǫrǫ bǫhǫk*, the head of a tortoise, Trionix gangeticus.

and after grinding the other 3 ingredients mentioned in (*a*) above foment her therewith. Then make a still fire of *mẹrǫm bhelaoṇḍi*, goats' dung, and blow the smoke into her.

274. *Gidrạ hoekate rǫg.* Complaints after childbirth.

Symptoms. This is when after childbirth the limbs and whole body are in pain as if broken and bruised.

Medicines: *Jạli siṅjǫ jǫ*, unripe fruit of Ægle Marmelos, Correa.

Tursi sakam, the leaves of Ocymum sanctum, Willd.

21 *gaṇḍa gol mạric*, 84 black peppercorns.

Adhẹ, ginger.

Grind these together and plaster her therewith; she will get well at once. Only the top of the flesh of the fruit to be scraped off and used.

275. *Siṭkạ.* Puerperal fever. (The name *siṭkạ* is used also about other fevers in women during pregnancy and after birth when the fever is accompanied by intense thirst and a dry mouth.)

Symptoms. This attacks women at childbirth. Sometimes the blood clots or collects in the abdomen and they have great pain there. The saliva thickens and dries up and they have intense thirst.

Medicines: (*a*) *Campa rẹhẹt*, the roots of Michelia champaca, Linn.

Sora, saltpetre.

Mix and prepare like tea; let the patient drink this and the thirst will be immediately quenched.

(*b*) If the blood is clotted in the abdomen, grind small the *jhiṅgur*, Arum campanulatum, tuber, heat it a little and apply it warm to the abdomen, when the blood will dissolve and come entirely away.

(*c*) *Gaḍa terel chal*, the bark of Diospyros montana, Roxb.

Gol mạric, black pepper.

Take some of the bark and reduce it to juice, and grinding it together with five peppercorns slightly warm it and make the patient drink it. Then taking more of the bark grind it fine and after heating it apply it over the abdomen. The blood will then dissolve. Then make the patient stand up and the liquefied blood will all flow out. *Note*, that saltpetre is added to the remedies in all kinds of *siṭkạ* except the following *Haga siṭkạ*.

(*d*) *Pọrọspoka jọ*,
20 *gol mạric*, 20 black peppercorns.
Dak ghoṛa lada rẹhẹt, the roots of Vitis tomentosa, Heyne.

Grind these three together and make about 21 pills (the size of goat's excrement) and give daily one in the morning, at noon, 3 P.M., evening and after supper, to be swallowed. This if the saliva fails to exude, and then it will flow.

(*e*) *Jiṭhimond*, Clerodendron Siphonanthus, R. Br.
Rạli, Piper longum, Willd.
Akọr kọra, Anthemis pyrethrum.
Thoṛa gan bọc, a little kalmus.
Darcini, cinnamon.
Kababcini, Cubeba officinalis, Miqu.
Mackundạ baha, Pterospermum acerifolium, Willd.
Gol mạric, black pepper.

Grind these 8 ingredients together and make into pills: one to be kept in the mouth all day long and the saliva will flow freely.

(*f*) *Tara* (like cotton in appearance and red) to be soaked in water.
Ulḍhạ da, root of a Nymphaea.
Dhiri kaṭkọm jaṅga, the leg of a certain crab found under stones.

Grind the last two together, then mix with the above water, strain and let the patient drink this daily for 4 or 5 days and she will certainly recover.

(*g*) *Kindet rẹhẹt sẹ chal*, the root or bark of the wild date tree.
Jaephọl, nutmeg.
Jāwān, Carum Ajowan, DC.

Soak all these together: to be drunk with spirit twice a day.

(*h*) *Sasaṅ bọhọk*, a knot of turmeric, Curcuma longa, L.
Mandargọm sakam, custard apple leaves, Anona squamosa, L.

Grind and apply as a plaster over where the pain is. If this does not remove the pain then grind the bark of the *ruhen* tree, Soymida febrifuga, Juss., and apply that as a plaster.

(*i*) *Murup poha rẹhẹt*, the roots of a seedling of Butea frondosa, Roxb.
Sọn pat rẹhẹt, the roots of Hibiscus cannabinus, Willd.
Darcini, cinnamon.

Gol maric, black pepper.
Sũṭ, dry ginger.
Jiṭhimond chal, the bark of Clerodendron Siphonanthus, R. Br.
Pipol, Piper longum, Willd.

Grind all together, make into small pills, cook in melted butter of cows' milk, and let the patient put one or two each hour in her mouth, so that she keeps swallowing the juice. Also once or twice grind *bir baraṅgom rẹhẹt*, the roots of , in fact the whole plant with water, and let her drink this water after warming it.

(*j*) *Campa rẹhẹt*, the roots of Michelia champaca, L.
Rạli rẹhẹt, the roots of Piper longa, L.
Cue cirola, Gentiana cherayta, Roxb.
Pipol, Piper longum, Willd.
Sũṭ, dry ginger.
Adhẹ, Zingiber officinalis, Roscoe.

Boil, add some *sora*, saltpetre, and give to drink. After the child is born, in order to obviate *siṭkạ*, boil some *Campa rẹhẹt*, roots of Michelia champaca, L., in water and give her to drink like tea.

(*k*) *Bele sinjo gabe lačtẹlko*, the entire contents scraped out of a ripe fruit of Ægle Marmelos, Correa.
Mit choṭak hao jạpulkom, 2 ounces of a kind of red ants, Oecophylla smaragdina.
Mare ul ạmsi, old dried inspissated juice of the fruit of Mangifera indica, L.
Thoṛa buluṅ, a little salt.

Boil in 2 lbs. of water of which give about 2 ounces to drink, which will clean the stomach. Then make her stand up and the blood will flow out, or if it fails to do so foment her a little.

(*l*) *Gạrunḍi aṛak rẹhẹt*, the roots of Acternanthera sessilis, R.Br.
Jera ạphim, a little opium.
Thoṛa phuṭiạ kạuḍi cun, a little lime from the shells used in India as money.

Mix and give to drink.

(*m*) *Gargạḍi rẹhẹt*, 1 *powa*, 8 oz. of the roots of Coix lachryma, Willd.
Mare backọm ghãs 1 *ạṭi*, 1 bundle of old Pollinia eriopoda, Hance.

Grind the first, boil the second down, throw the grass away, then mix the two and give to drink once in the morning.

(*n*) *Kadar rẹhẹt*, the roots of Bonnaya veronicæfolia, Spreng.
Gargạḍi rẹhẹt, „ „ „ Coix lachryma, Willd.

Jithimond chal, the bark of Clerodendron Siphonanthus, R. Br.

Cąulią rẹhẹl, the roots of Ruellia suffruticosa, Roxb.

Grind and give to drink.

(*o*) *Kitą mañj*, the heart of Phoenix acaulis, Buch.

Boil this in water, and let the patient drink this water for some two days.

(*p*) *Dak icąk rẹhẹl*, the roots of Jussiaea suffruticosa, L.

Tạṇḍi icąk rẹhẹl, " " " Woodfordia floribunda, Salisb.

Sọsọ chal, the bark of Semecarpus Anacardium, L.

Cąulią, Ruellia suffruticosa, Roxb.

Thoṛa orop da, a little of the tuber of Costus speciosa, Sm.

Grind all these together, mix with *cini*, sugar, and give to drink.

276. *Haga siṭką*.

Symptoms. This variety of childbed complaint is characterised by profuse diarrhœa.

Medicines: (*a*) *Niuri chal*, the bark of Elæodendron Roxburghii, W. and A.

Kawẹl rẹhẹl, the root of Abrus precatorius, L.

Gargąḍi rẹhẹl, the root of Coix lachryma, Willd.

Bhąbri rẹhẹl, the root of Embelia robusta, Roxb.

Poṇḍ peaj, white onion.

Corco chal, the bark of Casearea tomentosa, Roxb.

Rąsun, garlic.

Kasmar chal, the bark of Gmelina arborea, Roxb.

Tursi sakam, the leaves of Ocymum sanctum, Willd.

Meral chal sẹ rẹhẹl, the bark or root of Phyllanthus Emblica, Linn.

Adhẹ da, the tuber of ginger, Zingiber officinalis, Roscoe.

Rąli rẹhẹl, the root of Piper longum, Willd.

Paṛọ da, the tuber of Curcuma angustifolia, Roxb.

Grind all these together and after boiling the mixture with *mąhüt guṛ*, the refuse of molasses, give the patient to drink and then the diarrhœa will stop and she will recover.

(*b*) Take Nos. 1, 2, 3, 5, 11, 12 of above and *cąulią rẹhẹl*, the roots of Ruellia suffruticosa, Roxb., and prepare and administer as in (*a*) above.

(*c*) *Jhiṅgur da*, the bulb of Arum campanulatum, Roxb.

Grind to a pulp, warm and apply warm over the abdomen, which will liquefy the blood. Also take *kaera ḍąr*, the leaf-stalk of Musa paradisiaca, L., pound it to fibre, toast at the fire and take the juice thereof and after adding 5 *gọṭẹć gol mąric*, 5 black pepper-corns, give to drink.

(*d*) *Gaḍa terel chal*, the bark of Diospyros montana, Roxb.

Grind, warm and apply as an ointment over the abdomen. Take also 2 ounces of the juice, and after adding 5 black pepper-corns give to drink.

277. *Jolon sitka.*

Symptoms. In this there is pain in the abdomen and great thirst. In fact it may be classified with No. 275.

Medicines: (*a*) To cause the pain to cease and to liquefy and expel the blood:

Sinjo bele joto gabekoge, all the flesh of a ripe bael, Ægle Marmelos, Correa.

Hao ad chotak gan, about an ounce of a kind of red ants, Oecophylla smaragdina.

Mare ul amsi, old sundried, inspissated flesh of the mango.

Thora bulun, a little salt.

Boil all the above in some four pounds of water and let the patient drink this. Foment her over the abdomen, and a little later let her sit up. The abdomen will then make a noise and all the blood flow out. Afterwards boil the roots of *campa*, Michelia champaca, L., and give it her to drink. The blood will be completely staunched.

(*b*) *Kedar rehet*, the roots of Bonnaya veronicaefolia, Spreng.

Surukuc rehet, the roots of Salix tetrasperma, Roxb.

Grind together and apply under the navel on the abdomen where it pains her.

(*c*) When the flow of saliva is dried up:

Lilkathi rehet, the roots of Polygala crotalarioides, Buch. and Ham.

Tampar rehet, the roots of

Gol maric, black pepper.

To be ground and drunk by the patient.

(*d*) *Meral rehet ar sakam*, the roots and leaves of Phyllanthus Emblica, L.

Kedar rehet, the roots of Bonnaya veronicaefolia, Spreng.

Grind both these together, add some of her husband's *ado*, urine, and after mixing all together, tell her husband to rub it on her stomach, abdomen and buttocks; it will not do for any one else to rub it on.

278. *Toa anjedok.* The drying up of milk.

Symptoms. Sometimes women's milk does not flow after giving birth to a child, sometimes the same happens in fever or something similar.

Medicines: (*a*) *Pusi toa*, Euphorbia pilulifera, Linn.

Root up the entire plant and grind it small, strain off the water and let the patient drink it mixed with sugar or sugarcandy, which will cause the milk to flow. There are three varieties of this plant, any of which will do.

(*b*) *Chatni chal*, the bark of Alstonia scholaris, R. Br.

Dak catom arak, Marsilia quadrifolia, L.

Grind these two small together, give a little to the patient to drink and apply a little as a plaster to her chest till she gets well.

(*c*) *Moṭa baraṅgọm*, Vernonia cineria, Less., or Glossogyne pinnatifida, DC.

Take the leaves of this close to the ground, and after adding water make into pills which the patient should swallow till the milk flows.

(*d*) *Eraḍọm*, Ricinus communis, Linn.

Boil some three of the leaves and let her drink the water daily till well. In the evening plaster the breasts with the leaves all over except the nipples, leaving room for the child to suckle.

(*e*) *Loa banda*, the parasitical plant (a Loranthus) found on Ficus glomerata, Roxb.

Tie this on the patient, and her milk will certainly flow.

(*f*) *Aṇḍiạ koṅgat' rẹhẹl*, the roots of Dregia volubilis, Benth.

Grind these and make into pills. Then let her take some uncooked rice made from paddy that has been boiled, and masticate this well, and then chew one of the pills with that before swallowing. This to be done for some five days and you will see the milk is secreted.

(*g*) *Aṇḍiạ mọrọn aṛak rẹhẹl*, the roots of Gymnema hirsutus, W. and A., var. Decaisneanum, Wight.

Grind and give her some to drink and apply some to the chest.

(*h*) *Dud baraṅgọm*,

to be drunk.

(*i*) *Kamraj rẹhẹl*, the roots of Buettneria herbacea, Roxb.
Sakarkenda aṛak, the leaves of Ipomaea Batatas, Lamk.
Sasaṅ bọhọk da, the bulb of Curcuma longa, Roxb.
Kạliạ jirạ, Nigella indica, Roxb.
Puṭhi hako, small fish, Barbus stigma.

Mix and grind these, roast on hot embers wrapped in leaves and let her eat for four consecutive days. Also let her drink *nim dak mạṇḍi*, rice gruel with the addition of the leaves of Melia Azadirachta, L.

279. *Toa seteṅ ocoe.* To cause the milk to flow.

Medicines: (*a*) *Sunum muć*, a kind of black ant.

When these are on the move take three of those that separate to the right.

Chạtni chal, the bark of Alstonia scholaris, R.Br.
Bir mulạ,

Grind these three together and mixing thoroughly with *cini*, sugar, give to drink; and let her apply some to the breasts and chew *ạṇḍiạ mọrọn aṛak rẹhẹl*, the roots of Gymnema hirsutus, W. and A., var. Decaisneanum, Wight., slightly covered with dust.

If the mother's milk is drying up because the infant is suffering from atrophy, then add to above

Bhorkoṇḍ chal dare cetan reak, the upper bark of Hymenodictyon excelsum, Wall.

280. *Toa añjẹl ocoe.* To cause the milk to dry up.

Medicines : Let the woman extract her milk and bury it in a plough furrow, when the flow of milk will cease at once, but remember the woman herself will dry away to a stick.

281. *Toa haso sẹ bele tanak lenre toa añjẹl ocoe reak.*

To check the flow of milk when the breasts pain or suppurate.

Symptoms. Many women on giving birth to a child have a copious flow of milk which induces pain, and sometimes the breasts suppurate. If the flow is not checked, the breasts may be injured.

Medicines : (*a*) *Bana haṭak chal*, the bark of Oroxylon indicum, Benth.

Isor muli gọd rẹhẹt sẹ sakam, the roots or leaves of Aristolochia indica, Willd.

Ạsạrịạ chal, the bark of Capparis horrida, Linn. f.

Grind the second and warm it, heat the third, mix all three and plaster the mixture on and the pain will cease.

(*b*) *Corco sakam sẹ chal*, the leaves or bark of Casearea tomentosa, Roxb.

Grind fine, warm a little and smear it on: let her comb the breasts and she will certainly get quickly well.

(*c*) *Nahẹl sạmbhạuṛa hasa*, the earth heaped in front of a plough when ploughing.

Moisten some of this in water and apply daily till recovery.

(*d*) *Ọt dare japak rẹhẹt*, the roots of

Jugi ḍuriạ aṛak,

Grind, warm and apply daily, each medicine separately, and the flow of milk will be checked.

(*e*) *Arel dak*, melted hail.

Godo gẹlẹć hasa, earth excavated by rats.

Jurite jọk siñjọ, a pair of Ægle Marmelos, Correa, fruit growing two together.

Mix these and smear on her.

(*f*) *Ẹṭkẹć lore*, the exudation of Euphorbia antiquorum, Linn.

Pusi toa sakam, the leaves of Euphorbia pilulifera, Linn.

Ṭạṇḍi catọm aṛak, sakam, the leaves of Desmodium triflorum, DC.

Grind together and plaster her therewith.

(g) *Kidiṅ baha*, an entire Ipomaea Quamoclit, Willd.
Nanha pusi toa, an entire Euphorbia thymifolia, Burm.

Grind all together and plaster her with the whole.

(h) *Matkọm chal*, the bark of Bassia latifolia, Roxb.
Nanha pusi toa, Euphorbia thymifolia, Burm.
Turạm da, the bulb of

Grind all together and plaster her therewith.

(i) Apply *arel*, hail, and if it does not cease with that then
Eskar nahel reaǩ hasa, only the earth turned by a plough and
Arar̦ reaǩ mahadeb reaǩ, the scrapings of the centre of the yoke.

To be plastered on her.

(j) *Lọtọ sakam*, the leaves of Randia dumetorum, Lam.

Grind and apply as a plaster.

(k) *Jọnọǩ carẹcte jhar̦*, charm away by passing over a splinter of a broom.

Some people do this to a woman, and some women do it to themselves with the splinter from a house broom.

(l) *Kidiṅ baha rẹhẹt*, the roots of Ipomaea Quamoclit, Willd.
Corco bhiṭuạǩ, the leaf stem of Casearea tomentosa, Roxb.
Sẹkrẹc dọg, a leaf bud of Lagerstroemia parviflora, Roxb.

Grind together and after warming it slightly plaster on the breast.

282. *Dạtrạ jọmte bul họr̦ reaǩ ran.*

Remedy for stupor or intoxication induced by Datura.

Symptoms. In this cause also the lips turn black.

Medicines: (a) *Kasmar chal*, the bark of Gmelina arborea, Roxb.
Siṅ ar̦ak chal, „ „ „ Bauhinia purpurea, L.

Grind together and give to drink with stale rice water, recovery will follow.

283. *Ot jọmte bul họr̦ ar eṭaǩ eṭaǩ bul ran.*

Remedy for stupor or intoxication due to eating any of the following :—

Ot, mushrooms.
Janhe, Paspalum scrobiculatum, Linn.
Jera janhe, Panicum flavidium, Retz.
Jāhān ar̦ak, any pot herb.
Biṅ ot, a certain poisonous mushroom.
Biṅ ḍimbu,
Hạṇḍi ṅūte māyāmko uchlạu reaǩ, rice beer followed by the vomiting of blood.
Bubul ghās (*gạị sẹ họr̦ hõ*), any intoxicating grass (both cattle and human beings).

Medicines: (*a*) *Kasmar chal*, the bark of Gmelina arborea, Roxb.
Siń aṛak chal, „ „ „ Bauhinia purpurea, L.

Grind together and give to drink with stale rice water; they will recover.

284. *Mạhur bis reak ran.*

Remedy for stupor or intoxication due to a kind of Nematode worm.

Symptoms. The lips and tongue turn black.

Medicines: (*a*) *Kasmar chal*, the bark of Gmelina arborea, Roxb.
Siń aṛak chal, the bark of Bauhinia purpurea, L.

Grind together and give to drink with stale rice water.

(*b*) *Kasmar chal*, the bark of Gmelina arborea, Roxb.
Ul chal, „ „ „ Mangifera indica, L.
Siń aṛak chal, „ „ „ Bauhinia purpurea, L.

Take a pound of each of the first two, and 4 ounces of the last, and grind them with six pounds *kạńji dak*, stale rice water, and mix the whole together. Of this mixture give 2 to 4 ounces to drink at a time, and you will see no one will die from this cause. It should be given also to cattle or all animals when poisoned.

Whenever any one, human being or animal, is suffering from poison or the effects of *Jera janhe*, Panicum flavidium, Retz.
Ṭisi, Linum usitatissimum, Willd.
Eradọm, Ricinus communis, L.
Dạtrạ, Datura alba, Willd., or D. fastuosa, Willd., or D. Metel, L.
Biń ḍimbu,
Biń ol,
Jãhãn ol, any mushroom,

then give without delay to drink,
Kasmar chal, the bark of Gmelina arborea, Roxb.
Siń aṛak chal, „ „ „ Bauhinia purpurea, L.,

a little along with stale rice water, and all intoxication or stupefaction will disappear.

285. *Bhalok toyo sẹ bhalok seta gẹr bis ran.*

Remedy for the bite of a rabid jackal or dog, Rabies.

Medicines: (*a*) *Carọṛiń*, the longicorn beetle.
Mạṭha aṛak rẹhẹl, the roots on Antidesma diandrum, Tulas.
Ad choṭak gan ṗaurạ, about an ounce of spirits.

Grind the first two together and make him drink with the third. Then to increase the discharge of urine give him tea with sugar to drink, or, grind about 3 ounces of *orop' da*, the bulb of Costus speciosa, Sm., and give him to drink. As long as the urine is of a greenish colour, you will know the medicine has taken effect.

From the day he has taken the medicine let him urinate in a large potsherd so as to see it.

(*b*) *Icak rehel*, the roots of Woodfordia floribunda, Salisb.
Akaona rehel, " " " Calotropis gigantea, R. Br.
Sengel sin rehel, " " " Tragia involucrata, Jacq.
Etka rehel, " " " Mucuna pruriens, DC.

Grind these and give to drink daily.

(*c*) If bitten by a rabid jackal or dog then take the hair of a healthy jackal or dog and let him eat it with the ripe fruit of the plantain, Musa paradisiaca, Linn.

(*d*) *Saparom chal ros*, the juice of the bark of Nyctanthes Arbor-tristis, L.
Kärwät rehel ros, the juice of the roots of Carissa Carandas, Linn.

Mix these and give the patient to drink whether a human being or cattle.

(*e*) *Sengel sin rehel*, the roots of Tragia involucrata, Jacq.
Kalmeg, Andrographis paniculata, Nees.
Latha cip cirip rehel, the roots of
Garundi arak rehel, the roots of Actarnanthera sessilis, R. Br.
Corco chal, the bark of Casearea tomentosa, Roxb.
Kolo da, the bulb of Dioscorea daemonum, Roxb.
Etka rehel, the roots of Mucuna pruriens, DC.
Tursi rehel, " " " Ocimum sanctum, Willd.
Bharbhari rehel, the roots of Ocimum basilicum, Linn. or Ocimum canum, Sims.
Hat rehel, the roots of Holarrhena antidysenterica, Wall.
Gote rehel, " " " Croton oblongifolius, Roxb.
Jīoti dog pea tusa, 3 tips of a certain grass, Sesbania ægyptiaca, Pers.
Hin ar aphim, asafoetida and opium, as much as a pea of each.

Grind all the above into liquid and mix with a lb. or two of spirit and give an ounce of the mixture to drink daily. (Refer to the directions under (*a*) above.)

(*f*) *Hao*, a kind of large red ants, Oecophylla smaragdina.
Sengel sin rehel, the roots of Tragia involucrata, Jacq.
Nanha dudhi lota rehel, the roots of Ichnocarpus frutescens, R. Br.

Kill some of the first and with 2 ounces of them grind the other two together to make a dose, and give such a dose daily to be drunk.

(*g*) *Adhe*, ginger.
Gol maric, black pepper.
Bulun, salt.

Grind together; to be eaten three times every week for a year.

(*h*) *Kãṛwãl rẹhẹl*, the roots of Carissa Carandas, Linn.

Plaster him with this and give him daily a little to drink—after the second or third day subsequent to being bitten.

(*i*) *Kãṛwãl rẹhẹl*, the roots of Carissa Carandas, Linn.

Ḍhela chal, the bark of Alangium Lamarckii, Thus.

Make into a juice, cook in melted butter and anoint therewith the whole body from head to foot. For internal administration grind the first of these, make them into pills the size of goats' or sheep's excrement and give him to eat.

(*j*) *Maṭha arak rẹhẹl*, the roots of Antidesma diandrum, Tulas.

Carọṛiń, the longicorn beetle.

Mare naṅgle, an old leathern thong used for binding the yoke to the plough beam.

Grind the first two together, then roast the third to burning point and grind it, mix all three and make into pills, to be taken one at a time, thrice a day for three days. When the urine discharged in a potsherd has an oily film on the top know that a cure has been effected.

(*k*) *Carọṛiń*, one longicorn beetle.

Dare bọṅki sakam, the leaves of an epiphytic orchid.

1 *sim bele*, a hen's egg.

After squeezing the juice from the leaves of the second mix well together all three ingredients, roast in a leaf cup and let the patient eat it one day.

(*l*) *Akaona chal sẹ baha*, the bark or flower of Calotropis gigantea, R. Br.

Sẹkrẹć banda, parasitical plant growing on the Lagerstroemia parviflora, Roxb.

Carọṛiń, the longicorn beetle.

Mare sạuṛi reak guṇḍạ, the powdery refuse of old Heteropogon contortus, R. and S.

Grind all these together and give him to drink.

(*m*) *Bir baraṅgọm*, Glossogyne pinnatifida, DC.

Ḍuṇḍukil rẹhẹl, the roots of Gardenia turgida, Roxb.

Mare naṅgle rapak, old leathern yoke thong roasted.

Grind all together, mix and give him to drink.

Kolo rẹhẹl, the roots of Dioscorea dæmonum, Roxb.

To be ground and the whole body anointed therewith.

(*n*) *Carọṛiń*, one longicorn beetle.

Maṭha aṛak rẹhẹl, the roots of Antidesma diandrum, Tulas.

Grind together and make into pills; for an adult mix one pill with 2 ounces of water and give to drink daily and every two or three hours give tea to drink which will increase the discharge of urine, which should be passed into a potsherd so as to be seen. The dose for a child is half a pill and for an infant ¼ pill.

(o) *Saparom chal ros*, the juice of the bark of Nyctanthes Arbor-tristis, L.

Mare naṅgle rapak̄ roṅgo, an old leathern yoke thong roasted to burning point.

Mix and give to drink daily. This answers for cattle also.

(p) As soon as bitten give 2 ounces *kãṛwãl rehel*, the roots of Carissa Carandas, L., to drink which will cause the poison to be vomited out, and also plaster the whole body with the same which will neutralize the poison.

(q) *Laṭha cip ciṛip rehel*, the roots of

Sengel siṅ rehel, the roots of Tragia involucrata, Jacq.

Etka rehel, the roots of Mucuna pruriens, D.C.

Thoṛa kolo da, a little of the bulb of Dioscorea dæmonum, Roxb.

Thoṛa kalmeg, a little of Andrographis paniculata, Nees.

Aphim, ½ annas worth of opium.

Pound these and mix with four annas worth of spirits, and give to drink daily, preserving the urine as above, and you will see the larvæ come out like puppies.

(r) *Gidi jaṅ*, the bones of a vulture. } Both to be roasted
Mare naṅgle, an old leathern yoke thong. } to burning point.

Wash 12 pice in water and take the dirt. Then rub an unalloyed brass cup on a stone with water, and take this water and the other ingredients and put them in this cup and give the whole to drink daily. This is efficacious for both human beings and cattle or any animal bitten. Mix with the medicine also 2 ounces of the red ants that make their nests on trees. Recovery is certain.

(s) *Sengel siṅ rehel*, the roots of Tragia involucrata, Jacq.

Tejo mala rehel, „ „ „ Cissampelos Pareira, L.

Ḍodhar rehel, „ „ „ Adiantum lunulatum Burm., or A. concinum.

Aṇḍia koṅgat rehel, the roots of Dregia volubilis, Benth.

Bhadu chal rehel, the bark and roots of Vitex alata, Roxb.

Caroṛiṅ, a longicorn beetle.

Grind these and give to drink with *hanḍi*, rice beer, and he will get well.

(t) *Bir baraṅgom*,

Ḍahar tala reak̄ ḍunḍukit chal, the bark of a Gardenia turgida, Roxb., growing in the middle of a road.

Mare naṅgle, an old leathern yoke thong.

Barea caya, two Leptocorisa varicornis.

Half roast the last two, then grind all four together and give to drink.

Next day give the same as (s) above, save that there should be two longicorn beetles.

One "authority" says: When a person is bitten by a mad dog, the poison (the larvæ) grows like puppies to the size of red ants, and the person becomes "mad" gradually. If he becomes really "mad," there is no recovery. Some become "mad" in five days, others in 15 days, others in one month, or three months, or even six months.

286. *Bana gẹr ghao.* Wound from bears' bite.

Medicines: (*a*) *Dhubi ghãs*, Cynodon dactylon, Pers.
Adwa caole, rice that has been husked without boiling.

Grind together and apply as a plaster to the wound.

(*b*) *Bọd laṛ*, Vitis adnata, Wall.
Ṭipọc̣ da, the bulb of

Dry a little of each of these, grind without water and sprinkle on the wound.

To extract the pus:—

(*c*) *Turbitạ nãṛi*,

Pound and plaster on the wound.

287. *Cund gẹr bis reak ran.*

Remedy for the poison of the bite of the musk rat, Sorex caerulescens.

Medicines: *Kasmar chal*, the bark of Gmelina arborea, Roxb.
Siń aṛak chal, ,, ,, ,, Bauhinia purpurea, Linn.

Grind and give to drink with stale rice water, and plaster the whole body therewith. If there is no amendment, give some snake-bite medicine to take.

288. *Kul gẹr bis ran.*

Remedy for the poison of the bite of a tiger.

Medicines: (*a*) *Kasmar chal*, the bark of Gmelina arborea, Roxb.
Siń aṛak chal, ,, ,, ,, Bauhinia purpurea, L.
Sẹṅgẹl siń rẹhẹl, the roots of Tragia involucrata, Jacq.
Suruj mukhi ghãs rẹhẹl, the roots of Helianthus annuus, Willd.
Bir sọn rẹhẹl, the roots of

Make him drink a mixture of these with stale rice water.

(*b*) *Bạrsạ pakọṛ rẹhẹl*, the roots of Grewia sapida, Roxb.
Tarse koṭap rẹhẹl, ,, ,, ,, Grewia villosa, Willd.
Kamraj rẹhẹl, ,, ,, ,, Buettneria herbacea, Roxb.
Seta kaṭa rẹhẹl, ,, ,, ,, Grewia polygama, Roxb.

Grind whichever of these you can get and apply as a plaster to the wound.

(*c*) *Bọṛ chal*, the bark of Mimusops Elengi, L.
Kạuhạ chal, ,, ,, ,, Terminalia Arjuna, Bedd.

Grind together and apply as a plaster.

(*d*) *Khodę baha*,
Poha bod laṛ, a seedling of Vitis adnata, Wall.
Kamraj, Buettneria herbacea, Roxb.

Grind these three together and apply as a plaster; applicable for both human beings and animals.

(*e*) *Turam rẹhẹt*, the roots of
Ot ṭipoč rẹhẹt, ,, ,, ,,
Dare ṭipoč rẹhẹt, ,, ,, ,,

Grind together and apply as a plaster; apply the first of above quickly.

(*f*) *Baghut boṅgam ocok pahilkedea*, first of all exorcise the spirit who is supposed to be the herdsman of wild animals.

(*g*) *Bod laṛ rẹhẹt*, the roots of Vitis adnata, Wall.
Ot ṭipoč,
Turam,
Cip ciṛip rẹhẹt, the roots of Achyranthes aspera, L.

Grind these together and smear or plaster on.

N.B.—This remedy may also be used in bites of bears or jackals.

289. *Tayan gẹr bis ran.*

Remedy for the poison of the broad headed crocodile, Crocodilus trigonops.

Medicines: (*a*) *Kasmar chal*, the bark of Gmelina arborea, Roxb.
Siṅ arak chal, ,, ,, ,, Bauhinia purpurea, L.
Sẹṅgẹl siṅ rẹhẹt, the roots of Tragia involucrata, Jacq.
Etka rẹhẹt, the roots of Mucuna pruriens, DC.
Goṭe rẹhẹt, ,, ,, ,, Croton oblongifolius, Roxb.

Make him drink a mixture of these with stale rice water.

If cattle or animals are bitten, then

(*b*) *Jhol*, sooty cobwebs.
Caole, raw rice.
Maric, chilli or capsicum, Capsicum frutescens, Willd.
Gol maric, black pepper.
Poṇḍ peaj, white onions.

Grind these together and give to drink.

The remedies given in No. 288 for tiger bite may also be given advantageously in crocodile bite.

290. *Sanam lekan biṅ gẹr bis ran.*

Antidotes for the poison of all kinds of snake-bite.

Medicines: (*a*) *Siṅ arak*, Bauhinia purpurea, Linn.
Kasmar chal, the bark of Gmelina arborea, Roxb.

After grinding these two make him drink some with *kaṅji dak*, stale rice water, and anoint him with some of the mixture.

N.B.—If this remedy is given to drink in cases of intoxication from *kucla*, Strychnos potatorum, L. f., the intoxication will disappear.

(*b*) *Nim chal*, the bark of Melia Azadirachta, Linn.
Siṅjo̱ chal, „ „ „ Ægle Marmelos, Correa.

Take these from an old tree, grind them together and give him to drink, anoint him with a little, and drop some on the fontanel.

(*c*) *Kadar re̱he̱l*, the roots of Bonnaya veronicæfolia, Spreng.
Goṭe̱ chal, the bark of Croton oblongifolius, Roxb.

Grind these together, give him to drink and anoint him therewith.

(*d*) *Kumbiṛ chal*, the bark of Careya arborea, Roxb.

Grind and give him to drink and anoint him therewith.

(*e*) *Maraṛ baha chal*, the bark of Erythrina indica, Lam.

Give this to drink and wet a towel or some cloth in it and wrap him therein.

(*f*) *Jhiṅjiṭ chal*, the bark of Bauhinia retusa, Ham.

Grind this and give an adult not more than 2 oz. or a child not more than 1 oz. to drink. If he becomes intoxicated by this medicine, then mix *kasmar*, Gmelina arborea, Roxb., with sugar and let him drink it, the poison will not stay.

(*g*) *Moṭa go̱d*, the thick Aristolochia indica, Willd.

Grind all parts of the plant and give to drink, anoint also.

(*h*) *Isor muli go̱d*, Aristolochia indica, Willd.

Grind, give to drink and anoint.

(*i*) *Sisu go̱d*,

Grind, give to drink and anoint.

(*j*) *Iċ e̱we̱r da*, the bulb of Vitis latifolia, Roxb.
Candogaṛ go̱d,

Mix these and rub in or anoint therewith.

(*k*) *Hemca aṛak sakam*, the leaves of Enhydra fluctuans.

Grind and give to drink as well as plaster the body therewith.

(*l*) *Goṭe̱*, the roots of Croton oblongifolius, Roxb.
Kadar re̱he̱l, „ „ „ Bonnaya veronicæfolia, Spreng.

Grind together, give to drink and anoint ; he will certainly get well.

(*m*) *Se̱ṅge̱l siń re̱he̱l*, the roots of Tragia involucrata, Jacq.
Dudhi loṭa re̱he̱l, „ „ „ Ichnocarpus frutescens, R. Br.

Grind these together, give to drink and anoint the whole body therewith.

(*n*) *Etka re̱he̱l*, the roots of Mucuna pruriens, DC.
Se̱ṅge̱l siń re̱he̱l, the roots of Tragia involucrata, Jacq.

Mix, give to drink and anoint.

(*o*) *Tursi re̱he̱l*, the roots of Ocimum sanctum, Willd.
Bharbhaṛi re̱he̱l, „ „ „ Ocimum basilicum, Linn. or Ocimum canum, Sims.

Grind and mix these two and give to drink, and take the leaves of both, grind them and anoint therewith.

(*p*) *Sondhaeni sakam*, the leaves of Tylophora longifolia, Wight.
Grind, give to drink and anoint therewith.

(*q*) *Maraṅ catọm aṛak rẹhẹt*, the roots of Marsilea quadrifolia, L.
Grind, give to drink and anoint therewith.

(*r*) *Ạṇḍiạ koṅgat rẹhẹt*, the roots of Dregia volubilis, Benth.
Nanha toyo caṇḍbọl rẹhẹt, the roots of
Grind, give to drink and anoint therewith.

(*s*) *Nạṛī hund baha reak sakam*, the leaves of
Grind fine, give to drink and anoint therewith. Continue giving to drink till it tastes bitter.

(*t*) *Niuri chal*, the bark of Elæodendron Roxburghii, W. and A.
Grind, give 2 oz. to drink and plaster the whole body therewith. If he is quite unconscious, then grind together above and *bana haṭak chal*, the bark of Oroxylon indicum, Benth., stir together in a basin of water and wet a new piece of cloth or dip it therein. Then after anointing with the medicine, wrap him in the cloth; after an hour he will get well.

(*u*) *Orop' da*, the bulb of Costus speciosa, Sm.
Make him drink of this, and plaster the whole body therewith.

(*v*) *Tarọp chal*, the bark of Buchanania latifolia, Roxb.
Grind, give to drink and anoint the whole body therewith.

(*w*) *Lọpọṅ chal*, the bark of Terminalia bellerica, Roxb.
Pọpṛọ chal, „ „ „ Gardenia latifolia, Ait.
Grind these together and give to drink.

(*x*) *Bilạti thamakur*, imported tobacco.
Muṅga chal, the bark of Moringa pterygosperma, Gärtn.
Grind together and anoint therewith; and one gulp of the latter only to be drunk.

(*y*) *Gạbur chal*, the bark of Acacia Farnesiana, Willd.
Grind, give a little to drink and anoint therewith.

(*z*) *Adhẹ*, ginger.
Gol mạric, black pepper.
Thoṛa buluṅ, a little salt.
Grind these together and let him drink the mixture till he feels it pungent and plaster him with it also.

(*aa*) *Suruj mukhi ghas rẹhẹt'*, the roots of Helianthus annuus, Willd.
Laṭha cip' ciṛip' rẹhẹt', „ „ „
Gol mạric, black pepper.
Grind these together and give him to drink only.

(*bb*) *Boṅga bạri rẹhẹt'*, the roots of
Grind, give to drink and anoint the whole body therewith. When the patient feels cool it will show the medicine has worked.

(*cc*) *Kuclạ chal*, the bark of Strychnos potatorum, L. f.

Grind and give about a mussel shell full to an adult and half that quantity to a child. This is a powerful poison so only the amount should be given. Should there be any intoxication then let the patient drink No. (*a*) remedy given above and it will disappear.

(*dd*) *Utri dudhi loṭa*, Cryptolepis Buchanani, R. and S.
Hemca aṛak, Enhydra fluctuans.
Kuclą chal, the bark of Strychnos potatorum, L. f.
Isor muli gọd sakam, rẹhẹt', the leaves and roots of Aristolochia indica, Willd.
Candọgaṛ gọd sakam, rẹhẹt', the leaves and roots of
Ic̓ ẹwẹr nāṛī da, the bulb of Vitis latifolia, Roxb.
Bana haṭak' chal, the bark of Oroxylon indicum, Benth.
Moṭa gọd rẹhẹt', sakamko, the roots and leaves of the thick Aristolochia indica, Willd.
Jhiṅjiṭ chal, the bark of Bauhinia retusa, Ham.

After grinding all these together first plaster the whole body therewith. Then dip a clean cloth in the medicine and wrap the entire body in that cloth. Take notice, however, that if the evacuations contain blood or resemble mustard oil, you should take no further trouble, as he will not be saved.

(*ee*) *Ḍhela rẹhẹt' chal sẹ dare chal*, the bark of the root or stem of Alangium Lamarckil, Thws.

Grind, give a little to drink and anoint the whole body therewith.

(*ff*) *Saram lutur rẹhẹt'*, the roots of Clerodendron serratum, Spreng.
Sega rẹhẹt', the roots of Mimosa rubicaulis, Lamk.

Grind together and then to be drunk only.

If the bite is by a *bandphoṛa biṅ*, Bungarus fasciatus, then

(*gg*) let him drink some of the oilcake left after expressing oil from the kernel of the fruit of Bassia latifolia, Roxb., and put a plaster of the same over the navel, then something like the banded appearance of the snake will be voided in a thin form with the excreta, or he will vomit it up, or the medicine will dissolve.

When the poison of this snake takes effect it grows in the stomach like the snake that bit, and incantations and charms are of no use.

(*hh*) *Niuri chal*, the bark of Elæodendron Roxburghii, W. and A.
Bir hoṛẹc̓, Atyllosia scarabaedois, Benth.

The patient to be anointed with a mixture of these.

(*ii*) *Aṇḍią dhurup aṛak sẹ rẹhẹt*, the leaves or roots of Leucas cephalotes, Spreng.
Cip ciṛip rẹhẹtlẹt, the roots of Achyranthes aspera, Linn.

Grind these two together and plaster him therewith, or he may drink a little.

(jj) *Thamakur*, tobacco.
Cun, shell lime.

To be eaten.

(kk) *Bir gọd sakam*, the leaves of

Grind and rub him therewith and he may eat a little.

Poṇḍ dhubi ghãs, the white Cynodon dactylon, Pers. Apply as in the previous one.

Mare oṛak sạrim reak kana aṛaktẹl, Commelyna bengalensis, Linn., growing on the roof of an old house.

Poṇḍ rańgạini rẹhẹl, the roots of the white Solanum xanthocarpum, Schrad. et Wendl. Apply as in the first two above.

Thamakur, tobacco.

Hukạ dak, hookah water.

Muńgạ chal, the bark of Moringa pterygosperma, Gärtn.

Get quickly together as many of above as you can, grind all together, give him a little to drink and apply the rest as an ointment over the whole body.

(ll) *Niuri rẹhẹl*, the roots of Elæodendron Roxburghii, W. and A., to be dug and brought on the day of the Monsa or Hindu serpent goddess festival when they fast.

Grind and give half to the bitten person and anoint him with the other half. (This remedy was first given by a Dusad, and not a Santal *ojha*.)

(mm) *Lọpọń aṛak rẹhẹl*, the roots of Ærua lanata, Linn.

Grind, give him a little to drink and anoint his head therewith.

(nn) *Candọgaṛ gọd rẹhẹl*, the roots of

Grind and give to drink, and also grind the leaves of the same and plaster him therewith. If the poison has spread over the whole body, the medicine must be repeated three or four times. The leaves of this and the leaves of Vitis latifolia, Roxb. should be mixed, ground and plastered on him.

(oo) *Kumbiṛ chal*, the bark of Careya arborea, Roxb.
(pp) *Niuri chal*, „ „ „ Elæodendron Roxburghii, W. and. A.
(qq) *Corco chal*, „ „ „ Casearea tomentosa, Roxb.

These three should severally be ground and given to drink.

(rr) If the poison is latent to make it apparent:—
Duṇḍukil rẹhẹl, the roots of Gardenia turgida, Roxb.
Suruj mukhi rẹhẹl, „ „ „ Helianthus annuus, Willd.

Pound and give to drink about an ounce, when the action of the snake poison will at once become apparent. Then quickly give him *gọd*, Aristolochia indica, Willd.; make no delay.

(ss) *Isor muli gọd*, Aristolochia indica, Willd.
Candọgaṛ gọd,

Grind these together, or whichever of them may be obtainable and give to drink. If much poison has been absorbed the medicine will not taste bitter, so continue giving it till he feels it bitter, by which you will know the poison is overcome. Continue giving the medicine till he vomits, when you may know the medicine has taken effect, and the poison is gradually losing its effect. This rule is to be observed in many of the remedies.

(*tt*) *Moṭa gọd*, } to be applied in same way as (*ss*).
(*uu*) *Niuri chal*, the bark of Elæodendron Roxburghii, W. and A. } to be applied in same way as (*ss*).

(*vv*) *Kumbiṛ chal*, „ „ „ Careya arborea, Roxb.

Give 2 ounces of this to drink at intervals. This is a poison, so an overdose must be avoided; see that the first dose is ineffectual before giving a second, and so on.

(*ww*) *Jhiṅjiṭ chal*, the bark of Bauhinia retusa, Ham., to be used in same way.

(*xx*) The most powerful remedy is *kuclạ chal*, the bark of Strychnos potatorum, L. f., but it must be administered very carefully as if more of it is given than the poison absorbed it will prove fatal. If there is great stupefaction give 2 ounces. If he recovers consciousness after an hour give another 2 ounces, and if effectual, then give to drink

Kasmar chal, the bark of Gmelina arborea, Roxb., and

Siṅ aṛak rẹhẹl chal, the bark of the roots of Bauhinia purpurea, L.,

along with *kạṅji*, stale rice water, and all will be well.

(*yy*) *Maraṛ baha dare chal*, the bark of Erythrina indica, Lam.

Give to drink and also plaster therewith; he is sure to recover.

(*zz*) *Mil gọṭẹč lẹṇḍẹl*, an earthworm.

Grind and mix with about a dessert spoonful of water, and give the patient to drink without letting him know what it is, and he will get well at once.

(*a*1) First give to drink *kumbiṛ chal thoṛa*, a little bark of Careya arborea, Roxb., and five minutes later give him to drink about an ounce of *kuiṇḍi kaṛe*, the oilcake left after expressing oil from the kernel of the fruit of Bassia latifolia, Roxb. If this does not cause him to vomit, repeat the dose at intervals until he does vomit, when you will see the appearance of the snake in the stomach is brought up. Also warm this oilcake slightly and spread it thinly over the whole stomach from the navel downwards. This remedy is also good against the bite of the *tutri* (Eryx conicus, non-poisonous) snake. In fact give something to cause vomiting in all cases of snake bite, such as—

(*b*1) *Thoṛa bilạti thamakur*, a little imported tobacco.

Muṅga dare rẹhẹl chal, the bark of the roots of Moringa pterygosperma, Gärtn.

Prepare about 8 ounces, and give at intervals 1 ounce of it to drink, till he vomits.

(c1) Give in the same way *gọbur rẹhẹt*, the roots of Acacia Farnesiana, Willd.

(d1) „ „ „ „ „ *ḍhela chal*, the bark of Alangium Lamarckii, Thws.

(e1) *Baṛge reak laṭha cip ciṛipak rẹhẹt*, the roots of

Grind and smear on from the bitten spot and give a little too to drink; but be sure the poison has entered the system, otherwise it is not good to give this.

(f1) *Bir nim chal*, the bark of Melia Azadirachta, L., growing in forests.

Kumbiṛ chal, „ „ „ Careya arborea, Roxb.

Sirom chal, Andropogon muricatus, Retz.

(g1) Some 4 or 5 inches above the place where he was bitten smear all round some *jh inuk cun*, shell lime, such as is eaten with tobacco. This to prevent the poison from spreading through the body.

(h1) *Taroṕ chal*, the bark of Buchanania latifolia, Roxb.

Sirom rẹhẹt', the roots of Andropogon muricatus, Retz.

Grind and give to drink, and after grinding the latter smear it over the whole body.

(i1) *Etka jaṅ*, the seeds of Mucuna pruriens, DC.

Split these, wet them in water and make them adhere to the bitten spot, and when the poison is eliminated they will drop off spontaneously.

(j1) *Taroṕ chal*, the bark of Buchanania latifolia, Roxb.

Poṇḍ kọhu botke, Bryonia lacinosa, L., white variety.

Karla da, the tuber of Momordica muricata, Willd.

Sindrit, a fresh shoot of Bombax malabaricum, DC.

Make him drink these with water and smear him with *maraṛ baha*, Erythrina indica, Lam.

(k1) *Bheḍa dereṅ rẹhẹt'*, the roots of Cassia Tora, L.

Haṛhat' họtọt' rẹhẹt', the roots of a bitter Cucurbita lagenaria, Willd.

Grind these with *hukạ dak'*, hookah water, and give to drink. There is a variety of *suṛạ ghãs*, Cyperus tegetum, Roxb., which bears a white flower like a *kanphul*, ear ornament; pour that into his nose or make him smell it; break a *jọjọ jaṅ*, seed of Tamarindus indica, L., in two and apply so that it sticks fast.

(l1) *Salga chal*, the bark of Boswellia serrata, Wall.

Sondhaeni, Tylophora longifolia, Wight.

Grind and smear on him, or

(*mI*) mix with (*mI*) *Gọd sakam*, the leaves of Aristolochia indica, Willd. and

Ic̓ ẹwẹr hasa, the earth from Vitis latifolia, Roxb.,

and smear this on him while you give to drink after grinding them

Ic̓ ẹwẹr rẹhẹt', the roots of Vitis latifolia, Roxb.

Candọgaṛ gọd rẹhẹt', the roots of

Note.—There is no measure of the amount to be drunk of the above written medicines: one must exercise one's discretion in accordance with the way medicine is given. After giving one dose wait till it is assimilated before giving another. Two or three such doses should suffice.

Signs of the bites of snakes and other (supposed) poisonous reptiles:—

(1) *Ạmbạitar biń*, Vipera Russellii, Russell's viper (?). Their bite produces swelling and a splitting or bursting at the same time.

(2) *Boda biń*, Python molurus. A brown rock snake, a python: the whole body swells up in lumps.

(3) *Bandphoṛa biń*, Bungarus fasciatus, the banded Karait. The poison rises in the stomach of the victim with a banded appearance as in the body of the snake.

(4) Snake-bite causes the pulse to become less frequent and weaker.

(5) *Raekakaṛbak*, the chameleon. The chameleon's poison causes spots as in their own body to appear in that of the victim whose body sways.

(6) *Pọkọl rọṭẹ*, Bufo curinatus, the keiled nosed toad causes the body to appear spiky.

(7) *Kidiń kaṭkọm*, the scorpion's poison causes profuse perspiration of the whole body.

(8) *Sẹṅgẹl marmar*, Scolopendra versicolor or S. marsitans, causes the pulse to move with jerks and creeping like their gait.

To recognise when the snake was not seen to bite, and whether death is due to snake-bite or not:—

(1) If one has been bitten or breathed on by a snake then observe the person's or animal's eyes. You will see (*a*) he will be drowsy; (*b*) the eyes get blood red; (*c*) sometimes they look slate coloured; (*d*) the hair on the body stands on end, and comes out; (*e*) the body becomes cold as water; (*f*) the breath from the side on which he was bitten feels cold, the ears of animals become limp and the saliva dribbles from the mouth. By these signs you may know he has been bitten by a snake.

(2) The breath from the side on which the snake has bitten is cold, and warm from the other side.

(3) To know whether an unconscious snake-bitten person is alive or dead:—

(*a*) first feel the chest, if not dead it will be a little warm;

(*b*) put a little old cotton into the nostril, and if not dead it will move slightly by the breath;

(*c*) look at the tongue, if dead it will be drawn inside, i.e. it will be doubly thick and short;

(*d*) if dead the eyes will be turned over.

(4) To know that death is due to snake-bite: (*a*) blood and a fluid like mustard oil will issue from the mouth: (*b*) the same will issue from the nose: (*c*) if the excrementa have the same appearance, know that he is dead and give no medicine.

It might be remarked that the Santals believe that nearly all snakes and reptiles are poisonous. This influences them. Fear may bring on collapse. The following will show how fear works: A young and otherwise sensible woman had in the early morning heard a snake hiss not far from where she was. She had not seen the snake, but was sure it was a cobra. Some three or four hours later this happening fear took hold of her; she became frightened and was very near a collapse, showing quite alarming symptoms. We had great trouble in getting her round.

291. *Cẹrcẹṭẹċ aḍo.* Lizards' urine (causes blisters).

Medicines: Roast red hot *kuiṇḍi kaṛe*, the refuse in the oil press after extracting the oil from the kernel of the fruit of Bassia latifolia, Roxb., and then throw it into a basin of water. Steam the affected part with that water twice a day. If larvae appear it will get well.

292. *Ghirṛi gẹr bis reak ran.*

Remedy for the bite of the lizard Tiliqua rubriventris.

Medicines: *Laṭha cip ciṛip rẹhẹt*, the roots of
Gạruṇḍi aṛak rẹhẹt, the roots of Acternanthera sessilis, R. Br.
Suruj mukhi aṛak rẹhẹt, the roots of Helianthus annuus, Willd.

Mix these together and give to drink with stale rice water.

293. *Kakṛa gẹr bis ran.*

Remedy for the bite of a large lizard, Colotis veructor.

Medicines: *Laṭha cip ciṛip rẹhẹt*, the roots of
Gạruṇḍi aṛak rẹhẹt, the roots of Acternanthera sessilis, R. Br.

Grind and give to drink with stale rice water, also plaster him therewith and apply some as an ointment to the bitten spot.

294. *Kul sereń gẹr bis reak ran.*

Remedy for the bite of the lizard Uromastix hardwickii.

Medicines: (*a*) *Isor muli gọd*, Aristolochia indica, Willd.

Grind and give him to drink.

(*b*) *Kasmar chal*, the bark of Gmelina arborea, Roxb.
Siń aṛak chal, „ „ „ Bauhinia purpurea, Linn.

Grind and give to drink with stale rice water, and also plaster him therewith.

(*c*) *Udạl rẹhẹl*, the roots of Sterculia villosa, Roxb.
Karkaṭ rẹhẹl „ „ „ Zizyphus xylopyra, Willd.
Kaera rẹhẹl, „ „ „ Musa paradisiaca, L.

Grind together and give to drink.

295. *Pọkọl rọtẹ gẹr bis ran.*

Medicine for the bite of bufo curinatus.

Symptoms. The spiky appearance of their own bodies appears on that of the person bitten.

Medicines: Kasmar chal, the bark of Gmelina arborea, Roxb.
Siń aṛak chal, „ „ „ Bauhinia purpurea, Linn.
Kańji dak, stale rice water.

Mix the two former with the last, give him some to drink and plaster him therewith. If he does not get better use another snake-bite antidote.

296. *Raekakaṛbak gẹr bis ran.*

Medicine for chameleon's bite.

Symptoms. Spots appear on the body of the bitten person as on the chameleon's body.

Medicines: (*a*) *Kasmar chal*, the bark of Gmelina arborea, Roxb.
Siń aṛak chal, „ „ „ Bauhinia purpurea, Linn.
Kańji dak, stale rice water.

Mix the two former with the last, give him some to drink and plaster him therewith. If he does not get better try another snake-bite antidote.

(*b*) *Upạl baha reak da*, the tuber of Nymphaea rubra, Roxb.
Haṭ chal sẹ rẹhẹl, the bark or roots of Holarrhena antidysenterica, Wall.

Grind together and give to drink.

297. *Tọrhọl gẹr bis reak ran.*

Remedy for the bite of the guana, Varanus flavescens.

Medicines: Kasmar chal, the bark of Gmelina arborea, Roxb.
Siń aṛak chal, „ „ „ Bauhinia purpurea, Linn.
Laṭha cip ciṛip rẹhẹl, the roots of

Grind and give to drink with stale rice water, and plaster the whole body therewith.

298. *Bindi gẹr reak bis ran.*

Medicine for spider lick.

Medicines: (*a*) *Buru ghọṛa lada rẹhẹl*, the roots of Vitis tomentosa, Heyne.

Grind and plaster him therewith either hot or cold, and give him also a little to drink. The poison causes much swelling.

(*b*) *Edel poha rehel*, the roots of a seedling of Bombax malabaricum, DC.

Giru dhiri, a certain kind of red stone used as a pigment.

First rub the stone with an addition of water; then anoint him with the water thus obtained. Then grind the roots and plaster or anoint him therewith. The swelling will entirely subside.

If the spot attacked does not swell it will break out into an open sore, say on the hands or legs. Treatment:—

(*c*) *Latha cip cirip*,

Bhidi janatep, Urena sinuata, Linn., or Triumfetta rhomboidea, Jac.

Bir jhunka, Crotalaria calycina, Shrank.

Nanha dudhi lota rehel, the roots of Ichnocarpus frutescens, R. Br.

Andia moron arak rehel, the roots of Gymnema hirsutus, W. and A., var. Decaisneanum, Wight.

Buru ghora lada, Vitis tomentosa, Heyne.

Edel poha rehel, the roots of a seedling of Bombax malabaricum, DC.

Mare nangle, an old leathern thong used for binding the yoke to the plough.

Andia tale baha, the flower of the male Borassus flabelliformis, L.

Grind all these together and apply daily with a feather together with a little mustard oil, or if there is a watery discharge dust it on.

299. *Kul bindi ger.*

Bite of a large supposed poisonous spider, Mygale monstrosa.

Medicines: (*a*) *Gada terel chal*, the bark of Diospyros montana, Roxb.

Merom mel chal, „ „ „ Ixora parviflora, Vahl., or Olax nana, Wall.

Soso dare chal, „ „ „ Semecarpus Anacardium, L.

Grind together and apply as a plaster.

(*b*) *Ghora lada da rehel*, the roots of Vitis tomentosa, Heyne.

Give some to drink and apply some as an ointment.

300. *Ghugri ger bis reak ran.*

Remedy for the bite of the mole cricket, Gryllus gryllo-talpa.

Medicines: *Kasmar chal*, the bark of Gmelina arborea, Roxb.

Sin arak chal, „ „ „ Bauhinia purpurea, Linn.

Grind and give to drink with stale rice water.

301. *Kidiń katkom se jiol hako tor bis.*

The poison of the sting of a scorpion or of a certain fish.

Symptoms. The person stung at once gets hot, i.e. the perspiration drops from the whole body, and there is intense pain.

Medicines: (*a*) *Tarop chal*, the bark of Buchanania latifolia, Roxb.

Grind and make him drink some and smear him with some also.

(*b*) *Rangaini janum*, Solanum Jacquini, Willd.

Take 3 leaves, chew them small and retaining them in the mouth blow into both his ears till the pain is relieved. Do not let it be known you have anything in the mouth.

(*c*) *Rangaini janum rehel*, the roots of above.

Grind and give him to drink.

(*d*) *Rangaini janum*, same as above.
Bilati thamakur, imported tobacco.

Grind together and plaster him therewith.

(*e*) *Dhãi da*, the bulb of Grislea tomentosa, Willd.

Grind small and apply to the place stung.

(*f*) If he is intoxicated or the poison produces perspiration, the body turning into goose flesh:—

Sengel siń rehel, Tragia involucrata, Jacq.
Latha cip' cirip',
Suruj mukhi ghãs rehel, the roots of Helianthus annuus, Willd.
Dundukit rehel, the roots of Gardenia turgida, Roxb.
Kasmar chal, the bark of Gmelina arborea, Roxb.
Siń arak chal, the bark of Bauhinia purpurea, Linn.

Grind all these together, give to drink with stale rice water and smear over the whole body.

(*g*) Before the poison rises pass urine quickly on the spot.

(*h*) Get on the top of a termite hill and call out in imitation of a peacock's cry and apply the kernel of a tamarind seed, *jojo jań*, Tamarindus indica, L., so that it adheres to the spot.

(*i*) *Tarop chal*, the bark of Buchanania latifolia, Roxb.
Sauri rehel, the roots of Heteropogon contortus, R.S.

Grind together and plaster on the spot and chewing them quickly spit on the spot, or you may add to above, after grinding,

Pitua rehel, the roots of Spermacoce hispida, L.

(*j*) *Kasmar chal*, the bark of Gmelina arborea, Roxb.
Siń arak chal, „ „ „ Bauhinia purpurea, L.
Sengel siń rehel, the roots of Tragia involucrata, Jacq.
Etka rehel, the roots of Mucuna pruriens, DC.

Rạṅgạini rẹhẹl, the roots of Solanum Jacquini, Willd.
Tarọp chal, the bark of Buchanania latifolia, Roxb.
Laṭha cip ciṛip rẹhẹl, the roots of
Gol mạric, black pepper.
Adhẹ, Zingiber officinalis, Roscoe.

Grind all these together, stir in *kạṅji dak*, stale rice water, and give to drink.

302. *Kidiṅ kaṭkọm, sẹṅgẹl marmar, bindi emt. reak toṛ.*

The sting of scorpions, centipedes, spiders, etc. (see also No. 298, 300).

Medicines: (*a*) *Ẹdẹl chal*, the bark of Bombax malabaricum, DC.
Muṅga rẹhẹl, the roots, of Moringa pterygosperma, Gärtn.

Pound and apply to the stung part.

(*b*) *Rạṅgạini jạnum rẹhẹl*, the roots of Solanum Jacquini, Willd.

Grind and apply as a plaster to the stung part.

(*c*) *Sọsọ sunum*, the oil distilled from the seeds of Semecarpus Anacardium, L.

Dot this on, i.e. apply a drop or so.

(*d*) *Tarọp chal*, the bark of Buchanania latifolia, Roxb.

Grind and apply some as a plaster and let him chew some.

(*e*) *Arak peaj*, a red onion.

Squeeze the juice out into the eye on the opposite side to that on which he has been stung.

(*f*) *Sạṅci mạric*, black pepper.
Thamakur, tobacco.

Grind together and apply to the spot.

(*g*) *Kasmar chal thoṛa*, a little of the bark of Gmelina arborea, Roxb.
Siṅ aṛak chal, the bark of Bauhinia purpurea, L.
Sẹṅgẹl siṅ rẹhẹl, the roots of Tragia involucrata, Jacq.
Etka rẹhẹl, the roots of Mucuna pruriens, DC.
Rạṅgạini jạnum rẹhẹl, the roots of Solanum Jacquini, Willd.
Tarọp chal, the bark of Buchanania latifolia, Roxb.
Laṭha cip ciṛip rẹhẹl, the roots of

Pound all these and mix *adhẹ*, ginger, and *gol mạric*, black pepper, and then add *khub jọjọ kạṅji dak*, very sour stale rice water, and give to drink, applying some too as a plaster; he is sure to get well.

As soon as stung:—

(*h*) *Bilạti thamakur*, imported tobacco.
Rạṅgạini jạnum rẹhẹl, the roots of Solanum Jacquini, Willd.

Grind together and apply; he will get quite well.

(*i*) Grind and apply *dhại da*, the bulb of Grislea tomentosa, Willd.

(j) *Edhe rangaini janum sakam pea, janum salak*, 3 leaves, thorns included, of Solanum xanthocarpum, Schrad. et Wendl.

Put these with the thorns in your mouth and chew them slowly, and while they are in your mouth blow into both ears of the patient, and he will recover at once. Blow on till he is deaf. Spit on the stung spot and continue rubbing it with the medicine until it has become insipid and then spit it out. All the time until you have finished neither you nor the patient must let yourselves be seen by any one.

(k) *Tarop chal*, the bark of Buchanania latifolia, Roxb.
Sirom rehel, the roots of Andropogon muricatus, Retz.

Grind together and plaster on the spot.

(l) *Etka jan dalkate*, the split seeds of Mucuna pruriens, DC.

Wet in water, apply your spittle and make it stick to the stung spot.

(m) *Jojo jan dalkate*, the split seeds of Tamarindus indica, L.

Make these stick to the stung spot and squeeze out the juice of *arak peaj*, red onions and *bulun*, salt, into the eye on the same side as he has been stung.

(n) *Lonphul*, cloves.
Gol maric, black pepper.

Grind together and give to drink.

303. *Mahle kidiń ar sengel marmar bis ran.*

Antidote to the poison of two kinds of scolopenders.

Symptoms. The pulse of the person stung moves with jerks and a creeping or crawling sensation.

Medicines: (a) *Mare matkom*, the old dried flowers of Bassia latifolia, Roxb.

Grind and apply as a plaster.

(b) *Lendel hasa*, the earth thrown up by earthworms.

Daub or smear him over with this.

(c) *Ohoc arak rehel*, the roots of Boerhaavia procumbens, Herb. Banks.

Grind and apply as a plaster.

(d) Same as (a) above, only with the addition it should be warmed.

304. *Ńele tor.* Bees' sting.

Medicines: (a) Grind *mare matkom*, the old dried flowers of Bassia latifolia, Roxb., and plaster it on.

(b) *Rangaini janum rehel*, the roots of Solanum Jacquini, Willd.

Grind and plaster on.

(c) *Rasun*, garlic.

Grind and smear on the stung parts.

365. *Susurbaṅ, ṅẹlẹ, liṭạ tombṛe toṛ.*

The sting of wasps, bees and hornets.

Medicines: Mare matkọm, the old dried flowers of Bassia latifolia, Roxb. Grind and apply as a plaster.

V. I. *Gola Kanta.* Hæmorrhagic Septicæmia.[1]

Symptoms. The neck swells, the hair stands on end and falls off, the ears are limp and droop, the saliva drops and there is a little cough.

Medicines : (*a*) *Kasmar chal*, the bark of Gmelina arborea, Roxb.
Siṅ aṛak chal, the bark of Bauhinia purpurea, L.
Jhọl, soot covered cobwebs.
Rạsun, garlic.
Poṇḍ peaj, white onions.
Gol mạric, black pepper.
Caole mạric, a kind of capsicum resembling grains of rice.

Grind and give to drink.

(*b*) Apply the oil distilled from the seeds of *sọsọ*, Semecarpus Anacardium, L., var. cuncifolia, to the throat and between alternate ribs on the left side in three places.

(*c*) Thoroughly pound and crush the stem of the leaves of the palmyra palm, Borassus flabellifermis, L., dip in melted butter and after warming apply to the end of the tongue and set fire to it. Rub the remainder of the melted butter on the throat.

(*d*) *Caole mạric*, a kind of capsicum resembling grains of rice.
Kasmar chal, the bark of Gmelina arborea, Roxb.
Dare japak rẹhẹl sẹ nāṛī, the roots or tendrils of Scindapsus officinalis, Schott.
Sũṭ, dry ginger.

Grind together, mix in water and give to drink. Rub capsicum freely on the throat externally.

(*e*) *Kasmar chal*, the bark of Gmelina arborea, Roxb.
Siṅ aṛak chal, the bark of Bauhinia purpurea, L.
26 *gaṇḍa gol mạric*, 104 black pepper-corns.
20 *gaṇḍa caole mạric*, 80 of a kind of capsicum like grains of rice.
4 *chimbṛi rạsun*, 4 clusters garlic, or
Poṇḍ peaj sẹ inạ jọm peaj, white or the common onions will also do.
Ato piṇḍạ da, the bulb of Amorphophallus campanulatus, Blume.

[1] I am indebted to Mr. N. C. Roy, Veterinary Assistant Surgeon, Dumka, for the proper names of this and the four following cattle diseases.

Grind all these with *kạñji dak*, stale rice water, and stir the whole in that stale rice water and give it them to drink.

As a prophylactic, at the commencement of the symptoms:

(*f*) *Sọsọ jañ*, the fruit of Semecarpus Anacardium, L.

Wrap this in grass and give them to eat daily and it will stop the progress of the disease.

(*g*) As soon as you know a cow or buffalo has been attacked by this disease, apply a burning medicine, viz., *kạṭić tale ḍạr*, a small branch of the Borassus flabelliformis, L., or *kaera ḍạr ge*, or a branch of Musa paradisiaca, L. Take about four fingers' breadth from the top and pound and fray it, besmear it freely with *gại gọṭọm sunum*, clarified butter from cow's milk, and heat it over a glowing fire. Then pull out the animal's tongue and apply this 5 or 6 times to the swelling at the end of the throat and the end of the tongue, let the animal go and it will stand up. Smear the ramainder of the medicine on the outside of the neck. Be careful, however, to begin the burning from the inside, as otherwise it will die on the spot. If applied as directed it will be an immediate cure.

(*h*) *Laṭha cip ciṛip rẹhẹt*, the roots of
Tursi sakam, the leaves of Ocimum sanctum, Willd.
Malhan sakam, „ „ „ Dolichos Lablab, L.
Akaona rẹhẹt, the roots of Calotropis gigantea, R. Br., or C. procera, R. Br.
Sọsọ sunum, oil obtained from the seeds of Semecarpus Anacardium, L., var. cuneifolia.

Mix these and make them swallow the mixture. This remedy should be given promptly. Then obtain

(*i*) *Ghikuạri*, Yucca gloriosa.
Ato piṇḍe, Amorphophallus campanulatus, Blume.
Gol mạric, black pepper.

and mixing with the above (*h*) grind all together and make to drink.

V. 2. *Gại Khurạ*. Foot and mouth disease.

Medicines: (*a*) *Bandphoṛa biń jań*, the bones of the Bungarus fasciatus snake.

Tie these on the animal with yarn from the spinning wheel, and drive it daily into mud that no larvae may appear.

To prevent larvæ: pour kerosene oil on the diseased parts.

(*b*) *Kadam rẹhẹt*, the roots of Anthocephalus Cadamba, Benth. and Hook. f.

Pound and fray this. In one breath make passes over the animal three times, rub a little where the larvæ are, put the medicine on the ground, shake off, commencing from the head, anything from their whole body, and dry the medicine in the heat of the fire-place or in the sun. The larvæ will fall off in five days.

(c) *Suruj mukhi rẹhẹt*, the roots of Helianthus annuus, L.

Proceed in the same way with this. Do not tread in the footsteps of the animal, do not go to the house where it is. Let the person who administer the medicine continue chaste and have no intercourse with women until the larvæ have disappeared.

(d) First turn them into mud and let them trample about in this.

(e) *Sarjọm dạl*, the kernel of the fruit of Shorea robusta, Gärtn.

Make this into bran and sprinkle on the sores, which will dry them up.

(f) *Mẹrlẹċ chal*, the bark of Flacourtia Ramontchi, L' Herit.

Grind this to a powder and sprinkle it on.

V. 3. *Gại bọsọntọ*. Rinderpest.

Medicines: (a) *Salga chal*, the bark of Boswellia serrata, Wall.
Campa rẹhẹt, the roots of Michelia champaca, L.
Tarse koṭap rẹhẹt, the roots of Grewia villosa, Willd.
Sikuạr rẹhẹt, „ „ „
Huṭạr rẹhẹt, „ „ „
Bir muṅgạ chal, the bark of
Alagjạri, Cuscuta chinensis, Lamk.

Grind all these together, steep in an earthen pot and give to drink twice daily.

(b) *Karanat sim*, a fowl whose feathers, bones and skin are black.

Cut the throat of such and mix the blood in straw, and then give this straw to be eaten.

(c) *Ato piṇḍạ da*, the bulb of Amorphophallus campanulatus, Blume.

Grind and give to drink.

(d) *Bana haṭak chal*, the bark of Oroxylon indicum, Benth.
Bir họrẹċ sakam, the leaves of Atyllosia scarabædois, Benth.
Tạṇḍi baraṅgọm,
Atnak chal, the bark of Terminalia tomentosa, W. & A.
Sarjọm chal, „ „ „ Shọrea robusta, Gärtn.

Grind and mix these, steep in an earthen pot and give that water to drink.

(e) *Sadọm khurạ*, a horse's hoof.
Paḍer rẹhẹt, the roots of Stereospermum suaveolens, DC.
Bana haṭak chal, the bark of Oroxylon indicum, Benth.
Bidhạnta rẹhẹt, the roots of Entada scandens, Benth.

Grind and give to drink.

Before being attacked grind these and sprinkle it on straw daily so that they may be eaten with the straw. After being attacked mix these four ingredients in water in which *hoṛeč*, Dolichos biflorus, L., has been boiled and give to drink.

(*f*) *Soso chal ros*, the juice of the bark of Semecarpus Anacardium, L., var. cuneifolia.
Aphim, opium.
Hiṅ, asafœtida, Ferrula asafœtida, Willd.

Mix and give both sick and healthy cattle to drink.

(*g*) *Gabur baha rehet*, the roots of Acacia Farnesiana, Willd.
Bana haṭak rehet, „ „ „ Oroxylon indicum, Benth.
Bhalok seta reak ḍaṭa, the tooth of a mad dog.
Kul jomko sadom khura, the hoof of a horse killed by a tiger.
Kamarko dhukau reak hasa, the earth from a blacksmith's bellows.
Mẽrhẽt ič, iron rust.
Hesak banda, parasitical plant found on Ficus religiosa, Willd.
Caole maric reak banda, parasitical plant found on a variety of capsicum.

Grind these together and at cock-crow on Sunday morning bury them at the threshold of the cow house.

(*h*) When this disease attacks cattle tie them up for 9 days and do not let them leave the house. If allowed to graze at large they will drink water when they like and die off in heaps. Therefore tie them up for 9 days and give them only medicated water to drink twice or thrice daily, viz.

Bir malhan rehet, the roots of Atyllosia mollis, Bth.
Bir hoṛeč, Atyllosia scarabaedois, Benth.
Atore cas hoṛeč, Dolichos biflorus, L.
Babla chal, the bark of Acacia arabica, Willd.
Ul chal, „ „ „ Mangifera indica, L.
Hesak chal, „ „ „ Ficus religiosa, Willd.
Meral chal, „ „ „ Phyllanthus Emblica, L.
Kadam chal, „ „ „ Anthocephalus Cadamba, Benth. and Hook. f.
Ḍoka chal, „ „ „ Odina Wodier, Roxb.
Kasmar chal, „ „ „ Gmelina arborea, Roxb.
Siṅ aṛak chal, „ „ „ Bauhinia purpurea, L.
Ambṛa chal, „ „ „ Spondias mangifera, Pers.
Matkom chal, „ „ „ Bassia latifolia, Roxb.
Ạrmu chal, „ „ „ Bursera serrata, Wall.

Kọcbel chal, the bork of Feronia Elephantum, Correa.
Sega rẹhẹl, the roots of Mimosa rubicaulis, Lamk.
Makarkenda chal, the bark of Diospyros embryopteris, Pers.
Alagjạṛi nãṛĩ, Cuscuta chinensis, Lamk.
Pạni phọl, Trapa bispinosa, Roxb.
Gõṛẽ chal, the bark of Stephegyne parvifolia, Korth.
Karam chal, „ „ „ Adina cordifolia, H. f. and B.
Jhiṅjiṭ chal, „ „ „ Bauhinia retusa, Ham.

Collect all these, put them in an earthen pot to soak in water and give to drink daily in the morning.

(*i*) *Atnak chal*, the bark of Terminalia tomentosa, W. and A.
Terel chal, „ „ „ Diospyros tomentosa, Roxb.
Sọsọ chal, „ „ „ Semecarpus Anacardium, L.
Sahṛa chal, „ „ „ Streblus asper, Lour.
Saram lutur rẹhẹl, the roots of Clerodendron serratum, Spreng.
Hẹsẹl chal, the bark of Anogeissus latifolia, Wall.
Cạili chal, „ „ „ Morinda tinctoria, Roxb.
Ghoṛa lada da, the bulb of Vitis tomentosa, Heyne.
Ḍhalka hạtkạn rẹhẹl, the roots of Leea macrophylla, Roxb.

Collect all these and put them to soak in an earthen pot in water and give to drink daily in the evening.

(*j*) *Bana hataḳ chal sẹ rẹhẹl*, the bark of Oroxylon indicum, Benth., or its roots.
Paḍer chal, the bark of Stereospermum suaveolens, DC.
Moṭa sega chal, the bark of the thick Mimosa rubicaulis, Lamk.
Edẹl roṅga, the knots of Bombax malabaricum, DC.
Kuṛit rama rẹhẹl, the roots of Zizyphus Oenoplia, Mill.
Terel rẹhẹl, the roots of Diospyros tomentosa, Roxb.
Ọpọnọm, Angelica glauca, Edgew.
Ạmsi, dried pulp of mango.

Grind all these together, stir in *kạṅji dak*, stale rice water, and make to drink; also continually wash the mouth with *hoṛẹc̓ dak*, the water in which Dolichos biflorus, L., has been boiled; do not let it get dry.

As a prophylactic the two following:—

(*k*) *Edẹl chal*, the bark of Bombax malabaricum, DC.
Ḍoka chal, „ „ „ Odina Wodier, Roxb.
Ambṛa chal, „ „ „ Spondias mangifera, Pers.
Baṛe chal, „ „ „ Ficus bengalensis, L.
Pakaṛe chal, „ „ „ Ficus infectoria, Willd.
Jọm jạnum chal, „ „ „ Zizyphuz Jujuba, Lam.

Qmẹ chal, the bark of Miliusa velutina, Horask. fil. and Ths.
Kadar nāṛī rẹhẹl, the roots of Asparagus racemosus, Willd.
Karkaṭ chal, the bark of Zizyphus xylopyra, Willd.
Tilạ̣i chal, „ „ „ Wendlandia tinctoria, DC.
Sẹkrẹc̓ chal, „ „ „ Lagerstroemia parviflora, Roxb.
Sekra chal, „ „ „ Zizyphus rugosa, Lamk.
Jọm laṛ chal, „ „ „ Bauhinia Vahlii, W. and A.
Cihūṭ laṛ nāṛī chal, the bark of Spatholobus Roxburghii, Benth.
Sarjọm chal, the bark of Shorea robusta, Gärtn.
1 *sẹr dhūṛā*, 2 pounds of resin of Shorea robusta, Gärtn.

Soak all in a pot and give to drink.

(*l*) *Bana haṭak chal*, the bark of Oroxylon indicum, Benth.
Sinduạri sakam, the leaves of Vitex Negundo, L.
Sẹṅgẹl gidi im, the liver of the king vulture, Ologyps calvus.
Tayan bọhọk, the head of a crocodile.
Kul jāṅ sẹ bọhọk, the bone or head of a tiger.

Rub these on a stone and stir and mix with the juice of above bark, and sprinkle it on grass or straw which the cattle should eat and they will be immune. Make some sliding bars for the entrance to the shed of the wood of the Oroxylon indicum, Benth., so that they may step over them on entrance and exit.

V. 4. *Pilhoi*. Anthrax.

Medicines: (*a*) Mark with *cuạ sọsọ sunum*, the oil obtained by distilling the seeds of Semecarpus Anacardium, L., var. cuneifolia, from the left shoulder blade down to the spleen.

(*b*) *Pańjọt sakam*, the leaves of Clerodendron phlomoides, Willd.
Kasmar chal, the bark of Gmelina arborea, Roxb.
Kamraj, Buettneria herbacea, Roxb.

Pound these and give to drink.

(*c*) *Qrsọṛẹń da*, the bulb of Zingiber Cassumunar, Roxb.
Gargạḍi rẹhẹl, the roots of Coix lachryma, Willd.
Bana haṭak chal, the bark of Oroxylon indicum, Benth.
Kanda sạru da, the tuber of a certain variety of Celocasia antiquorum, Schott.
Mare jọjọ, old tamarinds, Tamarindus indica, L.
Cuạ sọsọ, distilled seeds of Semecarpus Anacardium, L., var. cuneifolia.

Grind all these, mix up with *kạńji dak*, stale rice water, and give to drink.

(*d*) *Sarjọm baha*, the flowers of Shorea robusta, Gärtn., brought by unmarried girls at the *baha porob*, or flower festival.

Kedar ręhęl, the roots of Bonnaya veronicæfolia, Spreng.
Sasaṅ baha, the flowers of Curcuma longa, Roxb.
Ręsun, garlic.
Peaj, onions.
Meral chal, the bark of Phyllanthus Emblica, L.

Grind and mix these and make to drink: also make dots between three of the ribs by applying the juice of the fruit of *sosǫ*, Semecarpus Anacardium, L., var. cuneifolia, with a bit of stick of the *nim*, Melia Azadirachta, L.

N.B.—This remedy is also used in *poca pilhoi*.

V. 5. *Gurmi janwarkore.* Black quarter.

Medicines: *Jhik poṭa*, the stomach of a porcupine.
Tirṛą da, the bulb of Pueraria tuberosa, DC.
Ahla chal, the bark of
Bir eraḍǫm da, the bulb of the wild castor oil plant.
Ghoṛa ladąuṛi da, the bulb of Vitis tomentosa, Heyne.

Grind these together, stir into stale rice water and give to drink.

V. 6. *Khaṛak muth janwarkore.* Gravel in cattle.

Symptoms. In this they double themselves up or the back is concaved and they are unable to pass urine.

Medicines: *Tǫlnǫpak chal*, the bark of Eugenia operculata, Roxb.
Kasmar chal, „ „ „ Gmelina arborea, Roxb.
Jiṭhimond, Clerodendron Siphonanthus, R. Br.
Jąnum ręhęl, the roots of Zizyphus Jujuba, Lam.

Grind all these together, stir in *mąhūt guṛ*, the refuse of molasses, and make to drink.

V. 7. *Tejoleko khan.* Larvæ in cattle sores.

Medicines: *Ḍhalka catǫm aṛak ręhęl*, the roots of

Scratch the inside of the ear with this without drawing your breath, and

Kadam ręhęl, the roots of Anthocephalus Cadamba, Benth. and Hook. f.

Pound and fray this and stroke the animal three times therewith, but do not touch the place and the larvæ will fall off of their own accord.

V. 8. *Gąiko udrilenre.* Dropsy in cattle.

Symptoms. As among human beings so also among animals, when sick, sometimes the body swells, or it may occur of itself.

Medicines: (*a*) *Patal rǫtę*, a white frog found deeply buried in the soil.
Tumbą ol, an edible form of mushroom.
Ąsąrią ręhęl, the roots of Capparis horrida, L. f.

Grind these and give to drink.

(*b*) *Buru ghoṛa lada ṛẹhẹl*, the roots of Vitis tomentosa, Heyne.
Grind, warm and plaster therewith.

(*c*) *Alagjạṛi sakam*, the leaves of Cuscuta chinensis, Lamk.
Sinduạri sakam, " " " Vitex Negundo, L.
Grind these, warm and plaster therewith.

V. 9. *Dhạki sẹ ninạ ṭipạ.*

Symptoms. This attacks cattle; the stomach swells up greatly, their legs tremble or they lie down and kick convulsively.

Medicines: (*a*) Take a leaf cup and urinate in it; then pour this into both nostrils, when the animal will breathe hard, and by degrees get well.

(*b*) *Meral chiṭkiṛic̃*, a switch of Phyllanthus Emblica, L.
Strip this of all its leaves, pass it three times over the animal in one breath, and after beating its stomach therewith quickly five times go straight home. Do not look back at all, and if on the way you meet any one who asks you anything, say nothing whatever.

V. 10. *Gại kaḍako kāṛālenre.* Blindness in cattle.

Medicines: (*a*) *Jiṭhimond*, Clerodendron Siphonanthus, R. Br.
Lọṅphul, cloves.
Grind these and drop the liquid thus obtained into the eye.

(*b*) *Simic̃*, the excrement of a fowl.
Arak̃ sindur, genuine red lead.
Karam ṭusạ, a tip of Adina cordifolia, H. f. and B.
Grind these together and pour into the eye.

(*c*) *Cip ciṛip ḍọg*, a sprout of Achyranthes aspera, L.
Chew this and spit into the eye.

(*d*) *Capol sakam*, the leaves of Desmodium cephalotes.
Chew this and spit into the eye.

(*e*) *Bir buṭ ṛẹhẹl*, the roots of Flemingia congesta, Roxb.
Chew this and spit into the eye.

V. 11. *Gại kaḍa jāhā ṭhen hasokore.* Pain in cattle anywhere.

Medicines: Rub him with kerosine oil and bathe him with hot water.

V. 12. *Gại kaḍa ṛạpuṭlenre.* Bone fractures in cattle.

Medicines: (*a*) *Bunum cetan reak̃ bọd laṛ*, Vitis adnata, Roxb., growing on a white-ant hill.
Suruj mukhi, Helianthus annuus, Willd.
Catọm aṛak̃, Marsilia quadrifolia, L.
Grind together, apply thickly as a plaster and affix splints.

(*b*) *Hãṛũ ãwãr*,

Grind, apply as a plaster and affix splints.

(*c*) *Haḍ joṛa* (*nãṛĩ*), Cissus quadrangularis, Willd.

Grind, apply as a plaster and affix splints.

(*d*) *Ḍahu chal*, the bark of Artocarpus Lakoocha, Roxb.
Pusi toa sakam, the leaves of Euphorbia pilulifera, L.
Ṭampuṛ bindi 5 *goṭęć*, 5 long legged spiders.
3 *golmaric*, 3 black pepper-corns.

Grind and apply as a plaster.

(*e*) *Moṭa alagjaṛi*, a thick Cuscuta chinensis, Lamk.
Miru baha rẹhẹt, the roots of Abutilon indicum, Don.
Icạk rẹhẹt, the roots of Woodfordia floribunda, Salisb.
Bọd laṛ rẹhẹt, „ „ „ Vitis adnata, Wall.

Grind with water and apply as a plaster.

(*f*) *Bunum cetanre tahẹn bọd laṛ rẹhẹt*, the roots of a Vitis adnata Wall., growing on a white-ant hill.
Ḍhalka hạtkạn rẹhẹt, the roots of Leea macrophylla, Roxb.

Grind together, warm slightly, apply to the fracture and then splints.

(*g*) *Gạrunḍi aṛak rẹhẹt*, the roots of Acternanthera sessilis, R. Br.
Suruj mukhi rẹhẹt, the roots of Helianthus annuus, Willd.
Sim kaṭa aṛak rẹhẹt, the roots of Vitex peduncularis.
Catọm aṛak rẹhẹt, the roots of Marsilia quadrifolia, L.
Hãṛũ ãwãr nãṛĩ,
Etka rẹhẹt, the roots of Mucuna pruriens, DC.
Kawẹt rẹhẹt, „ „ „ Abrus precatorius, L.

Grind all these together, warm and apply, affixing splints on top.

(*h*) *Ghoṛa lada da*, the bulb of Vitis tomentosa, Heyne.
Ić ewer da, „ „ „ Vitis latifolia, Roxb.

Warm these and apply, and then splints.

(*i*) *Bunum cetan bọd laṛ rẹhẹt*, the roots of Vitis adnata, Wall. growing on a white ant hill.
Suruj mukhi rẹhẹt, the roots of Helianthus annuus, Willd.
Turạm rẹhẹt, the roots of
Sim kaṭa aṛak rẹhẹt, the roots of Vitex peduncularis.
Catọm aṛak rẹhẹt, the roots of Marsilia quadrifolia, L.

Grind together, warm and apply. Five days afterwards remove it and give a fresh application of the same, replacing the splints. We consider this the most efficacious remedy.

(*j*) Apply *haṛ joṛa*, Cissus quadrangularis, Willd., in the same way.

V. 13. *Bajra jomte gaiko bul ran.*

Remedy for cattle intoxicated by eating Sorghum vulgare, Pers.

Medicines: *Kasmar chal*, the bark of Gmelina arborea, Roxb.
Siń arak chal, „ „ „ Bauhinia purpurea, L.

Grind and give to drink with stale rice water; plaster them therewith and they will recover.

V. 14. *Er eradom se ato eradom sakam jomte bullenre ran.*

Remedy for intoxication caused by eating the castor oil plant leaves, Ricinus communis, L.

Symptoms. They run round and round, and if medicine is not given quickly the eyes will burst and death ensue.

Medicines: *Kasmar chal*, the bark of Gmelina arborea, Roxb.
Siń arak chal, „ „ „ Bauhinia purpurea, L.
The root of the tree that they ate from.

Grind and give to drink with stale rice water.

V. 15. *Tisi se cikna jomte bul gai kada ran.*

Remedy for cattle who have been stupefied by eating the linseed plant, Linum usitatissimum, Linn.

Medicines: *Kasmar chal*, the bark of Gmelina arborea, Roxb.
Siń arak chal, „ „ „ Bauhinia purpurea, L.
Pond peaj, white onions.
Jhol, thora, a little sooty cobwebs.

Grind all these and give to drink with stale rice water.

V. 16. *Cas basko reak ran.*

To preserve the crops.

Sometimes flies suck the young ears of paddy; to obviate this :—

(*a*) On Sunday bury *kahu botke*, Bryonia lacinosa, L., in three corners, and naming the spirit *Garbhu Kũãr* make marks with *sindur*, red lead, and they will suck the ears no more.

(*b*) To prevent thieves stealing your crops, name the same spirit, and whatever wish you express will be fulfilled; if you say, Let a snake bite the thief, it will come to pass; or Let him stay here till morning, and that will happen; or whatever your wish may be he will bring it about.

PART III

HOW THE SANTALS LIVE

NOTE.

The Introductory Remarks give details regarding the genesis of the present work, and nothing needs to be added, except to make my excuses that a non-professional man has taken upon himself the responsibility of editing anything of this kind.

There are, however, a few matters that I wish to emphasize or to mention here.

My aim has throughout been to give a faithful record of what the Santals have in the way of medicine and how medicine is practised by them. There is just the possibility that among the many ingredients used by them some few might be found that are not known to western science as medicines. Apart from this possibility what has to the writer been of paramount interest is the anthropological value of what has been recorded. We get a glimpse of how an aboriginal people lives and attempts to face and fight the real or supposed enemies of life, with the help of magic, invocation of spirits, suggestion and natural remedies, or, generally, these combined. The work is a literal translation of what I have received from the Santals, the only exceptions being the Introductory Remarks and a few easily recognized explanatory remarks. When words like 'this is a sure cure' or something similar is met with, I trust it is understood that it is the opinion of the medicine-man, not that of the writer.

As is to be expected, much nonsense and superstitious matter are found. All this has been kept on account of the anthropological and psychological interest attached to it.

Some doubt might perhaps be entertained, whether my informants have given me all the ingredients of their recipes, or have kept something back, or substituted something else in stead of what they really use.

The possibility is there; but the way in which the information has come to me will not make this likely as a general rule. I have in many cases received the same recipes from sources separate and independent in time and place. On the other hand, it has, so far as I can remember, thrice happened that ojhas have been unwilling to divulge a 'professional' secret; they have said so and not attempted to deceive me, in spite of the offer money.

Naturally the Santals have recipes that the writer has not succeeded in getting. In so far the present work is incomplete; but I believe most of the ingredients made use of by them will be found here.

There must also be complaints that have not been mentioned. On p. 142 it is stated that diphtheria is practically unknown among them; it may be of interest to state that quite recently we have had a limited epidemic of this disease in a children's home belonging to the mission, happily without any deaths, all having been treated with serum.

So far as it has been possible to me I have given the scientific names of the ingredients made use of. In the case of trees I trust all names are correct. As regards several plants I am not so sure. It will also be seen that a number stand without identification. If any research worker should wish to investigate the properties of these or, for that matter, of any of the ingredients mentioned, it would as a rule be practicable to get a supply of the stuff itself.

Before closing I feel the need of expressing my deepfelt gratitude to the Council of the Asiatic Society of Bengal for having published this work and for the generous way in which it has been done.

P. O. Bodding.

A LIST

of the plants and other various stuffs used by the Santal medicine-men and mentioned in this work.

In the first column the Santal names are given, alphabetically arranged. In the second column the botanical, etc., names will be found, when known. The third column gives the number of the disease, etc., where the ingredient is mentioned as used by the Santals.

The writer is greatly indebted to Miss I. Gahrn (now Mrs. O. Eie) for first preparing this list.

Santal name	Botanical, etc., name	Disease number
Adagạthiạ	*Panicum repens, L.*	66, 90, 93, 96, 97, 99, 100, 138, 201, 203, 208, 221, 241, 244, 247, 249, 250, 251, 252, 253.
Adhẹ ..	Ginger, *Zingiber officinalis, Roscoe.*	90, 93, 94, 96, 99, 136, 147, 166, 219, 222, 224, 238, 244, 247, 252, 253, 265, 274, 275, 276, 285, 290, 301, 302.
Aḍo ..	Urine ..	277.
Adra cip ciṛip		51.
Adwa caole	Rice husked from sun-dried paddy	7, 61, 191, 201, 206, 244, 247, 266, 286.
Ạgạire ..	*Dillenia scabrella, Roxb.*	155.
Ahla ..		V. 5.
Ak̄ ..	A bow ..	110, 123.
Akaona ..	*Calotropis gigantea, R. Br.* or, *C. procera, R. Br.*	31, 45, 60, 62, 66, 67, 68, 70, 75, 84, 88, 93, 94, 96, 100, 107, 111, 112, 123, 124, 127, 131, 136, 150, 163, 167, 173, 185, 188, 189, 191, 193, 197, 198, 207, 242, 244, 245, 255, 270, 285, V. 1.
Akaona tejo	The caterpillar found on above shrub	101, 102, 107.
Akaṛ baha ..	*Limnophila Roxburghiana, G. Don.*	35, 51, 85, 182, 244.
Akọṛ kora ..	*Anthemis pyrethrum (?)*	266, 275.
Alagjạṛi ..	*Cuscuta chinensis, Lamk.* or, *Cassytha filiformis, Roxb.*	75, 82, 208, 268, V. 3, V. 8, V. 12.
Ạlu ..	Potato ..	245.
Amaegọm ..		192.
Ạmbạitar biṅ[1]	*Vipera Russellii*	85, 101, 110.
Ambṛa ..	*Spondias mangifera, Pers.*	10, 61, 86, 209, 240, 241, 244, 245, V. 3.
Amsam dhiri	Stone beads, generally made of agate, of various colours, found in the ground, used as amulets against dysentery	245.
Ạmsi ..	Dried pulp of mango	275, 277, V. 3.
Amsopori ..	*Psidium Guava, Raddi.*	198.
Amṭha ..	Old inspissated juice of certain fruits	12, 193, 250.
Ạṇḍiạ dhurup	*Leucas cephalotes, Spreng.*	7, 290.
Ạṇḍiạ ghaṛwa	Male sparrow ..	260.
Ạṇḍiạ goṅgha	Shell of a male snail	247.
Ạṇḍiạ koṅgaṭ	*Dregia volubilis, Benth.*	75, 197, 278, 285, 290.
Ạṇḍiạ morọn arak̄	*Gymnema hirsutus, W. & A., var. Decaisneanum, Wight.*	50, 75, 117, 163, 171, 192, 193, 195, 197, 203, 207, 208, 242, 245, 252, 253, 255, 260, 278, 279, 298.
Ạṇḍiạ tale ..	The male *Borassus flabelliformis, L.*	160, 165, 166, 171, 173, 176, 195, 298.
Ạphim ..	Opium ..	60, 65, 66, 68, 80, 90, 94, 100, 101, 102, 103, 111, 113, 117, 123, 130, 136, 148, 157, 161, 173, 200,

[1] The writer has never succeeded in getting a specimen from the Santal Parganas district of the snake called ambaitar by the Santals. It is very rare here and much feared on account of its supposed poison. The description given has led me to think that it is the Russell's viper. Quite lately I have received a specimen of the ambaitar from Assam (Goalpara district). This is the Russell's viper (stated by Col. F. Wall in 1917 as not known from the Brahmaputra Basin).

Baṛu ..	*Schleichera trijuga, Willd.*	51, 61, 87, 93, 244, 255, 257.
Baṛu banda	A parasitical plant found on do. (*Loranthus vestitus, Wall.*)	94, 244.
Basok (=*bakos*)	*Justicia Adhatoda, Willd.*.	253.
Batapi sindur	A preparation of red lead	10, 25, 38, 64, 258.
Bayaṅ ..	*Dioscorea crispata, R.*	80, 245.
Bele ..	An egg ..	110.
Beṅgar ..	*Solanum Melongena, L.*	245.
Beṅgar betahel	*Solanum stramonifolium, Jacq.*	31, 111, 138, 247, 250, 252.
Berdor ..	*Combretum nanum, Hamilt.*	66, 232, 239, 244, 245.
Bet ..	*Calamus Rotang, L.*	110.
Bhabri ..	*Embelia robusta, Roxb.*	78, 196, 198, 206, 244, 255, 267, 276.
Bhadoria ..		117.
Bhadu ..	*Vitex alata, Roxb.* (?)	285.
Bhaloḱ seta (data)	(The tooth) of a mad dog	V. 3.
Bharbhari ..	*Ocimum basilicum, L.*, or *O. canum, Sims.*	57, 61, 75, 100, 101, 107, 110, 131, 147, 206, 244, 285, 290.
Bharwa tejo	Large caterpillars, as of *Attacus atlas* and *A. Selene.*	115.
Bhauri mala	A vertigo necklace, made from certain fruits	4.
Bhaya bhagwa	*Polygonum plebejum, Br.* (the same as *muć araḱ*)	266.
Bheda bohoḱren tejo	Worms found in a ram's head	101.
Bheda dereṅ	*Cassia Tora, L.*	107, 166, 198, 290.
Bheda jel ..	Ram's flesh ..	142.
Bhedwa ..	*Hibiscus cancellatus, Roscoe, var. fusiformis, Willd.*	206, 245.
Bhelaondi ..	Sheeps' or goats' dung	261, 273.
Bhelaoṅja ..	*Caesulia axillaris, Roxb.*	2.
Bherṇḍa ..	*Jatropha Curcas, L.*	35, 40, 75, 85, 110, 147, 173, 193, 255.
Bhidi achim	*Centifida orbicularis, Lour.*	101, 207.
Bhidi janatep	*Urena sinuata, L.*, or *Triumfetta rhomboidea, Jac.*	40, 41, 85, 112, 298.
Bhidi toa ..	Sheep's milk ..	33, 35.
Bhorkond ..	*Hymenodictyon excelsum, Wall* or, *H. thyrsiflorum.*	58, 77, 85, 178, 191, 208, 244, 279.
Bhudalore ..		35.
Bhuku chata	A termites'nest	45, 76, 208, 253.
Bidam ..		259.
Bidhanta ..	*Entada scandens, Benth.*	75, 82, 92, 101, 222, V. 3.
Bilati thamakur	Imported tobacco	40, 101, 181, 193, 207, 290, 301, 302.
Bindi ..	A spider ..	54, 110, 116, 125, 151, V. 12.
Bindi ..	A straw ring ..	262.
Biṅdimbu ..		22, 283, 284.
Bindi mutha ghās	*Fimbristylis monostachya, Hassk.*	160, 171, 173, 176, 195, 198, 206, 244, 245, 247, 252, 261.
Biṅ kaṅcur	The slough of a snake	23.
Biṅ ot' ..	A poisonous mushroom	283, 284.
Bir baraṅgom (=*baraṅgom*)	(see *baraṅgom*)	195, 245, 247, 275, 285.
Bir barni (=*barni, q. v.*)		110.
Bir but ..	*Flemingia congesta, L.*	66, 68, 191, 238, 244, 245, V. 10.
Bir campa ..	*Ochna squarrosa, Willd.*	48, 51, 61, 253.
Bir camuk ..		245.
Bir catom araḱ'		229, 239, 241.
Bir god ..		290.
Bir dimbu ..		124, 244.
Bir eradom	The wild Ricinus	45, 244, 245, V. 5.
Bir goṅgha ..	A certain snail	176, 207.
Bir hat ..	*Holarrhena antidysenterica, Wall.*	205.

	R. Br., and *Saccolabium caerulium.*	
Dare japak'	*Scindapsus officinalis, Schott.*	82, 166, 192, 193, 195, 220, 231, 239, 244, 255, 256, 257, V. 1.
Dare katkọm jaṅga	*Viscum attenuatum, DC.*	99.
Dare murup'	*Butea frondosa, Roxb.*	245.
Dare piṇḍạ	*Randia uliginosa, DC.*	12, 23, 42.
Dare ṭipọc'	(*Loranthaceæ* ?)	146, 235, 288.
Darka ristu	*Sapindus detergens, Roxb.*	252.
Dạru ..	Gun powder ..	139.
Daṭạuni ..	A tooth brush, made from a twig of *Shorea robusta, Gärtn.*	50, 54, 262.
Dater mañjọn	Tooth powder	32.
Daṭrạ ..	*Datura alba, Willd.* or *D. fastuosa, Willd.*, or *D. Metel, L.*	6, 23, 35, 39, 60, 75, 80, 90, 94, 96, 97, 89, 99, 100, 101, 103, 105, 110 113, 136, 152, 156, 173, 191, 192, 207.
Ḍẽt' cẽṛẽ ..	A humming bird	208.
Ḍhadra haṭak'	An old worn out winnowing fan	209.
Dhạ̃i ..	*Grislea tomentosa, Willd.*	25, 117, 301, 302.
Ḍhạkni aṛak'		238.
Ḍhalka catọm aṛak'		88, 187, 241, 266, V. 7.
Ḍhalka haṭkạn	*Leea macrophylla, Roxb.*	60, 68, 87, 245, 255, 256, 257, V. 3, V. 12.
Dhạnia ..	*Coriandrum sativum, Willd.*	65, 175, 176, 192.
Ḍhela ..	*Alangium Lamarckii, Thws.*	70, 75, 117, 229, 237, 238, 239, 244, 252, 285, 290.
Dhiri banda (ghās)		196, 198, 206, 247.
Dhiri ghās ..		194.
Dhiri kakṛa	A lizard ..	110, 149.
Dhiri kaṭkọm	A crab found under stones	77, 210, 275.
Dhonantori	A certain bird	88.
Dhọnọsọr cẽṛẽ	The same as *cama cakọr, q. v.*	126.
Dhubi ghās	*Cynodon dactylon, Pers.*	6, 7, 110, 140, 198, 286, 290.
Dhũṛạ̃ ..	Resin of *Shorea robusta, Gärtn.*	82, 83, 90, 100, 109, 123, 165, 173, 182, 191, 193, 195, 207, 238, 244, V. 3.
Dhurup aṛak'	*Leucas cephalotes, Spreng.* or, *Leucas Clarkii, Hook.*	9, 19.
Ḍimbu baha	*Ocimum Basilicum, var. thyrsiflorum, L.*	25, 136.
Ḍodhar ..	*Adiantum lunulatum, Burm.* or *A. Concinum.*	81, 89, 241, 285.
Ḍoka ..	*Odina Wodier, Roxb.*	133, 164, 198, 205, 241, 244, 245, V. 3.
Ḍọmkọ dọkọc'		
Dud barañgọm		156, 173, 245, 278.
Dud bilạsi ..		238.
Dudhiạni ..	*Asclepias rosea, Roxb.*	68.
Dudhi loṭa ..	*Ichnocarpus frutescens, R. Br.*	70, 290.
Dumur rasa	Honey of the small honey bee	10, 58, 78, 146, 158, 206, 214, 247.
Ḍunḍukit' ..	*Gardenia turgida, Roxb.*	51, 101, 107, 131, 156, 181, 189, 205, 243, 244, 245, 255, 285, 290, 301.
Ḍurạ ..		245.
Ḍurạ sañ ..	*Dioscorea pentafylla, Willd.*	75.
Ḍuriạ haṭkạn	*Leea hirta, Herb. Banks.*	61, 87, 96, 99, 201, 245, 255, 256, 257.
Ẹdẹl ..	*Bombax malabaricum, DC.*	30, 31, 35, 45, 53, 61, 81, 156, 181, 188, 191, 198, 200, 205, 244, 255, 266, 268, 298, 302, V. 3.
Ẹdhẹ campa	*Ochna* (?) ..	267.
Ẹdhẹ cip-cirip'	*Achyranthes* (?)	93.
Ẹdhẹ raṅgaini jạnum	*Solanum xanthocarpum, Schrad. et Wendl.*	98, 250, 253, 302.

Ekasiṛạ ..	*Crataeva religiosa, Forst.*	2, 174, 180, 207.
Elaci ..	*Alpinia cardamomum, Roxb.*	252, 253.
Eraḍọm ..	*Ricinus communis, L.*	75, 88, 136, 180, 182, 209, 278, 284.
Etka ..	*Mucuna pruriens, DC.*	41, 56, 75, 80, 82, 152, 163, 189, 193, 247, 257, 268, 285, 289, 290, 301, 302, V. 12.
Etkẹċ ..	*Euphorbia antiquorum, L.*	22, 40, 75, 173, 192, 193, 218, 245, 252, 281.
Eṭko hasa ..	Burnt clay from inside the fireplace	5, 108, 110, 111.
Gabla ..	*Acacia arabica, Willd.*	3, 26, 244, 258.
Gabla tejo ..	A caterpillar found on *gabla.*	
Gạbur ..	*Acacia Farnesiana, Willd.*	80, 85, 103, 114, 136, 178, 244, 264, 290, V. 3.
Gaḍa cańcir	*Motacilla luzoniensis.*	260.
Gaḍa gā̃ṛī ..	A certain water insect	104, 195, 198.
Gaḍa icaǩ ..	*Woodfordia floribunda, Salisb.* (growing near rivers).	268.
Gaḍa kasmar	*Gmelina arborea, Roxb.* (growing near rivers)	76.
Gaḍa suṛạ ..	*Cyperus tegetum Roxb.*	81.
Gaḍa terel ..	*Diospyros montana, Roxb.*	55, 204, 206, 255, 257, 266, 275, 276, 299.
Gadha iċ ..	Donkey's excrement	123, 173.
Gạị ado ..	Cow's urine ..	68.
Gạị dahe (uruľ oḍok nạinu)	(The butter obtained by churning) curds of cow's milk	90, 252.
Gạị ghuṛạ aṛaǩ	*Polygala chinensis, L.*	4, 21, 59, 80, 146, 235.
Gạị ghurbạị		107.
Gạị gọtọm }	} Butter of cow's milk	2, 35, 83, 97, 207, 238, 250, V. 1.
Gạị gọtọm nạinu }	} Butter of cow's milk	90.
Gạị mulạ ..		245.
Gạị phọl ..		253.
Gạị toa ..	Cow's milk	64, 191, 208, 225.
Gạndhạri aṛaǩ	*Amaranthus gangeticus, var. angustifolia, L.*	245, 253.
Gạṅgiṭ cun ..	Lime from nodular or Hydraulic lime stone	85, 181.
Gańja ..	*Cannabis sativa, Willd.*	101, 103, 110, 111, 113, 123, 136, 173, 250, 251.
Ganthar ..	A filmy substance	171.
Gargạdi ṛẹhẹḷ	*Coix lachryma, Willd.*	63, 191, 227, 245, 275, 276, V.4.
Gā̃ṛī (bọhọǩ)	A monkey (head)	110, 133, 135.
Gạrundi aṛaǩ	*Acternanthera sessilis, R. Br.*	11, 21, 27, 50, 131, 238, 241, 245, 275, 285, 292, 293, V.12.
Gạtur baha ..		264.
Gẹḍẹ māyām	Ducks' blood	253.
Gẹgẹtẹreń ..	*Lẹndọń* whilst small	65, 68, 175.
Ghańgra ..	*Vigna Catiang.*	191.
Ghā̃rā ghā̃ṛī		144.
Ghikuā̃ri ..	*Yucca gloriosa.*	96, 163, 196, 197, 245, 252, 258, V.1.
Ghuṛi ..	*Tiliqua rubriventris.*	
{ *Ghoṛa lada*		9, 68, 156, 181, 255, 299, V.3, V.12.
{ *Ghoṛa laḍạuri*	*Vitis tomentosa, Heyne.*	9, 60, 65, 68, 75, 181, 245, 255, 257, V.5.
Ghugri ..	*Gryllus gryllotalpa.*	133, 155, 169, 172, 202, 244.
Gidi ..	A vulture	258, 285.
Giru dhiri ..	A certain kind of red stone used as a pigment	298.
Gitil gā̃ṛī kaḍa	*Gryllus monstruosus.*	79, 85, 101, 103, 202.
Goboria dudhi lota		244.
Gọd ..	*Aristolochia indica, Willd.*	51, 75, 82, 244, 290.
Gọdo gẹlẹċ hasa	Earth excavated by rats	281.
Gọeṭha ..	Dried cow dung	191.

Golmaṛic ..	Black pepper	7, 36, 38, 61, 67, 68, 75, 80, 94, 96, 98, 99, 100, 101, 103, 105, 107, 110, 111, 112, 113, 117, 119, 120, 124, 125, 132, 136, 142, 144, 145, 147, 151, 152, 161, 188, 191, 192, 200, 202, 206, 207, 209, 219, 221, 222, 223, 224, 225, 227, 236, 244, 245, 247, 248, 249, 252, 253, 255, 256, 258, 266, 270, 274, 275, 276, 277, 285, 289, 290, 301, 302, V.1, V.12.
Gọndhọk ..	Sulphur	166, 167, 176, 188, 206.
Goṅgha ..	A snail	
Gõṛẽ ..	*Stephegyne parvifolia, Korth.*	21, 51, 71, 73, 198, 244, V.3.
Goṭe ..	*Croton oblongifolius, Roxb.*	6, 51, 55, 61, 67, 68, 80, 98, 101, 112, 128, 188, 192, 195, 196, 197, 207, 213, 223, 236, 240, 242, 244, 245, 255, 285, 289, 290.
Gotọm ..	Melted or clarified butter	10, 12, 20, 30, 84, 85, 94, 123, 127, 161, 168, 182, 207, 238, 253, 258.
Guạ ..	*Areca Catechu, L*	191, 192, 237, 244, 245.
Guihạ gạndhạri ..		110.
Gujhạ kạudhạri		110.
Gukhur kaṭa		259.
Guklạ ..	*Hygrophila spinosa, T. Andres.*	82.
Gulạṅj baha	*Plumeria acutifolia, Poiret.*	225, 244.
Guli paṭhi ..	A brown female kid	
Gundli ..	*Panicum miliare, Lamk.*	198.
Guṇḍri gẹrvẹl		110.
Guṛ ..	Molasses	21, 191, 193, 204, 225, 266.
Gurič ..	Cowdung	80.
Gurič gaṇdar	Beetle *larvae* found in middens of cowdung	208.

Gurli ..		80, 145, 195.
Gurli jaṅ ..		111, 160.
Haḍ joṛa ..	*Cissus quadrangularis, Willd.*	46, 184, V. 12.
Haḍ pạṅglạ		61.
Hako ..	Fish	245.
Hako itil sunum ..	Cod liver oil	21.
Hạliạ kũãri mulạ ..		245.
Hạlim ..	*Lepidium sativum, L.*	87, 88, 201, 206, 227, 229, 239, 245, 252, 256, 257.
Hạṇḍi ..	Rice beer	61, 142, 283.
Hạṇḍi kuṇḍi	*Physalis minima, L.*	22.
Hạṇḍi mera	The refuse after brewing rice beer	155.
Hao ..	A kind of red ant. *Oecophylla smaragdina*	275, 277, 285.
Harba ..	*Manis pentadactyla*	190.
Haṛhaṭ sisir	Gall	21.
Haṛ joṛa ..	*Cissus quadrangularis, Willd.*	V. 12.
Hãṛũ (bọhọk̄)	(The head of) a baboon	122, 166, 196, 207.
Hãṛũ ăwăr ..		163, 166, 173, 272, V. 12.
Hasa aṛak̄ ..		252.
Haṭ dare ..	*Holarrhena antidysenterica, Wall.*	51, 66, 67, 68, 86, 101, 117, 131, 200, 206, 223, 229, 239, 240, 241, 244, 245, 246, 249, 253, 266, 285, 296.
Hạti (ič) ..	Elephant's excrement	35, 81, 123.
Hạti (suṇḍạ)	*Heliotropium indicum, Willd.*	12.
Hạtkạn ..	*Leea macrophylla, Roxb.* and *Leea hirta, Herb. Banks.*	255
Hẹhẹl ..	*Millettia auriculata, Baker.*	31, 68.
Hemca aṛak̄	*Enhydra fluctuans*, or *Limnophila conferta, Benth.*	75, 171, 290
Hẹmsagọr ..	*Cotyledon laciniata, Willd.*	51, 54, 55, 212, 220, 252.

Hẹndẹ buluṅ	Black salt	252.
Hẹndẹ horo	Black paddy	101.
Hẹndẹ mẹrọm (māyām) ..	(Blood) of a black goat	21, 238, 244, 253, 261.
Hẹndẹ sim māyām	Blood of a black fowl	253.
Hẹnjẹl ..	*Solanum stramonifolium, Jacq.*	188, 250, 251, 253.
Hẹrẹm tij ..	Anything sweet	245.
Hesak ..	*Ficus religiosa, Willd.*	23, 35, 61, 81, 96, 156, 191, 198, 200, 201, 206, 222, 226, 244, 245, V. 3.
Hesak banda	Parasitical plant found on above	191, V. 3.
Hẹsẹl ..	*Anogeissus latifolia, Wall.*	31, 70, 82, 198, 204, 241, 244, 247, 250, V. 3.
Hiṅ ..	*Ferrula asafoetida, Willd.*	65, 66, 68, 80, 90, 100, 101, 110, 117, 285, V. 3.
Hiṅjọṛ ..	*Barringtonia acutangula, Gärtn.*	244.
Holoṅ ..	Meal or flour	
Hondro ..		
Hopo baha..	*Cochlospermum gossypium, DC.*	175, 181.
Hoṛ (ạḍo, ič)	Human (urine, excrement)	80, 101.
Hoṛẹč ..	*Dolichos biflorus, L.*	83, 159, 161, 173, 182, 190, 191, 204, 238, 245, 255, 258, V. 3.
Horo bohok	Head of a tortoise	29, 192, 199, 238, 266, 273.
Horo itil ..	The fat of a tortoise	95.
Hoṛo caole ..	Rice	218.
Hoṛo rọṅgo	Burnt paddy	54.
Hoṛ toki ..	*Terminalia Chebula, Retz.*	253, (same as rọl)
Hotọl ..	*Cucurbita lagenaria, Willd.*	70, 75, 86, 123, 125, 136, 160, 178, 182, 253, 290.
Huḍiṅ catọm arak	*Desmodium triflorum, DC.*	
Hukạ dak ..	Hookah water	65, 117, 166, 181, 193, 290.
Hund baha	*Jasminum arborescens, Roxb.*	51, 61, 80, 175, 252, 290.

Hūṛ huṛạ ..	*Cleome viscosa, Willd.*	7.
Hutạr ..	*Indigofera pulchella, Roxb.*	V. 3.
Huter baha	*Indigofera pulchella, Roxb.*	101, 201, 266.
Icạk banda	A parasitic plant found on *icak*, *Loranthus Buddeoides, Wedd.*	244.
Icạk dare ..	*Woodfordia floribunda, Salisb.*	21, 44, 61, 63, 68, 81, 89, 155, 165, 169, 171, 172, 175, 178, 192, 193, 196, 198, 245, 266, 267, 275, 285, V. 12.
Icạk gotẹ dare		26.
Icạk hako ..	A prawn	117.
Ič ẹwẹr ..	*Vitis latifolia, Roxb.*	88, 173, 198, 256, 290, V. 12.
Im ..	The liver	21.
Iṛi ..	*Panicum Crus-galli, L.*	198.
Isạbgul ..	*Plantago ispaghala, R. Fleming*	88, 249.
Isor muli gọd	*Aristolochia indica, Willd.*	244, 281, 290, 294.
Jaephọl ..	Nutmeg, *Myristica moschata, Willd.*	253, 275.
Jạmbir ..	*Citrus medica, L.*	117, 210.
Jambṛo biṅ	*Zamenis mucosus.*	95, 98, 182.
Janhe ..	*Paspalum scrobiculatum, L.*	198, 283.
Janhe naṅjom	*Polycarpaea corymbosa, Lamk.*	81.
Jạnum ..	*Zizyphus Jujuba, Lam.*	6, 173, 178, 230, 231, 241, 244, 245, V. 6.
Jạnum arak	*Amaranthus spinosus, Willd.*	210.
Jao ..	*Hordeum vulgare, L.*	244.
Jạphir phọl		253.
Jāwān ..	*Carum Ajowan, DC.*	103, 192, 250, 253, 275.
Jāwān jirạ..	*Carum Ajowan, DC.* and *C. Carui, L.*	81, 219, 238, 253.
Jel ..	Meat	245.
Jel dẹreń ..	A deer's horn	110, 129, 138, 255.
Jera janhe..	*Panicum flavidium, Retz.*	283.

Kalia kũãr mulạ		245.
Kalmẹg ..	*Andrographis paniculata*, *Nees*.	66, 68, 117, 124, 222, 223, 229, 232, 239, 241, 244, 252, 253, 285.
Kalọṭ ..	A pullet	243.
Kamar dhukạu hasa	Earth from a blacksmith's bellows	121, V.3.
Kamraj ..	*Buettneria herbacea*, *Roxb.*	46, 173, 184, 187, 195, 206, 244, 245, 247, 266, 278, 288, V. 4.
Kana aṛak̓	*Commelyna bengalensis*, *L.*	23, 155, 290.
Kanda sạru	Var. of *Colocasia antiquorum*, *Schott.*	253, V.4.
Kạñji dak̓ ..	Stale rice water	85, 90, 97, 191, 196, 198, 229, 239, 284, 290, 295, 296, 302, V. 1, V. 3, V. 4.
Kanṭa kucạ / *Kanṭa kucạ aṛak̓*	*Mimosa rubicaulis*, *Willd.*	252, 253.
Kanṭa sạru	*Lasia heterophylla*, *Schott.*	252, 253.
Kanṭa siris	*Albizzia myriophylla*, *Bl.*	252.
Kantha aṛak̓	*Euphorbia granulata*, *Forsk.*	252
Kanṭhaṛ ..	*Artocarpus integrifolia*, *L.*	31, 142, 154, 191, 198, 261, 272.
Kaphọr ..	Camphor	253.
Kạpu ..		206.
Kạr ..	*Argemone mexicana*, *Willd.*	
Karam ..	*Adina cordifolia*, *H.F.&B.*	21, 197, 198, 237, 244, V. 3, V. 10.
Karam hoṛo	A variety of paddy	
Karanat sim	A fowl whose feathers, bones and skin are black	11, 21, V. 3.
Karbolik ..	Carbolic acid	193.
Karhani hoṛo	A variety of black paddy	68, 101, 207, 244, 266.
Karkaṭ ..	*Zizyphus xylopyra*, *Willd.*	245, 294, V. 3.
Karla ..	*Momordica dioica*, *Roxb.*	7, 9, 70, 119, 137, 145, 245, 252, 290.
Kāṛwāṭ' ..	*Carissa Carandas*, *L.*	75, 80, 94, 96, 100, 101, 103, 107, 129, 131, 136, 145, 147, 149, 163, 197, 285.
Karsaṛe / *Kasaṛe* ..	*Thysanolaena acarifera*, *Nees.*	252, 253.
Kạsi ghās ..	*Saccharum spontaneum*, *L*	182, 201, 244, 247, 252, 253.
Kaskọm ..	*Gossypium arboreum*, *L.*	25, 68, 80, 149, 191, 273.
Kasmar (chal) ..	*Gmelina arborea*, *Roxb.* (bark)	38, 61, 75, 90, 96, 97, 98, 99, 105, 113, 117, 136, 152, 191, 193, 197, 220, 244, 252, 276, 282, 283, 284, 287, 288, 289, 290, 294, 295, 296, 297, 300, 301, 302, V. 1, V. 3, V. 4, V. 6, V. 13, V. 14, V. 15
Katkọm careċ ..	*Rottboellia perforata*, *Roxb.*	81, 89, 102.
Katkọm jaṅga ..	*Viscum attenuatum*, *DC.*	45, 71, 81, 83, 99, 195.
Kaṭ kọrọñj	*Cæsalpinia Bonducella*, *Roxb.*	
Kaṭlạ jẹr ..		194.
Kaṭ oṭ ..	An edible *fungus* that grows on wood	25.
Kạuḍi ..	The shell used as money in India	235, 244, 275.
Kạuḍi diạṅ ..	A black winged kite	135.
Kạuhạ ..	*Terminalia Arjuna*, *Bedd.*	42, 60, 86, 133, 204, 255, 258, 288.
Kawet̓ (rẹhẹt̓)	*Abrus precatorious*, *L.* (root.)	21, 32, 88, 92, 149, 201, 206, 276, V. 12.
Kedar ..	=*Kadar*, *q.v.*	
„ *nā̃ṛī* ..	=*Kadar nā̃ṛī*, *q.v.*	
Kedok̓ aṛak̓	*Argyreia speciosa*, *Sweet.*	142, 176, 191, 195, 241, 245.
Kelhaṭ ..	A broken bit of pottery	178.
Kerasin sunum ..	Kerosine oil	
Kesari ..	*Lathyrus sativus*, *L.*	45.
Kesari dạl ..	The *dal*, split bean of above	142, 245.
Kẹsọr ..		150.
Khạḍi tọrọċ	The ashes of Indian corn cobs	223.

Kuṛi tukuć	*Lobivanellus goensis*, or, *Sarciophorus bilobus.*	268.
Kuṛmbi aṛak		142, 245.
Kũs ..	*Themuda gigantea, Haskel.*	59, 66, 75, 81, 163, 200, 206, 229, 239, 244, 247, 252, 253, 260.
Lag joṛ ..		51, 71, 73.
Lạli guṛ ..	Refuse of molasses	15, 61.
Laṭha cip ciṛip		7, 35, 40, 50, 51, 68, 93, 167, 188, 191, 195, 209, 223, 224, 225, 238, 244, 249, 270, 285, 290, 292, 293, 297, 298, 301, 302, V.1.
Lebeḍ cenḍeń jạnum	Trodden down *Zizuphus Jujuba*	
Lenḍeṭ (hasa)	(The earth thrown up by) earth worms	7, 125, 290, 303.
Lenḍoń ..	A centipede, *Spirocystus cilcylindricus.*	68, 207.
Lilibichi ..		237.
Lilkạthi ..	*Polygala crotalarioides*, *Buch.* and *Ham.*	7, 8, 31, 72, 101, 117, 190, 237, 247, 248, 277.
Loa ..	*Ficus glomerata, Roxb.*	84, 88, 159, 161, 188, 191, 200, 207.
Loa banda ..	The parasitical plant (A *Loranthus*) found on *Ficus glomerata, Roxb.*	278
Lọbọń ..	Cloves	195.
Lodam ..	*Symplocos racemosa, Roxb.*	253.
Lọńphul ..	Cloves (*Eugenia caryophyllata, Willd.*)	7, 10, 17, 30, 101, 107, 206, 244, 250, 252, 253, 258, 261, 302, V.10.
Lọpọń ..	*Terminalia bellerica, Roxb.*	51, 61, 89, 109, 130, 190, 204, 244, 250, 252, 253, 258, 261, 290, 302, V.10.
Lọpọń aṛak	*Aerua lanata, L.*	201, 212, 244, 290.
Lọtọ ..	*Randia dumetorum, Lam.*	42, 110, 156, 223, 281.
Lubui jirạ ..		81, 253.
Lumạm ..	A silkworm	110.
Lumạm tejo	A silkworm	80, 115, 123, 136.
Luti rasa ..	The honey of the *luti*	10, 146.
Luṭni tuṛi ..	A var. of *Brassica campestris, L.*	256.
Mackunḍạ baha	*Pterospermum acerifolium, Willd.*	266, 275.
Mahabạri bọc	*Zingiber zerumbet, Roscoe.*	201, 252, 253.
Mahadeb jala	A certain variety of the rice plant; or, a small shrub	12, 17, 19, 142, 191.
Mạhũt guṛ ..	Refuse of molasses	61, 79, 200, 201, 202, 205, 206, 237, 266, 269, 276, V.6.
Makaṛkenda	*Diospyros embryopteris, Pers.*	206, 244, 245, 266, V.3.
Malhan ..	*Dolichos Lablab, L.*	21, 25, 38, 70, 101, 191, 202, 205, V.1.
Malhanreko tahẹn tejo	Caterpillars found on do.	101, 102, 107, 205.
Mandargọm	*Anona squamosa, L.*	94, 192, 198, 275.
Mạṅgri hako baha	The gills of *Macropherotus magur* (a fish)	263.
Mạnikjọṛ ghās dare		165, 171, 196.
Mạńjur jhuṭi		35, 51, 61, 63, 99, 195.
Man saru ..	A variety of *Lasia*	31.
Marak ..	A peafowl	130, 132, 214.
Marań catọm aṛak	*Marsilea quadrifolia, L.*	156, 168, 173, 196, 290.
Maraṛ baha	*Erythrina indica, Lam.*	111, 112, 127, 156, 266, 290.
Maṛic ..	*Capsicum frutescens, Willd.*	6, 8, 10, 21, 89, 159, 167, 179, 249, 250, 289.
Masri ..	*Ervum Lens, L.*	245, 258.
Maṭ ..	Bamboo	110, 123.
Maṭha aṛak	*Antidesma diandrum, Tulas.*	40, 41, 75, 85, 88, 161, 206, 245, 255, 285.
Matkọm ..	*Bassia latifolia, Roxb.*	32, 61, 81, 156, 181, 184, 204, 244, 252, 253, 281, 303, 304, 305, V. 3.
Maṭọr ..	Peas	245.
Mera ..	The refuse after brewing rice beer	155.

Rạtcora ..	*Locusta viridissima.*	50.
Rereń ..	A *cicada* belonging to the species *Platypleura*	133.
Rẹthẹ ghoṛa lada		159.
Riḍe ..	*Casearia tomentosa, Roxb.*	237.
Risạ sim ..	A fowl with bristling or up standing feathers	253.
Rọ ..	A fly	103, 110, 117, 149.
Rọkọč (dak, jel)	Small molusces or periwinkles	10, 11, 21, 42, 195.
Rọkọt cọndọn	Blood coloured sandal-wood, *Santalum album, L.*	174, 201, 245, 253, 265, 266, 267.
Rọl	*Terminalia Chebula, Retz.*	12, 35, 66, 68, 190, 204, 205, 241, 247, 253.
Rolani jọ		253.
Rọndọč ..	*Blumea Wightiana, DC.*	134.
Roṛa ..	*Mallotus philippinensis, Mull. Arg.*	173.
Rọs mạnik ..		253.
Rọsọ kapur	A white sublimate or muriate of mercury	193, 195.
Rọsọ muni ..		193, 244, 258.
Rọs sindur	A sort of factitious cinnabar made with zinc, mercury, blue vitriol, and nitre fused together	193, 253, 258.
Rot ..	*Ougeenia dalbergioides, Benth.*	241, 244, 245.
Rọtẹ capal ..		
Ruhen ..	*Soymida febrifuga, Adr. Juss.*	60, 244, 255, 257, 275.
Ruhi hako ..	The fish *Cyprinus denticulatus, Buch*	126.
Sadọm ič ..	Horse dung	240.
Sadọm jhin	Horse's iron bit	110, 135.
Sadọm khurạ	Horse's hoof	V. 3.
Sạgu dana ..	Sago	245.
Sahar ..	*Dillenia pentagyna, Roxb.*	175, 181, 198, 255.
Sahẹt sakam		120.
Sahṛa ..	*Streblus asper, Lour.*	75, 78, 82, 145, 178, 206, 229, 239, 241, 244, 245, 266, V. 3.
Sahraj (bele)	(Egg of) the Indian crane	10.
Sakarkenda aṛak	*Ipomaea Batatas, Lamk.*	278.
Salga ..	*Boswellia serrata, Wall* or *B. thurifera, Colebroke.*	101, 254, 290, V. 3.
Salọk misri	A kind of sugar candy	253.
Sạluk baha ..	The flower of *upạl*, q.v.	266.
Sạńci mạric	Black pepper	7, 102, 122, 302.
Sạṇḍi saba ..	*Briedelia stipularis, Bl.*	257.
Sạṇḍi hạtkạn	A *Leea.*	255, 257.
Sańkha ..	A shell bracelet	15.
Saoraj / *Sãoraj* ..	*Vernonia anthelmintica, Roxb.*	195, 222, 223, 226, 244.
Saparọm ..	*Nyctanthes Arbor-tristis, L.*	78, 81, 82, 165, 176, 196, 245, 266, 267, 285.
Sạpin / *Sạpiń* ..	*Opuntia Dillenii, Haw.*	156, 173, 193.
Sạphur ..		253.
Sar ..	*Saccharum Sara, Roxb.*	110, 147, 195.
Saram ..	*Rusa aristotelis*	253.
Saram babea	*Herpestes moticolus.*	149.
Saram lutur	*Clerodendron serratum, Spreng.*	51, 61, 75, 94, 96, 100, 163, 197, 238, 244, 270, 290, V. 3.
Sarjọm ..	*Shorea robusta, Gärtn.*	10, 40, 51, 58, 61, 82, 155, 169, 172, 173, 181, 191, 192, 193, 195, 198, 204, 206, 231, 239, 241, 244, 245, V. 2, V. 3, V. 4.
Sạru ..	*Celocasia antiquorum, Schott.*	31, 81, 186.
Sasań ..	*Curcuma longa, Roxb.*	11, 12, 21, 36, 43, 49, 69, 81, 90, 94, 96, 99, 108, 128, 144, 166, 188, 193, 197, 198, 208, 218, 220, 238, 244, 247, 249, 250, 252, 275, 278, V. 4.

HOW THE SANTALS LIVE.

By THE REV. P. O. BODDING.

INTRODUCTORY.

As an appendix to what has already been related in the previous parts of this volume, it might be of interest to learn something about the way in which the Santals live, especially about what they use as foodstuffs and how they prepare them. This has a direct bearing on hygiene.

Many years ago now, when we in our part of the country had had a bad year, with resultant scarcity bordering on famine, the writer tried to find out what the Santals had been living on, in addition to their ordinary foodstuffs. The Santals had apparently been able to come through the hard times better than had people of other races, living in the same locality and similarly circumstanced as regards income.

A Santal undertook to write down a list of all the articles of food that he knew his people would eat. The list has been added to from several sources, and what is mentioned below may be taken as comprising most, if not all, that a Santal uses or may use for food. It will naturally be understood that the Santals have not all these foodstuffs available for use as they like. It is only intended to give the gastronomic range of the Santals in as complete a form as possible.

Instead of merely giving a list, the writer considers that it is of greater anthropological interest, so far as these affect hygiene, to furnish information of the every-day life of the Santal people, of the way in which they procure their foodstuffs, and prepare them for eating, when they are not eaten raw.

The present-day condition of the Santals is of note. They have, according to their traditions, (and these have been verified as far as possible) always been a wandering people, and they are so even now. This nomadic state may be due to several causes. They have been, and are still, very much behindhand in regard to civilization, and have consequently not been able to compete with their neighbours and maintain their position amongst other communities. At the same time they are a very prolific people. The families grow, and before very long they reach a stage, when their means of supporting themselves become hopelessly inadequate. The problem of economic existence must then be faced. Some may try to learn from their neighbours; but this will, with most of them, go very much against the grain. Consequently they seek other localities where they may be able to support themselves and live in their customary manner.

In a few cases all members of the race have, according to their traditional record, migrated to save themselves and preserve their freedom. But the writer's impression is, that as a rule only part of the people have moved and kept up their old customs and practices to some extent in their new locality, while those remaining have gradually adapted themselves to what they find most suitable in their immediate environment. Something similar may be seen to-day. On reaching new spheres they will naturally be affected by the influences which they find there, and may, to some extent, adopt some of the local habits, customs and practices, so that they may not be regarded as entirely alien. Those on the move manage somehow to maintain their individuality as a separate people. The writer has often wondered, whether some of the many untouchable low-caste Hindus in Northern India may not have originally been some of the ancestors of the present-day Santals and other Muṇḍa peoples, that have remained behind and have formed themselves into fresh castes.

The Santals are not, by any caste rules, restricted or bound to follow a fixed occupation. It can, however, now be stated that they are well on the way to becoming settled agriculturists. According to the standards of others, e.g., of the neighbouring Bengali agriculturists, they are at present much behindhand. They do not know how to get the maximum benefits from the soil and their methods are still most primitive. To improve in this direction they will have to alter many of their ingrained habits as well as their mode of life. Also they must learn the value of money. It may be said that they have learnt the value of a pice, but, not the value of a rupee. This seems to be far beyond their capacity, and they suffer for it. In their forest life they naturally use barter and not money.

On the other hand the Santals are second to none in India, so far as clearing the jungle is concerned, also, except in manuring, in making the soil ready for cultivation, a fact recognized and taken advantage of by other people. As an example and proof of this the following fact may be mentioned. When the managers of the Lutheran Santal Mission, now nearly sixty years ago, impressed by what they saw of the wanderings of the people, were wishing to find a place, where part of the superfluous Santal population might settle down, they ultimately decided on a spot in the western part of the Goalpara district in Assam. Here was a tract of land that people in the near neighbourhood, both Hindus and Mohammedans, had attempted to bring under the plough, but had never succeeded. A tract of land, some 25 to 30 square miles was, with the permission of the Government of India, set aside for Santals' or others' cultivation. The soil was absolutely covered by what the Santals call *bir*, i.e., forest, not, however, of trees, but of an impenetrable kind of grass, measuring some 25 feet in height. It cost much, both in lives and labour, to clear the land; but the Santals stuck to it and succeeded where others had failed. At one time it seemed as though success would not be achieved, but in spite of the none too friendly attitude of Lieutenant-Governor of Eastern Bengal and Assam, the goal was reached. Where formerly no human being could live, we have now a population of some 7,000 Santals (and some others); where Government formerly had no income, they now receive many thousands of rupees in annual rent.

The time when the Santals relied on hunting, or on what they might find in the forests for their food, is not so far distant as to be forgotten. Anything even remotely resembling a hunt is still enthusiastically enjoyed. The first thing that a Santal father makes for his boy to play with is a bow and arrow, a sure sign of the old mode of obtaining food supplies. They no longer think of, or rely on, hunting as a means to this end; but the glorious fascination of the chase and its possibilities hold a prominent place in their minds. The sports are deemed their greatest delicacies, and these they divide or send as presents to their relatives, even the female ones. They have retained much of their former knowledge of the edible products that are to be found in the forests and elsewhere wild. Their taste is apparently also less discriminating than that of their neighbours of other races, with some rather curious exceptions.

Many of the things found in the forests are constantly used, others only occasionally sometimes for a change of diet or for what they consider a delicacy, sometimes for genuine sustenance, when nothing else is available.

The Santal Village.

The Santals always live in villages, that is collectively; they are never found dwelling in isolation. As this in some respects is relevant to the subject dealt with here, it will be of interest to describe how the Santals set about selecting the site for, and building and establishing a new village. What follows has special reference to places where there is forest land. This description has mainly been based on what an old Santal sage, Kolean *guru*, related to the late Rev. L. O. Skrefsrud nearly 70 years ago.

Three or four men proceed with a leader to inspect a site in a forest, which has been reported to be a likely one. If, after entering the forest, any of three kinds of quails are seen flying, they say: 'Some day in the future a village established here will be deserted'. But if they see these birds sitting quietly on their eggs, or if they meet a tiger or see the footmarks of a tiger, they say: 'Some day in the future a village founded here will thrive and become prosperous, and we shall settle down here contentedly'. Continuing to investigate they select a site of the following nature, viz., a place where there is dry ground, where there will be room for good highland and homestead fields, where rice-fields can be prepared, and where water is readily accessible. Satisfied with what they have discovered they return home. (There is in all this a curious mixture of superstition and common sense.)

Later a day is fixed for testing the omens. They take with them one speckled and two white fowls, a little sun-dried rice, oil, *sindur* and water in a new *ṭhili*[1] (a *ṭhili* is a narrow-necked earthenware pot). The leader goes in the evening to the place where he intends to build his house and makes five *sindur*-marks. Close to the *sindur*-marks small heaps of sun-dried rice are made; the *ṭhili* containing the water is set down; the fowls are tied in a row, just far enough away to be unable to reach the rice. They then make an invocation as follows:—' Oh *Siṅ bonga* (Sun-god) in Heaven, like a bamboo mat thou art spread; the four corners, the four worlds thou hast covered; and ye, the Five, the Six of the earth (some *bongas*), in your name, as ye see here, in the virgin soil, the virgin forest, we are seeking omens; show these to us, the milk as

[1] *Ṭhili* in Bengali—*Ed*

milk, the water as water; having judged show them to us'. After this they depart to spend the night elsewhere.

Next morning they return and investigate. If a big fowl-feather has fallen, they say: 'A few grown up persons among us will die'. And if small feathers have fallen they say: 'Children will die here in the future'. And if no feathers at all have fallen: 'This is excellent, no one will die here soon'. And if the fowls have left droppings round about the place, they say: 'All in the village, well-to-do and poor, will thrive here'. If the birds have left droppings in a heap in one place, they say: 'The headman alone will become wealthy'. If the same is seen in two places, they say: 'The headman and his deputy will become wealthy'. And if in three places, then in addition to the headman and his deputy one of the villagers will also become wealthy. In the directions in which rice has been carried off by ants, in so many directions will it be necessary to discover the *bongas* and establish them. If the water in the *ṭhili* has dwindled a little, they say: 'After two years there will be scarcity of water'. And if the water has not dwindled at all, they say: 'There will be no scarcity of water'. If the fowls have disappeared, if there is no rice, and if the water in the *ṭhili* has dried up, they say: 'This place is ill-fated', and they leave it and will not found a village there.

But if there are good omens from the fowls, the rice and the water in the *ṭhili*, they dig a small four-cornered hole; on three sides of this hole they place the dug-out earth. With this earth they again fill up the hole. If it is filled with the earth lying on two sides, they say: 'We shall get full crops here'. But if no earth is left in filling the hole, they say: 'It is inauspicious here'. They then seek omens on another high place within the boundaries that they have set up, and in the name of another headman. They continue to act in this way, until all the omens have proved propitious. Ultimately such is bound to happen.

At a later date they return and put up some sticks against each other to make a shelter for the leader. The leader, who is to become the headman of the village, cuts down the first tree. Nowadays after they have investigated and fixed on the site in the forest, they ask the landowner for permission; formerly, before landowners made their appearance, there was no need for anything of this kind.

In consultation with the headman they now divide homestead fields amongst themselves. On each homestead field a hut for the family, and also a pen to keep the cattle in are erected. They then return to their old homes and call on each other, saying: 'When shall we start?' Taking their children and all they possess along with them they proceed to the new village. The exodus takes place during the months of Phalgun and Chait (from the middle of February to the middle of April, when there is little or no rain). All of them set to work to clear the jungle on their homestead fields; the trees cut down serve them for house-timber. Any timber left is burnt. Houses are built. Running along the middle of the site a clear space is left for the village street, and near the end of this is found the sacred grove, that is to say, a number of men become possessed by the national *bongas* and in this state show where the grove is to be.—So far old Kolean.

Before proceeding further, a few words about the houses of the Santals will be of value. They naturally build their own houses. Their original and also now not uncommon way of building a house is as follows: Nine wooden posts are required; formerly, as mentioned above, these were taken from among the trees cut down on the spot; now they have to be brought from elsewhere and paid for. The nine posts are fixed in the ground in three rows, three posts in each row, those in the middle being higher than those on the two sides. On the top of each of these three rows a heavy pole or beam (called *pạṛ*), as long as the house is to be, is fixed. Next cross-beams are set up, one end resting on the outside posts and the other end being tied securely to the posts in the middle row. The rafters are then put in position; the old rule was twenty rafters (called *sẹnẹr*) on each side of the roof. To keep these in place three sets of laths (called *bata*) are used, one set being tied at the top, another set in the middle, and a third set at the lower, the eaveṣ', end of the rafters. On the rafters a framework of saplings (called *chaṭãṛ*, nowadays mostly of split bamboo) is tied, and finally the roof is thatched with grass (*sạuṛi*, Heteropogon contortus *R. & S.*). This grass which is excellent for thatching grows in abundance in the forests. Nowadays one may see fairly large fields of this grass on the outskirts of the forests guarded against the cattle. This *sạuṛi* is much stronger and more lasting than the paddy straw, that, for want of *sạuṛi*, is coming into use in many villages. When the roof is ready, the walls are made by placing branches or anything suitable between the posts and filling in with earth, the branches, etc., furnishing the necessary strength for the thin walls. The women finally plaster the wattle-walls with clay or earth that is kneaded into a dough. A layer of earth is spread on the ground inside the one-roomed house; this is trampled down hard, smeared with a dough of earth and made smooth with mud mixed with cow-dung. To complete the house a low earthen wall is built in one corner to provide a separate dwelling place for the ancestors (called *bhitạr*). In this closet rice and beer are offered to the *bhitạr* and to the house-bonga. No outside woman, (in some families not even a married daughter of the house,) is permitted to enter this closet. There is only one entrance to the house, generally with a mere apology for a door. A Santal house has no windows and only a few small holes high up in the walls, to let out the smoke. A fireplace of earth is also made inside, and along one or two of the walls contrivances are put up to accommodate paddy-bundles, or other possession. The inside of a Santal house is consequently quite dark. Except during the cold season, when the inside is warm, the Santals generally stay outside, both day and night. The inside of a Santal house cannot be either pleasant or healthy.

The form of the house mentioned is what the Santals call a *baṅgla oṛak*, or gable house. It is rectangular in form, its breadth being two-thirds of its length; the original size is said to have been 9 by 6 cubits, but it is now generally considerably larger. Another form of house is called *catọm oṛak*, lit. umbrella house, having a four-sided roof. The different Santal septs must have one or the other form of house mentioned, in which to live and have their *bhitạr*, the closet for the ancestors. Except where this type of house is necessitated by custom any other form of house desired may be erected. It is now quite common to find houses with walls of earth, the earth being mixed with water and kneaded. When ready, it is formed into large blocks. It takes some time to build the walls properly and get them thoroughly dried. This kind of house will most likely become almost universal as they are cheap and easy to construct. For this kind of house small tiles, instead of thatch are now being used, an idea adopted from other races. It might be added, that the hole from which the earth for the walls is obtained is generally utilized as a dumping pit for all kinds of offal.

In the course of time more houses are built round the courtyard, a shed for the cattle and one for the buffaloes (if the family have any), sheds for goats and sheep are erected, and, when the family grows, more dwelling-houses—these, however, have no *bhitạr*. For the pigs a small sty is made. The fowls live inside the dwelling-house at night. A few Santals have a dove-cot, generally in the middle of the courtyard. On the side of the courtyard, where there are no buildings, a fence, or sometimes a wall is built. One opening, with or without a door, leads out to the village street (called *chaṭka duạr*, *chaṭka* being their name for the part of the street just outside the courtyard); another opening leads out to the *baṛge*, the homestead field.

As regards water, the Santals will always be on the look-out for natural springs and fetch water from these or from pools with constant water, or from tanks, streams or rivers. They may also dig wells to be used by the individual families, or by a number of people. While the men gather in the evening, (especially at the *mạñjhi than*, the place erected for the spirit of the original headman,) to have their talk, the women will meet in the afternoon (at *dak̓ lo ber*, i.e., the water-drawing time, about five o'clock) at the place from which they fetch water to gossip and discuss everything. They always have large earthenware pots (broad-mouthed, called *ṭukuć*, or narrow-necked, called *ṭhili*) standing on a special stand, or, more commonly, on a raised level surface at the base of the house-wall outside the house.

When visitors come, they are met at the entrance of the house with water and have their feet washed. A bridal pair going from house to house in the village to be regaled with molasses, have their feet washed at the entrance to every house. Before taking food, all Santals wash, especially their hands and mouth. In this connexion it may be mentioned, that they are careful with their teeth. When getting water to wash, before taking food, they also get a toothbrush, i.e., a twig of some suitable wood, more especially Sal. The end of this the user chews, so that it becomes like a brush, and then vigorously brushes his teeth. When this is done, he splits the twig into two, and with one of these he scrapes his tongue, and finally throws the twig away; it is used only once. All eating is done with the right hand. It would be dishonourable to use the left hand for this purpose or to offer it to anybody; it is used for washing parts of the body, and always after stooling.

Before commencing to describe what the Santals eat and how the foodstuffs are produced or obtained a few other matters connected with the life of the Santals may be mentioned. According to their traditions their ancestors must in former times have had a peculiar communal organization. It appears that each man occupied and owned as much land as he could cultivate in any one season. At the end of the season all lands were given up to the village community, for redistribution for the next season. A part of this custom is still formally kept up.

In the month of Magh, i.e., the latter half of January and the first half of February, they have in every village what is called *Mag sim*, Magh fowls. The headman's messenger, the village *goḍet*, one of the village officials, collects from every Santal house one fowl and half-a-seer of rice with some salt and turmeric. On a fixed day he takes all that has been collected to the village priest to a place near water. After having had a bath (a bath is ordained before a sacrifice) the priest sacrifices the fowls to the national *bongas* and to a few *bongas* of the neighbourhood. (*Bonga* is the Santal name for the spirits or godlings, believed to be living on hills, in rivers, pools, tree-stumps, everywhere, and practically all believed to be malevolent and dangerous.) The sacrificed fowls are cooked with rice into a hash and eaten by the men present; they also drink beer brewed for the occasion. A formal meeting is then held. The village headman says: 'Now, Sirs, as is seen, we are at the end, the month of Magh. There is a month of Magh for the thieves (an expression that is explained as referring to the fact that there is nothing to be found in the fields or on the threshing floors by persons who would take anything, the only kind of thieving, viz., of foodstuffs, that occurred among the Santals of old); there is a month of Magh for the cultivators; there is a month of Magh for the village headman and his deputy; there is a month of Magh for servants male and female. We have consequently all got a month of Magh, so please, if any of you will become our village headman I will also resign in the month of Magh'. All the village officials formally resign in the same way. Thereupon the cultivators say: 'Also we, Sir, have finished. We give our agricultural lands and possessions into your hand, Sir, headman, for the hot season. We shall retain in our possession only our old sites; these we do not give into your hands. Our houses we shall also keep'. The 'sites' are explained as being their wives.

The whole of this nowadays is only a customary ceremony without any reality behind it, except as regards matters that are annually ended or renewed, as, e.g., the engagement of servants. For a few days after the ceremony bouts of beer-drinking are indulged in the village houses. Thereafter all is, as it was before. This is mentioned here as an interesting point marking a stage in the development of the Santals, when from being only jungle-dwellers and hunters they became also cultivators. This was before they became tenants of a landlord and subjects of a State.

The Santal Agriculture.

We have no record of how the Santals actually went about their first attempts at cultivation. It is just possible that one of their first attempts to get something out of the soil may have been something like what is now called *kuṛā̃u*, a mode of cultivation that is said to have been used also by Santals in former years, but is not practised by them at the present time, so far as is known. It is, however, still kept up by the Paharias living on the hills of the Santal country. A piece of jungle is cut down high up on a steep hill-side; when the wood of the felled trees is dry, generally towards the end of the hot season, it is burned. In this way the ground is cleared, and when the rains set in, the seed is sown without any ploughing. The present-day Paharias make small holes with a crow-bar and drop the seed into the holes, especially of *bajṛa*, Sorghum vulgare *Pers.*, of maize and of a few other kinds. This is all, except that they may pluck away weeds. It is said that when the Santals in former times followed a similar mode of cultivation they simply sowed the seed (especially *bajṛa*) at the top of the cleared hill-side, the spreading being left to the water of the rains flowing down; in some cases, a branch of a Thorn-tree (Zizyphus Jujuba *Lam.*) is said to have been pressed into a flat shape and dragged over the ground to spread the seed.

The present-day Santals have naturally progressed further than this. They are, however, as already remarked, lacking much to make them good farmers. They have not as yet learned the need for and the benefits of weeding and manuring or of changing the crops, and much more. For example, they do not take proper care of their cattle. These are mostly herded by children who use much of the time for their own games and pleasures. When the paddy is harvested, the cattle are permitted to roam about. A direct result of this is that it is impossible for people to have any crops standing after the middle of December or thereabouts; the cattle would eat all; and the Sạntals only very rarely fence anything in.

They are on the way to become agriculturists, but are, as yet, far behind.

Rice has become the staple food of the peoples living in North-East India, where the majority of the Santals have their present home. Consequently rice is a food-stuff that the Santals have taken to. Rice is not their only nor their principal cereal; but they consider rice the best and most desirable, to such an extent, that if they cannot get rice, they now feel they have not had proper food. A Santal once expressed himself as follows: 'For us in this country rice is the finest agricultural product, because while all other cereals when eaten get the better of us, we never become tired of rice'. By this he meant that they were satisfied with rice and nothing was left over after a meal, whereas before, when they had eaten all they wanted of other cereals, something was always left over.

The cultivation of rice will be mentioned first on account of the rôle it plays amongst the present-day Santals.

The founding of a new village has already been described. It will be remembered, that when on the look-out for a site for the new village one of the main deciding factors is the suitability of the ground for the establishment of rice-fields.

A Santal considers it his birthright to fell trees; it has become an instinct with him to cut down. It is a pity that they have not learnt also to plant trees. Occasionally they have begun to form the habit of planting certain kinds, especially fruit-trees, in their villages, and to let some trees stand; but there is very much left for them to learn in this respect.

The present-day Santals prepare three kinds of agricultural fields; what they call *baṛge* (their homestead field), *goḍa* (highland fields, some distance away from their houses) and *khẹt*.

Khẹt[1] is a word borrowed from Hindi or Bengali, and is the name for a rice-field.

[1] *Khẹt* means agricultural field in Bengali and is not confined to rice-fields—*Ed.*

The origin of the word is a sure proof that the Santals have adopted the cultivation of rice from others.

The Santals apparently enjoy preparing rice-fields. In a country like that in which the bulk of the people live at the present time, it takes no little work to do it. As is well known, the paddy plant must stand in water, or in moist soil, until it ripens. A rice-field must consequently be prepared so as to make this possible. The field itself must be absolutely level and furnished with ridges to prevent the water from running away. In a flat country, as in large tracts of Bengal, little work is required; in the parts where the Santals live, it is different. The country is hilly, and the surface only very rarely fairly level. The nature of the surface, combined with the necessity of having sufficient water, makes it natural for them to commence making rice-fields as low down as possible. These low-lying rice-fields where they may be fairly sure of having a sufficiency of water, are by the Santals called *bạihạṛ*, i.e., first class or *aul* rice-fields. If there happens to be a spring with flowing water or a tiny rivulet in such places, they make what is called an *ahar* or a *hiṛ* (both expressions borrowed, *ahar* from Hindi, and *hiṛ* from Desi).[1] A small ridge or dam is thrown across the lower side of the depression to keep the water standing inside up to a certain height. The draw-back to such rice-fields is prolonged inundation that may spoil the plants.

With certain restrictions the owner or tenant of a *bạihạṛ khẹt* has a right to the uncultivated land lying directly above this, and a Santal will, as soon as he conveniently can, commence to make rice-fields there also. *Khẹt* situated on fairly flat, higher lying land are called *bạd*. These rice-fields become less and less valuable for cultivation, the higher up they lie. Only in these years when there is an exceptionally heavy and late rainfall, do they get fair crops in these higher fields. Other crops than rice might well be profitably cultivated in these *bạd*, if they would only learn how to go about it.

A special kind of rice-field is made in what is called *sokṛa*, a depression in the land running downwards like a tiny narrow valley. Here fields are comparatively easy to make. A ridge is thrown across the 'valley', the ground is levelled, and the field is practically ready.

The method of preparing a rice-field amongst the Santals is of interest. After having selected a suitable site they proceed to clear it of all vegetation. During this process the size of the field is decided upon. The land generally slopes a little, so that a ridge or ridges have to be made on the lower side. These ridges are roughly made at the time of levelling the ground, and when all is ready, they are properly dressed with the help of a *kuḍi*, a kodali, a kind of spade. The ridges have to be trimmed and repaired annually.

If there is little to be done, the whole may be finished with a plough and a *kuḍi*. To level the ground they generally use what is called a *karha*, a wooden earth leveller, drawn by a pair of bullocks or buffaloes.[2]

---

[1] Lowland Bengali—*Ed.*

[2] The *karha* is a piece of wood, some 1·5 m. (more or less) long, some 0·3 to 0·4 m. broad and some 10 cm. thick at the top side, and gradually sloping down to a broad edge. As they have no saws, the Santals (who make all such things

The final levelling is done when the rains set in and the *khẹt* is filled with water, just before the planting of the rice. Considerable work is needed to get the field ready for the transplanting.[1]

---

themselves) fashion the *karha* with axe and adze. It is made of some strong and heavy wood (Sal, Mahua, etc.). In the middle of the top side a handle (the *karha kạrmba*) is fixed in a hole cut for the purpose. It is a straight piece of wood. The size of the *karha* varies according to need; the smaller one is called *ḍaṅgra karha*, bullock-leveller, and the larger one *kaḍa karha*, buffalo-leveller. At each end there is ordinarily what is called *nạkic*, comb, having one, two or three 'teeth', called *sulạ*, on which an iron ring, called *halka*, is slipped down, when the *karha* is to be used. This form is called *nạkic karha*. In one form of *karha* there is no *nạkic*, but two rectangular holes are cut through the wood, one near each end. In this kind of *karha* the *halka* is put through the hole and kept in position by a piece of wood inserted, to prevent the *halka* from slipping through. This form is called *rọtọk karha*, cut-through leveller (from *rọk*, to cut). There is a third form called *rọtọk nạkic karha*; this is so large that it would not be convenient to have the *nạkic* at the two ends. Two large holes are therefore cut in the body of the *karha*, equidistant from each end; on the inner side of each hole a *sulạ*, 'tooth', is made to slip the *halka* in. The *karha* is, as stated, dragged by a pair of bullocks or buffaloes. To join the *karha* to the yoke a *karha ḍạṇḍil*, a leveller-beam, is used, corresponding to the ploughbeam (*isi*). It is a piece of wood, frequently bamboo, some 2 m. long, or a little more. It is split in two at the *karha* end, with a hole at each end. Into each hole an iron hook, to which a *halka* is attached, is fixed. There are naturally two *halka*. At the yoke end the *ḍạṇḍil* is whole; where the split commences (some 0·7 to 1 m. down) a cord is tied to prevent the beam from splitting higher up. In the case of a bamboo *ḍạṇḍil* the *uṭi* or joint serves the same purpose as the cord. When in use the man in charge puts the *karha* down into the earth that is to be removed, like one would put in a spade; when the bullocks drag the *karha* along with the earth, the man holds the handle firmly to prevent the *karha* from turning over. When he has reached the spot where the earth is to be deposited, he lets go the handle, and then the *karha* automatically turns over. The earth is left lying there and the bullocks drag the *karha* back to the place where they started. On a new *karha* with three 'teeth', the *halka* is placed on the lowest *sulạ*; when the *karha* becomes worn, the *halka* is put on the middle or the top *sulạ*. Some well-to-do Santals have instead of the *ḍạṇḍil* two iron chains with a *halka* at the *karha* ends. Loose earth is naturally necessary for the operation. The use of a *karha* is therefore practically restricted to the autumn or just after rain in the dry season. Ploughing is often resorted to preparatory to using the *karha*.

[1] The Santal plough is a very primitive kind of implement, the wooden part of it being made by the Santals themselves. It consists of a piece of wood, bent a little naturally, so fashioned as to have an angle of 130° to 140°, each side of the angle being some 50 cm. long, and about 20 cm. broad at the thickest. The under- and back side is cut flat, while the upper side tapers towards the middle. The different parts of the plough have separate names: *nahel bọhọk*, the plough head, is the top back to which the handle (*kạrmba*) is fixed. The part below the 'head' is called *nahel koṛam*, the plough breast; the bottom, bending part is called *nahel ḍẹkẹ*, the plough buttocks; the two sides of the front part are called *nahel bulu*, the plough thighs, and the front point is called *nahel ṭoḍa*. In the middle of the front top a groove is cut for the ploughshare (the *pal*). This *pal* is a piece of flat iron, some 40 to 50 cm. long and some 3 cm. broad and up to 1 cm. thick. It is fixed in the groove (called *pal oṛak*, ploughshare house) by an iron staple. This, the common Santal ploughshare, is called simply *pal* or *nanha pal* (a narrow ploughshare). Some Santals, especially those living near the Bengal lowland (*dẹs*), have commenced to use what is called *dẹs pal*, *dhalpa pal* or *khonta pal* (*dhalpa* means broad, and *khonta* is their name for a wooden bar with a flat iron head). This kind has a broad front, protruding a little from the wooden part. Just above the bend in the lower part of the 'breast' a hole is cut. Into this the *isi*, the ploughbeam, is inserted. The *isi* may be what is called simply *isi* or *họṛ isi* (a Santal ploughbeam); this has three notches on its underside, where it is to be joined to the yoke. Some use what is called *baṅgla* or *dẹs isi*, a ploughbeam of the shape used in the Bengal districts, having no notches. Every plough has naturally a handle, *kạṛba* or *kạṛmba*. According to shape this is called *baṅgla k.* (Bengal ploughhandle), resembling the *cạṇḍi pạṭi k.*, that is nailed to the front side of the rear part of the plough, the top of the handle being pared so as to bend backwards; another shape is the *gạṛ boṭa k.*, a handle that is fixed on the rear side of the plough so far down that the *isi* goes through a hole cut in it (this is also called *pẹnd laṭka k.*); a further kind is *rọk* or *rọtọk k.*, a handle fixed in a hole cut in the back part of the plough. *Ṭir k.* is any kind of handle that has a grip fixed on its top. The part where the handle is fixed is called *họtọk*, neck. The ploughbeam is fixed to the yoke *arạ̃ṛ*, (quite a work of art with the Santals) by a bit of twisted leather thong called *naṅgle*.

A plough of the kind described can, as remarked, be used only when the soil is soft, just after a shower of rain or during the rainy season and some time after. It will not enter more than three to four inches into the soil. Santal ploughing is consequently no particularly hard work. A boy some ten years of age is called 'fit for ploughing'. It is one of their ways of stating the age of a boy. As a rule they plough in elipses; if they have more than one plough they follow one after the other. The Santals commence ploughing at about sunrise and continue for some four hours, rarely longer, and then only when they are pressed for work.

A Santal as a rule ploughs a rice-field four times before transplanting. The first ploughing of the season is called *paṛak*, lit. splitting. The soil is broken up and opened out for air and moisture. After some time it is ploughed a second time, the furrows running across those of the first ploughing; this ploughing is called *dẹć*, lit. mounting, i.e., ploughing on top of the first furrows. These two ploughings are used for all kinds of agricultural land. In the rice-fields after *dẹć* comes what is called *lạhut* or *si lạhut*, lit. powdering, or ploughing into powder. This is done shortly before the last ploughing operation, called *lọsọt*, lit. muddying. The object of this last operation is to get the water standing in the field thoroughly mixed with earth. The surface of the field becomes a kind of thick mud-soup, suitable for planting the paddy-seedlings in. Sometimes the third ploughing may be omitted; it depends on the situation and the amount of water.

When, as frequently happens, it is seen that the field is not quite level, they attempt to put this right during the two later ploughings, especially the last one. For this purpose they use an implement called *raksa* or *rakhsa*.[1]

As regards the cultivation of rice the following may be noted: Except for one kind all paddy is transplanted. It is sown, generally in a rice-field, broadcast. The seedlings (*gạchi*) stand there until they reach a size suitable for transplanting, when they are pulled out (this is done by women, often helped by men) and planted in the prepared fields. The ploughing is done by men alone, and the planting practically always by women. The seedlings, generally two or more together, are stuck into the mud-soup at a suitable distance from each other. It is quick work. One woman will without difficulty plant one-third of an acre during the day, or even somewhat more.

With the Santals in the eastern parts the paddy is generally sown during *ruhni*, the 13th *Jhẹṭ* and the following six days, i.e., approximately during the last days of May and the first days of June (Dr. Campbell says it is a period of 13 days but this is not so in the Santal Parganas). They have heard from Bengalis that this is the proper and most auspicious time to sow, and they try to follow the Bengali custom. They have an immense number of varieties, all named (I have 143 different names of varieties [2]). They have three classes of transplanted paddy (*hoṛo*, as they call it). The earliest varieties are called *bhạdoi hoṛo*, ripening in September (the name is derived from Bengali *bhādui*, ripening in the month of Bhadra). Next comes *bạd hoṛo*, ripening

---

When taking their ploughs out to the field they fasten the plough to the yoke carried by the bullocks, the *isi* during the transportation standing straight up in the air. When the ploughing is done for the day the plough is carried back in the same way, or the plough may be left in the field, the ploughshare alone being taken out and carried home.

[1] The *raksa* resembles the *karha*. It is a piece of wood some two to three mm. long and 15 to 20 cm. broad, slightly thinner than a *karha*. The *raksa* is slightly curved and has an edge. It has two holes cut equidistant from the centre for the *halka*, and has a handle (*raksa kāṛmba*) fixed in the middle. It resembles the *rọtọk karha* and is worked very much like a *karha*. It is used only for levelling rice-fields just before the planting, and as it is used in watery mud, there is no need for the same strength as in the *karha*. Only few men in a village have a *raksa*. They willingly lend it to those who need such an implement.

[2] According to the traditions the Santals are divided into 12 septs and each sept (traditionally) into 12 subjects. There should be as many kinds of paddy; but there is one kind less. If there had been the same number or even one more, the paddy would have gained on the people and 'eaten' them. Now the people gain on the paddy, according to Santal talk.

about October, a little richer crop than the one previously mentioned (the name is derived from *bạd*, Desi *bader*, the high-lying land). Finally *bạihạr hoṛo*, the heaviest and best crop, ripening in November and December (the name is derived from *bạihạr*, the low-lying rice-fields).

As already mentioned they have one variety that is not transplanted, but sown broadcast. It is called *goḍa hoṛo*, (highland paddy), sown in May and ripening in August in the Santal Parganas. Here it is very rare; but, in Assam it is fairly commonly cultivated by the Santals living there. The name (*goḍa*) shows it is not cultivated in rice-fields, but in fields generally some distance away from their houses.

It might be further mentioned that wild rice, called by the Santals *uṛi*, Oryza sativa *L.*, may be found growing on the edges of water, and is eaten by the people.

When the paddy has been harvested, it is threshed. This is done on what is called *khạrai*, a threshing-floor,[1] a roundish piece of ground, some 5 to 10 mm. across, plastered with earth and cow-dung. The threshing cattle walk round and round in the spread-out straw. The grain is cleaned and stored in large bundles covered by straw-rope (called *boṛ*).[2]

---

[1] To prepare a threshing-floor the ordinary Santals have not only to find a suitable place and to do the necessary digging and plastering but they have to make sure that the place chosen is lucky or the opposite. They have a curious superstition that the place itself has something to do with the amount of grain they obtain from threshing. They go about it as follows: When they have found a place that seems suitable, they go there, some on the *bel bọrọn* day (a day of the Durga festival, as celebrated in their neighbourhood), others on the last day of the Jithia festival, and others again on a Sunday morning early (generally in the months of September or October). With a *kodali* they clean a small place and here make a cross-mark, what they call a *ḍhera dag* (the *ḍhera* is a hand-spindle having two pieces of wood fixed across each other in the middle). The cross-mark is sufficiently large, the two ditches of the cross being each about two cubits long, one running North and South, the other West and East. In the middle they dig a square hole, putting the earth dug out on the four sides of the hole. Next they again fill this hole up with the earth dug out. If it is filled up with the earth, well and good; it will be advisable to have the threshing-floor there. (Compare what is told above about a similar proceeding when choosing a site for a village.) But if not all earth goes into the hole, it will not do to have it here; they must find another place. Some Santals put the dug out earth on only three sides of the hole. Many Santals do not now, however, take such precautions. They simply chose a place haphazard. They go to the place chosen on one of the days mentioned above and with a *kodali* make a cross-mark. At the crossing they put *sọsọ* (Marking-nut, Semecarpus Anacardium *L.*) leaves and a bit of a thorn-tree branch (some place a full branch). At the crossing they place the leaves turned upside down and put a small stone on each of them to keep them there, until the paddy ripens. When people see this, they understand that somebody has taken steps to make a threshing-floor there. As it is deemed safe to have several together, they will often arrange to have their threshing-floors adjoining. Besides, it is a pleasure so to arrange them as when watching during the nights; they can keep each other awake by telling stories, folktales, singing, etc.

[2] If they have more grain than they need for immediate future, they store it in what they call *bạndi* (bundles). These are made in the following way: A rope of straw (called *boṛ*) of sufficient length is made; with this they make a ring on the ground; on the top of this they put a layer of straw, and on this a basket (that is later on taken away) filled with grain; the *boṛ* is wound round this, more straw is added round the whole, and gradually more grain is filled in. When the required quantity of grain is reached the straw-rope is arranged in a ring (like it was done at the bottom), and the whole is tied up with some thin straw-rope (called *sikol*). This keeps the *bạndi* tight. A *bạndi* as a rule is made to hold some ten to twelve maunds (of 40 seers), but may be larger and also much smaller (e.g., when used for storing seed).

These bundles are naturally kept inside their houses; they have no other safe place for them. To keep them properly they always put these bundles on an erection called *ḍhulạ*. This has two solid pieces of timber placed besides each other a foot or thereabouts apart, resting on crossbars on top of some solid poles fixed in the ground; nowadays they have often supports, made of earth, for the parallel pieces of timber; these are about a cubit above the ground. The bundles are brought in and lifted up and placed in position on them. It is a practical arrangement, at a safe distance from the wall and the floor, safe against wet and animals. When some of the contents are wanted, it is easy to get a hand in between the layers of rope, without pulling the bundle to pieces.

We shall now hear how the Santals treat and use the paddy and rice.

The first is to husk the paddy; this is done either in a *ḍhiṅki*,[1] the common husking machine, generally by two persons, a man or a woman treading the one end, and a woman sitting at the mortar end, handling the grain; or in an *ukhuṛ*, a large wooden mortar, found all over the tropics and subtropics.

Before husking the paddy may be boiled and dried, or simply dried. It makes a very great difference in the nutritive value of the rice, whether it is boiled in the husk or not. When boiling the paddy in the husk, they proceed as follows: To start with they first soak the paddy in water in a large earthenware vessel for one or preferably two days. When thoroughly soaked, it is taken out and put into a suitable cooking vessel with a sufficient quantity of water and boiled. It is carefully watched with eyes and ears, with ears to be sure that the paddy is not scorched, and with eyes to see the steam rising, by which they know when the boiling is completed. When ready the cooking vessel is taken down and its contents spread out in any suitable place to dry. This takes two days. The paddy must not be exposed to the sun for any considerable length of time, as this, according to Santal experience, would cause it to become brittle, in which case it will break when husked, become like ant-heads, as a Santal woman expressed herself; and such rice is not satisfactory.

When properly dried the paddy is stored away until needed for food and then husked. To get properly clean rice the Santals husk it three times. The first operation, called *sẹṭẹć*, removes the *hẹṛẹ*, the husk itself; the husk separated from the grain is all placed in a *haṭak*, a winnowing-fan (made by the Mahles of bamboo), and sifted. The grain, being heavier, gathers at the back of the *haṭak* (kept lower down) while the husk by proper manipulation is gradually brought to the outer brim of the fan and thrown out. The husk is given to animals to eat.

After this the grain is pounded once more to remove impurities; this is called *tala*, middle (or second) husking.

To make the rice ready for cooking, it is pounded a third time; this is called *sọk*. The result of this operation is pure rice, from which all impurities have been removed, called *sọk caole*, finally cleaned rice.

Santal women are clean and careful when preparing the food. When cooking rice they proceed as follows: First the cooking vessels and the fireplace are carefully cleaned; water, sufficient for the rice to be cooked, is poured into the cooking vessel and put on the fireplace with the mouth covered to prevent any impurities falling into it. The rice is put into another vessel filled with water, the object of this being to get all possible impurities removed. When the water in the cooking vessel is seen to be boiling, the rice is transferred to that vessel. The cooking is watched to ensure that all goes well and that the rice is properly cooked. An experienced woman will know this at sight; otherwise they test it by pinching. They must be sure that it is not overcooked, i.e., that the rice retains its shape and does not become a soft mass. When all is ready, the vessel is taken off the fire, the water is drained off, and something

[1] Bengali *Dhẽṅki*—*Ed.*

is put on the mouth of the vessel to prevent flies or impurities reaching the rice. When still suitably warm the cooked rice (now called *daka*) is served out in heaps on a plate (of brass, or, made generally, of leaves) and eaten together with curry (by the Santals called *utu*). Mention of this will be made later.

As is well known, rice treated in the manner described contains certain vitamins found in the husk, making the rice a healthy and nourishing food, whilst rice husked without having been previously boiled is inferior as food. Rice of the kind described is the ordinary food of the present-day Santals. Well-to do Santals will eat a little above half-a-seer of this rice daily. When providing food for our boarding schools we have found that this amount daily is quite sufficient, naturally with curry added. In the villages a family that can provide so much per individual per day is considered well off.

Daka is specially prepared for two meals daily, for a mid-day meal (called *mañjan*) and for *kedok*, the evening meal, which is the principal one. Chance visitors of a family may partake of the *mañjan* meal; if anyone is invited as a guest (except to family festivals that occupy the whole day or part of a day, as the case may be), it is to partake of *kedok*, the dinner,—as with many other races. They have a saying that poor people have their *kedok*, as soon as it is evening, because they are hungry after the day's work, while wealthy people have it much later, sometimes even when ordinary people get up the first time after sleep, i.e., at about 1 A.M. They say that these people have had enough food during the day and have not worked on an empty stomach, if they have worked at all.

What is left of the rice, from the *kedok*, is kept until the following morning and then eaten cold or together with *dak mạṇḍi*, rice-gruel, at about 9 A.M. This meal is called *baskeak*, lit., what is stale, a kind of breakfast.

The *dak mạṇḍi* just referred to, lit. translated 'water-food', is the rice already mentioned, boiled in a quantity of water into a kind of rice-gruel. It may be the form of food used when they have little rice. It is also the form of food taken out in the forenoon to people engaged in agricultural work to enable them to continue without interruption. It may also be taken along (in a brass-cup) as food for the day or part of it, when any work takes one away from home.

It should further be mentioned, that they also use rice for what they call *khir* [1], a kind of rice-porridge [2]. The rice is boiled in water, and milk is added, when it is on the boil. No salt is used for this; but sugar or molasses may be added. This form of food is, however, not common.

Naturally they also have rice husked of unboiled paddy; this is called *adwa caole*, sun-dried rice, and is used for a number of purposes. The above-mentioned *khir* is prepared from this kind. They further make it into a kind of flour and use this for different kinds of cakes or bread (called *piṭhạ* [3], that will be described later on), for small rice-balls and sweetmeats of sorts. The last-mentioned comestibles may be prepared

[1] Bengali—thickened milk—*Ed.*
[2] Rice Porridge in Bengali—*Pâyash*—*Ed.*
[3] From Bengali—*Piṭhâ*—Cake—*Ed.*

by the Santals themselves, but are mostly bought from Hindus. A curious point worthy of mention is that the *adwa caole* is the only kind of rice used in connexion with their spirit worship. They put this down on the magic circle or square, and the animal or fowl to be sacrificed is made to eat from it. When an *ojha* or the priest of the outskirts has to perform what is called *bul māyām* (offering of one's own blood), it is also this kind of rice that is used. The man pricks himself with a thorn, so that a little blood oozes out. He smears this blood on the rice and strews it as an offering to certain *bongas*. This rice is also used when seeking omens. The last-mentioned use of *adwa caole* might be thought due to the fact, that there is less work in connexion with preparing it; but it must not be forgotten, that its use is ordained, and that the use of the other kind is forbidden.

In connexion with rice *khạjạṛi* and *taben* have to be mentioned. Both are generally bought from Hindus, but are also prepared by Santal women.

Khạjạṛi (the *muṛi* of the Bengalis) is parched rice. Santals prepare it as follows: The boiled rice is well cleaned, and some salted water is sprinkled on it; thereupon it is dried. Sand is then put in a shallow earthenware vessel, that is placed over the fire. When the sand becomes burning hot, the rice is put into the sand, and it is stirred with a small 'broom' made of split bamboo. The rice is in this way quickly parched. It is eaten with molasses. Nowadays Santals will also eat it soaked in tea. It is also often taken along to serve as food on the road.

Taben is flattened rice. The Santals prepare this as follows: The rice is soaked in hot water and boiled a little, thereupon roasted a little and finally pounded in a *taben ḍhiṅki*. This has a broad pestle and no iron ring. The bottom of the mortar is also broad and level, so that the rice is pounded flat. One person treads the *ḍhiṅki*, while a woman works at the mortar. With her left hand she roasts one handtul of rice, while with her right hand she keeps the rice in the mortar, until the portion there is ready flattened, and she continues in this way, until all is ready. *Taben* is used much like *khạjạṛi* and is considered more substantial and sustaining.

The *khẹt* is primarily made for the rice; but occasionally other crops may be seen cultivated in these fields, e.g., a kind of bean, that is sown among the paddy when the latter is fairly well developed. Mention of this is made later. During the cold season, after the paddy has been harvested, *guhum*, wheat, is cultivated by a very few Santals in the western parts, also barley (*jao*); but both these cereals play no rôle in a Santal household.

Let us now turn to what is cultivated on the *baṛge*, the homestead field. As already stated, the *baṛge* is the plot of land that is first cleared by a Santal settler. While the Santals never live singly, apart from each other, they will on the other hand, when there is sufficient room, not build their houses in a continuous row along a narrow street, as is often to be seen in the villages of other races. They will arrange a fairly broad and straight stretch of land (that ultimately becomes the village street), and on both sides of this each settler acquires a plot of land on which to build his house or houses. These plots may naturally vary in size, from half-a-*bighạ* up to two or even more *bighạs* (one *bighạ* is about one-third of an acre, regularly 120 feet square). Each occupier will have his private field, with fixed boundaries. Besides giving privacy it is a sanitary arrangement, although this last-mentioned fact has likely had little to do with the procedure, as is shown by the way in which they nowadays build their houses in many places, after having seen what other more civilized peoples do.

The *baŗge* is always a fairly level plot of ground, unsuitable for the cultivation of rice. How unpleasant and insanitary it would be to have rice-fields too close to one's living quarters!

Except for the space actually occupied by the houses, the land of the *baŗge* is all cultivated. As regards ploughing the two first ploughings are the same as for rice-fields (viz., *paŗak̇* and *dẹč*); then comes a final ploughing called *uṭhạu* (raise, start, break up). While all other fields are simply only ploughed, the *baŗge* is manured with cow-dung, ashes or whatever other manure they may have.

The first and most important crop on the *baŗge* is *joṇḍra*, as the Santals call the maize or Indian corn (Zea Mays *L.*). The sowing of the maize is done by the Santals in the following way: A furrow is ploughed; a man goes along and drops the maize grains, one after the other, into this furrow at suitable intervals, closely followed by the ploughing bullocks. The earth thrown up by the plough covers the sown maize. Fresh furrows are then ploughed, and the sowing goes on in the same way but only in alternate furrows. To plant the maize in every furrow would make the plants grow up too close together. The Santals very often sow hemp seed in the furrows left without maize. This hemp, mostly what is called *jāŗī* or *kudrum jāŗī* (Hibiscus cannabinus *L.*) is generally ready in October.

They have quite a number of varieties of maize, named according to the size and appearance of the cobs and the corn, or according to early or late ripening, and so on. The following varieties may be mentioned. *Bagha joṇḍra*, lit. tiger-maize, having dark coloured grains between light coloured ones, the same also being called *kabra joṇḍra*, lit. spotted maize; *buru* (or *bạru*) *joṇḍra*, lit. hill-maize, the cobs being so high that jackals cannot reach them (also called *moṭa joṇḍra*, lit. thick maize); *dudhiạ joṇḍra*, lit. milk-maize, also called *poṇḍ joṇḍra*, lit. white maize, the name being due to the colour of the grain *ḍhibri joṇḍra* puny maize, one of the earliest varieties with cobs so low that jackals can reach them (another name for this variety is *ṭoṭẹ joṇḍra*, *ṭoṭẹ* being a small gourd); *hạrdiạ joṇḍra*, the yellow maize; *muṇḍạ joṇḍra*, the *Muṇḍa* maize, so called, because this variety is cultivated on the hills by the *Muṇḍas*, i.e., the Mal Paharias; *nanha joṇḍra*, lit. thin maize, cultivated by Santals in Assam and near water; finally *satoliạ joṇḍra*, very rare, said to have acquired its name from commencing to fruit when it has seven leaves.

In the Santal Parganas maize is generally sown in June, so that they can hoe the plants when there is a short break in the rains in July. This hoeing is of great importance for the growth. If too much rain prevents proper hoeing, there will be no, or only a very poor, crop. In other parts (as, e.g., in the Santal colony in Assam) the maize is sown at other times. I remember I once took a photograph in the colony of a field containing full-grown and half-grown maize and maize just sprouting, all at the same time.

As soon as the cobs commence to ripen, some are torn off. The covering leaves are removed, and the whole is suitably roasted, and they commence to gnaw off the grains. All Santals do this, especially boys may be seen occupied in this way with a cob. It takes some time to bite off all the grains. It is really a very tasty food, and comes to many as a great relief from hunger.

Most of the cobs are naturally left until fully ripe. As there is always the danger of cobs being stolen by people or taken by animals (by jackals and also by dogs, who at this time may often be seen with a long stick tied to their necks to make it impossible for them to get in among the maize plants), when the maize is grown in a place some distance away from their dwelling houses (in some old *baṛge* or some otherwise suitable field) they erect a *macan* [1] somewhere in the field. The *macan* is a kind of scaffolding, generally a small platform, resting on four slender posts, so high above the ground as to give the watcher a full view of the field. To guard against rain, etc., the posts are high enough above the platform to allow a kind of sheltering cover. Up here a man will stay during the night and keep watch. It is not pleasant to stay there alone. One may hear a Santal say, that he is going to be a bait there for a tiger.

When the ripe cobs are harvested (called *ọṛẹć*, tear off), they remove the covering sheaths (this operation is called *sala*, remove impurities), that is to say, the covering sheaths are not torn off, but turned back, so that the grains are bare. If not needed for food at once, generally sets of four cobs (one *gaṇḍa*) are tied together by the turned-back sheaths, and these sets are again slung together, mostly in aggregates of 80 cobs (one score of *gaṇḍa*, called *pọn*). The cobs are then hung inside on the crossbeams to dry and remain there, often discoloured by smoke, until needed. The Santal idea is that maize is best as food during the hot season, and if they can, they will keep it until April or even May. The Indian corn is calculated by the Santals to keep them in food from one to nearly two months.

In the *baṛge* and in the *goḍa* they also cultivate *bajra*, Sorghum vulgare *Pers.*; this is very commonly cultivated by the Paharias living in the hills in the Santal country, and is possibly one of the oldest grains cultivated by the Santals. They have the following varieties: *bandọrneja* or *bandọrleja b.*, lit. monkey-tail *bajra* (in Assam they call it *kạuniạ b.*); *bhạdriạ* or *bhadọriạ b.*, so called because it ripens in Bhador [2] (Aug.-Sept.); *kubạ b.*, having drooping (*kubạ*, ears); and *sisuạ b.*, that ripens in Aghaṛ [3] (Nov.-Dec.). This last one is, however, not botanically the same as the *bajra*; it is a Pennisetum typhoides *Stapf* et *Hubbard*. The grain is pounded after having been damped (this makes it easy to remove the husk of the grain). When made into a kind of flour, cakes (*piṭhạ*) are prepared from it; otherwise it is cooked like *daka*. It is said to have a sweetish taste and is eaten warm. When it is cold, it has no taste at all, they say.

When the crops mentioned are harvested, the *baṛge* is cleaned and ploughed for some cold-weather crops, certain pulses (*họṛẹć*, *ghaṅgra* and *buṭ*) and oil giving plants (*tuṛi*, *tilmiṅ*, *surguja* and others). Mention of these will be made later.

---

[1] Bengali meaning platform—*Ed.*

[2] Bengali—*Bhādra*—*Ed.*

[3] Bengali—*Agrahayana*—*Ed.*

In connection with the *barge* one special matter should be mentioned. As *barge* fields belonging to separate tenants lie beside each other, it is necessary to have something to show the boundary. They generally have a small ridge, on which some plants grow. The most common of these is what the Santals call *sirom*, Vetivaria zizanioides *Stapf.* (It is from the roots of this that the still common *khas khas* tatties are made, although not by the Santals.) The culms are used for making the commonest broom that the Santals have. The culms are plaited together at the root end, the top ends being free. When this is rolled up, it makes an excellent broom.

The third class of land cultivated by the Santals is what they call *goḍa*, a piece of high-lying ground, generally a little distant from the houses. Officially it is called second class *baṛi* land. It is a piece of ground not suitable for rice. It is cleared of jungle and cultivated like the *barge*, but not manured. If, as sometimes happens, it is manured, it is called *baher barge* or *goḍa barge*.

The *goḍa* naturally represents the oldest attempts of cultivation amongst the Santals. Here they have a large variety of jungle corns that ripen early and help them through the hard times before the rice is ready. Santals often speak of one special advantage of these jungle corns: a mahajon (money-lender) will not take these to recoup himself.

The *goḍa*-crops are the following:—

Iṛi, Panicum Crus-galli *L.*, a millet, formerly very commonly cultivated by the Santals, now only occasionally. They have the following varieties: *sama iṛi* and *se mãyãm iṛi* (lit. louse-blood millet, from the colour of the seed); *kọkọr jaṅga* or *kọkọr kaṭa iṛi* (lit. owl-leg millet), Echinochloa colona *Link.*, var. frumentaceum. *Ọhọe*, Panicum miliaceum *L.* These millets are treated very much like *adwa caole*, i.e., dried, pounded and cooked. Then, too, a wild plant, *ọhọe iṛi*, is also used as food, but not cultivated.

Erba, Setaria italica *Beauv.*, a jungle grain cultivated like *iṛi*, but treated like *teke caole*, i.e., it is first boiled in the husk, then dried, pounded and cooked. What has been said about *iṛi* also applies to *erba*. It is not so commonly cultivated now. A curious point is that, in certain ceremonial talks, *iṛi* is used metaphorically about girls and *erba* in the same way about boys.

Gundli, Panicum miliare *Lamarck*, is a commonly cultivated millet, ripening by the end of August or the beginning of September. To thresh the *gundli* the Santals make small threshing-floors, quite separate from what they have for the rice. Their name for this (*gundli kharai*), it is curious to note, is used metaphorically about a circular hairless area on the crown of the head. The *gundli* millet is, like paddy, first boiled in the husk after having been soaked. It is then dried and finally husked. When being prepared for eating it has to be carefully cooked, so as not to be spoilt. A sufficiency of water is put on the fire, and when this is heard to have reached boiling point, the grain is put in. *Gundli* is said to be quite satisfying. They name two varieties, one *layo gundli*, that will be mentioned further on, and *por gundli*, lit. bush millet, Echinochloa colona *Link.*, var. frumantacea *Fischer*.

Janhẹ, Paspalum scrobiculatum *L.*, a commonly cultivated millet. There are two varieties, one called *bhadọr* (or *bhadoriạ*) *j.*, ripening in Bhador, and another *aghãṛ* *j.*, ripening in Aghaṛ. *Janhẹ* is treated like paddy. It is sometimes boiled in the husk, dried and then pounded; or it is simply dried and husked. The husk is much less substantial than in *gundli*, and may be removed even in a hand-mill. The sun-dried husked grain is said to be what is commonly eaten, and to be sweet and tasty. The grain boiled in the husk, dried and then husked, is mostly used for brewing beer, and is considered by the Santals the best grain they have for brewing intoxicating beer. Even gruel prepared from it is believed to be intoxicating. I remember that, when I once wished to taste such gruel, they seriously warned me not to eat too much, otherwise it might make me drunk. They have a curious belief, that if a cobra or a rat-snake has been in the *janhẹ* field, this will cause the *janhẹ* there to become especially intoxicating.

Besides the cultivated *janhẹ* there is a wild variety, called *jera janhẹ*, Panicum flavidum *Retz.* This may be eaten, specially in times of scarcity.

Kukrạ is a grass, Setaria pallidifasca *Stapf* et *Hubbard*, found growing together with *gundli* and *janhẹ*, and is harvested and the grain eaten along with these; another name for the same is *ciprạ*.

Kọde, Eleusine coracana *Gaertn.*, is a millet, of which they have four varieties: *aghọniạ k.*, ripening in Aghaṛ (end of Nov.); *bhạdriạ k.*, ripening in Bhador (Aug.-Sept.), *dasãe k.*, ripening in Dasae (Sept.-Oct.) and *kọkọr jaṅga k.*, lit. owl-leg *kọdẹ*, because the ears are reminiscent of the leg of an owl. *Kọdẹ* is cultivated somewhat like paddy, sown broadcast, the seedlings being pulled out and planted in a high-land field, a *gọḍa*, or a *baṛge*. It is harvested and threshed like paddy. It is pounded into a powder, that is eaten in the form of cakes or together with rice or other cereals. *Kọdẹ* is not considered to be very good, but is said to be a food that will keep people in a fair condition during times of scarcity, and is consequently cultivated by most Santals.

Layo, Panicum antidotale *Retz.*, is a millet commonly cultivated on high-land fields. Sown in June, some transplant it, but generally it grows where it is sown. It is harvested in November and treated like *gundli*.

In connection with the cereals mentioned there are two kinds of grass, that in times of need may be used for food. One is the *sama ghãs* [1], Echinochloa colona *Link.*, often found growing as a weed in the rice-fields. The grass is an excellent fodder. In times of scarcity it is used as food, prepared into a kind of gruel (*dak̓ mạṇḍi*). In addition *sumtu bukuć ghãs*, Dactyloctenium ægyptiacum *Beauv.*, may be used like *sama ghãs*. Children use the ears as toys.

Different forms of cereals prepared.

Before going further mention may be made of what the Santals call *piṭhạ*, that is translated cake or bread. They have a large number, all differently named after the ingredients, the method of preparing, or the shape. Meal or flour, mostly of rice (always sun-dried, *adwa*) [2], but also of other grain, is made into a batter mixed with one

[1] From Bengali meaning Grass—*Ed.*

[2] From Bengali—'ātap'—meaning sun—*Ed.*

or more kinds of other foodstuffs and then fried or cooked. The different kinds of *piṭhạ* here follow in alphabetical order.

Aṛsạ piṭhạ is made of flour, milk and raw sugar and is cooked in mustard oil. It is allowed to rise a little. Not common. Probably adopted from low-caste people. The name is derived from Desi *aṛsa*.

Chọr piṭhạ, the same as *dul piṭhạ*, the name being descriptive of the sound heard when the batter is thrown into the boiling oil.

Dul piṭhạ, lit. cast cake or bread, made of rice-flour and molasses mixed in milk or water. The batter, flattened between the hands, is thrown into the boiling mustard oil. It is very hard to digest, but is considered to be the finest 'pastry' the Santals have.

Ḍombok piṭhạ, a ball-formed cake, made of flour and molasses. Cooked in water. (*Ḍombok* is a name for a round ball.)

Guṛ[1] *piṭhạ*, a cake made from the molasses of the Date palm.

Jel piṭhạ, meat cake. Sun-dried paddy is husked and cleaned, soaked in water for a little while, then dried and made into a coarse flour and sifted. The flesh is cut into small bits. Turmeric, pepper and other spices and salt are ground fine. All is well kneaded and mixed into the flour, that has been moistened. The whole is then pressed down on a leaf-plate. Another leaf-plate is with the help of straw-pins fixed on as a cover. The whole is placed into a fire-place, where there are live coals, and on top more live coals are put. When ready the whole is taken out and eaten. This is much relished. The flesh used is mostly that of pigs or of fowls, also of sacrificed animals.

Joṇḍra piṭhạ, a bread made from Indian corn and fried.

Jhinuk[2] *piṭhạ*, lit. mussel-cake. Two thin pieces of batter are made, or one large piece is folded over. Molasses and some *lobok* (bran of mustard or other stuff) are put in. The whole is then cooked in water. This is made for festivals, especially the *Sakrat*[3]. The name is descriptive of the shape, which is reminiscent of mussels.

Kọdẹ piṭhạ, bread made from the flour of *kọdẹ* millet. Fried.

Khapra piṭhạ, made from rice-flour. The flour is made into a batter with water, nothing being added, except sometimes a little salt. Some batter is put into a shallow earthenware dish (*karahe*); a little oil being rubbed on the batter to prevent it from sticking to the dish. An earthenware lid is pressed down on the batter; and the dish is then put on the fire-place and heated. When ready fried, the *karahe* is taken off and turned, so that the cake falls out, and fresh batter is put in. This *piṭhạ* is fairly large. *Khapra* is the Santal name for a roofing tile or a large potsherd.

Ol piṭhạ, mushroom cake, prepared like *jel piṭhạ*, with mushrooms instead of flesh or meat. If the opening of the fire-place is small, a large potsherd is placed on the fire. When this is sufficiently heated, the *paṭra*[4] (leaf-plate) with its contents is placed on

---

1 From Bengali meaning molasses—*Ed.*

2 From Bengali meaning mussel—*Ed.*

3 From Bengali '*Śankranti*', the last day of *Paus*, when cakes are eaten—*Ed.*

4 In Bengali *Pātra* means vessel—*Ed.*

this. When baked on the underside, the whole is turned over with a twig to get the other side baked.

Parwa pitha is the same as *jel pitha*, but made with the flesh of pigeons.

Patra pitha is any flour-batter placed between two leaf-plates (*patra*) and baked like *jel pitha*.

Sakam pitha, the same as *patra pitha*, except that instead of a leaf-plate one large leaf (*sakam*) is used.

Sim pitha is the same as *jel pitha*, the flesh of fowls (*sim*) being used. This is especially used by ojhas, when they have sacrificed fowls.

Serving of food.

The Santals have no tables, no chairs, no knives, forks or spoons, and no dining room. People belonging to the family may take their food inside or on the verandah, if they have one. As a rule they will sit down on the ground in the courtyard. This is generally plastered with cowdung and carefully swept and cleaned, before they sit down, or mats are used. The food is served in whatever utensils they may have. Nowadays they generally have one or more brass-plates and brass-cups. These are, however, of fairly recent introduction and bought from other races, especially Hindus. When they have no such vessels, or if these are insufficient, they have to use their old plates and cups, all made of leaves. These are invariably used only once and then thrown away. To use these on more than one occasion, even by the same person, would be considered a terrible thing, opposed to all rules of cleanliness and quite impossible.

The leaf-plate (*patra*) is made of any kind of leaf that is large enough (especially leaves of the Sal, Shorea robusta *Gærtn.*, and of the Mahua, Bassia latifolia *Roxb.*). To make a leaf-plate a dozen or more leaves are used, always of the same kind, not different ones mixed together. The leaves are pinned together with bits of hard dry straw. This work is done by women, although a few men have also learnt how to make them. Leaf-plates are especially made at the commencement of the hot season in large numbers. The women collect leaves that have fallen and are in good condition. If too dry, they are wetted during the operation. Santals keep high piles of ready-made leaf-plates to have for use during the coming rains, their working season, or for guests. A leaf-plate is round and up to about 30 cm. across.

The leaf-plate is used for *daka*, cooked rice, which is served on it in heaps. Cooked rice is nowadays the principal food of the Santals, and consequently *daka* is a term commonly used for food in general, something like the English use of the word 'meal'.

As previously remarked *daka* is not eaten alone, something has to be added that, having value as a foodstuff, also imparts taste to the otherwise insipid rice. This is curry, called by the Santals *utu*, i.e., pulses, meat, flesh, or practically anything eatable, that can be made into *utu*. *Utu* is described in detail later.

Utu is served in brass- or leaf-cups. The brass-cups need no description; they are small bowls bought in the bazar. The leaf-cups (*phuruk*, as the Santals call them) are made of the same kind of leaves as the *patra*. The Santals have several kinds of leaf-cups, named according to their form or use. All leaf-cups naturally have the leaves so turned up and folded, that they form a cup which is compact enough to retain fluids. As it is of some ethnological interest, a list of the Santal leaf-cups is given here.

Aṭal phuṛuk, lit. layer-leaf-cup, is made of two Sal-leaves placed side by side with two others on top of these, all stitched together with straw-pins. Sometimes double leaves are used.

Boṅga bhą̃utić ph., made of one leaf, with straw-pins at four corners, used for drinking milk, also for keeping sun-dried rice, sindur, etc., at the time of sacrifices.

Bhą̃utić ph. is made of two leaves placed one across the other, and is used for any kind of *utu*, also for fish curry (then called *hako jọm bhą̃utić ph.*), and also for curds.

Cuṭiul ph., lit. pigtail leaf-cup, made of one leaf. It is used for serving out beer and is very small. Its use is considered niggardly.

Ḍangra jọm ph., lit. ox-eating leaf cup, is made like the *aṭal ph.*, but of very large leaves, and is used for meat curry.

Ḍhoṇḍra ph., a large leaf-cup, made of one leaf. (Desi *dona.*)

Ḍhoṇḍra khalak, a large leaf-cup, made of two leaves. *Tale ḍhoṇḍra*, made of the leaf of the Palmyra palm, especially used for drinking *taṛi*, liquor (toddy) made from the Palmyra or Date palms.

Haṇḍi[1] *ph.*, lit. beer leaf-cup, made of one leaf, both ends pinned. As the name shows, this is used for drinking beer. The same kind is also used for water or milk when given to children.

Jel ph., the same as *aṭal phuṛuk*, but used for meat or flesh curry.

Khalak ph., a large leaf-cup, made of four leaves (Sal) pinned together, used for certain foodstuffs, such as tripe.

Paṭra khalak ph., very large, pinned like the *paṭra*, leaf-plate.

Soṛha ph., the same as *aṭal ph.*, of large leaves, used for any kind of curry, also for *dak maṇḍi* and *nim dak maṇḍi*, the rice-gruel with nim added. It is also called *soṛwa.*

Utu ph., the same as *aṭal ph.*, except that as the name implies it is used for curry.

Tale ph., a leaf-cup, made of the leaf of a Palmyra palm (made by men only), used for drinking or for carrying flesh, etc.

Cọkọrhat, a leaf-cup made from one leaf, the stalk end of the leaf being folded on both sides of the midrib. If there is sufficient stalk, this is used as a pin; otherwise a bit of stiff straw is employed. This is used for serving out dry, especially parched, food.

Cukṛũć, a leaf-spoon; the leaf is folded from the tip twice over, so that the tip comes round to the stalk on one side and is there fastened with a straw-pin. This is used for *dak maṇḍi* and water.

Dolkha, the same as *khalak*; the word is seldom used by the Santals, but by the Mahles.

---

[1] Bengali jug—*Ed.*

CULTIVATED VEGETABLES.

Curry, called in Santali, as already stated, *utu*, is never eaten alone, but always with *daka*, cooked grain, mostly rice. It is an important part of the Santal diet, and also imparts taste to the otherwise somewhat insipid *daka*. *Utu* is prepared separately, and either cooked with turmeric, spices and salt, or cooked in oil. Vegetables are also cooked in water, when no oil is available.

The Santals cultivate the following vegetables and pulses, and these are mostly used for *utu*:—

In parenthesis, it may be noted, that the Santals prepare what they call *dạl*[1], split pulse (of all dicotyledonous fruits), for use in their *utu*. The *dạl* is prepared in a hand-mill, the kernel being generally (but not always) roasted before being ground. When being prepared for *utu* the *dạl* is first boiled long enough to dissolve it and spices and salt are then added with the oil.

Raheṛ[2], Cajanus indicus *Spreng.*, is one of the most commonly cultivated pulses of the Santals. It is frequently sown together with the maize in the *baṛge*, but also alone. They have several varieties, mostly named in accordance with the time when they ripen, thus:—

> *Aghãṛ raheṛ* (or *aghoniạ*), ripening in Aghaṛ (Nov.-Dec.), *mạṅghi* (or *mạghi*) *raheṛ*, ripening in Magh (Jan.-Feb.), *cạitạli raheṛ*, ripening in *Cạt* (March-Apr.), and *lạprạ raheṛ*, so called on account of its large and broad pods.

Buru raheṛ is quite another plant, Cyamopsis tetragonoloba *Taub*, not cultivated by itself, but sown along the borders of a field together with some other crop. It is considered a crop for times of scarcity. There is also a wild plant resembling the *raheṛ*, that in times of scarcity is eaten raw.

Kesari[3] (or *kisạri*), Lathyrus sativus *L.*, is sown in rice-fields in Aghaṛ (Nov.-Dec.) when the heavy paddy has ears. It is left, when the rice is cut and is harvested in *Cạt* (end of March). This plant is not to be confounded with *lal kisạri*, Eclipta alba *Hassk.*, var. prostrata, or with *lạu* (or *ṭạṇḍi*) *kisạri*, Eclipta prostrata *L.*, used in Santal medicine, but not eaten; both these are wild plants.

Ghaṅgra, Dolichos iat Jang, *Linn.* is a commonly cultivated bean. The Santals distinguished a number of varieties: *Aghanuạ* (or *aghoniạ*) *gh.*, ripening in Aghaṛ, *bhadọr* (or *bhạdriạ*) *gh.*, ripening in Bhador, *cihṛi gh.*, (acc. to Dr. Campbell, not known in the Santal Parganas), *boḍa gh.*, having large beans, *dasãe* (or *dạsmi*) *gh.*, ripening in Dasãe, *ḍaṅ gh.*, grown on wooden supports (cultivated like *malhan*, q.v.), *moṭa* (also called *buru*) *gh.*, having small beans, and *sutri gh.*, having small thin legumes.

Ghạṅgri, a variety of *ghaṅgra*, ripening in Bhador.

Hoṛẹċ, Dolichos biflorus *L.*, largely cultivated during the cold season, are beans used for *utu* and *sạtu* (a kind of flour or meal). Women who have borne a child are allowed only *hoṛẹċ utu*, until they are cleansed. *Hoṛẹċ* is also used medicinally. Water

---

[1] *Dâl* is also used in Bengali and Hindi for cooked pulse—*Ed.*

[2] Arhhar (Bengali)—*Ed.*

[3] Bengali—*Khesâri*—*Ed.*

in which *hoṛeč* has been boiled is used to wash the mouth of animals suffering from mouth disease. A mixture of crushed *hoṛeč*, salt and pigeon excreta is put on boils to ripen them. The Santals distinguish between *poṇḍ* (white) and *hende* (black) *hoṛeč* in accordance with the colour of the beans, but they are not botanically different. Besides they have *disom hoṛeč*, lit. land-*h.*, Glycine Soja *Lieb* and *Zucc.*, cultivated, eaten parched (*ata*, *saṭu* or *khicṛi*, cooked with rice), and *bir disom hoṛeč*, a wild variety of the preceding, used in Santal vet. medicine; also *bir hoṛeč*, Attylosia scaraboides *Benth.*, a jungle plant, not cultivated, but sometimes eaten. It may be noted that this plant is successfully used by Santals against foot and mouth disease.

Rambṛa, Phaseolus radiatus *Roxb.*, is commonly cultivated. Also, *Ghasuạ rambṛa*, (?) Phaseolus Max *Roxb.*, a variety planted on rice-field ridges, having black beans.

Alpạluạ, Phaseolus aconitifolius *Jacq.*, is sown with *janhe*, or cotton, or alone. It is not extensively cultivated and is used for *dạl*.

Buṭ, gram, Cicer arietinum *L.*, is cultivated, where the soil is suitable, perhaps more now than formerly. *Bir buṭ*, Flemingia congesta *Roxb.*, a jungle plant, of which the fruit is eaten. The fruit resembles *buṭ*, hence the name.

Sutri, Phaseolus calcaratus *Roxb.* is cultivated together with maize or *ghaṅgra* and is called *sutri ghaṅgra*.

Tiri riti, a kind of pulse, is found growing in the rice-fields in the cold season together with *kisạri*. The *dạl* is eaten. Its leaves are also used for curry.

Maṭor, Pisum sativum *L.*, and Pisum arvense *L.*, the pea, is very rarely cultivated by the Santals but is bought in the shops.

Masri [1], a pulse, Lens esculanta *Moench.*, is cultivated in certain parts.

Muṅ [2], a cultivated pulse, Phaseolus Mungo *Linn.*, var. Max., is commonly grown.

Malhan, Dolichos Lablab *Linn.*, the common bean, is cultivated in gardens or near the houses. They have a number of varieties: *Ato malhan*, lit. village bean; *arak m.*, having reddish pods; *bilạti m.*, lit. Europe-bean, any bean introduced from Europe or America and cultivated in gardens; *dūṛi m.*, a bean having long and roundish pods (so named because the pods are reminiscent of the eel-like *dūṛi* fish); *ḍuriạ m.*, a variety having more than one pod from the same raceme; *gele m.*, a variety of Dolichos Lablab *L.*, having the legumes on an erect spike; *hende m.*, a variety of Dolichos Lablab with blackish legumes; *kurse m.*, a variety with purple-coloured flowers and legumes; *lạpṛạ m.*, a variety with broad legumes; *poṇḍ m.*, a variety with white flowers and legumes and white beans; *rethe m.*, a variety of Dolichos lignosus *Linn.*, having small pods and leaves (also called *tuṛi m.*, mustard beans); *uṭi m.*, a variety of Dolichos Lablab, having pods at 'joints'. Beans are naturally also eaten raw. From beans the Santals also prepare what is called *malhan suṛe*, a bean hash. The ripening pods are cleaned and cut into two or three pieces and then boiled; when sufficiently soft, rice is added and the whole cooked into a hash that is eaten instead of rice and curry.

---

[1] Bengali *Mūsūri*—*Ed.*

[2] Bengali *Mug*, Hindi *Mung*—*Ed.*

In times of scarcity the seeds of *bheḍa dereń*, lit. Ram's horn, Cassia Tora *L.* (also called *cakaoḍa*) are eaten boiled together with mahua flowers. The tender leaves may also be used in curry.

Besides the leguminous plants mentioned the Santals cultivate a number of plants, the fruits of which are used for curry or otherwise eaten. These plants are mostly kept growing singly or a few together, near the houses, often so that they run up and have fruits lying on the roofs.

Beṅgaṛ [1], the egg-plant, Solanum Melongena *L.*, is commonly cultivated. They recognize the following varieties: *Barǫmạsiạ* [2] *b.*, so called, because it is fruiting the whole year (also called *barse b.*); *ḍhuḍuạ b.*, having large round fruits (so named because the fruits resemble a *ḍhuḍuạ*, an oil container of leather); *hẹndẹ b.*, having blackish fruits; *jhompa* [3] *b.*, having two or three fruits from a common stalk (*jhompa* means 'in clusters'); *kạjri b.*, having greyish fruits (*kạjri*, having dark spots); *kǫṛcẹ* (or *kuṛcạ*) *b.*, the tomato, now commonly called *belati* [4] *b.*, European egg-plant, recently introduced and not as yet commonly cultivated by Santals; *pạilạ b.*, lit. seer egg-plant, having large round fruits; *sǫela b.*, having long fruits (*sǫela* means long and sharp pointed). The fruit is cooked in oil.

Jhiṅgạ [5], Luffa acutangula *Roxb.* The Santals recognize the following varieties: *Cạr sirạ jh.*, lit. four-edged *jh.*, fruit having sharp ridges; *ḍuriạ jh.*, bunch *jh.*, having several fruits from one stalk; *jhompa jh.*, cluster *jh.*, the same as *ḍuriạ jh.*; *nirǫn jh.*, hot weather *jh.*, cultivated during the hot season; *kạilạ jh.*, lit. light-coloured *jh.*, resembling the *ḍuriạ jh.*; *jhiṅgi*, the same as *jhiṅgạ*, but having only small fruits. In addition: *Porol jh.* (also called *pǫtǫl* [6] *jh.*), Luffa aegyptiaca *Mill.* ex *H.f.*, uncommon; and *Ram jh.*, Hibiscus esculentus *L.*, lady's finger, commonly cultivated.

Hǫtǫl, the bottle gourd, Lagenaria vulgaris *Ser.*, is largely cultivated by the Santals, both on account of its fruit, which is used for curry, and for the shell of the ripe and dried fruit, which is used for all kinds of vessels, and, formerly, was practically their only kind of vessel. The Santals distinguish several varieties, according to the shape of the fruit: *Jante* [7] *h.*, fruit resembling a mill-stone (*jante*); *jeleń h.*, the fruit being long; *lạuạ* [8] *h.*, having a more or less globular fruit (*lạuạ* is a name for cup); *bhạriạ* [9] *h.*, having only one fruit (*bhạriạ* is the word for carrying on the shoulder on a yoke, bangy pole); *pǫnḍ h.*, fruit white; *hạriạṛ h.*, fruit green when ripe; *mare h.*, having only one fruit (also used about an old, last year's fruit). The varieties mentioned are what they call *sebel*, meaning tasty, eatable. There is one variety called *haṛhal h.*, bitter bottle gourd. This is not eaten, but its shell is very serviceable for making cups, ladles, water-bottles, etc. *Bokak̄ hǫtǫl* is of this bitter kind. The fruit has a peculiar form, being narrow close to the stem and having a round head at the other end. When this is cut with a sickle made red-hot along the middle, two serviceable

---

1 Bengali *Begun*—*Ed.*

2 From Bengali *Bāro*=12; *Mās*=month—*Ed.*

3 In Bengali also called *Belati Begun*—*Ed.*

4 Bengali *Jhinga*—*Ed.*

5 Bengali *Jhāṛ*—*Ed.*

6 Bengali *Patol*—*Ed.*

7 From Bengali *Jānta*—*Ed.*

8 From Bengali *Lāu*—*Ed.*

9 From *Bhār* in Bengali meaning 'load'—*Ed.*

ladles are obtained. To do away with the bitter taste the ladle thus prepared is filled with cow-dung and ashes and left for about a fortnight; then all is scraped out with a mussel-shell. These are used for ladling out rice and curry. Implements made from the bottle-gourd are supposed not to become defiled. (*Bokak* means ladle.)

Kohṇḍa[1], pumpkin, Cucurbita moschata *Duchesne*, is cultivated everywhere by the Santals, and its fruit eaten as curry. They differentiate varieties in accordance with the shape of the fruit and the season when cultivated. *Jante k.*, fruit resembling a mill-stone; *jeleń k.*, fruit being long; *ṭukuć k.*, having fruits shaped like a *ṭukuć*, an earthenware water-pot; *poṇḍ k.*, having light-coloured fruits; *nirọn k.*, cultivated during the hot season.

Karla[2], several creepers are so called. *Deko karla* (also called *haṛhaṭ k.*), Momordica Charantia *Linn.* and Momordica muricata *DC.*, is commonly cultivated; the *haṛhaṭ k.* has a bitter fruit. *Ghi* (or *sebel*) *karla*, Memordica dioica *Roxb.* ex *Willd.*, the fruits of which are used in curry, before they are ripe. They also recognize *ato karla*, the cultivated kind, and *bir karla*, lit. forest *karla*, that is wild. The leaves of this are edible and are called *kacan aṛak*. These are often found when they are out hunting and are used in curry.

Kundri; there are two kinds, *ato kundri*, Cephalandra indica *Naud.*,=Coccinia cordifolia (L) *Cogn.*, commonly cultivated; and *bir kundri*, Melothria heterophylla *Cogn.* The fruit and tuber (called *at*) are used in curry. The plant is dioecious, the male creeper being called *ạṇḍiạ kundri*, the fruiting one *eṅga kundri*. The tubers of both are eaten boiled or roasted.

Pọṭọl, Trichosanthes dioica *Roxb.*, is only rarely cultivated by the Santals, but is very common amongst Bengalis. The ripe fruit is much used in curry. Dr. Campbell mentions two varieties, *genḍ pọṭọl* raised from tubers, and *palta pọṭọl*, raised from cuttings. These distinctions are not known among the Santals in the Santal Parganas, most likely because there is little cultivation.

Ato piṇḍe, Amorphophallus campanulatus *Blume.* Cultivated; the tuber is peeled, steamed and eaten with mustard and *amtha*, the inspissated juice of the tamarind or the mango. The tamarind is soaked, the stones pressed out, and the pulp kneaded, This is then dried and made into balls that are preserved for use as a condiment with curry (especially fish curry). There is also a *bir piṇḍe*, a small forest tree, Randia uliginosa *DC.*, the fruit of which is eaten as curry.

Sạru, the Taro plant, Arum Colocasia *Linn.*, or Colocasia Antiquorum *Schott.*, is commonly cultivated. The tuber or corm is eaten, also the stem and leaves (all in curry). The Santals recognize a number of varieties: *Aṛak sạru*, of which only the leaves are used; *bir sạru*, a wild Taro, the leaves of which are eaten in curry (Roxb. considers this only a variety of Arum Colocasia); *bhạluk liṇḍhi sạru*, lit. bear-hindquarters Taro, a variety; *bhoṇḍa sạru*, a variety with large corms (*bhoṇḍa*, fat, unwieldy); *deko sạru*, a variety cultivated by Dekos; *họṛ sạru*, a variety especially cultivated by Santals; *kanda sạru*, Arum Colocasia *Linn.*, a variety with one large corm; *mukhi sạru*, cultivated; *picki sạru*, cultivated (the two last varieties are mentioned by Dr. Campbell);

1 Bengali *Kumra—Ed.*

2 Bengali *Karala—Ed.*

rọhọe sạru, any planted variety may be so named (*rọhọe*, to plant). Besides the *sạru* already mentioned they have two different plants, also called *sạru*, viz. *kaṇṭa sạru*, Lasia spinosa *Thv.*, that is planted near water for the medicinal use of its corm, and *man kanda sạru*, also only used for its medicinal properties (the corm being applied to painful spots).

Kaera, the plantain, Musa sapientium *L.*, or Musa paradisiaca *L.*, is fairly commonly planted near the courtyard, but as a rule only the coarser varieties are grown.

In connection with the plants just mentioned the following may be noted:—

Ạk[1], the sugarcane, Saccharum officinarum *L.* The Santals distinguish a number of different kinds which, however, are not botanically different:—

Bajṛa ạk, resembling the *bajṛa*, Sorghum vulgare *Pers.*; sown in June, cut in Nov.-Dec., not irrigated.

Basta ạk, white, planted and cut like *kạjri ạk*, q.v.

Bombae ạk, reddish, thick, planted in June, cut in April, irrigated.

Kạjri ạk, reddish, planted in June, cut in March; requires irrigation.

Pạchiạri ạk, also called *raonda ạk*, whitish, planted in November, cut in Oct.-Nov. the following year.

Poṇḍe ạk, white, planted and treated like *kạjri ạk*.

Rẹṭhẹ ạk, a stunted kind.

Formerly an implement called *maha sal*, drawn by bullocks, was used for pressing the cane. This is now very rare, and instead the Santals use a *rạksi*, two heavy rollers, fixed on two solid posts and worked by hand. Two men sit at either end, pulling one end of the turn-pole towards them by the hand, whilst pushing the other end away with the foot. The product is then boiled in a large pan. In this way they make *guṛ*[2], molasses or treacle, the form of raw sugar that is most commonly used.

Ạlu[3], the potato, is very rarely cultivated by Santals, except where they are in contact with Europeans. Potatoes are bought in the bazar and used for curry.

Asẹr, a climber; the root is eaten boiled.

At, the edible root of *bir kundri*; v. *kundri*.

Bayaṅ, a creeper, Dioscorea hispida *Denns.* The root is eaten.

Cạmuạ, a creeper. The root is eaten. The Santals have possibly obtained this from the Paharias, as the name is borrowed from them (*camua*).

Kolo, a variety of Dioscorea hispida *Denns.* The tuber is bared and a number of incisions made in it. It is then boiled and placed in a water-pool for one night, taken out, again boiled and eaten. The tuber is also used for making beer intoxicating.

Kuclạ, the clearing-nut tree, Strychnos potatorum *L.* fil. The pulp is eaten.

Kunạm, a plant, the tubers of which are eaten. There are two varieties, *gại kunạm*, having small tubers, and *nāṛī kunạm*, having large tubers. They have a saying that the tubers of this plant in former times grew to the size of a kettle-drum.

Piskạ, a climbing plant, Dioscorea oppositifolia *Linn.* The tuber is boiled and then treated as *kolo*, q.v.

---

[1] Bengali—*Āk—Ed.* [2] Bengali—*Gūr—Ed.* [3] Bengali—*Ālu—Ed.*

Sahṛa, a small tree, Streblus asper *Lour.* The leaves are placed in milk to make it coagulate.

Sãṅ (or *saṅ*) is a Santal name for various plants or bushes having edible tubers. They have *bir sãṅ*, a wild species, Phaseolus mungo, var. radiatus *L.*; *dare sãṅ*, Dioscorea alata *L.* Cultivated; *ḍurạ sãṅ*, Dioscorea pentaphylla *Linn.*; *jọ sãṅ*, Dioscorea pubera *Bl.* Cultivated; the fruit and tubers are eaten; *nạṛī sãṅ*, the male plant, the same as the female *jọ sãṅ*; the tubers are eaten. The Santals are very fond of these tubers when cooked in oil.

Sakarkenda (also called *sẹkẹrkenda*), Ipomæa Batatas *Poir.*, a kind of sweet potato, is commonly cultivated.

Susni, Dioscorea esculenta *Burkill.* Commonly found wild, but it is also planted. The tubers are eaten.

Taher, Cucumis sativus *L.*, is commonly cultivated.

Phuṭ taher, a kind of Melon, Cucumis Melo *L.*, var. momordica. The fruit is much relished. When young, it is a good substitute for the common cucumber; later it will burst, and with sugar added it is excellent.

Tarbuj (or *tạrbuj*), the Melon, Cucumis Melo *Linn.*

Culinary oils and other oils.

We will now deal with the oils and spices, etc., that are used in connection with the preparation of curry. Of oil and similar cooking media they have several kinds.

Gọtọm, ghee or clarified butter. When churning, the unsalted butter (*nạinu*) is collected, put in a vessel over a fire and boiled. In this way they prepare what looks like a kind of oil that remains fluid, so long as the air temperature is high. During the cold season it is liable to coagulate, but this does not affect its quality. It is the same kind that is used all over India. Made from cow's milk it is called *gại gọtọm*, and from buffalo-cow's milk *bitkil gọtọm*. It should, however, be noted that very few Santals are sufficiently well-to-do to use ghee when preparing their curry.

Sunum is the Santal name for oil in general. Among Santals the oldest they have is probably what they call *kũiṇḍi sunum*. This is prepared from the kernels of *kũiṇḍi*, the fruit of the Mahua tree. These kernels (*kũiṇḍi jaṅ*) are split into *dạl*, and the split kernels are dried and pounded into a kind of flour (called *kũiṇḍi họlọṅ*). This is first washed and dried and then put into a small basket, that is placed on the mouth of an earthenware pot not quite half full of water, standing on the fire. When the flour has in this way been sufficiently 'steamed' (this is tested by seeing whether oil comes out when it is pressed between the fingers), it is put in a straw cover that is tied up with a string. This cover is then placed in an oil-press, and the oil pressed out.

The Santal oil-press (*sunum lẹnok* (or *lẹlẹn*) *paṭa*) consists of two heavy logs of wood fixed on two solid posts, one near each end of the logs. These logs are planed on the sides that meet, and in the lower log's surface a ring (*candwa*) is cut, sufficiently large to take the oil. This finally runs out over a small spout called *luṭi* (lip). To press the oil out a rope is taken round the logs at one end, a piece of wood is inserted through the upright post at the other end, to keep this end down, and with the help of a solid belaying-pin the two logs are pressed together. Occasionally one comes across another, probably older, form of oil-press, called *cuṇḍuć paṭa.* This consists of a large piece of stone, the surface of which is made plane and has a circular ring and a channel cut in it. This stone is placed at the foot of a large tree (g., a Mahua), a fairly large hole is cut in the stem of the tree, and into this the end of a long piece of timber is inserted for pressing out oil from a wrapper prepared as described above. The weight of the timber on which people lean or sit provides the necessary pressure.

The oils so obtained are used for many purposes, anointing, lubricating, as medicine, as well as for preparing curry. The various kinds of oil are generally utilized separately and are seldom mixed together. The oil-cake (*kaṛe*) left is used as a hot fomentation, as a fish-poison, and to drive away snakes. In this last case it is burnt on a fire and the smoke drives the snakes away.

Other oils, extracted by the Santals for culinary purposes, are produced from: *Boṅga sarjọm,* a large climbing shrub, Ventilago calyculata *Tulasne.* Oil obtained from the fruit is used for culinary purposes.

Dare kudrum, Hibiscus cannabinus *L.* Oil is extracted from the fruit kernel, which is husked, made into flour and eaten in curry.

Kujri, a climbing shrub, Celastrus paniculata *Willd.* Oil is extracted from the seed (in a similar way as from *Kũiṇḍi*) and is used in medicine as well as for frying parched Mahua flowers.

Surguja, Guizotia abyssynica *Cass.* Very commonly cultivated, this yields the Niger seed and oil, which is largely used. Nowadays it is a common practice for the seed to be sold to Hindu oilmen (*tili*), and the oil bought from them. The same is the case with the following, viz.:—

Tilmiń, Sesemum indicum *Linn.* Commonly cultivated. They distinguish *hẹndẹ*, black, and *poṇḍ*, white *tilmiń*, in accordance with the colour of the seed.

Tuṛi, the mustard plant, Brassica campestris *L.* Very commonly cultivated. The Santals distinguished the following varieties: *Badam* (or *badọm*) *tuṛi* and *luṭni* (*tuṛi*), both having black seeds, *man tuṛi*, *rại tuṛi*, giving small yellow seeds, and *ṭhạḍia* (or *ṭhạṛiạ*) *tuṛi*, having yellow seeds. The Santals cultivate these also for sale to obtain money to pay their agricultural rent. The leaves are used in curry.

The oil that is now probably most commonly used in preparing curry is what they call *utiń sunum*, lit. barter oil. It is so named from the way in which this oil was originally obtained from the Telis, i.e. by paying for it in kind (all kinds of oil seed). It is mustard oil mixed with oil of other seeds.

As it is of some ethnological interest, the oils extracted by the Santals for other than culinary purposes may also be mentioned. They are obtained from:—

Aṭkuṭi, a prickly annual, Argemone mexicana *L.* Oil extracted from the seeds is used in lamps.

Bando, a creeper, Spatholobus Roxburghii *Benth.* Oil is obtained from the fruit.

Bạru, a tree, Schleichera trijuga *Willd.* Oil extracted from the seeds is used against skin diseases.

Bhẹrṇḍa[1], a small tree, Jatropha Curcas *L.* Oil obtained from the seeds is used both in lamps and as a laxative.

Eraḍọm, Ricinus communis *L.* Fairly commonly planted. Oil extracted from the fruit is used for lamps as well as a laxative (castor oil).

Kọrọṅj, Pongamia glabra *Vent.*, a large forest tree, is also grown. Oil from the kernels is used against scabies.

Musnạ, Linum usitatissimum *L.* The oil is used in Santal medicine. In some parts of the country they use *ṭisi* or *ṭhisiạ* a very similar plant. This plant is cultivated but not in any great quantity.

Nim[2], the Neem tree, Azadirachta indica *Jus.* Oil is extracted from fruit kernel and has a very bitter taste.

Sọsọ, the Marking nut tree. Oil, distilled from the drupe, is much used as a vesicant on animals, to paint numbers on houses, and for other purposes.

The ingredients used by the Santals in connexion with preparing the curry are, besides the oils, the following:

Sasaṅ, turmeric, Curcuma longa *Linn.* This is very commonly cultivated and used when preparing all kinds of curry, except those made from leaves. The Santals have a saying: What pleases the mouth is salt; what pleases the eye is turmeric; what pleases the nose are spices; what pleases the lips is pepper and when you combine all these things, the result is most agreeable. What they say seems to show that they have little understanding of the value of turmeric in their food. Turmeric is also used in Santal medicine, both externally and internally, it is largely used as a temporary yellow dye, and, mixed with oil, as an anointment. When women wear a new piece of cloth, it is almost invariably dyed yellow by the application of turmeric but the first washing removes it.

Peaj[3], onion, Allium ascalonicum *Linn.* Fairly commonly cultivated by the Santals. They recognize the following varieties: *Arak peaj*, the red (common) onion, and *chimbṛi peaj*, the same, but so called when growing in clusters; *sãci peaj*, Allium odorum *L.*, and *kaḍa peaj*, lit. Buffalo onion, Allium Cepa *Linn.*, a very large onion. It is curious that the beautiful Pancratium verecundum *Ait.* is also called *kaḍa peaj* by the Santals. *Poṇḍ peaj*, white onion, is only another name for garlic.

Rạsun[4], Garlic, Allium sativum *Linn.*, is not commonly cultivated.

Mạric[5], pepper. The Santals have a number of varieties: *Caole mạric*, lit. rice-pepper, Capsicum minimum *Roxb.*; *dare mạric*, lit. tree pepper, Capsicum annuum *L.* (also called *ḍiṇḍi mạric*, *ḍiṇḍi* being their name for the boll of cotton); *dimbo mạric*, Capsicum grossum *Willd.*, or Capsicum cerasiforme *Lamk.*; *sakwa mạric*, lit. horn pepper, Capsicum frutescens *Linn.*, so named from its long pods; *siṅghin mạric*, lit. spiny pepper, botanically the same as the *sakwa mạric*, but so named from the pods

---

[1] Bengali *Bherenda*—*Ed.*
[2] Bengali *Nim*—*Ed.*
[3] Bengali *Peãj*—*Ed.*
[4] Bengali *Rasun*—*Ed.*
[5] Bengali *Marich*—*Ed.*

growing upwards; another name for the same is *sim saba mạric*, lit. fowl spur pepper, also *suruj mukhi mạric*, the sun-flower pepper. All the above varieties are cultivated by the Santals and used in preparing curry. Often these are also eaten like chillies. Besides the varieties mentioned they have *gol maric*[1], lit. round pepper, Cayenne pepper, that is used in their curry, but not cultivated by the Santals. They have two other names for the same, *sạnthi mạric* and *sạńci mạric*.

Buluṅ, salt. They have: *Biṭ buluṅ*, a factitious salt containing sulphur; *hẽndẽ buluṅ*, black salt; *paṅga buluṅ*, a white salt. Many Santals know how to make *hẽndẽ buluṅ* into white salt. It might be mentioned that they call an arsenical stuff used for preserving hides *harta buluṅ*, lit. hide-salt; this is naturally not used by the Santals, except when supplied to them by those who buy the hides. In former times the Santals are said to have produced a kind of salt. A Santal has given me this description of the process: In rice-fields or in low-lying spots in forests saline clayish soil that had cropped up, whitish in colour, looking like the leavings of earth-worms was occasionally discovered. This was collected by means of a broom or with their hands. Any stones or grass were removed. Pouring water in an earthenware pot in which the soil was kept they boiled it and then took it off the fire and allowed it to cool. This was to remove all dirt and extraneous matter. This water was then poured into a cooking vessel, and the whole was boiled, until nearly all the water had evaporated. The vessel was then removed from the fire, and the salt deposit obtained. Salt produced in this way was not like the salt bought nowadays. It was not tasty but had a disagreeable flavour.

In preparing *utu*, curry, they use a number of spices, *mọsọla*[2], of which some are called *gọrọm mọsọla*[3], i.e., hot, pungent spices. The following are in constant use: *Adhẹ*[4], Ginger, Zingiber officinale *Roscoe*, cultivated by the Santals; *dar cini*[5], cinnamon, the bark of Cinamomum Tamala *Nees & Eberne.* (or of other cinnamon trees) bought in the shops; *dhạnią*[6], Coriander seed, Coriandrum sativum *Linn.* (name adopted from Hindi); *elaci*, Cardamoms, Alpinia Cardamomum *Roxb.* (name through Bengali from Persian); *jirą*[7], Cummin, Cumimum Cyminum *Linn.* (name from Hindi); *kạlią jirą*[8], Nigella sativa *L.* (the name is from Hindi); *loṅphul*, Cloves, Eugenia caryophyllaea *Willd.* (name adopted from Bengali). With the exception of *Adhẹ*, Ginger, Zingiber officinale *Roscoe*, the plants of these spices are unknown to the Santals and are not grown by them and they buy the spices from the shops.

LEAVES AND PLANTS.

Let us now turn to what the Santals call *ạṛak*, i.e., leaves, pot-herbs, of plants and bushes and even trees, that are eaten, mostly as curry. Some of these are

---

[1] In Bengali *Gôl Marich* means also Cayenne pepper—*Ed.*

[2] Bengali *Masalâ* means spices—*Ed.*

[3] *Garam Masalâ* in Bengali means cardamom, cinnamon and cloves and together as spices in meat and other curries—*Ed.*

[4] Bengali *Ãdà*—*Ed.* [5] Bengali *Dàrchini*—*Ed.* [6] Bengali *Dhane*—*Ed.*

[7] Bengali *Jeerâ*—*Ed.* [8] Bengali *Kàla Jeerâ*—*Ed.*

cultivated, but most of them are found growing wild. We shall take them in alphabetical order.

Apaṅgir aṛak, lit. eloping vegetable; leaves of a pot-herb found in Assam and on the hills. Not commonly known.

Ạlu aṛak, leaves of the potato plant, used as curry but rare.

Ạtkuṛạ aṛak, the tender leaves of a small forest tree, Wrightia tomentosa *Roem.* et *Schultes*, used in curry. The bark of the stem and the root are used in Santal medicine.

Bambaṛo aṛak (also called *ambaṛo*), the Roselle plant, Hibiscus Sabdariffa *L.* The Santals recognize two varieties, *poṇḍ*, white, and *arak*, red, in accordance with the colour of the stalk and flowers. They are not botanically different. These are commonly cultivated. The flesh of the fruit is used as a curry; the kernel is roasted and ground and used with *matkom laṭhe*, a dough made of the mahua flowers, especially taken along as a food when they go hunting. *Laṭhe* is prepared as follows: The dried mahua is soaked in water and then roasted on a large potsherd. When this is ready it is mixed with one of the following substances: roasted maize, *surguja* (the Niger seed), *tilmiṅ* (the Sesame seed), the seed of hemp or of *bambaṛo*, and finally pounded in the *ḍhiṅki* [1]. When ready it is made into balls and put into leaf-cups. For the annual hunt they take a number of these balls along with them in a large leaf-cup. (It might be mentioned that memsahibs use part of the calyx for making jellies and juice and find it very good for the purpose.) The *bambaṛo* ripens in December.

Banda rukhi aṛak, not known to the writer. *Banda* is the name of parasitical plants, belonging to Loranthaceæ; *rukhi* means a bit.

Baṛe loa, v. *baṛe*.

Bạhu ṭuṭuri aṛak, the leaves of a small plant, Veronica cinerea *Less*, used in curry. The meaning of the name is the head-covering of a bride.

Bạru aṛak, the leaves of Schleichera trijuga *Willd.*, a large forest tree, the tender leaves of which are used in curry. An oil is extracted from the seeds and used in Santal medicine, as also are the bark and root.

Boebindi aṛak, Randia dumetorum *Lam.*, a thorny tree. The leaves are used in curry, the fruit is eaten and the bark and roots used in Santal medicine.

Buc aṛak, the tender leaves of Cordia Myxa *L.*, used in curry. The fruit of the tree is also eaten.

Buṭ aṛak, the leaves of gram, Cicer arietinum *L.* (also called *bhuṭ*), used as curry.

Bhạbri, a shrub or small tree, Embelia robusta *Roxb.* The young shoots are eaten raw.

Bhạtuạ aṛak, the leaves of Chenopodium album *Linn.*, a wild plant, used in curry.

Bhedwa, a plant, Hibiscus cancellatus *Roxb.*, var. fusiformis *Willd.* The tubers are eaten raw, after having been scraped.

---

[1] Bengali *Dhenki*—*Ed.*

Bhorkonḍ aṛak, the leaves of Hymenodictyon excelsum *Wall.*, a forest tree, used in curry. The bark is used medicinally; the wood is used by the Santals for making fiddles, yokes, etc.

Cakaoḍa (or *cakaonḍa*) *aṛak*, the young leaves of Cassia Tora *L.*, a small plant, are used in curry, but are not considered first class.

Catọm aṛak, lit. umbrella vegetable; several plants are so called, and these are used in Santal medicine. One variety is *dak catọm aṛak*, Marsilea quadrifolia *L.* It grows near water and its leaves are used in curry.

Coṭo lutur aṛak, lit. field-mouse-ear vegetable, Ipomæa Pes-tigrides *L.*, a creeper. The fruit is also eaten (i.e., the kernel).

Cọrọ mọkọć aṛak, the leaves of the *bambaṛo*, Hibiscus Sabdariffa *L.*, used in curry.

Cunḍuć aṛak, a small plant, Commelina communis *L.*, used in curry.

Dare japak aṛak, a climber, Scindapsus officinalis *Schott.* The leaves may be used in curry. It is also used in Santal medicine.

Dhurup aṛak, there are two species, one called *ạnḍiạ dhurup aṛak*, a plant, Leucas cephalotes *Spreng.*, the leaves of which are used in curry, but not often, as they are bitter. It is also used in Santal medicine. The other is called *eṅga dhurup aṛak*, a plant, Leucas Clarkei *Hook. f.*; used in curry and considered very savoury, it is also fried wrapped in leaves.

Ḍaṅgra kaṭa aṛak, a wild plant. The leaves used in curry.

Ḍimbu aṛak, a creeper, the leaves of which are used in curry (? Ocimum Basilicum *Linn.*). Two varieties are recognized, one called *baṛge ḍimbu aṛak*, found in the *baṛge*, and one called *họṛ* (or *jọm*) *ḍimbu aṛak*.

Ḍunḍukil aṛak, a forest tree, Gardenia turgida *Roxb.* The leaves are used in curry and the bark in Santal medicine.

Gargạḍi, a grass, Job's tears, Coix Lacryma-Jobi *L.* Eaten in times of scarcity.

Gạndhạri aṛak, Amaranthus gangeticus *Linn.*; commonly cultivated, and used in curry. They recognize these varieties: *Arak* (red) *gạndhạri*, *dare* (tree, i.e., high) *gạndhạri* and *eḍhẹ* (low, with branches down to the ground) *gạndhạri*.

Gạrunḍi aṛak, a plant found growing in rice-fields and moist ground. The leaves are used in curry, as a rule together with *dạl*, split peas. Too much of it is said to cause diarrhoea. The botanical name is Aeternanthera sessilis *R.Br.*

Sā̃ṛī hataṅ, lit. monkey-brain, Ampelocissus tomentosa *Planch.* The shoots are eaten to quench thirst during the hot season. Also called *buru ghoṛa lada* (or *lạdạnri*).

Gitil aṛak, lit. sand vegetable, Leucas mollissima *Wall.* The leaves are eaten boiled, in times of scarcity.

Hasa aṛak, a plant, a Ruellia. Used in curry.

Hạpuk aṛak, a small plant. The leaves are eaten as curry.

Hemea aṛak, the *dak* h.a. variety, a plant, Enhydra fluctuans *Lour.* The shoots are roasted in leaves and eaten.

Hendasạri aṛak, the same as *boebindi*, q.v.

Hesak aṛak, the tender leaves of Ficus religiosa *L.* Used in curry with *dạl*, split peas, it is also roasted and cooked together with rice.

Huṛ huṛa̜ a̜ṛak, a plant (also called *seta kaṭa*). The Santals recognize two varieties: *a̜ṇḍia̜ huṛ huṛa̜*, that has red flowers and is not eaten, and *eṅga huṛ huṛa̜*, Cleome viscosa *L.*, that has white flowers, the leaves of which are eaten in curry.

Ica̜k aṛak, a wild pot-herb, Pouzalzia pentandra *Benn.*

Ja̜num aṛak, a thorny plant, Amaranthus spinosus *Linn.* The leaves are used in curry and considered excellent. The fruit of the *ja̜num* tree (Zizyphus Jujuba *Lam.*) will be mentioned later.

Jo̜rmo̜ṭ aṛak, lit. violence vegetable, Verbescum Thaspus *L.*; the leaves are eaten in curry, when there is a scarcity of food.

Jhiṅga̜ aṛak, the leaves of *jhiṅga̜*, q.v., used in curry.

Jhiṅgur, a plant, Amorphophalus lyratus *Kunth.* This is eaten, but it must be well boiled and cleaned, otherwise it is considered poisonous.

Jhun jhunia̜ aṛak, the leaves of Crotalaria calycina *Shrank.*, so named from the rattling sound of its pods. This plant is also called *bir jhunku̜*.

Kacan aṛak, the leaves of *karla*, q.v., used as curry.

Kana aṛak, Commelina benghalensis *Linn.* Used in curry with *da̜l*, split peas; but as this is often difficult, it is sometimes eaten roasted or cooked into a hash with rice.

Kantha aṛak a common wild plant, Euphorbia granulata *Forsk.* The leaves and the whole plant are crushed in a mortar, before being prepared for curry. This is greatly relished.

Kedok aṛak, lit. supper vegetable, a creeper, Argyreia speciosa *Sweet.* This is sweet and is used as curry.

Kohn̥ḍa aṛak, v. *kohn̥ḍa*. Generally eaten as curry with *da̜l*, or with fish, it is also roasted.

Kubi aṛak, Cabbage. Any form of this eaten, when they can get it.

Kundri aṛak, v. *kundri*.

Kuṛbi (or *kuṛmbi*) *aṛak*, a plant, used as curry.

Loa aṛak, lit. fig vegetable; the unripe fruits of the tree, Ficus glomerata *Roxb.*, are gathered and steamed, and when dried pounded in a mortar. A small vessel is heated and some oil poured in; when this is boiling the figs are thrown in, and salt and spices added. When ready this is eaten as curry.

Lo̜po̜ṅ aṛak, a plant, Ærua lanata *Juss.* This is baked with flour and eaten, specially valuable as a medicine.

Makaṛkenda aṛak, the tender leaves of a forest tree, Diospyros Embryopteris *Persoon*, are used as curry. The fruit is also eaten.

Malhan aṛak, v. *malhan*.

Matko̜m aṛak, a plant, Hygrophila angustifolia (R.Br.) *Nees.* Used as curry.

Maṭha aṛak, the leaves of a small deciduous tree, Antidesma diandrum *Roth.*, used as curry with *da̜l*, it is also roasted or cooked into a hash with rice.

Me̜ro̜m cuṅci, a plant; the tubers are eaten raw.

Mo̜ro̜n aṛak, lit. death vegetable. The Santals recognize two varieties: *a̜ṇḍia̜ mo̜ro̜n aṛak*, Gymnema hirsutum *W. & A.*, var. Decaisneanum *Wight.* of which the leaves and fruits are eaten raw, and the *eṅga moṛọn aṛak*, of which the leaves and flowers are eaten, also without boiling.

Muć aṛak, lit. ant vegetable, a plant, Polygonum plebejum *Br.* The whole plant (except the roots) is eaten as curry. Too much of this is said to cause diarrhoea.

Mulạ[1] *aṛak*, the leaves of the radish, used as curry. The Santals distinguish the cultivated radish (called *ato mulạ*, Raphanus sativus *L.*) from the wild variety called *bir* (or *dud*, or *ṭaṇḍi*) *mulạ*. These are also eaten raw.

Mungạ aṛak, the leaves of the Horse-radish tree, Moringa pterygosperma *Gaertn.*, =Moringa olcifera *Lam.*, eaten in curry, with *dạl*, they are also roasted or cooked into a hash with rice. The *mungạ* tree is one of the few trees that are commonly planted. Besides the leaves the flowers and fruits also are eaten. It has many other uses. The bark, crushed and moistened, is used as a remedy against headache. When the bark is crushed, mixed with water and poured into a snake's hole it is said that it will drive out the snake. The root is crushed, mixed with *jọ̃ti* grass and then thrown into water to poison the fish.

Olaṅ mocaṅ aṛak, lit. voracious vegetable; the leaves are used as curry.

Onol aṛak, lit. wattle-wall vegetable, a small plant, eaten raw or as curry.

Oṛsa (or *ọṛsa*) *aṛak*, a plant having white flowers. The leaves eaten as curry.

Ọhọć aṛak, lit. potsherd vegetable. The leaves of this small creeper, Boerhaavia diffusa *L.*, are eaten as curry. The root is used medicinally.

Palaṅ (also called *palọṅ*) *aṛak*, Beta benghalensis *Roxb.* (or, Beta vulgaris *Linn.*). It is cultivated, but only rarely by Santals.

Paṭ aṛak, plant, Corchorus olitorius *Linn.* and Corchorus capsularis *Linn.* Cultivated. The leaves and shoots are used in curry.

Piṭuạ aṛak, a plant, Spermacoce hispida *K. Schum.* This is eaten as curry in times of scarcity. The plant is also called *piṭuạ ghãs* and *ṭaṇḍi piṭuạ*.

Purại aṛak, a twining plant, Basella rubra *Linn.* The whole plant is used as curry. They distinguish two varieties: *Moṭa purại*, having large leaves, and *nanha* (or *kaṭić*) *purại*, having small leaves.

Rọṭẹ capal aṛak, an aquatic plant, Ottelia alismoides *Pers.*

Rọṭẹ capal, another aquatic plant, also called *cala bulạ*.

Sạru aṛak, the leaves of *sạru*, q.v., used as curry.

Sạuṛi aṛak, a plant, Polygonum glabrum *Willd.* Eaten in curry.

Seta kaṭa aṛak, lit. dog-leg vegetable, a plant, Gynandropsis pentaphylla *DC.* The leaf-buds are eaten boiled or in curry.

Siṅ aṛak, lit. day (or sun) vegetable, a tree, Bauhinia variegata *L.* (possibly also B. purpurea *L.* is so named). The young shoots are eaten as curry, but are said to cause loose stools. Also they are eaten as curry with *dạl*, or roasted or cooked as a hash with rice.

Sirgeṭi (or *sirgiṭ*) *aṛak*, a plant, Celosia argentea *Linn.* The leaves are eaten as curry.

---

[1] Bengali *Mulā*—*Ed.*

Tabẹn aṛak, a plant found especially in rice-fields. This is eaten as curry, mostly with *dạl*, split peas.

Tagol aṛak, a plant, Gnaphalium indicum *L.* Eaten as curry.

Toa aṛak, a plant, eaten as curry. So named from the juice which exudes when the plant is broken, and which looks like milk.

Tuṛi aṛak, the leaves of the *tuṛi*, Brassica campestris *L.*, eaten as curry.

Ṭhuiạk aṛak, a plant, Melochia corchorifolia *Linn.* The leaves and buds are eaten as curry.

Ulić alaṅ aṛak, a small plant, Portulaca oleracea *L.* Eaten as curry and much relished.

To gather wild vegetables and leaves is the work of women. When going to the forest, they will not go alone, for several reasons, but always in a body at the time agreed upon. When entering the forest, also when they start plucking, a kind of invocation is made:—'Be quiet in the row, be quiet in the rows; I have put my babe in the niche and left it there; may the eyes of those who have seen me leaving burst, be squeezed out; may I quickly find; my child will cry; may I quickly return; may my basket be filled, be filled to overflowing'.

On returning from the forest they arrange at once for the food to be cooked. They give the leaves and vegetables, the mushrooms, and whatever else they may have found, over to the cooking woman, after having cleaned them. The cook takes a little in her hand, and waving it over the fireplace and the cooking vessel she says: 'May a spell be thrown on it; may it get warm!' Thereupon she throws what she has in her hand into the fireplace through the front opening.

In connexion with the use of vegetables by the Santals the following is of interest. They warn people not to eat any amount of vegetables, as too much will be bad for the stomach by causing loose bowels. Vegetables, they say, are not for those who eat for satisfaction, but are the poor man's food. Well-to-do Santals, however, will also eat vegetables to avoid being called haughty (according to Santal ideas).

Besides the ordinary curry (*utu*) they have two other ways of cooking their food. One is called *kohṛa*, a kind of frying or roasting. The food is placed in a pot, with salt and spices added, if they have any. The pot is then put on the fire and whilst the contents are being cooked they are stirred with a ladle. When ready it may be eaten alone or together with *dạl*, split peas, i.e., with curry of split peas (or any pulse so prepared).

Another way is what is called *suṛe*, i.e., as a hash of the foodstuffs cooked together with rice.

A Santal once expressed himself thus:—'Vegetables are mostly eaten *kohṛate*, i.e., prepared by frying or roasting. During the "poor", "hunger" times (i.e., when there is a scarcity of food) we eat one cup (*bokak*, the shell of a gourd, *hoṭol*, cut in two and used as a cup) of rice-gruel and one leaf-plate of vegetables; in this way we manage to live. During "hunger" time we are not able to procure salt, or only a very little. Parents will often say to the children: "Listen, little ones, don't plunge salt in the rice-gruel; it will not be properly seasoned, if you do. Just put in a pinch". In this way they economize.'

MUSHROOMS.

Especially during the rainy season mushrooms are much in evidence. The Santals have an idea that thunder causes the fungi to sprout cf. M. A. Henry, 'Scientific American', vol. 124, No. 16, April 16, 1921, p. 318, where he has shown that continual discharges of artificial 'lightning' produced by a large static machine caused a very marked effect on speed of growth and size of the cultivated mushrooms. This experiment thus confirms the Santals' popular belief. The edible mushrooms are much used in curry, and some of them are very much relished. The Santals somehow have no difficulty in distinguishing the edible from the poisonous varieties. The writer has never heard of a Santal having eaten poisonous mushrooms. This may be accidental; but on the other hand he has heard of cattle having died from eating such.

Here follows a list of the varieties of mushrooms eaten by the Santals. The probable botanical names are given side by side.

Biṅ ol, snake mushroom (so named from shape) (*Lepiota mastoides* probably).

Bunum ol, lit. white-anthill mushroom (*Entoloma macro-carpum*); so called because it is found on white-anthills. Considered delicious.

Busuṗ ol, lit. straw mushroom (*Volvaria terastrius*); found growing on old, often decayed, straw. Considered good.

Dak mạṇḍi ol, lit. rice-gruel mushroom. Considered savoury (*Entoloma micro-carpum*).

Gopha ol, a very large kind of edible mushroom (*Collybia albuminosa*).

Guṇḍri gopha ol, a mushroom, said to be intoxicating, but sometimes eaten (a var. of *Collybia albuminosa*).

Hasa ol, lit. earth mushroom. Eaten boiled. Found in Asāṛ and Bhador (*Agaricus campestris*).

Hạti ol, lit. elephant mushroom (*Boletus sp.*), large, bad smelling. Rare, said to be eaten only by old people.

Hurul ol, lit. tree-stump mushroom. Eaten boiled. There are two species: *Sisir hurul ol*, lit. dew tree-stump mushroom, also called simply *sisir ol*, found after the rains have ceased; and *poṇḍ ol*, lit. white mushroom (*Lentinus subnudus*), found during the rains. Both are eaten boiled.

Kaṭ ol, lit. wood mushroom, found growing on tree-stumps (*Pleurotus ostreatus*).

Kạṛnạ ol, lit. bitter mushroom (*Puff-ball*); name due to the taste. Eaten raw or as curry. Found in Bhador.

Kạṛnạ paṭka ol, v. *paṭka ol*. (Var. of *puff-ball*).

Kod ol, so called on account of its black colour, resembling the fruit of the *kod*, Eugenia Jambolana *Lam.* (*Coprinus comatus*).

Mat ol, lit. bamboo mushroom (*Collybia sp.*), because it is found growing on stumps of the hill bamboo. Considered very savoury.

Motam ol. Besides being eaten as an ordinary food, it is given to persons suffering from smallpox, because it is believed to bring out the eruption. (Var. of *Collybia albuminosa*).

Muci ol, lit. the Muchi's mushroom (a var. of *Entoloma micro-carpum*).

Murum ol; this is taboo to Santals of the Murmu sept. Possibly so named owing to its colour, as *murum* means reddish. The Santals connect the name with the name of the sept. (*Clavaria sp.*).

Ọr tol ol, lit. pulled out mushroom, so called, because the whole of the mushroom (rooting *Collybia albuminosa*) is pulled out of the ground. Found in abundance in July and August. It is eaten raw or boiled in oil as curry. The Santals consider this one of the finest varieties.

Ọtẹc ol, lit. burst open mushroom (var. of *Collybia albuminosa*). It is white in colour, and commonly found in August. It is eaten as curry, but sometimes also raw, though it is then somewhat pungent in taste.

Paṭka ol, (*Puff-ball*) growing together with *kaṛnạ ol*, possibly the same, but of a different colour.

Piskạ ol, not poisonous, but it has a bitter taste, and is therefore not commonly eaten.

Bonḍ kaṭ ol, lit. white wood mushroom, a variety of *kaṭ ol* (*Pleurotus sp.*).

Ponḍ tormaṛ ol, a whitish variety of the *tormaṛ ol*, q.v. (a var. of the *Geaster*).

Puṭkạ, the puff-ball, a fungus of the *Lycoperdaceæ*. The Santals recognize the following edible varieties: *Ẹrok puṭkạ*, lit. sow puff-ball, so called because it appears at sowing time, earlier than the other *puṭkạ* it is also called *hoṛ puṭkạ*, *Lycoperdon giganteum*, *Calvatia sp.*, *Geaster sp.*, lit. man puff-ball, and *ruhni puṭkạ*, because it may be gathered during *ruhni*; *rọṭẹ puṭkạ*, lit. frog puff-ball, a small kind; *seta puṭkạ*, lit. dog puff-ball (*Truffle*) which has a rough surface. The Santals very much relish eating these naturally in their early stage of growth. It is curious that the Santals regard the puff-balls as animate, as shown by their language.

Rọṭẹ ol, lit. frog mushroom. (Small puff-ball).

Sagak ol, lit. awn mushroom (mentioned by Dr. Campbell).

Seta ol, lit. dog mushroom; the same as *seta puṭkạ*, q.v., the commonly used name. (*Truffle*).

Sim ol, lit. fowl mushroom, reddish in colour. (*Cantharellus aurantiacus*).

Sisir ol, lit. dew mushroom, found growing on stumps of the *Sal* tree (*Lentinus subnudus*).

Tormaṛ ol. Eaten, but not very common. (*Geaster sp.*).

Tumbạ ol, lit. gourd-shell mushroom, of a large round shape. (*Bovista gigentia*).

As regards mushrooms a Santal writes: 'Mushrooms sprout from decayed leaves or straw, and from white-anthills and cow-dung. We boil them in oil adding spices, add a little *rase*, sauce, soup, and eat them. Sometimes we also make a hash of them, cooking them with rice. A few kinds we also eat raw.'

RESINS.

We will now consider the kinds of food obtained by the Santals from trees, fruits, resins, etc., which are used either in the form of curry or in the raw natural state.

Amongst the resins, i.e., exudations from trees, called by the Santals, *jer*, the following may be noted:—

Atnak jer, the exudation of Terminalia tomentosa *W. & A.*=T. alata *Heyne* ex *Roth.*

Ḍoka jer, the exudation of Odina Wodier *Roxb.*

Hesel jer, the exudation of Anogeissus latifolia *Wall.*

Hopo jer, the exudation of Cochlospermum Gossypium (L) *DC.*

Lopon jer, the exudation of Terminalia bellerica *Roxb.* The gum is eaten together with the edible part of the marking nut (*soso*, Semecarpus Anacardium *L.f.*) and is said to be very sweet.

Tarop jer, the exudation of Buchanania latifolia *Roxb.*=B. Lanzan *Spreng.*

Terel jer, the exudation of Diospyros tomentosa *Roxb.*

All these are eaten raw. A Santal once said: 'We eat resin whenever we find it. Those who love children will take some home to give to them'.

FRUITS.

The names of the trees or climbers whose fruits are eaten, are given in alphabetical order.

Ambṛa [1], the Hog-plum, Spondias mangifera *Willd.* The fruit is eaten raw or cooked when used with curry it gives this an acid flavour. The panicles and the tender leaves are also eaten raw or with curry. This refers to the planted tree (called *ato ambṛa*, village Hog-plum; and not to the wild, *bir ambṛa*, that is not used for food, being far too bitter).

Amrit [2], the Papaw tree, Carica Papaya *L.* (Also called *ambrit.*) The fruit is excellent.

Amrud (or *amrut*; or *amsophori*, the most common Santal name), the Guava tree, Psidium Guajava *Linn.* Very common.

Bakṛe, the flesh of the *kũiṇḍi*, rind included; v. *matkom.* Said to have a good taste when roasted.

Baṛe, the Banyan tree, Ficus bengalensis *L.*

Bad janum, v. *janum.*

Bai bindi, v. *boi bindi.*

Barsa pakoṛ, a small bush, Grewia sapida *Roxb.* (also Grewia Campbellii *Watt.*).

Baru, Schleichera trijuga *Willd.* Oil is obtained from the seed.

Boi bindi, Randia dumetorum *Lam.* The ripe fruit is eaten; and the leaves are used in curry.

Bhadu, Vitex altissima *L.f.* The Santals distinguish between *buru bhadu*, hill *bhadu*, and *gada bhadu*, river *bhadu.* The fruit of both is eaten.

---

[1] Bengali āmṛā—*Ed.*

[2] *Amrita* in Sanskrit means nectar—*Ed.*

Dan banda, several parasitic shrubs, belonging to Loranthacea.

Ḍabha, the Shaddock tree or Pomelo, Citrus decumana *Linn.* Rare amongst the Santals. The fruit is excellent.

Ḍahu, Artocarpus Lakoocha *Roxb.*, generally found wild, but it is also planted. The fruit is eaten and the flowers sucked by children.

Ḍiḍhauṛi, the planted *janum*, q.v. The fruit is much relished.

Dunḍukil, Gardenia turgida *Roxb.* The fruit and the bark are used medicinally.

Ḍhela, Alangium salviifolium (L.f.) *Wenger.* The fruit is eaten. The bark is used in medicine.

Edel, the Cotton tree, Bombax malabaricum *DC.* The calix is eaten together with steamed Mahua. The tender fruit is eaten as curry. The roots are crushed and given as a drink with the scum of boiled sugarcane or sugar. This is especially eaten in times of scarcity.

Guḍu lerel, Diospyros montana *Roxb.* Fruit eaten.

Gua, the Betel Palm, Areca Catechu *L.* Nut used by a few, imitating the Dekos.

Ghoṛa lada (or *ladanri*), climbers, *buru* l.gh. Ampelocissus tomentosa *Planch.* The fruits are eaten to quench thirst in the hot season.

Hesak, the Pipal, Ficus religiosa *L.* The tender leaves are used as curry. The fruit may be eaten. They say about eloping people, that they have gone to eat Pipal fruit. Another expression is: *hesak sakam lekan hoṛ*, a person like a Pipal leaf, i.e., one who is a coward, or who always changes his mind. The leaves are large with a long slender petiole and are turned by the slightest breeze.

Icak, a shrub, Woodfordia fruticosa (L) *Kurz.* The flowers are sucked, as they contain much honey.

Jambir, the Citron tree, Citrus acida *Roxb.* The fruit is eaten. Cultivated. They also have the wild Citrus medica *L.*

Janum, lit. thorn, Zizyphus Jujuba *Lam.*, both wild and cultivated. The fruit is much relished. They distinguish several varieties of the wild bush: *Jom janum*, lit. eaten thorn, which is called *bad janum*, when ripening in Aghaṛ, and *baihaṛ janum*, when ripening in Pus and Magh. One variety is called *edhe janum*, a small bushform with low-spreading branches. This is also called *toyo janum*, lit. jackal thorn, because jackals eat the fruit. *Ḍiḍhauṛi janum* is the same when cultivated and has larger fruits. The ripe fruit may be dried and pounded, and used in curry or in drinks.

Jojo, the Tamarind, Tamarindus indica *L.*, very common in Santal villages. The ripe fruit is eaten. Taken with warm water it acts as a laxative. The inspissated juice of the fruit is used in curry. The leaves are dried, pounded and eaten in gruel or with curry.

Jhiṅjiṭ, a tree, Bauhinia retusa *Roxb.* The fresh leaves are chewed to quench thirst.

Kadam, Anthocephalus Cadamba *Miq.*=A. indicus *Rich.* The fruit of this large tree is eaten raw, as well as in curry.

Kaera, the Plantain, has already been mentioned.

Kanthaṛ[1], the Jack tree, Artocarpus integrifolia *L*. Very commonly cultivated. The fruit is commonly eaten, but is forbidden to people suffering from certain diseases. The wood does not crack, and is therefore used for making drums and other articles.

Kãṛwat, a large shrub, Carissa Carandas *L.* The fruit is eaten.

Kạri, a large climbing shrub, Erycibe paniculata *Roxb.* The fruit is eaten. It is also called, *kạri dare, kạri jhạuạ, kạri jhõṇḍ* and *kạri nạ̃ṛī*, according to the shape.

Kiṭạ, Phoenix acaulis *Ham.* The fruit is eaten.

Kod, the Jam, Eugenia cumini *Druce.* The fruit is eaten. They recognize the following varieties of the wild tree: *Cuḍuk kod*, having small round fruits; *gaḍa kod* lit. river Jam, growing near rivers; and *seta kod*, lit. dog Jam, having (according to Dr. Campbell) small astringent fruits. The cultivated *kod* is called *sọ*, q.v.

Korkoṭ, a tree, Dillenia indica *L.* The flesh and the leaves of the calyx surrounding the ripe fruit are eaten raw or cooked together with mahua flowers.

Kũiṇḍi, the fruit of *matkọm*, q.v.

Kurse, a creeper, Mucuna pruriens *DC.* The fruit is eaten together with mahua flowers.

Kuṛit rama, lit. kite talons (so named from the hooked talon-like form of the thorns), Zizyphus Oenoplia *Mill.* The fruit is eaten.

Khijur[2], the wild Date tree, Phoenix sylvestris *Roxb.* The fruit is eaten. A juice is extracted from near the top of the tree and this is fermented into a kind of toddy and drunk. It is also used for yeast.

Khiṛuạ[3], water melon, Citrullus vulgaris *Schrad.*

Lamak jaṅ, the kernels of the pods of *jọm laṛ*, Bauhinia Vahlii *W. & A.*, gigantic climber. The kernels are eaten roasted. This climber is much used. Its fibre is used for bowstrings, halters, slings, etc. and from the leaves they make waterproofs, (used, when pulling out paddy seedlings), also leaf-plates and leaf-cups.

Lẹmbọ, the Lime tree and its fruit, Cirtus medica *L.* (also called *nẹmbọ* and *nimbu*).

Loa, the Fig tree and its fruit, Ficus glomerata *Roxb.* The ripe fruit is naturally a common form of food. As regards the curry made from the unripe fruit, v. *loa aṛak*.

Makaṛkenda, a forest tree, Diospyros Embryopteris *Persoon.* The fruit is eaten raw, the tender leaves are used for curry, and the juice of the ripe fruit is used as a gum.

Mandaṛgọm, the Custard apple, Anona squamosa *L.* and Anona reticulata *L.* The fruit is eaten raw when ripe. Before ripening the fruit is boiled and eaten.

Matkọm, a large tree, Bassia latifolia *Roxb.* and Diploknema butyracea (Roxb.) *Lamk.* (The latter is very rare, but otherwise is treated like the commoner one.) The *matkọm* or Mahua is found widely spread throughout the country, and each tree is allotted to one of the tenants of the village. It is a tree of the greatest importance to the people. The corolla of its flowers falls at the commencement of the hot season,

---

1 Bengali *Kānthāl—Ed.*

2 Bengali *Khejur—Ed.*

3 From *Khirā* in Hindi meaning cucumber—*Ed.*

before the fresh leaves come out. The ground at the foot of the tree may be quite covered by these corollas that are picked up and dried. When dry they are beaten with a stick to remove the *matkọm sọhọe*, the stamens of the flower. The dried corollas are used for food boiled, roasted or parched, alone or together with other foodstuffs (especially pulses). At the commencement of the rainy season this is for many their only daily food. Of the dried corollas they prepare what is called *lathẹ*, a kind of dough. They soak the dried Mahua in water and then roast it on a potsherd. When properly roasted, they mix it with roasted maize, *surguja* (Niger seed), sesame seed (*tilmiṅ*), the seed of the Roselle plant (*bambaṛo*) or hemp (naturally only one of these) and pound it in the *ḍhiṅki*. It is then made into balls and taken along as food when away from home, e.g., on the annual hunt. The Mahua is very sweet and is also used in the distillation of country liquor, both by the authorities and those who distil illicitly. The fruit is called *kũiṇḍi*, that has already been mentioned.

Mat, bamboo. There are several varieties. The common wild bamboo is Dendrocalamus strictus *Nees*. The seed of the bamboo, resembling wheat, is cooked and eaten. The young shoots are also used for food. The Santals take a foot or two of this (called *helta*) and slice it, grind it in a mortar, and put it in an earthenware pot, that is covered, and allowed to stand for two or three days. It is then taken out and spread on a mat or a flat stone and dried in the sun. This is called *haṇḍuạ*, and may be kept for months in pots. It may be eaten raw with salt or be made into curry; in the latter case it is generally cooked with spices in *ạṛic̆ dak maṇḍi*. It is now a very rare article of food, as Government have forbidden them to gather *helta* in the forests. It might further be mentioned, that the bamboo flowers after very long intervals, one whole cluster at the same time, the whole cluster thereupon dying. None of the other varieties have been mentioned here, as they are practically all cultivated and used, not for food, but for a number of other purposes.

Maṭha suṛạ, a small tree, Antidesma Ghesaembilla *Gaertn*. The fruit is eaten, also the fresh leaf-buds. It is also called *maṭha suṛạ*.

Mẹrlẹc̆, a tree, Flacourtia indica (Burmf.) *Merrill*. The fruit is eaten and the bark used in Santal medicine.

Mungạ, the Horse-radish tree, Moringa olcifera *Lamk.*, v. *mungạ aṛak*, where the tree has been described.

Murup' (also *Murut*), a tree, Butea frondosa *Roxb*. The flowers are sucked as they contain honey.

Nạrkọr, Cocos nucifera *L*. Sometimes found cultivated but does not bear fruit in the country. The cocoanut is eaten and the shell used as a hookah bowl.

Nim, a tree, Azadirachta indica *Juss*. Common. The leaves are used in gruel, and this is considered a tonic. At the name-giving festival *nim dak maṇḍi* is always used; it is further customary to drink *nim dak maṇḍi*, when the sower comes home after having sown the first paddy; all of the household drink this, it is believed that then the ears will be bitter, so that flies will not "drink" them. It is also used as a remedy against certain stomach troubles, especially worms.

Nũṛũc, the Indian Laburnum, Cassia Fistula *L.* The flowers are eaten in curry and the fruit is used in Santal medicine.

Olat, there are two trees so called, *jaṅ olat*, Grewia asiatica *L.* and *poska olat*, Kydia calycina *Roxb.* Dr. Campbell mentions also simply *olat* as the Santal name of Grewia vestita *Wall.* and of Grewia tiliæfolia *Vahl*, not known in the Santal Parganas.

Ọmẹ, a large forest tree, Saccopetalum tomentosum *H.f. & Th.* (According to Dr. Campbell, Miliusa velutina *H.f. & Ths.*) They have *hoṛ ọmẹ*, lit. man *ọmẹ*, Saccopetalum longiflorum *H.f. & Th.*, and *seta ọmẹ*, Saccopetalum tomentosum *H.f. & Th.* The fruit of both is eaten.

Pakaṛe, Ficus infectoria *Roxb.* The fruit is eaten.

Papitạ, the same as *ạmrit*, g.v.

Piṇḍe, a small tree, Randia uliginosa *DC.* The unripe fruit is cooked and eaten in curry or with Mahua.

Pọḍọ, two varieties: *hoṛ pọḍọ*, Ficus Cunia *Ham.* the fruit of which is eaten, and *seta pọḍọ*, dog *pọḍọ*, Ficus hispida *Linn.* fil., which is not used as food.

Pọ̃pṛọ̃, a tree, Gardenia latifolia *Aiton.* The fruit is eaten. Bells are made from the wood, and give a good sound.

Sahar, a tree, Dillenia pentagyna *Roxb.* The fruit is used as a condiment in curry. The bark is used in Santal medicine.

Sarjọm, the Sal tree, Shorea robusta *Gaertn.* The most common tree found in the forests, where the Santals live. It must be found in their sacred grove. The fruit is eaten. Parts of it are used in Santal medicine.

Sekra, a small tree, Zizyphus rugosa *Lam.* The fruit is eaten and the bark has medicinal properties.

Seta ãṇḍga, a small bush, Grewia pilosa *Lam.* (or Grewia polygama *Roxb.*). The fruit is eaten, and the roots are used in Santal medicine. Besides *seta ãṇḍga* (lit. dog scrotum) the following names are used for the same bush: *seta ãṇḍir*, *seta ãṛga*, *seta kaṭa* and *seta peska*.

Siṅjọ, the Bael, Ægle Marmelos *Correa.* Commonly grows wild but is also cultivated. The fruit of the cultivated variety is much larger than that of the wild one. The fruit is excellent as a sherbet, and is much esteemed as a specific in stomach disorders (such as dysentery). The leaves, bark and roots are used in Santal medicine.

Sọ, the Black Plum tree, Eugenia cumini *Druce.* Generally cultivated but it is also found wild (v. *kod*). The fruit is eaten and is very good. The juice of the fruit is squeezed out and used as a medicine.

Sọsọ, the Marking Nut tree, Semecarpus Anacardium *L.f.* The orange coloured hypocarp is eaten. An oil is distilled from the drupe that is much used in Santal medicine as a vesicant for animals. The drupe (*sọsọ jaṅ*) is also widely used as a vesicant against pain for human beings. When the oil is daubed round the stems of trees on which silkworms are feeding, it acts as a preventative against climbing ants.

Sunum jhor, Ficus Rumphii *Bl.* The fruit is eaten. Not common.

Tale [1], the Palmyra palm, Borassus flabelliformis *Murr.*, the most common palm in the Santal country, planted on embankments, boundaries, and so on. The fruit is eaten, and the pulp, when the fruit is ripe. The seeds are eaten by children, the hard shells of these being used for bells hung on goats. A sweet sap runs from the peduncles that are cut before flowering. The sap is collected in pots and fermented into toddy. The wood is used and the leaves are utilised for many purposes (thatch, umbrellas, rain-hats, etc.).

Taroṗ, a tree, Buchanania Lanzan *Spr.* The fruit is eaten.

Terel, the Ebony tree, Diospyros tomentosa *Roxb.* (or, Diospyros Melanoxylon *Roxb.*). Common. The fruit is eaten. The kernel of the unripe fruit is also taken out, rubbed, washed and eaten. The ripe fruit is further squeezed open, spread, out to dry, and when dry, pounded into a kind of flour, that is mixed with water into a sherbet and drunk.

Tiṅhon, a creeper, Canavalia ensiformis *DC.* The fruit is eaten in curry.

Toinopak, a tree, Eugenia operculata *Roxb.* The fruit is eaten.

Ul, the Mango, Mangifera indica *L.* The excellent fruit is much relished. The unripe fruit is also sliced, the slices being dried in the sun (this is called *amsi* [2], and is a custom adopted from the Hindus) and used as a beverage. The unripe fruit is also used for curry.

Upal baha, the Water Lily, Nymphæa Lotus *Linn.*, Nymphæa rubra *Roxb.* and Nymphæa versicolor *Roxb.* The tuberous root of all these (called *uldha*, and treated as being animate) is eaten both raw and boiled. These and the flowers are also used in Santal medicine.

Poraeni, the Lotus, Nelumbium speciosum *Willd.*=Nelumbo nucifera *Gaertn.* The tender shoots are eaten boiled or in curry, whilst the seeds are eaten raw, roasted or boiled.

In connexion with fruits a few facts may appropriately be given about what the Santals call *rasa* [3], a word used for juice, must and honey, and also for wine (though this is not known to the ordinary Santals). The juice of most fruits or plants is not kept, but is sucked when found, mostly perhaps by children, but also by grown-up people. The following are the most commonly found:

Icak rasa, the juice of the *icak* flowers, Woodfordia fruticosa (L) *Kurz.* This is much relished.

Khijur rasa, the juice of the wild date, Phœnix sylvestris *Roxb.* This is fermented and used as a liquor.

Matkom rasa, the juice of the flowers of the Mahua. The expression is also used of the liquor distilled from the dried mahua flowers.

Murup rasa, the juice of the flowers of the Butea frondosa *Roxb.* Sucked especially by children.

So bele rasa, the juice squeezed out of the fruit of Eugenia cumini *Druce.* is used as a medicine.

---

1 Bengali *Tāl—Ed.*

2 Bengali *āmsi—Ed.*

3 *Rasa* in Bengali means juice—*Ed.*

Tale rasa, the juice or sap of the Palmyra palm, obtained from the out peduncles and used for making toddy.

Ul rasa, the juice of the mango fruit.

Darkha rasa, must or grape-juice, and now, commonly, wine. The Santals have no grapes.

Fowls and Birds.

The Santals eat the flesh of a great variety of birds. Fowls are kept by every Santal family and their flesh is much relished and probably eaten more commonly than any other kind of flesh, especially when fowls are sacrificed to the bongas, or when they wish to give visitors a treat. Fowls and any birds eaten as curry are always cut into small pieces. The Santals always use their fingers when eating, having no spoons or forks; everything, therefore must be cut up into pieces that are easily handled. Eggs of all birds and fowls are boiled and eaten.

So far as is known to the writer the following is a complete list of the birds that may be taken for food. It should be noted that most of the scientific names given are the result of a visit to the Indian Museum in Calcutta where a number of Santals were taken to point out the birds they recognized. Where a query is written, it is intended to show that the Santals were not quite sure whether the bird seen was the one they know, and use as food.

Askal, a kind of partridge, said to live among stones on the hill sides; ? Francolinus vulgaris.

Bãk, the Paddy bird, Heron, Herodias alba. For varieties v. sub *kõk*.

Barǫmąsią, the Green Bulbul, Chloropsis jerdoni. So named from its varied call.

Baṭa, a Quail, Coturnix communis. They recognize a number of varieties of snipe called *baṭa*, viz. :—

- *Bhoṇḍa baṭa*, a fairly large snipe.
- *Dak̓ baṭa*, the Painted snipe, Rostratula capensis, or Totanus glottis.
- *Dhinuąr baṭa*, the Fan-tailed snipe, Capella gallinago gallinago.
- *Guṇḍri baṭa*, small, coloured like a *guṇḍri*, q.v.
- *Kũk̓ baṭa*, middle sized. So named from its call heard at night like *kũk̓ kũk̓*, said to forebode rain.
- *Khedra baṭa*, the smallest snipe known to Santals.
- *Khes baṭa*, a small kind.
- *Laṇḍha baṭa*, a small kind.
- *Ṭiṛuič̓ baṭa* a small kind; its call sounds like *ṭič̓ ṭič̓*.
- *U guṇḍri baṭa*, another name for *dak̓ baṭa*, q.v.

Bẹč̓ bẹḍrẹč̓, a small waterfowl, Nettapus coromandelianus (its call is said to sound something like its name).

Biṅ cẹ̃ṛẹ̃, Iynx torquilla. So named from its long, thin tail. The *laṅtiti* may also be so called.

Bir sim, the Jungle Fowl, Gallus bankiva. Fairly common.

Bǫrǫriṅ, the Indian Magpie, Dendrocitta vagabunda. So named from its call.

Bhąlųą, the Swallow. The Santals distinguish:

Kaṭić bhaluạ, the Palm-roof Swift, Collocalia fuciphaga, or Cypselus infumatus.

Laṭu bhaluạ, the common Indian Crested Swift, Macropteryx coronata.

Buru bhaluạ, Hill swallow; known, but not seen in the country.

Cama canọp (or *cama cakọr*), two birds are so called, viz., Anthracoceros coronatus and Lophoceros birostris.

Cạńcir, several birds are so called:

Care (or *cạri*) *cạńcir*, the Forest Wagtail, Dendronanthus indicus.

Cirhọć cạncir, the Titlark, Anthus rufulus (so named from its call, which sounds like *cirhọć*).

Dak cạńcir, the Deccan Wagtail, Motacilla dukhunensis, or M. leucopsis. Feeds near water.

Dhạkuć cạńcir and *Gạda cạńcir*, other names for *Dak cạńcir*.

Gại cạńcir, the wagtail, Motacilla flava.

Ṭạndi cạńcir, a species of Wagtail.

Cirhọć, the same as *Cirhọć cạńcir*, v. supra.

Ciṛić cọṛọń, a sparrow-like bird.

Citri, a Partridge. The Santals distinguish:

Kẹṛọ citri, the Grey Partridge, Francolinus pondicerianus.

Muṇḍhạl citri, the Black Partridge, Francolinus vulgaris.

Dak baṭa, v. sub *Baṭa*.

Dak sim, the Cormorant, Phalacrocorax javanicus (or P. fuscicollis). The feathers of the tail and neck of this bird, tied to a piece of bamboo to form a kind of tuft, are stuck into the hairknot or turban of men dancing at marriages or at the Pata festival, are believed to be a safe preventative against *ban pạthri*, sudden illness, caused by witches, or swooning.

Dundu, an Owl. The Santals distinguish:

Kẹ dundu, a small owl, so named on account of its call *kẹ kẹ*.

Khedra (or *kheṛra*) *dundu*, a small owl.

Lal dundu, Asio accipitrinus.

Pọlọm dundu, a large owl, Bubo bengalensis.

Sakam dundu, a small owl.

U dundu, so named on account of its call *u u u u*.

Ḍạk, a water-hen, Gallinula phoenicura (so named on account of its call *ḍạk ḍạk*).

Ḍẹrẹl, a small bird; name due to its call which sounds like *ḍrrel ḍrrel*.

Ḍẹl cẽṛẽ, a very small bird, also called *sãuṛi cẽṛẽ*.

Ḍheṅka, a species of Crane, Tringa platyrhyncha.

Band ḍheṅka, besides the same as for *ḍheṅka*, this name is also used for the Red-footed Pecked Ibis, Ciconia alba.

Bạd ḍheṅka,? Pseudotautalus leucocephalus; fairly common.

Ḍhipcui, the Racket-tailed Indian Drongo, probably Dissemurus paradiseus. Also called the chowkedar of the birds.

Eṛe, a Woodpecker.

Bhoṇḍa eṛe, a large species, Liopicus mahrattensis.

Goenṭha eṛe, a small kind.

Kabra eṛe, the Striped Woodpecker, Brachypternus aurantius.

Seṅgel eṛe, Tigra shorei.

Eṛe kisni, v. *kisni*.

Galoć, the Hawk Cuckoo, Hierococcyx varius. This word is not used before women.

Gaṛuṛ, the Adjutant bird, Leptoptilus dubius.

Baḍ gaṛuṛ, the Bald-headed Adjutant, Leptoptilus javanicus.

Dheṅka gaṛuṛ, a Stork, a little larger than *baḍ ḍheṅka*.

Thailak gaṛuṛ, Ardea argala.

The Adjutant and any part of the bird or its feathers are believed to be the death of snakes.

Geḍe, a Duck, the domestic duck.

Dak geḍe, a wild kind, able to fly; also called *arna geḍe*.

Nãi geḍe, the Ganges Duck.

Gunḍri, a Quail. The Santals distinguish:

Gadle gunḍri, the Blue-breasted Quail, Excalfactoria chinensis.

Ghura gunḍri, the Female Indian Bastard Quail, Turnix taigoor, or Turnix sykesi.

Huker gunḍri, the Painted Bush-quail, Microperdix erythrorhynchus.

Kàsi gunḍri, the Little Button Quail, Turnix dussumieri.

Kho gunḍri, a Quail, so called on account of its call (*kho kho*).

Ṭira gunḍri, the male of *ghura gunḍri*.

To catch quails the Santals keep a female bird as a decoy in a cage placed on the ground, with a number of snares arranged round the cage.

Gutrul, two species of Barbets, Megalaima caniceps and Xantholæma indica; one of these is also called *gaḍa gutrul*. So named from their call sounding like *gutrul gutrul*.

Ghardidi, a certain humming bird, the Tailor bird, Orthotomus sutorius.

Ghaṛwa, the Sparrow, Passer indicus.

Hapuk, the Nightjar, Caprimulgus monticolus, or C. asiaticus.

Huć bir, the Indian Pitta, Pitta brachyura.

Huhaṛ, the Green Pigeon, Crocopus chlorigaster.

Huker, v. *gunḍri*.

Jejeveṛ, a small bird, the size of a sparrow, but having a longer tail.

Jiam (or *Jien*), the same as the *ghardidi*, so called on account of its call, sounding like *jiam jiam*.

Jihu, two kinds:

Bhoṇḍa jihu, the Bengal Babbler, Malacocercus terricolor.

Janum jihu, the Green Babbler, Chaltorius striatus.

Jhọrọjhọċ, the Pied Crested Cuckoo, Coccystes jacobinus. They believe that when this bird calls *phiṛiphiċ* it will be fine weather, and when *jhọrọ jhọċ*, there will be a spell of rain; *jhọrọ jhọċ* means drenched.

Kạhu, a Crow. They eat all young crows, before they can fly, but not full-grown ones, because these feed on anything. They distinguish the following kinds:

Buru Kạhu, a large kind, a Raven; also called *gaḍa kạhu*.

Bhoṇḍa kạhu, the Bow-billed Corbie, Corvus levaillantii.

Kuilạ Kạhu, a wholly black Crow.

Kheḍra kạhu, a small kind.

Pọṇḍ kạhu, a white Crow, said to be a crow, but very rare.

Kạlạia, the Cuckoo Shrike, Graucalus macei; also called *kạlọi*.

Kāṛī, Cuculus canorus. Very voracious; it eats chickens and silkworms. Also called *pirthi cẹṛẹ*.

Kạsi jera (or *kạsi jerak*), the same as *kạsi gunḍri*, v. *gunḍri*.

Kẹrkeṭa, the Brown Shrike, Lanius cristatus, also called *jhaṭa kẹrkeṭa*.

Baghe kẹrkeṭa, Lanius melanocephalus.

The name is due to its call sounding like *kẹr kẹṭẹ kẹṭẹ*; when this is heard, it is a sign that the cold season is setting in.

Kikir, the Kingfisher. The Santals distinguish three kinds:

Bhoṇḍa kikir, the large Kingfisher, Halcyon fuscus.

Ḍuċ kikir, the little Kingfisher, Alcedo bengalensis.

Kamar kikir, the medium-sized Kingfisher, Alcedo ispida.

Kẹhẹ̃, the Maroon-backed Kite, the male is called *arak kẹhẹ̃* and the female *heṛak kẹhẹ̃*.

Kisni, the Myna, Sturnopastor contra. They distinguish:

Care kisni, Sturnopastor contra, the Pied Starling; also called *ẹrẹ kisni* and *naṅgar kisni*.

Ḍọḍhọr kisni, Gracula religiosa; also called *ḍọṇḍhọr kisni* or *bhoṇḍa kisni*, the first name being due to their having their nests in the hollows in trees (*ḍọḍ ọr*).

Kol, the Indian Cuckoo, Cuculus indicus.

Korkoṭ marak, a small kind of peafowl or possibly a pheasant common in Assam.

Kọkọr, an Owl. They distinguish:

Dereń kọkọr, the Collard Scops Owl, Scops bakkamoena, or Scops lettia.

Lat kọkọr, Scops spilocephalus, also called *dundu kọkọr*.

Bhuk kọkọr, an owl nesting in a hollow in a tree. This name is used of women who do not go out and who are reserved.

Kō̃k, a Paddy-bird. The Santals distinguish:

Bak kō̃k, Herodias alba.

Bakoli kō̃k, the same as *ńindạ kō̃k*, q.v.

Bitkil kō̃k, the samè as *gại kō̃k*, q.v.

Ḍheṅka kō̃k, a very large kind with a black beak.

Gạị kǫ̃k, the Cattle Egret, Bubulcus coromandus. So named because it is often seen perched on cattle.

Laṛ kǫ̃k, Bubulcus coromandus.

Lobok kǫ̃k, Ardeola leucoptera (?).

Lọbọe kǫ̃k, the same as *bak kǫ̃k*.

Ńindạ kõk, Nycticorax griseus, called Night Paddy-bird, because it feeds at night.

It might be noted that the name *kǫ̃k* is a near reproduction of the call of most of these birds.

Kuhi besra, an Osprey, Spilornis melanotis.

Kuṛi ṭukuć, two birds, the Lapwing, Sarcogrammus indicus, and Sarciophorus malabaricus. So named from their call as heard by the Santals.

Kuṭạm dạblạ, the Indian Hoopoe, Upupa epops, or Upupa indica.

Khẹṛ guńjạ, a small bird about the size of a sparrow, Orthotomus longicauda.

Lańtiti, the Paradise Fly-catcher, Terpsiphone paradisi.

Laṇḍha, the same as *pọt ḍọdọ*, q.v., called *laṇḍha*, because it is found among paddy stubble; also called *laṇḍha galọć*, a word not used before women.

Lipi, the following birds are so called:

Bhoṇḍa lipi, the Indian Corbie, Corvus macrorhynchus.

Gõẹṭha lipi, the Ashy-crowned Finch Lark, Pyrrhulauda grisea.

Kumbạ lipi, the Madras Bush Lark, Mirafra affinis.

Lọbọe ḍạk, the long-tailed water-hen, Hydrophasianus chirurgus.

Macreńka, a tern, Sterna melanogaster.

Marak, the Peafowl, Pavo cristatus. This is fairly commonly found wild. *Pińcạr marak* is the peacock and *Mạtu marak* the peahen.

Korkoṭ marak, v. *korkot*.

Pọṭọm marak, a large kind of bird; some say it is a name for the peahen.

Mạhkạl, the Indian Crow Pheasant, Centropus sinensis.

Heṛak mạhkạl, likely the female, others say it is the same as the *galọć*.

Mạnikjọṛ, the White-necked Stork, Ardea leucocephala. Rare.

Ńokor, a small bird, ? Arogetes sachatilis. It is eaten by old people, but not by young folk as they believe this will cause "the trembles". *Ńokor* is their name for paralysis agitans, St. Vitus' dance. The name of the bird is due to its trembling movements.

Ọṛe, the Bush-quail, Perdicula asiatica. This is caught in many ways, as well as by using decoy females.

Pajhaṛ, an Eagle.

Buru pajhaṛ, the Hill-eagle, Aquila imperialis.

Hako sap pajhaṛ, a Fish-eating Eagle (also called *dak pajhaṛ*, Water-eagle), ? Spizætus limnætus.

Parwa, the common Pigeon, Columba livia intermedia. There are many varieties, named according to their shape and habits.

Bạji parwa, tumbles in the air.

Jhańga parwa, has feathers down its legs.

Khiṛki parwa, stays in openings in the wall.

Oṛak parwa, house pigeons.

Rajmoholia parwa, a large kind, named after Rajmahal.

Ṭaungi parwa, kept in lofts.

Pio, the Golden Oriole, Oriolus melanocephalus (*Linn.*).

Potam, a Dove. The Santals distinguish the following:

Baṛge potam, small, brown, Turtur cambayensis (*Gmel.*), or Turtur orientalis (*Lath.*).

Bosko (or *bhosko*) *potam*, large like a pigeon, colour variegated.

Guṛughum (or *guḍrugum*) *potam*, the same as *mala potam*, q.v. So named from its call.

Huhu potam, the Imperial Dove, Carpophaga aenea (*Linn.*). So named from its call.

Kĕndrŏ potam, the Spotted Dove, Turtur suratensis (*Gmel.*).

Keke ḍeber, a small kind, Turtur orientalis (*Lath.*).

Kisāṛ potam, the same as *huhu potam*. Said to be so named from its habit of collecting grain in small "bundles" of earth.

Kuḍbur potam, the same as *mala potam*.

Mala potam, the Ring Dove, Turtur risorius (*Linn.*).

Peṭer potam, the same as *bosko potam*; name due to its call, heard as *peṭer duk*.

Pondhaṛ potam, a large kind, Chalcophaps indica (*Linn.*).

Saṇḍi kakar potam, the same as *baṛge potam*; name due to its call; also called *suṇḍi kukur potam*.

Tilai potam, the same as *mala potam*.

Toyo ḍeḍger (or *toyo hoḍgoṛ*) *potam*, the same as *baṛge potam*.

Thekro potam, the same as *kĕṇḍrŏ potam*.

Ṭhikri potam, the same as *baṛge potam*.

Pol ḍoḍo, the Flamefronted Flower-pecker, the same as *laṇḍha*. So named from its call sounding like *pol pol*.

Rici, a kind of Falcon, the Pale Harrier, Circus macrurus (*Gmel.*). Sometimes it is also kept for hunting purposes.

Sahraj, the Sarus Crane, Megalornis antigone (*Linn.*).

Sãk, the Goose. Rare amongst the Santals.

Sasaṅ cĕṛĕ, the Grey-headed Fly-catcher, Culicicapa ceylonensis (*Swain.*).

Sasaṅ galoč, a small bird. The name is not used before women.

Sasaṅ pio, the same as *pio*, q.v.

Sauṛi cĕṛĕ, a very small bird, so called because they generally make their nest in a thatching-grass field; they are also called *ṭheč ṭheč cĕṛĕ*, because their call sounds like *ṭheč ṭheč*.

Serale, a wild Duck, fairly common and much relished.

Sim, the common domestic Fowl. The Santals distinguish:

Belati sim, a large kind; so named because believed to have been brought from Europe.

Gede sim, having short legs like those of the ducks.

Jhaṅga sim, having feathers down the legs.

Karanat sim, having black feathers, black skin and black bones; used as medicinal food in certain diseases.

Duci sim, having some feathers standing out on the neck.

Kulạm sim, a large kind.

Khaṛku sim, a very tall kind.

Kheḍra sim, having scanty feathers.

Ọṛẹ sim, a fowl resembling the *ọṛẹ*, the Bush-quail.

Risạ sim, having reverted feathers.

Sạuriạ sim, a kind that lays many eggs and produces many chickens.

The cocks are called *sim sanḍi* and the hens *sim eṅga*.

Besides the domestic fowls mentioned the following are also called *sim* by the Santals:

Bir sim, that has already been noted.

Dak sim, a kind of wild duck smaller than the *serale*.

Ṭhu ṭhukur sim, the Turkey, very rare amongst the Santals.

Suċ, the Purple Sunbird, Cyniris asiaticus (*Lath.*), also called *sakwa suċ*. Another small bird is also called *suċ* or *gadle suċ* and *jugi suċ*. The name is due to the call of these birds, heard by the Santals as *suċ suċ*.

Tạrjuạ, the Black Ibis, Inocotis papillosus (*Temm.*). Fairly common.

Tirmuti, v. *ṭirmuṭi*, the common name.

Tuṭ, the Crimson-breasted Barbet, Xantholæma hæmacephala (*P. L. S. Müller*). So named from its call sounding like *tuṭ tuṭ*.

Ṭiċ ṭọṛọk, the Bengal Bulbul.

Ṭikmiṅ, a kind of Falcon, ? Cerchneis tinnunculus (*Linn.*).

Ṭirmuṭi, a small kind of Falcon, Falco severus (*Horsf.*), or Tinnunculus alaudarius (*Linn.*). Kept to catch birds, esp. by Hindus.

Ṭirọm, the Indian Bee-eater, Merops viridis (*Linn.*).

Ṭiṭiṛhiċ, also called *ṭeṭẹ ṭẹṅgọċ*, two species of Lapwing, Sarciophorus malabaricus (*Bodd.*), and Sarcogrammus indicus (*Bodd.*) (acc. to Dr. Campbell). One of them is also called *gõeṭha ṭiṭiṛhiċ*.

Ṭoya, the Indian Blue-jay, Coracias indica (*Linn.*).

Uṛiċ, two small birds, called *hạti uṛiċ* and *tope uṛiċ* (the Indian Shama). So named from its call *uṛiċ uṛiċ*. To hear the call of an *uṛiċ* on the left hand side, when going to do business, e.g., to arrange a marriage, is a bad omen, hearing it on the right hand side is a good omen.

Animals eaten.

Let us now speak about the animals that the Santals eat, taking them in alphabetical order.

Bana, the Indian Black Bear, Melursus ursinus (*Shaw*), also called *parkọm bana*; fairly common in the forests.

Banwaṛ, a Jungle Mouse.

Barduṛuč, a Bat. The Santals distinguish the following:

Coṭo barduṛuč, Nycticejus kuhli (*Leach.*).

Cuṭia̦ barduṛuč, lit. the mouse bat, the smallest kind.

Goḍo barduṛuč, Cynopterus marginatus (*Geoff.*).

Ho̦n barduṛuč, lit. rat bat; a fairly large kind.

Ka̦hu barduṛuč, the Flying Fox, Pteropus medius (*Temm.*).

Po̦ṭo̦m barduṛuč, a species so called.

Boyo bana, the Indian Badger, Mellivora indica (*Kerr*).

Bhiḍi, an Ewe, sheep. A ram is called *bheḍa*[1], but the name of the female is used as a name for sheep in general, just like *ga̦i* for cattle in general. Sheep are commonly kept by Santals for food, not for their wool.

Gaḍo̦r bhiḍi, a kind of Sheep with a very heavy tail; not ordinarily kept by Santals but often seen by them.

Bhiḍi jel, a kind of Deer, Ovis vignei (*Blyth.*).

Ce̦me̦ń, the Mongoose, Herpestes auropunctatus (*Hodgs.*). Often kept by the Santals because of their usefulness in connexion with the catching and killing of snakes and rats.

Cund, the Musk-rat, Crocidura caerulea (*Kerr*). They distinguish two varieties, *bhoṇḍa cund*, large, and *re̦the̦* (or *reṭhea*) *cund*, a small kind. Snakes are believed to avoid houses where there are musk-rats. Some Santals will eat them, after having cut away the head, but generally only when there is a scarcity of other kinds of food.

Cuṭia̦, a Mouse, Mus musculus (*Linn.*).

Ḍaṅgra, an Ox; v. *ga̦i*.

Ẹrgo, a Field-rat (coloured like a hare).

Gaḍo̦r bhiḍi, v. *bhiḍi*.

Ga̦i[2], a Cow; word used for cattle in general. Bullocks and often also cows are used for ploughing and carting. The Santals have no objection to eating the meat of cows and bullocks, in fact they relish it, but owing to the landlords and their Hindu neighbours they have to exercise restraint, and they will mostly go about obtaining, preparing and eating it at night. Bullocks may be sacrificed. The writer once came across a large number of Santals who had cut up a couple of cattle who had died from some disease. He tried to warn them not to eat such meat; but they had no fear of anything happening to them; and so far as is known no harm came to them. The milk is used, but Santal cows give very little.

Goḍo, a Rat. The Santals distinguish the following:

Bhus goḍo, the Bandicoot Rat, Nesocia bandicota (*Bechs.*) (or, Mus malabaricus *Shaw*, or Mus giganteus *L.*). This rat digs holes in embankments, near rice-fields, etc. The Santal believes that they gather food, sufficient for a whole year at a time and store it in their holes.

Caole goḍo, the common House-rat.

---

[1] Also Bheḍa in Bengali—*Ed.*

[2] Also Gai in Hindi and Bengali—*Ed.*

Dander goḍo, living near rice-fields where they burrow holes and collect quantities of paddy. The same is also called *khẹt goḍo*, *piṇḍhe goḍo* and *ṭaṇḍi goḍo*.

Murup̣ goḍo, a small light-grey rat, also living near rice-fields, burrowing there.

To catch rats a number of Santals will go to a place where they have found that rats have burrowed. They dig them out and kill them, and if they cannot reach them in this way, they fill the hole with water, which will drive them out. They wrap the head, the intestines and the legs up in separate leaves and put each on burning coals to fry, with salt, spices and oil added, if they have such; or they may cook it with rice into a hash. They will either eat this on the spot or, dividing it into equal portions, each take one portion home. The flesh is divided in the same way and taken home, where it is made into curry. Before being cut up such small animals are hammered with a stone, and then singed.

Hạti,[1] the Elephant. The writer's informant stated that Santals will eat elephant flesh and they may have done so in olden times, but nowadays they never get an opportunity.

Họn, a Rat. The *họn* has, except as mentioned, hair on its tail. It is not hairless like the tail of the *goḍọ*. The Santals distinguish:

Cãuriạ họn, the same as *urič họn*, q.v.

Kheḍra (or *kherṛa*) *họn*, a small rat with a bare tail.

Oṛak̓ họn, a rat commonly found in houses.

Saṅga họn, Mus rattus (*Linn.*).

Urič họn, the Gerboa-rat, Gerbillus indicus (*Hardw.*).

Hunted like *goḍo*, but smoked out, when necessary.

Họrọ, a Tortoise. The Santals distinguish the following:

Buru họrọ, lit. Hill-tortoise.

Catọm họrọ, the same as *lapra họrọ*.

Dak̓ họrọ, Trionyx gangeticus (*Cuvier*) (?).

Lapra họrọ, Kachuga dhongoka, found in the Ganges and in the Eastern parts. It has a soft edge round the leg openings.

Raj họrọ, lit. King-tortoise.

Ṭaṇḍi họrọ, a small kind, Morenia ocellata (*Dum. & Bibr.*).

Ṭoklak̓ họrọ, a kind of tortoise living in water. The name is said to be due to its resemblance of a *ṭoklak̓*, a small earthenware vessel used for cooking curry.

Ṭukuč họrọ, a kind of tortoise.

Jel, a Deer. All kinds of deer are called *jel*, perhaps because the only meat (*jel*) the Santals originally had was that of the deer. They know a number of different kinds, the names being often different for the male and the female of the same species, the word *jel* is very often omitted.

Badaṛ selep̣ jel, the buck of the Ravine Deer, Gazella bennetti (*Sykes*).

---

[1] Also Hati in Hindi and Bengali—*Ed.*

Bhăuṭiạ jel, the Indian Black Buck.

Ghọṭrẹt (or *ghoṭra*) *jel*, the hind of the *badaṛ selep jel*, Gazella bennetti (*Sykes*).

Jhaṅkar, the buck of the Spotted Deer, Cervus axis (*Erxl.*). They distinguish:

Paḍa jhaṅkar, an old buck the horns of which have fallen off; and *ponḍa jhaṅkar*, having whitish horns.

Also *Icạk jhaṅkar*, Cervus porcinus (*Zimmer*).

Kuṛmbi selep jel, the hind of the *badaṛ selep jel*. Some Santals say that this is the same as *badaṛ selep*.

Mẹrọm jel, lit. Goat-deer, the same as *ghọṭrẹt jel*.

Murmu, the Nilgai, Boselaphus tragocamelus (*Pallas.*) Tabu to people of the Murmu sect.

Mŭṛghos (also *munḍghos*) *jel*, a small species, not known in the Santal Parganas.

Posta, the hind of the *jhaṅkar*.

Pọṭrẹt jel, the same as *ghọṭrẹt jel*.

Saram, the Sambar Stag, Cervus unicolor (*Besch.*), also called *gadle saram*. *Gutrut saram* is a stag that has not as yet got horns; *paḍa saram*, is an old stag, the horns of which have fallen off.

Sạl, the Gaur, Bibos gaurus (*Ham. Smith*) (Gavæus gaurus of *Blyth*); also *bir kaḍa*, lit. forest buffalo. The cow is called *sạl bitkil*.

Sosam, the hind of the *murum*.

Tanḍi selep, the same as *badaṛ selep*.

It should be noted that, except in the reserved forests, deer are now practically extinct in the Santal Parganas.

Jhĭk, the Indian Porcupine, Hystrix leucura (*Sykes*).

Kaḍa, the Buffalo; the cow is called *bitkil*. They have quite a number of prefixes, varying according to the appearance of the animal and its horns. The Buffalo is now fairly common among the Santals, at least among well-to-do people. They will eat the flesh, but very rarely can afford to do so. The milk is also used.

Kul, the Tiger, Panthera tigris (*Linn.*). The tiger is now fairly rare in the Santal Parganas. The Santals enjoy eating it, when they get an opportunity.

Kulại, the Bengal Hare, Lepus ruficaudatus (*Geoff.*). Fairly common and much hunted. They distinguish:

Buru kulại, lit. Hill-hare; a large kind found in the hills.

Eṛgo kulại, found in Assam. These look like ordinary hares, only their ears are small.

Khedra kulai (also called *rẹthea kulại*), a small thin kind.

Saphọn kulại, the Coney.

Khikṛī, the Bengal Fox, Vulpes bengalensis (*Shaw*).

Laṛ togo, the red Squirrel.

Maṅgaṛ, the Alligator, Crocodilus palustris (*Less.*). Now very rare in the Santal Parganas, and only seen in the great rivers.

Mahla, the Palm Civet, Paradoxurus hermaphroditus (*Pallas*), var. niger (*Blanf.*) (or Paradoxurus musanga (*Jerdon*)).

Merom, a Goat, also used as a general name for male and female animals; *mihũ merom*, lit. calf-goat, is used for cattle in general, including cows and bullocks, goats and sheep. *Boda* or *merom boda* is the Santal name for an uncastrated he-goat. *Merom khasi* is a castrated goat, the flesh of which is considered excellent as curry, and constantly used.

Odam, the Indian Otter, Lutra vulgaris (*Erxl.*), and Lutra leptonyx (*Horsf.*).

Runda, a Jungle Cat. The Santals distinguish:

Badar runda, the Jungle Cat, Felis chaus (*Gülden.*), about the size of a domestic cat.

Boas (or *boak*) *runda*, the large Tiger-cat, Felis viverrina (*Bennett.*). So named from their call, sounding like *boas boas.*

Kubra runda, a species of jungle cat.

Sagak runda, the same as *badar runda*.

Sila runda, a species of wild cat.

Saram babea, a kind of Mongoose, Herpestes smithi (*Gray*), large.

Selep, v. sub *jel.*

Sogol, the Civet Cat, Viverra zibetha (*Linn.*) (or Vivericula indica (*Hodgs.*)).

Sukri,[1] a Pig. Most Santals prefer the flesh of pigs to that of any other kind of animal, although a few will not touch it on account of the way pigs feed. Most Santals keep pigs. Practically all male pigs are castrated (they are called *sukri badhia*). A boar is called *kudu sukri*. Besides the domesticated pigs wild ones are also found:

Bir sukri, the wild Pig, Sus indicus (*Gray*). These are still found, where there are forests. Pigs, also domestic ones, are killed by shooting them with arrows.

Tayan, the Broad-headed Crocodile, Crocodilus palustris (*Less.*). What has been said about the *mangar* also applies to the *tayan.*

Tarup, a Leopard. The leopards are rather plentiful in the country, and are not only eaten, but their whiskers and claws are used as amulets, giving the wearer luck and strength in certain matters. They distinguish several kinds of leopards. It may be remarked that even tigers are called *naprak* or *maran tarup*, lit. big leopard.

Kurse baha tarup, the largest kind, so named from its colour like the *kurse* flower. It is as large as a small tiger; the writer once measured one killed outside his station; it measured seven feet. It was cut up and eaten.

Lar sakam tarup, large, of a light colour.

Potea tarup, the small kind (also called *degra tarup*).

Sona cita tarup, of medium size, probably the most common in the country.

Ad baghin tarup, lit. half-tiger leopard; a large kind.

Tor, a Squirrel, Sciurus tristriatus (*Waterh.*) (or Sciurus palmarum (*Linn.*)). Common.

Toyo, the Jackal, Canis aureus (*Linn.*). Very common, plays the same rôle in Santal folklore as the fox in European folklore.

---

[1] Bengali 'Sükar'.—*Ed.*

Ṭikmiń (or *kiṭmiń*), a small tree-rat.
Urič hon, v. sub *hon*.

THE CATCHING, TREATMENT, ETC. OF ANIMALS AND BIRDS.

Hunting is the great delight of Santal men. Anything that can be hunted is fair game and is eagerly pursued. The Santals have their annual hunt in which all men of the countryside are expected to participate, so much so that if they without good reasons do not follow the others, they are called "women". The annual hunt is the highest social function amongst the Santals. The scene of the hunt may be anywhere, where they have reason to believe that animals may be caught. When hunting they have certain customary rules which must be followed and which are of a communal character. The one who on the annual hunt first hits an animal, whether he kills it or not, has a right to the felled animal; but he must give certain parts to others, and he has to divide what is left with the men of his own village, only keeping certain parts for himself.

At other hunts the hitter and killer have their rights; but here also all participating get an equal share of the flesh, that is not prepared and eaten on the spot, to take home with them.

Of the head of sacrificed animals and fowls a hash is cooked with rice. Only men eat this; no woman is allowed to partake of it. When parts of killed animals or birds are brought back from a hunt, any man, whose wife is enceinte, must not be given any portion, to take home with him, in which there is a part of the head. If such a woman should eat this, it would mean something bad for her child, especially if it should be a boy when grown up he would be unable to kill any animal, when out hunting. People suffering from disease also must not eat the head.

If the skin of a killed animal is wanted, they naturally flay it. Otherwise it is singed. The animal is put on burning coals, and all hairs are singed off. Birds are similarly treated to singe off the feathers.

Small animals are to start with, frequently, beaten with a stone or an axe-head, to pulp, and are then put on live coals to be singed. Hares are similarly treated, but only the four legs and the head are beaten not the whole body.

Anything intended to be eaten as curry is, before cooking, cut up into small pieces. The Santals have no knives, forks or spoons and have to use the fingers of the right hand to convey the food to the mouth; hence the need for cutting it all up.

If meat of oxen or cows is brought, the Santals do not take this inside their houses, nor the vessels in which it is cooked. It is hung under the eaves at the rear of the house or under the eaves of the cowshed. When cooking it they put in salt, turmeric, seed of the Roselle plant, hemp seed, Niger seed and Sesame seed, all partially roasted and pounded. Men (not women) boil this meat, and men also serve it out. It is eaten in the courtyard.

The liver, lungs and intestines of larger animals are prepared separately.

Under the influence of their Hindu and (so far as pigs[1] are concerned) their Mohammedan neighbours some Santals have ceased to eat the flesh of many animals. They will not eat the meat of bullocks, cows and buffaloes and of pigs. It is not up to their standards of culture. Some folk say they feel disgusted at eating meats which their ancestors enjoyed. But, as a saying of theirs has it "If you become wealthy you will give up eating all kinds, but if you become poor you will eat everything".

Nowadays the Santals are compelled to rely mostly on agriculture. Except where there are reserved forests, where hunting is greatly restricted, the real forests have mostly disappeared, and the spoils of the chase are extremely poor, very much so when compared with what is said to have happened in former times. Hunting now, it seems, gives a good deal of enjoyment with but little spoils. They will hunt for hares and for rats, and for single animals that they have seen or heard about; and they will use snares or traps to catch certain animals and birds. Otherwise the game is only what they happen to come across accidentally and kill.

CURRY.

A few words in connexion with the way in which the Santals prepare their *utu*, curry, may suitably find a place here. The procedure is naturally somewhat different for the different foods used, and all working cooks do not act in the same way. They have no recipes.

To prepare meat or flesh curry they generally proceed in the following manner:— Turmeric, leaves of Laurus Cassia *Willd.*, coriander seed, salt and spices are placed in oil in a vessel that has been heated; the vessel is then put over a fire, and when the oil boils, they add onions and pepper, and finally the flesh. It is then cooked until ready. Some do not use turmeric in all cases, especially is this the case when they make curry from hares.

With curry of fish, mushrooms, vegetables and split pulse (*dạl*) they proceed in almost the same way, but in many cases they omit turmeric. When making *dạl* curry, they first put the dal into hot water to make it into a soft mass, and turmeric and spices are added. Oil is poured into a heated vessel and made to boil, and onions and pepper are put in. When the onions have been boiled so as to look reddish, the *dạl* is poured in. When cooking certain vegetables only salt is added; no oil and no spices are used.

The Santals fear the evil eye. To guard against this some women will take in their hand a little of the food that is to be made into curry and holding it over the vessel used they will say: "May it have a spell cast on it, may it get teeth". The meaning of this is said to be, that if any woman with an evil eye has looked upon it, no spell may be cast on the food, and it may be eaten and digested without any resultant stomach-ache, vomiting or diarrhoea.

MILK.

Before closing this section a few words may be added about the use of milk among the Santals. The cows, buffalo-cows and goats, that the Santals have, give, according

[1] Pig is taboo to the Hindus also.—*Ed.*

to our ideas, very little milk. If a cow gives one seer daily, it is considered extraordinary. It is significant, that, when being milked, a cow must have its calf (or, anyhow, a calf) standing at its head; otherwise it will not give any milk according to Santal experience. The Santals do not drink much milk. They will give fresh milk to their children, when the mother has too little or has died. They may also boil rice in milk and enjoy eating it in this way.

Dahe,[1] Curds, is not generally eaten alone, but together with parched and flattened rice (this is considered a great treat) or with Mahua. It is further used for churning butter. It is boiled and then poured into an earthenware vessel and kept there, more milk being constantly added. It soon becomes sour, but this does not matter.

The churning is done in the following way:—the vessel in which the *dahe* is kept is, when there is a sufficient quantity, placed at the foot of a post. They have a churning-staff, a staff of wood, generally bamboo, some five feet long, split at the lower end into four parts, that are kept apart by fixed cross-pieces. This churning-staff is put into the *dahe*, its top being kept in position by a loop of cord running round the post and the stick. Another long cord is taken three or four times round the churning-staff, and by alternately pulling this cord at each end, the staff is made to revolve. This may be done by either a man or a woman. The result is *nạinu*,[2] unsalted butter. They do not know how to make this into butter, but make it into ghee.

The *dahe*, from which the *nạinu* has been extracted is called *ghọr*,[3] butter-milk. This is considered very savoury and a very nourishing food.

Forbidden Food.

It may be of interest to state what Santals will not eat. They will not eat any kind of monkeys, as may be quite naturally supposed. Their traditions tell that the present-day *Bir họr* (lit. forest men), a now very small tribe, originally belonged to the ancestors of the Santal people; but they were "outcasted", in every way ostracised, because they would kill and eat *hãṛũ*, the Hanuman monkey, Presbytis entellus. Strangely enough they have no objection to using the skin of these monkeys, bought from the *Bir họr*, to cover the narrow end of their *tumdak*, dancing drum.

Santals will not eat horse-flesh. On two occasions the writer has been obliged to kill a pony. The Santals were on both occasions offered the flesh for food, but they absolutely refused to take it, and were apparently horrified at the offer.

They will not eat hyenas, seemingly on account of the way in which they feed. Some Santals will, for the same reason, refuse to eat pigs, although to most Santals their flesh is the best they know.

As regards birds, they will not eat any that are known to touch anything putrefying, e.g., practically all the vultures and the *jalo* falcon. Crows they will eat before they are able to fly, but not after they are full-grown ones; nor will they eat parakeets.

[1] In Hindi Dahi, in Bengali Dai.—*Ed.*

[2] In Bengali Nani.—*Ed.*

[3] Bengali Ghōl.—*Ed.*

CRUSTACEANS, MOLLUSCS AND REPTILES EATEN.

Boḍa, a Python, Python molurus (*Linn.*). Fairly rare in the Santal Parganas, but common in the Eastern parts and Assam. The Santals distinguish the following:

Dudhią boḍa, lit. milk-python, so called on account of its whitish colour.

Dhimą boḍa, lit. the mild-tempered python, it is marked somewhat like a Russell's viper.

Dhanwa boḍa, and *dhinuąr boḍa*, the same snake, kept by people, because it is believed to bring wealth.

Ramnat boḍa, a python that has rudimentary legs.

The flesh is considered excellent. Quite recently the Santals caught a python near to the writer's station. They brought it in to let people see this rare snake. Next day word was sent down to the village that the writer wanted to buy the skin, but the messenger came back saying that they had cut it to pieces and eaten it. They said it was fat and very good.

Jambṛo, the Dhaman or Rat-snake. The Santals distinguish:

Kod jambṛo, Ptyas mucosus; so named from its dark colour, like the colour of *kod* fruit.

Man baha jambṛo, having a yellowish colour.

Sǫsǫ jambṛo, black like *sǫsǫ*, the Marking-nut.

Tǫrngǫṛ jambṛo, light-coloured.

The *jambṛo* is treated as follows: When they have killed it they tie it to a tree by its head. One man takes hold of its tail and keeps it stretched out, while another man starts skinning it. The skin is cut along the backbone and torn off. Having made a cut at the neck they tear the flesh of one side off, and when this is done, the flesh on the other side is torn off in the same way. The flesh is next cut into pieces and collected on a leaf-plate. They thereupon beat the backbone with a stone and also do the same to the ribs. The tail is singed, and when all this has been sufficiently beaten, it is cut up into bits and mixed with the flesh on the leaf-plate. They put all in a small vessel or a large piece of broken earthenware, and cook it on a piece of rock or on a fireplace made of three stones. When they are cooking it, they take a ball of the stuff and break it into two; throwing one half in, they say: 'This is salt', and throwing the other half in, they say: 'This is turmeric'. And they who eat it find it savoury, as though salt and turmeric had been added. They say to the children, that they must eat with care, or they may get something sticking in the throat. The ancestors have said, that if you get a bone of a *jambṛo* sticking in your throat, and then do not find and kill and eat its mate, you will never get rid of the choking matter. To divide the flesh they make leaf-cups of one leaf, the leaf-stalk being used to keep the leaf in a proper position.

They have a curious superstition in connexion with the *jambṛo*. To see a *jambṛo*, before taking any seed out to sow is unfortunate, because the *jambṛo* is a being that attracts all luck to itself. To obviate this bad influence some people will, before they see a *jambṛo*, roast some Mahua, Sesame and Niger seed, pound this and eat it. Every member of the household will each eat one ball of it.

So far as the writer has been able to find out, the Santals do not eat any snakes other than those mentioned. A Santal once told the writer that he had one day seen a snake entering a hole; thinking it was a *jambṛo*, he had taken hold of its tail and tried to pull it out. He did not get the whole out; it broke, and the head was left in the hole. The man prepared and ate what he had got; but next day he felt very queer. He then went and dug out the head of the snake and found that it was the head of a cobra. Many cobras look very much like a *jambṛo*, so that the mistake is understandable. The Santals have an idea that all cobras are female, and that they copulate with these rat-snakes. They have often seen them copulating, they say.

Dak gongha, a large snail, living in water. The flesh is eaten.

Icạk,[1] a Prawn. Very common in the Santal country; eaten as curry. Also called *rẹthẹ icạk*, small prawn, to distinguish it from the *sole icạk*.

Sọlẹ icạk, a large kind of prawn, not so common as the *rẹthẹ icạk*.

Jhinuk,[2] a Mussel. The flesh is eaten.

Kaṭkọm,[3] a Crab. The Santals distinguish the following, the flesh of which is eaten as curry:

Bạd kaṭkọm, common in the higher rice-fields.

Bạihạṛ kaṭkọm, the same as *bạd kaṭkọm*, but found in the low-lying rice-fields.

Buru kaṭkọm, a small black kind, found in hill streams.

Des kaṭkọm, the same as *bạd kaṭkọm*.

Dhiri kaṭkọm, found under stones in rivers, a large kind.

Patal kaṭkọm, the same as *dhiri kaṭkọm*.

Pọkọl kaṭkọm, the same as *bạd kaṭkọm*.

Rega kaṭkọm, a small kind.

Rẹthẹ kaṭkọm, another small kind.

Sọdọk kaṭkọm, a crab found in rivulets, resembling *buru kaṭkọm*, but not so black.

Toa kaṭkọm, white and soft, found in rice-fields.

Rọkọc̓, a Periwinkle, Whelk. The flesh is eaten as curry. The Santals distinguish the following:

Coelo rọkọc̓, a small periwinkle having a thin tapering shell.

Jọm rọkọc̓, any periwinkle that is eaten, the most common is Melanoides tuberculatus. A number of *rọkọc̓* are not eaten.

Rọtẹ, a Frog. Of frogs the Santals eat:

Bạruḍaṅ, the Bull-frog, Rana tigrina *Daud*.

Hạrdiạ bạruḍaṅ rọtẹ, the yellow Bull-frog.

Other frogs than these they do not eat; rather they express horror at the mention of some of them.

---

[1] In Bengali Ichā.—*Ed.*

[2] Also Jhinuk in Bengali.—*Ed.*

[3] Kāṅkrā in Bengali.—*Ed.*

Tọrhọt, the Iguana. The Santals distinguish:

Bạd tọrhọt (also called *ṭaṇḍi tọrhọt*), Varanus flavescens *Gray*.

Bạihạṛ tọrhọt (also called *piṇḍhạ tọrhọt*), Varanus monitor(?). The flesh of both is very much relished. They are now becoming rare in the country. The skin is used for covering part of the Santal fiddle.

HONEY.

It should be mentioned that the Santals collect and use the honeys of different kinds of wild bees and insects. They naturally have not yet reached the state of keeping bees. Their name for honey is *rasa*.[1] They distinguish:

Dumur rasa, the honey of a wild bee called *dumur*.

Kaṭ uru rasa, the honey of a large black wasp, also called *rasa uru*; from this they also prepare a kind of small sweet balls that are eaten.

Luti rasa, the honey of the now very rare *luti*, Trigona terminata.

Ṅẹlẹ rasa, the honey of the *ṅẹlẹ*, Apis dorsata *Fabr*. This bee is fairly common and often seen. When they are swarming they make their hives shaped like a large rudder suspended from trees. The Santals eat the young *ṅẹlẹ* bees.

Tẹrọm rasa, the honey of the *tẹrọm*, Apis florea.

FISHES.

Where not otherwise stated, the fish mentioned below all live and are caught in the rivers. They are eaten mostly as curry.

Aṛ,[2] a not very common fish, Macrones aor (*Ham. Buch.*).

Badhọṛ, Notopterus chitala (*Ham. Buch.*), a fish full of bones (hence probably the name, *badhọṛ* meaning twisted, crossgrained).

Bãspata,[3] Chela bacaila (*Ham. Buch.*). The word literally means bamboo leaf.

Bạmbi, Anguilla elphinstonei (*Sykes*), an eel. Specially applicable to large specimens. *Bạm*[4] is also used by itself.

Bạslạ hako, lit. adze-fish. Large, not common.

Boaṛ,[5] two kinds of fish; the one called only *boaṛ* being Wallago attu (*Bloch.*).

Raghọ boaṛ (also called *raghọp*[6] *boaṛ* or *rạghu boaṛ*). It might be mentioned that the *raghọp boaṛ* is mentioned in the Santal traditions as the fish that was called on to raise earth from the sea to make land; but all the earth melted for this fish.

Siṭkạ boaṛ, is a name used for the Wallago attu (*Bloch.*) when still young.

Bumbuć, Lepidocephalichthys guntea (*Ham. Buch.*). When large it is called *buḍhi bumbuć*. Considered excellent food.

Caole bumbuć, a small fish, often found in rice-fields.

Kaḍa bumbuć, possibly only another name for *bumbuć* when dark-coloured.

---

1 Rasa in Bengali means Juice.—*Ed.*
2 Also in Bengali Ār.—*Ed.*
3 Same in Bengali.—*Ed.*
4 Also in Bengali.—*Ed.*
5 Cf. Boāl in Bengali.—*Ed.*
6 Same in Bengali.—*Ed.*

Kul bumbuć, Botia dario (*Ham. Buch.*).

Coć bumbuć, a fish so called, because it gives a kind of squeak (*cọć*) when caught.

Bheḍa hako, lit. ram-fish. Not common.

Calha, Barilius bendelisis, var. cocsa, *Ham. Buch.*, considered very good food, especially during the cold season.

Rodo calha, a certain fish.

Calka, probably the same as *calha* (name not known in the Santal Parganas).

Citol,[1] Notopterus chitala (*Ham. Buch.*), a broad, flat and spotted fish. Sometimes kept in tanks.

Coḍa, the same as *cọḍgọć*, q.v. Large specimens caught in rivers are often called *gaḍa coḍa*.

Cọḍgọć, Ophiocephalus gachua *Ham. Buch.* Found also in rice-fields. (Divorced girls and this fish are said to be of the same nature, always moving about.)

Dūṛī, also called *bạihạṛ dūṛī*, *lọsọt dūṛī* (from the places where they are found, in low-lying rice-fields or in mud) or *mal sakam dūṛī* (lit. bamboo-leaf, from its shape), Rhynchobdella aculeata (*Bloch*).

Gaḍa dūṛī, lit. river *dūṛī* (because it is found in rivers); also called *kabra* or *lạṭu dūṛī* (*kabra* means spotted, *lạṭu* big). Mastacembelus armatus (*Lacép.*). Very slippery, eel-like.

Ḍạṇḍkạ, Perilampus laubuca (*Ham. Buch.*) (also called *maraṅ ḍạṇḍkạ*, big *ḍ*.). Common during the rainy season.

Kạṭić ḍạṇḍkạ, Danio (Brachydanio) rerio *Ham. Buch.*

Sadọm ḍạṇḍkạ, Esomus danricus (*Ham. Buch.*). Considered good food. *Ḍaṛkạ* and *ḍhạṇḍkạ* are the same as *ḍạṇḍkạ*.

Gajal[2] (or *gadjal*), a fish found in shallow lakes or marshes.

Gạṛại,[3] Ophiocephalus gachua (*Ham. Buch.*). They bury themselves in mud and are considered one of the best for eating. They are another kind of *cọḍgọć*.

Gendlaṅ, a small kind of fish. This word is also used for small fish in general (also *geṅjlaṅ*).

Ilsạ,[4] the Hilsa or Sable fish, Clupea ilisha (*Ham. Buch.*). Not found in the Santal Parganas, but in the big eastern rivers.

Jiọl,[5] a certain fish, having spines on the sides of the head.

Kakṛa hako, a certain fish found in rivers.

Kal bạgus,[6] Labeo calbasu (*Ham. Buch.*). (Also called simply *bạgus*, or *kal bokos*.)

Kara ghakor, a certain fish (found in Manbhum).

Kāṛā, lit. blind, has very small eyes, Glyptothorax botia (*Ham. Buch.*).

Katla, Catla buchanani (*Ham. Buch.*), very large, kept in tanks. The fry are annually brought from the Ganges or other large rivers.

Koṭro hako, a certain fish (found in Manbhum).

Kuclạ[7] (also *kucilạ* and *khucilạ*), an eel-like fish.

---

[1] Also in Bengali.—*Ed.*
[2] Also in Bengali.—*Ed.*
[3] Also in Bengali.—*Ed.*
[4] Also in Bengali.—*Ed.*
[5] Also in Bengali.—*Ed.*
[6] Compare Kāl Baus in Bengali.—*Ed.*
[7] Compare Künche in Bengali.—*Ed.*

Linḍa, Garra lamta (*Ham. Buch.*). Also called *pathọr caṭa*. Considered excellent food.

Lituṛ, a certain eel-like fish, Amphipnous cuchia (*Ham. Buch.*).

Matkọm hako, lit. the Mahua fish, Gobius giuris (*Ham. Buch.*).

Mal sakam hako, v. sub *duṛī*.

Mạṅgri, a certain fish, Clarias batrachus (*L.*). It has no scales and is kept in tanks.

Miṛik, a certain fish; kept in tanks.

Paṅgas [1] *hako* (also called *paṅgas boaṛ*), a certain fish found in eastern rivers. Considered bad for sick persons.

Poṭea gạṛạị, a fairly common kind of fish.

Poṭha hako, the same as *puṭhi hako*, when grown to a certain size. Also called *buḍhi puṭhi*.

Puṭhi [2] *hako*, Barbus stigma (*Cuv. & Val.*); small, often found in rice-fields. Also called *kạṭić puṭhi*.

Raghọ boaṛ, v. sub *boaṛ*.

Rẽṛẽl hako, a certain fish, Macrones tengara (*Ham. Buch.*). Considered excellent food. They have thorn-like barbs on their back and head, the sting of which is considered poisonous.

Ruhi (also called *rui* [3]), Labeo rohita (*Ham. Buch.*); one of the best kinds for eating. Kept in tanks.

Siṅghin hako,[4] a species of fish, so called on account of its spines. Not found in the Santal Parganas.

Sirhọć hako, a certain fish, said to be so called, because its head reminds one of the head of the *sirhọć* bird.

Siṛiń hako, a certain fish without scales. Said to be very savoury.

Sisiń hako, a certain fish, Amblyceps mangois (*Ham. Buch.*). Certain filaments on the head are said to be poisonous.

Siṭkạ boaṛ, v. sub *boaṛ*.

Sọl,[5] Ophiocephalus striatus (*Bloch.*).

Sọrọć, a short, thick and round fish, Barilius bendelisis, var. cocsa (*Ham. Buch.*). Considered excellent food.

Su [6] (or *sũh*), a dolphin, Platanista gangeticas (*Lebeck*). Said to be so named from sound like *su*, heard when they rise to the surface.

Tale hako, Anabas scandens (*Daldorf*). Said to be so named from a belief that during rain they will mount a *tale* (Borassus flabelliformis).

Ṭeṅgra,[7] Macrones vittatus (*Bloch.*).

Ṭirom hako, a certain fish.

FISHING.

As it is of ethnological interest, something may be related of how the Santals catch fish. Like hunting the catching of fish is said to be one of the real joys of the people.

---

1 Also in Bengali.—*Ed.*
2 Same in Bengali.—*Ed.*
3 Same in Bengali.—*Ed.*
4 Compare 'Singhi' in Bengali.—*Ed.*
5 Same in Bengali.—*Ed.*
6 Compare 'Sisuk' in Bengali.—*Ed.*
7 Same in Bengali.—*Ed.*

A man may naturally go alone to angle; but this is very rare and likely of fairly recent introduction, as it is only of late years that they have been able to get serviceable fish-hooks. As a rule a number of men go together to a spot where they know that there are fish. If one or several of the party have no rights to the surrounding land, they will always have to come to an arrangement beforehand with the owner, but this does not apply to the big rivers. To catch the fish they employ different kinds of nets.[1]

At certain times the Santals hold a kind of public fishing festival, in which the whole neighbourhood, and anyone wishing to do so, participates. It is quite a social event. In such cases even the women may be seen accompanying the men. The women will naturally not enter into the deep water, but standing on or moving along the edge they will try to catch what they can with their hands. They apparently enjoy the fun.

The headman of the village, inside the boundaries of which the fishing is to be, makes a public announcement that on such and such a day there will be a public catching of fish. If believed necessary, they make sacrifices to the *bongas* (spirits) to remove possible impediments. They use their nets or hands to catch the fish. All fish caught are collected in the nets (in the *bukạ*), the big fish being cut into pieces. When the fishing is over, they collect half of the big fish from every net. This portion is for the people of the village. They divide this half into three portions; one portion for the owner of the place, the two other portions for the village people.

If the public fishing is held in a river, the village headman of the boundary gets his one portion; but if the place is within the boundaries of two villages this portion is divided into two equal parts, and the two village headmen each get one of these parts. The remaining two portions are divided among the people of the two villages.

---

[1] The following are the nets used (called *jal* [Same in Bengali.—*Ed.*] or *jhạli*) by the Santals: *Cạbhi jal* (or *jhạli*), shaped like a spoon-net, but has no handle. The wide circular opening is fixed to a ring of bamboo, and to this ring four pieces of bamboo or other suitable saplings are fixed tent-like and joined together above. The user takes hold of the thin end of the net (called *bukạ*, lit. navel), that is not tied. When he thinks there are fish to be caught, he carefully presses the net down, so that the bamboo ring is firmly pressed against the ground. Letting go of the *bukạ* he feels for the fish with his hand and takes them out. This kind of net is used in the larger rivers and in what is called *ahar*, low rice-fields that have a small dammed up rivulet.

Gạnạri, small round net, like a hand-net, with or without a handle.

Gitoe jal, a net up to 10 m. long and 1 m. broad with floats; only used in still water. Very rare amongst the Santals.

Huṇḍạ jal, the most common fishing net of the Santals. It is made like a big bag, tapering towards the centre, and the *bukạ* is long and narrow. It is fixed to three poles which give it a triangular form. One of the poles protrudes and serves as a handle. When using it the man, keeping the *bukạ* in his hand, presses one side down and moves it along the ground. Any fish caught are kept in the *bukạ*, until the fishing is over.

Lebda jal, a casting-net, fairly common and used in shallow water. It has a wide circular form, tapering, with a long cord fixed at the top. At the border it has weights of iron or anything suitable fixed so as to make the net sink quickly. Practice and skill are needed to use this effectively.

Or jal, made of thick string with large meshes. It has weights of iron or stones at the bottom and floats (wood or straw-bundles) at the top. It is 3 to 4 m. deep and very long. It is used in large tanks, being dragged along the bottom to catch fish that are otherwise difficult to get. Very rare amongst the Santals.

Rạṅki jal (or *janalọm*), a very large net, consisting of a netting fixed to four poles, some 3 to 5 m. long, and tied together so as to form a square. To each corner a rope is tied. Four men are needed to work this. Standing one on each corner they press the frame down to the bottom. After a short while they raise the frame by pulling the ropes. If any fish are brought up in the net, they kill them with a stick. It is used in water some five feet deep. It is rare amongst the Santals, and not found in all districts.

The Santals also have a way of catching fish by poisoning. They obtain noxious substances from the forest, crush them and throw them into the water. The fish are drugged thereby, float to the surface and are caught. The substances most commonly used for this purpose are the following: The roots of *kiṭą*, Phœnix acaulis *Roxb.*; the fruit of *corco*, Casearia tomentosa *Roxb.*; *jiọti*, a grass growing in rice-fields and moist places; the bark of *kumbiṛ*, Careya arborea *Roxb.*; the fruit of *lọṭọ*, Randia dumetorum, *Lam.*; and the bark of a tree called *sạkri phọl*. This poisoning can only be done in still water (in tanks, pools and certain parts of rivers).

Another very common way of catching fish, especially the smaller kinds, is by using a *ṭọrọḍaṅ*, a weir-basket, a kind of fish trap. The *ṭọrọḍaṅ* is made of wicker-work, either circular or oval, and up to some 80 cm. long. The lower end is tightly closed. Water will run through, but no fish can pass. The 'mouth' is broad and furnished with 'teeth' to prevent the fish from getting out again. The *ṭọrọḍaṅ* is placed in running water where there is a narrow passage. It may be set in a river, but more commonly in an opening in the lower ridge of a rice-field. Here it is usually employed towards the end of the rainy season. Small fish may frequently be seen in the water of the rice-fields, and when the water is led out through the gap, the fish are carried along and fall into this trap. Practically every Santal uses this. A Santal makes something like the real *ṭọrọḍaṅ*, except that it is of straw, for his children to play with. It might be added that the name of the material from which they make the *ṭọrọḍaṅ* is generally combined with this word, thus *icạk ṭọrọḍaṅ*, when made of the twigs of *icạk*, Woodfordia floribunda *Salisb.*, *mat ṭọrọḍaṅ*, when it is made of split bamboo, *tale ṭọrọḍaṅ*, when made of the leaves of *tale*, Borassus flabelliformis *L.*, and so on.

SMOKING AND DRINKING.

In connexion with the hygiene of the Santals smoking and drinking must be mentioned for they play an important part in the lives of the people, especially of the men.

Santals may smoke tobacco. Their national way of smoking is to take a dried tobacco leaf or part of one and make it into a kind of cheroot by wrapping a Sal-leaf round the tobacco and then smoking it like a cigarette. This way of smoking is not very common. The writer has, in quite recent times, seen Santal girls smoking modern machine-made cigarettes.

The use of the hookah is rare; but some Santals have adopted it from the Hindus. The hookah used by the Santals never has any flexible tube attached to it. It is made from a cocoa-nut shell, or the emptied kernel of the Palmyra palm, with a wooden stem attached, on top of which is the *cilim*,[1] the earthen bowl in which the tobacco and the fire are placed. The tobacco used in the hookah is generally mixed with some other substance. The *cilim* is frequently used alone, removed from the hookah-stem, the lower empty end of it being put to the mouth. The Santal name for smoking is *ñũ*, to drink.

---

[1] Same in Hindi.—*Ed.*

The manner in which tobacco is most commonly enjoyed by the Santals is, however, by chewing[1] it. As this is a social custom of considerable importance among the men, it must be fully described. Pieces of a dried tobacco leaf are mixed with mussel-lime. Holding this in the palm of the left hand they pound it with the thumb of the right hand into a solid mass. When ready a pinch is given to each one present who puts it into his mouth and commences to chew it. It is kept in the mouth until the tobacco can no longer be tasted, (this is said to take one to two hours), then it is spat out. This chewing does not hinder speech, but on the contrary, gives them an excuse for conversation. If two Santals meet, even though they do not know each other, and one of them wants to have a talk, he will ask the other for tobacco. If the other one says he has nothing, he will himself offer it. In this way all kinds of conversation are started and kept up. Nearly every Santal man carries pieces of a tobacco leaf and some lime with him. This lime is burnt from mussel or snail shells. The shells are put in a small bundle together with chips of wood, bark, etc., and wrapped up with a straw-rope, like a small *ba̜ndi* (paddy-bundle). This is placed in a crate of branches. A rope is tied in one end, and after having set fire to the chips the man takes the rope and commences to swing the bundle round himself to keep it burning. This operation is continued until no more smoke is seen, when the lime is considered to be ready. This task is usually performed in the evenings. Sometimes they make a bundle too large to be swung in this manner. In that case they suspend it by a long rope from a tree and swing it to keep the fire burning by pulling a cord attached to the bundle. A Santal carries this lime with him in a small receptacle, made of brass or some other metal, or in the kernel of certain fruits, tied to his loin-string. Otherwise it is stored in the house.

A few Santals have commenced to cultivate tobacco, but as a rule, the dried leaves are bought in the shops.[2]

---

[1] This practice is also common among the Hindus of Bihar.—*Ed.*

[2] They have a folktale about the origin of tobacco. It is as follows:

"In olden times, it is said, there was a Brahmin girl who did not get a husband, and died an old unmarried woman. They say that no one applied to marry her, and no one was willing to become a *house-son-in-law either* [means a son-in-law who lives in the home of his bride and is maintained by her family. A common practice with richmen in former times who did not like to send their daughters to their husbands' houses when they were not well off. A term of contempt.—*Ed.*].

Then Chando (a name for the Supreme Being, also for the sun) said: 'Strange, I sent this person into the world and no one was pleased with her. Very well, I shall give this person a blessing, in order that people of the whole world may ask for her all day long'.

Now, truth to tell, they cremated this girl by a river. When this was done, all the village men went back home from the river. Next day, they say, Chando sowed tobacco where they had put the ashes into the water. Tobacco sprang up, grew big and produced very fine leaves.

Now a Mahra (a Goalla, a man of the Hindu cow-keeping caste) was in the habit of daily herding his cattle there. While he was tending his cattle, he saw these leaves. They looked very fine, and he said: 'I wonder what plant has grown up here?' It was very wonderful in his eyes.

One day he saw some goats eagerly eating these leaves, and he drove them away; but the goats came there again to eat. The Mahra then said: 'I wonder why these goats find these leaves so good to eat'. With this thought he tore off a piece of a leaf and chewed it to taste it for himself. He found it bitter and spat it out.

A few days afterwards the Mahra had a toothache. He applied some medicine, but it would not stop. He had intense pain. Then he remembered that the leaves of this newly found plant were very bitter and he said to himself: 'I will try chewing these leaves'. And thinking this he tore off a leaf. Having chewed it into a mass he stuffed it into his mouth and kept it on the spot where the pain was. The pain at once stopped, and he said: 'Wonderful, this is an ex-

Pan,[1] the leaf of Piper Betle *L.*, mixed with lime and certain spices, so commonly chewed by Hindus, is very rare among the Santals. It is bought from Hindus.

Santals do not smoke opium.

Gańja,[2] the hemp plant, Cannabis sativa *Willd.*, is on the other hand used by a few who have learnt to smoke it from other races. The plant is secretly cultivated by some few people. The leaves of the male plant and the flowers of the female plant are dried and mixed with tobacco for smoking, but only very rarely by Santals. The ojhas may teach their disciples to smoke *gańja*, when they are to be 'possessed'.

Now let us consider what the Santals drink, apart from what has already been mentioned among the foodstuffs. The Santals have no wines. To buy them would be more than any ordinary Santal could afford.

Liquor, *pauṛa*, as they call it, is used by some. When Santals take to using this, they soon become addicted to it, and become spoilt and unfit for ordinary work. The liquor is distilled from dried Mahua flowers. It is illegal for Santals to distil *pauṛa*, and is now but rarely done in very primitive apparatus. So far as the writer can remember, he has only once seen what they use, and this was something confiscated by the police.

What may be called the national intoxicating drink of the Santals is their *haṇḍi*, beer, brewed from cereals, rice or other grain. They distinguish a dozen different kinds, in accordance with the name of the cereal used, putting the name of the grain in front of *haṇḍi*, such as *hoṛo haṇḍi*, beer brewed on rice, *janhẹ haṇḍi*, beer brewed on *janhẹ*, a millet, Paspalum scrobiculatum *L.*, and so on. They use besides nearly fifty other prefixes in accordance with the social or festival events, when beer has to be used. It may be noted that Santals drink, not to enjoy the taste, but to become more or less intoxicated, so as to forget the troubles of this world. The Christian

---

cellent medicine'. After that he always had a leaf of this plant with him when he was herding his cattle. Whenever he felt any pain, he chewed this and kept it in his mouth.

Then one day, it is told, he found some bones that had been burnt to ashes there, or perhaps it was some limestone that had been burnt to ashes. When he saw this, he said: 'I wonder, what this white stuff is'. He picked some up and crushed it between his fingers, and taking this and tearing off a piece of the tobacco leaf he chewed them together and felt them very enjoyable. Afterwards he became so accustomed to eating tobacco with lime that he was unable to give this up.

When anyone has a toothache they crush a tobacco leaf, place it in the mouth where the pain is, and the pain ceases. And from that time, they say, other people also became accustomed to chewing tobacco and lime. The Santals call this tobacco *thamakur* (Hindi *tamākū*).

Thus very many people adopted this habit. Even people who have no toothache feel an intense longing for it, if they do not chew. 'In this way', they say, 'people have learnt to chew tobacco, and as is seen, also now we are chewing. Our ancestors have told this; whether it is true or not, we cannot say. We have learnt it from our forefathers."

The Santals have generally excellent teeth. It should be mentioned that what in the above story has been translated by toothache, is in Santali expressed by *reṅgoṭ jom*, lit. a kind of microbe, called *reṅgoṭ*, eating the teeth. They believe that there are two kinds, one that eats holes in the teeth and another kind that causes the pain. The ojhas pretend to be able to get the *reṅgoṭ* out by smoke. When blowing the smoke into the mouth of the sufferer, the ojha uses the hollow stem of a plant and if some small particle of this become detached, he will point to them and tell the spectators, that he can see the *reṅgoṭ* !

[1] Bengali Pān.—*Ed.*

[2] Bengali Gānja.—*Ed.*

missions have, for this reason, been obliged to prohibit the use of Santal beer, and Santals now frequently use tea in its stead.

As beer plays such a prominent part in Santal life, we shall describe how they brew *hanḍi*. This has already been related in a note to one of the Santal Folktales, edited by the Norwegian Institute for sammenlignende kulturforskning, and is repeated here.

When a Santal is going to brew beer, his first act is to prepare the pot in which the beer is to be manufactured. Any earthenware pot with a fairly large mouth will do; they generally use what they call *ṭukuć* or *hanḍha*. The pot is filled with dry leaves, straw, etc., and this is set fire to in the morning of the day when they are going to start brewing. It takes some hours before everything is burnt. The pot is generally placed a short distance away from the house, as there is much smoke. When the pot has cooled down, the ashes are taken out, and the brewing ingredients are put in. This is all got ready in the afternoon. They take rice boiled in the husks and afterwards husked (what they ordinarily use for their food, and not the sun-dried rice) and roast this a little. This roasting is said to impart a certain flavour to the beer. The rice is then boiled and afterwards spread out to dry. The quantity of rice used depends on the number of people for whom the beer is being made. It varies from four to six *pại* [1] (half-seers), or it may be as much as ten *pại*, and the quantity will also naturally depend to a certain extent on the economic state of the house. The *pại* is very nearly equal to half a kilogram.

When the rice is fairly dry, it is mixed with *rạnu*, a vegetable fermenting substance, which is rolled and ground. *Rạnu* ordinarily consists of some four or five different vegetable products. Generally it is bought in the market prepared in small white balls, although most Santals know how to prepare it. As the primary object of the Santal in drinking beer is to get drunk, certain vegetable poisons are frequently added to the *rạnu* to make the beer intoxicating. When a number of deaths had occurred after drinking beer, the writer was once asked by the Subdivisional Officer, Dumka, what ingredients the Santals had used. On investigation it was found that twenty-three different vegetable substances had been utilized. These were naturally not all used at one time, but only one or two were added to the fermenting medicine for the purpose mentioned. People of the *Sunḍi* [2] caste, who manufacture and sell beer in the Santal country, make special use of these poisons, to make their clients drunk in a short space of time. When a Santal is drunk he continues to drink, and the proprietor of the place is said to give him practically nothing but water in the last cups sold. It has several times happened that people who have been to such shops and have become drunk have died from the effects of these poisons on their way home.

When the rice and the *rạnu* have been properly mixed, all is put into the brewing pot, prepared as described above, generally in the evening. The boiled rice has swollen, so that the pot will be fairly full. The contents of the pot are covered with a leaf-plate

---

[1] Compare 'Poah' in Bengali.—*Ed.*

[2] In Bengal also people belonging to Sundi caste manufacture and sell wine.—*Ed.*

pressed down on the rice. Another leaf-plate is placed on the mouth of the pot, and a *ḍhạknić*,[1] an earthenware lid, or a small cooking vessel is put on top, to keep it all intact. There is now nothing more to be done for some days, and the brewing pot is put aside in some place where people do not ordinarily go, commonly in the *bhitạr*,[2] the closet for the worship of the ancestors. As it must not tumble over the pot is placed on a *biṇḍi*,[3] a ring of straw used as a stand for round-bottomed vessels.

The rice takes some five days to ferment (*isin*, as it is called, the word that is ordinarily used for the act of cooking). When the fermentation is complete it can be heard outside the pot. There is an exudation from the rice (called *jhar*), which looks like brown water. This is ladled out with a leaf-spoon, and is said to be the most intoxicating part of the beer. It is generally drunk mixed with a little water and it may be kept, they say, up to one month, before it goes bad. As a rule it is quickly consumed.

To obtain the real beer hot water is poured on to the rice from which the *jhar* has been extracted. During fermentation the rice contracts a little. If insufficient hot water is available, cold water may be added, until the pot is full. The beer when ready looks like milk-water, a little brownish in colour. It has a peculiar acid-sweet smell. Any one who has drunk a little may be detected by the smell, a considerable distance away.

Before drinking, libations are made to *Marañ buru*, the principal national godling of the Santals, possibly, because he belongs to the ancestors. (The Santal traditions tell that our first parents lived holy and happy lives until one day a being came to them, saying he was their grandfather. He was pleased to see them so happy, he said, but there was one joy that they did not know. He then taught them to brew beer, showed them the vegetable poisons they should use to make it good, and made them drink. They became drunk and fell into sin, i.e., had sexual intercourse. This 'grandfather' is the same as *Marañ buru*). They also offer libations to the ancestors, to each, one after the other, so far as they are known. This is done by pouring a little beer onto the floor inside the house (but not in the *bhitạr*) for each ancestor.

They take a broom, made from the straw of *sirom* (Andropogon muricatus *Retz.*) that has not been used to sweep the floor, consequently generally a new one or one specially kept for this purpose, and place it in the mouth of the pot with the broom portion downwards, so as to prevent the rice from coming out when the pot is tilted to let the beer run out.

The beer is poured out into brass-cups, with rims (these make it easy to pour from the cup). If there are enough cups, they drink from these; otherwise the beer is poured out from the brass-cups into leaf-cups. Of such they have one kind called *haṇḍi phuṛuk*, beer leaf-cup. As the name implies, this is specially intended for drinking beer, but also used for any other household purpose for which it is suitable. This leaf-cup is made from one Sal (Shorea robusta *Gærtns*) leaf. Both ends are plaited, once on each side of the midrib, which is covered by the plaits, the plaits being kept

---

[1] Compare 'Dhâkni' in Bengali.—*Ed.*

[2] 'Bhitar' in Bengali means 'inside', inner part of the house, etc.—*Ed.*

[3] Compare 'Biṇḍa' or 'Biṇḍé' in Bengali.—*Ed.*

in position by a pin of stiff straw, a thorn, or the like. Filled up to just below the holes made by the pins at each end such a cup will take about two to four ounces of fluid. It should be mentioned that the beer is stirred with a wooden ladle before being poured out. The leaf-cups are filled over and over again. It is said that it will take some twenty of these cups to make a person drunk.

When the first 'edition' is finished, fresh hot water is again poured on the rice. This is called *doja hạṇḍi*, second brew beer. It is, of course, not so strong as the first *taṅ hạṇḍi*, poured out beer, as it is called (*taṅ* means to pour out by tilting the container). For the second brew the pot is not filled to the brim.

The same rice may generally also serve for a third brew, called *bọḍọc̣ hạṇḍi*, lit. squeezed out beer. The rice is taken out of the pot and put into a *pạṭiạ*, a small basket made of bamboo. A little water is poured on, and the rice is squeezed with the hand. Another way is to put the rice inside paddy-straw, a hole being left at the top for the purpose of putting the right hand in. Water is then poured on, and the rice squeezed. The 'beer' that trickles down is caught in a cup and drunk.

The rice, or rather the refuse, is given to pigs to eat. If they eat too much, they get drunk, it is said.

As remarked above, the Santals drink beer to become drunk. No description is needed of a drinking bout. According to what has been told to the writer, they pass through all the stages, some becoming hilarious, others melancholy, some scold and become abusive, others sing and tell stories; some become vile, lascivious and pugnacious, others moral, amiable, religious, and so on. The avowed object is to be able to forget for a few hours the miseries of this world and feel like kings, as they put it. Drunkenness is one of the great obstacles to Santal development.

The above description refers to the manufacture of beer from rice. It is manufactured in the same way from *janhẹ* and other cereals that are husked. It is also manufactured from maize and *bajra* (Sorghum vulgare *Pers.*) in the same manner, only omitting the roasting at the start.

It might further be remarked that they prepare a kind of beer from *matkọm*, the dried flowers of Bassia latifolia *Roxb.* These are steeped for three days in water, that is then strained, *rạnu* is added to the water, and is allowed to stand for five days, when it becomes thoroughly fermented and is then ready to be drunk. This 'beer' is called *duhli*, not *hạṇḍi*.

The beer has to be 'watered' and drunk when fermentation is complete. They say that the fermented grain may be allowed to stay for one day and then have the water poured on. If it is left longer, it turns very sour and is unfit for use.

One might well say that *hạṇḍi* is absolutely essential at all social functions amongst the Santals.

Santals may occasionally drink *tạṛi*, a kind of toddy, the fermented juice taken from the Palmyra or Date palms. The peduncles of the *tale*, the Palmyra palm, Borassus flabelliformis *L.*, are cut before flowering. The freely running sap is collected in pots and kept until fermented, when it is drunk. This *tạṛi* is prepared during the hot season. The *tạṛi* of the Date palm (*khijur*, Phœnix sylvestris *Roxb.*) is obtained during the cold seasons. The sap is extracted from the tree near the top after having removed a couple of leaves. It is prepared in the same way as the *tạṛi* of the Palmyra palm. As mentioned, *tạṛi* is only occasionally drunk by the Santals.

Santal clothing.

In an account like this of Santal life some mention of their clothing must find a place.

The Santals cultivate sundry varieties of the cotton plant, especially Gossypium herbaceum *L.* and Gossypium arboreum *L.* When ripe the fruit is collected and the seeds cleaned out (generally done by women) in a *cạrkhi*,[1] an instrument that has two wooden rollers between which the cotton is made to pass, the seeds being extracted by the pressure of the rollers. The ginned cotton is called *tulạm*.[2] This is teased with a bow of peculiar shape, made of bamboo. The portion held in the hand is whole, whilst the upper portion is split and bent into a shape which resembles a mark of interrogation. The string is of catgut and 'played' with the thumb and index finger of the left hand. The cotton is afterwards spun into thread on a spinning wheel. To prepare for the weaving, a man fixes a number of sticks, always two and two together, in a sufficiently long row along a path or a straight border, and runs the thread on these sticks. The thread is cut, rolled up on a piece of wood, and finally arranged as the warp through a comb. The Santals have no permanent ready-made looms, these are always makeshift arrangements. Poles are fixed in the ground. On these the different working parts are hung, and the weaver (invariably a man) sits on the ground with his legs in a hole dug out for the purpose. With his feet he works the heddles from the hole. Only cotton cloth is woven by the Santals.

It should be noted that whilst formerly it was a fairly common sight to see men weaving cloth, it is now very rarely that one sees a Santal occupied in this way. Nowadays the Santals mostly buy what they use, partly from the local weavers, especially from the Mohammedan Jolhas,[3] partly from the Hindu Tantis (from these especially certain silk cloths), and partly, and now much more frequently, from the shops. In Assam they buy a kind of rough, strong silk cloth from the local Meches, or Boros, as they prefer to be called.

Santal children wear no clothing for the first few years. At the name-giving festival just after the birth of a child the 'midwife' ties a thread that has been soaked in turmeric round the waist of the child. This remains on the child as long as possible and is then replaced by a fresh one. A girl continues to wear this loin-string (called *ḍora*) until she commences to wear clothes. After that time girls and women only occasionally use a *ḍora*. With males it is otherwise, they always wear a loin-string. There are several kinds, named after the pattern or the makers. A *ḍora* generally has a knot at one end, called *ḍora bọhọk*, lit. loin-string head, and at the other end a loop, called *ḍora gạli*, lit. loin-string noose, which is easily fixed. Besides its use in

---

[1] Compare Çarkhâ in Bengali and Hindi.—*Ed.*

[2] Tulâ means cotton in Bengali and Hindi.—*Ed.*

[3] Usually the term Jolha is applied to Moslem weavers in Bengal as against the term Tânti to Hindus.—*Ed.*

connexion with male clothing the *ḍora* is of help in carrying articles that can be tied to it with a string. The ordinary Santal attire has no pockets.

The first piece of clothing that a boy puts on is the *bhagwa*, a strip of cloth just sufficient to cover the private parts. It is passed between the thighs and tucked into the loin-string in front and behind. Also grown-up men may wear a *bhagwa*. This is some three cubits long and up to one cubit broad (the Santal cubit is the distance from the elbow to the tip of the middle finger and may consequently vary a little in accordance with the size of the person; it is used here as a translation of the Santal *moka*). It is very commonly the only piece of clothing that men wear when out ploughing or doing earth-work that might soil the clothes. It is also used as a bathing costume. Curious to relate the writer once met on the highroad the reputed wealthiest Santal of that part of the Santal country his only attire being a *bhagwa*, a bit of cloth round his head, and a pair of native shoes. Parsimony shows itself in similar ways everywhere.

Very poor men use what is called a *kupni*, really the same as a *bhagwa*, only smaller, two cubits long and half-a-cubit broad.

The regular male attire consists of a loin-cloth and something wherewith to cover the upper part of the body. A common name for the several kinds of loin-cloth is *ḍeṅga* (or *ḍeṅganak̃*) with a word prefixed to show what kind it is. The oldest form is probably what is called *kaca ḍeṅga* of merely *kaca*.[1] It is a piece of cloth that is taken round the loins, passed between the legs and tucked in behind. For a grown-up man the regular size is a cloth five cubits long and one cubit broad. Formerly the Santals wove this cloth themselves. Nowadays they generally buy what they need from the shops, the loin-cloths being both longer and broader, and often dress somewhat like the Bengalis, so far as this part of the body is concerned. This loin-cloth is generally called *dhuti*. Especially well-to-do Santals use this kind.

To cover the breast and shoulders they have a piece of cloth, called *pichạuṛi*, some five cubits long and three cubits broad, two or three pieces being sewn together, the number of pieces depending on the original breadth of the cloth used. Sometimes even four pieces are sewn together, in which case it is called *bạrki*. *Cadọr*[2] is a name also applied to the overcloth; but this word is considered foreign. This cloth is wrapped round the body as a protection against cold, and it is also worn at social and festive gatherings. It may also be used as a covering at night by both sexes. When at work, and when it is hot weather, the men generally wear nothing above the waist.

It should, however, be noted, that present-day Santals have very commonly taken to wearing jackets, which are almost invariably white. A few Santals may be able to make them but as a rule they are bought in the bazars. Boys and young men may also be seen in khaki-coloured shorts, which are apparently much appreciated.

A Santal man will occasionally wear a long narrow piece of cloth on the head as a protection against the sun. A turban is not essential part of a Santal man's dress. When attending Hindu festivals young men may adorn themselves with large wheel-like turbans. A turban is a ceremonial form of headdress in connexion with betrothal

[1] Same in Bengali.—*Ed.*

[2] Same in Bengali.—*Ed.*

and marriage. The relatives of the bride go to the bridegroom's home and put a turban on him. At the marriage ceremony, before the *sindrạdan*[1] (the application of sindur on the bride's forehead by the bridegroom, the binding ceremony) the bridegroom puts what is called *sara dạhṛi* on the head of the younger brother of the bride (or the one who represents him). It is yellow, having been soaked in turmeric. The bridegroom himself and his *lumti* (best man) wear a peculiar kind of turban during the ceremony. It has part of its cloth pulled out and twisted so that it stands up like a peak. The Santal use of a turban may point towards its Hindu origin.

The Santals generally go barefoot. Some may occasionally be seen wearing a very heavy kind of shoe when fording a river, or when walking along a sun-burnt road, and so on.

They have quite a number of different shaped clogs or wooden sandals called *badha.*[2] These all have a wooden sole, flat on the top and cut on the underside to form a wooden 'heel' at the back and something similar in front. These are kept on the foot with the help of strings. A very common form has a toe peg of metal or wood in front, the peg being narrow at the bottom and having something resembling a small wheel at the top. When in use this peg fits between the big and the second toes. These clogs can naturally not be used for walking any distance. The Santals use them during the rainy season to avoid trampling in mud with their bare feet; when moving about at night, to avoid treading on thorns and stones that cannot be seen; and also to avoid treading on snakes and to frighten these away by the noise that the clogs make. They have some ten different shapes of *badha*, besides the *ṭheṅga badha*, stilts, that are used to wade through deep mud. These are made much like ordinary stilts, but when the Santals use them, they put their feet along the piece of flat wood that is fixed in a hole in the pole and keep this between the big and the second toes.

We shall now describe how Santal women are dressed.

When a Santal girl commences to wear clothes—i.e., when she is between three and six years old, she puts on what is called a *putli*, a piece of cloth about two cubits long and one cubit broad. It is tied round the waist, the upper edge ends being tucked together. When the child begins to run about, it is now quite common to see a smaller *putli* being worn. When about eight years old, the girl wears what is called a *pạṅci*, a cloth one and a half cubits broad and four to six cubits long. This cloth is put on like the *putli*.

When a girl approaches maturity she wears a piece of breast-cloth. The end of this is fixed on both sides in the *pạṅci*, or *paṛhāṇḍ*, as this 'skirt' is called, and then taken up over the left shoulder and fixed in the *paṛhāṇḍ* behind. This breast-cloth is called *gọgọk* or *gọnọk*. It may be used by women at any time, more especially during the rainy season when they work in the fields. Poor women will often clothe themselves in this way daily, for obvious reasons.

The ordinary full dress of a Santal woman is a piece of cloth, commonly called a *khạṇḍi*. This is a locally woven (mostly by the Mohammedan Jolhas) rough kind

[1] Compare 'Sindurdân' in Bengali.—*Ed.*

[2] In Bengali it is called Khaṛam.—*Ed.*

of cotton cloth, white, generally with a red border. Up to about a generation ago it was two cubits broad and twelve cubits long, the length being the same as what *Pilcu Buḍhi*, the first human mother, measured round her waist, according to Santal lore. Nowadays this length is not considered necessary; it may be only nine or ten cubits long. This is considered ample. The breadth is the same, two cubits.

The cloth is put on in the following manner:—The woman pleats the cloth at one end, and taking the cloth round her waist passes it firmly over the pleated part on her left side and tucks in the upper side of the cloth, just beyond where the pleats are, the ends of these rising just above the upper border of the cloth. In this case the pleated end is taken round the back of the waist. The rest of the cloth is then taken back across the front, one edge being fastened on the right side of the 'skirt' so formed, and then taken up over the breast and the right shoulder, the end of the cloth hanging down the back, loose or tucked in at the waist. This is called *gọgọk* or *gọnọk bande*. *Bande* is the name for a cloth worn by a woman. Another method is to take the cloth, after having tied the 'skirt', up over the back to the right shoulder, then to take it down over the breast to the right side and tuck the end of the cloth into the 'skirt' on both sides. This procedure is called *gọgọk japak bande*.

Besides the *khạṇḍi* mentioned any suitable cloth of the requisite size may be used. One special kind may be mentioned. It is called *doal*, woven by the local Jolhas. The *doal* is twelve cubits long and two cubits broad. Both warp and weft are of double thread. It has red and white stripes in pairs across the entire length, and broad red borders. At each end there are broad red stripes across the cloth. It is now comparatively rare. On the occasion of his marriage the bridegroom must give such a cloth to the mother of his bride. Nowadays, however, money is more commonly given instead.

Cotton cloth, bought in a shop, is now very often used.

Against cold and for coverings at night the women use the same kind of overcloth as the men. A good many women now use a kind of jacket or blouse. This is naturally due to European influence. It should be noted that Santal women are not by custom obliged to keep their heads covered, they go bare-headed, except when required by custom or necessity to wear a headdress.

The position of the Santal women is very different from that of the women among the neighbouring Hindus and Mohammedans. Theoretically the Santal woman is inferior to man. She may not have landed property, must not be present at religious sacrifices, and so on; but as often as not she rules the house, the household and the family, and when she is the wife of the headman, the whole village.

The man naturally represents the family outwardly. He is the tenant of the landlord (only recently have the settlement people recorded certain females as tenants). The man is the head of the family and is expected to do everything in connexion with money-lenders, and so on. Men alone prepare the different agricultural fields, make them ready for the plough, sow all kinds of seed, and (except the planting of rice, that is solely the work of women), they may do everything in connexion with growing crops, but may be assisted by the women folk. They prepare the threshing floor and do the threshing, they also do everything connected with the storing of the seed. To quote the words of the old Kolean guru, 'From the month of Phalgun to the end of Baisak (i.e., from the middle of February to the middle of May) is "sitting time" (there is no agricultural work). During this time the men make implements for their own use and gather provisions for the household. They make plough-beams and yokes, ploughs and clod-crushers, earth-shovels and cart-wheels, cart-shafts and -axles, neck-ropes and yoke-leather-thongs, hide-straps and ropes, spinning-wheels and cotton-cleaning machines, handles for the spades and pick-axes, axes and adzes, bedstead-legs and frames, stools and wooden slabs to sit on, wooden ladles and spoons, bows and arrows, flutes, wooden pestles and mortars and weaving implements; they weave cloth and string bedsteads and they bring firewood and wood for the house, and they repair the house'. The men build the houses and thatch them.

As already stated, Santal women are deemed inferior to men. There is certain work that they must not do, whilst on the other hand there are many kinds of work that the women must do, because the men would consider these tasks *infra dig*. The Santals say that the women are constantly working, and this is more or less true. They get up at cock-crow (about 4 A.M.), clean and put the house in order, throw the dung out of the cowshed, fetch water, pound grain (a woman always works the mortar, but a man may tread the *ḍhiṅki*) and prepare the food. (It should, however, be noted that, if there is any special feast, the men may act as cooks.) The women pull out the paddy-seedlings (often assisted by men) and plant the rice, cut it when ripe (in this often assisted by men), and hoe the maize (also assisted by men). They pull out the cotton plants and clean the cotton and make thread for the men to weave. They make leaf-cups and leaf-plates. They plaster the floor and the walls and make all smooth, especially when the rainy season rain has caused damage. The women folk never singly but always in a body gather leaves and small firewood from the forest, and vegetables. They never take part in hunting, but may do so in fishing. The women do not partake of food along with the men. They serve the men and children first, and when they have fed, the women sit down to eat.

Conclusion.

In conclusion the following effusion of a Santal may be quoted. 'We Santals pass our life in much hardship, because we have no means of earning our livelihood other than by ploughing. We may wish to trade and do business, but we are unable to use the language of the other races properly, and it is with them that we must trade. For this reason we are unable to enter into commerce. Besides, mostly due to foolishness and laziness, indolence and slothfulness, we have no wish to work and to learn any real craft, and we have no time for anything. On the other hand, we are always eager and always find the needed leisure for dancing and attending festivals. At such times we say: "Who knows whether I shall die or live, I must go and meet the people of the country". Saying this we at once turn our back on any work and run off to attend a festival. A few of us have realized that all this is due to laziness, and that it is in this way that we Santals have become so poor.

From olden times our ancestors have said and we also now say, that five months of the year are extremely difficult. From the month of Chait until San (i.e., from the middle of March until the middle of August) we name it "the hunger period". In villages where they have Mahua they are fairly well off for one or two months; but for three or four months we exist with great difficulty. The cultivation of rice is mainly for the benefit of the Hindu money-lenders; these people rob us of everything.'

What the Santal said is a fairly correct synopsis of the attitude of a great many of the Santal people. It takes a long time to change a nomad race to one of settled agriculturists. Something is being done to help the people, but much more is sadly needed.